D0602478

# The Theory and Practice of Therapeutic Massage

by Mark Beck

New Revised Edition

Bobbi Ray Madry
*Editor/Curriculum Specialist*

*The original THEORY AND PRACTICE OF BODY MASSAGE by Frank Nichols has been revised and expanded to include new techniques while retaining the quality of the original text.*

**Milady** Publishing Corporation
(A Wiley Company)
3839 White Plains Road, Bronx, N.Y. 10467-5394

AUTHOR: Mark Beck

EDITOR: Bobbi Ray Madry

EDITORIAL DIRECTOR: Mary Healy

PRODUCTION MANAGER: Jan Lavin

ART DIRECTOR: John P. Fornieri

TYPSETTER: Barbara Cardillo

GRAPHIC ARTISTS: Pat Miret, Mark Stein, Pat Genova

ILLUSTRATIONS: Shiz Horii



MILADY PUBLISHING CORPORATION,
BRONX, NEW YORK

Library of Congress Cataloging in Publication Data:
ISBN 0-87350-800-9



Printed in the United States of America

# Preface



Massage, when properly applied by qualified practitioners, is of positive value in building and maintaining a healthy, vigorous body for men and women. The strain and stress of modern living tends to contribute to a decline in physical vigor, and creates stress and its attendant ills. There has never been a greater need for therapeutic massage. The public is beginning to appreciate the many benefits of regular massage as a means of enjoying more vibrant health, for offsetting the tensions of modern living and for getting more out of life.

Athletic clubs, health clubs, and full service salons throughout the country are employing practitioners who are trained in the art and science of massage. Those trained in the fundamentals of massage will be able to take advantage of the many opportunities awaiting them in this promising field. Many practitioners are also opening their own businesses and operating them successfully.

Leading schools, instructors, and businesses employing massage practitioners were consulted during the preparation of this textbook. Their valuable advice, as well as the needs and interests of practicing and prospective massage practitioners were constantly kept in mind. No effort was spared to include all the information essential for the successful practice of therapeutic massage. It was not possible within the scope of this book to include all the excellent therapies in the depth they deserve, however, a booklist is available from the publisher for those who wish to pursue further study and to expand their reference libraries.

Men and women engaged in associated fields such as cosmetology, healthcare, and physical fitness will find a wealth of valuable information in THE THEORY AND PRACTICE OF THERAPEUTIC MASSAGE. Those who are contemplating careers in the practice of massage will find that it is a dignified and lucrative profession. It also offers personal satisfaction in serving the health needs of the public.

Mark Beck

# Acknowledgments

The author and publisher of THE THEORY AND PRACTICE OF THERAPEUTIC MASSAGE wish to express their appreciation to the many professional people who contributed their valuable time and counsel during the preparation of this text. We would also like to thank the following people for contributing to the chapters dealing with their special areas of expertize.

Susan Beck whose background in consumer science, her experience and knowledge as a certified myomassologist and instructor, added so much to the research and development of materials of interest to the professional massage practitioner.

Gail A. Drum, R.N. and specialist in patient care, who contributed her valuable knowledge and advice to the chapter on massage in nursing and healthcare.

Joel Gerson, author and educator in the field of esthetics, whose contributions include the chapters dealing with skincare and facial massage techniques.

The members of AMTA, American Massage Therapy Association and IMF, International Myomassethics Federation, for their continued efforts in promoting the massage profession and for their support and encouragement of high standards of education for massage practitioners.

# Contents

# PART I THE HISTORY AND ADVANCEMENT OF THERAPEUTIC MASSAGE

# Chapter 1 Historical Overview of Massage

## LEARNING OBJECTIVES

After you have mastered this chapter, you will be able to:

1. Explain why massage is known as one of the earliest remedial practices for the relief of pain and discomfort.
2. Explain why massage is a natural and instinctive remedy for some illnesses and injuries.
3. Explain the use of massage from ancient to modern times as an aid to physiological and psychological well-being.
4. Describe the basic differences in massage systems.
5. Explain why it is important for legitimate practitioners to be licensed.

## INTRODUCTION

Massage (ma-sazh), also called massology, is defined as the systematic manual or mechanical manipulations of the soft tissues of the body by such movements as rubbing, kneading, pressing, rolling, slapping, and tapping, for the purpose of promoting circulation of the blood and lymph, relaxation of muscles, relief from pain, restoration of metabolic balance, and other benefits both physical and mental.

The massage practitioner is referred to as a massologist, or massage technician. A male massage practitioner is often called a masseur (ma-sur), and a female practitioner is called a masseuse (ma-sooz). Today, most professionally trained men and women prefer to be called practitioners or massage therapists. For practical purposes, *massage practitioner* will be the term used throughout this book.

The word *massage* is from the French word *masser,* meaning to shampoo. The word *shampoo* is from the Hindu word meaning to press. In Greek, *massage* means to knead with the hands. The origin of the word is attributed to the Arabian *mass* or *mash,* which means to press softly. Both the Bible and the Koran mention the use of aromatics to lubricate and annoint the skin.

## MASSAGE IN ANCIENT TIMES

Massage is one of the earliest remedial practices of humankind and is said to be the most natural and instinctive means of relieving pain and discomfort. When a person has sore, aching muscles, abdominal pains, or a bruise or wound, it is a natural and instinctive impulse to touch and rub that part of the body to obtain relief.

Artifacts have been found in many countries to support the belief that in prehistoric times men and women massaged their muscles and rubbed herbs, oils, and various substances on their bodies as healing and protective agents. According to research reports, in nearly all ancient cultures some form of touch or massage was practiced. In many groups a special person such as a healer, religious leader, or doctor was selected to administer healing power. These ancient civilizations used therapeutic massage not only as a pain reliever but also to improve their sense of well-being and their physical appearance.

### Chinese Amma Techniques

In the British Museum, records reveal that as early as 3000 B.C., massage was practiced by the Chinese. *The Cong Fau of Tao-Tse* was one of the ancient Chinese books containing lists of exercises and movements used in massage techniques. The Chinese continued to improve their massage techniques through a special procedure they called *amma.* This massage technique was developed over many years of experience in finding the points on the body where various movements such as rubbing, pressing, and manipulations were most effective.

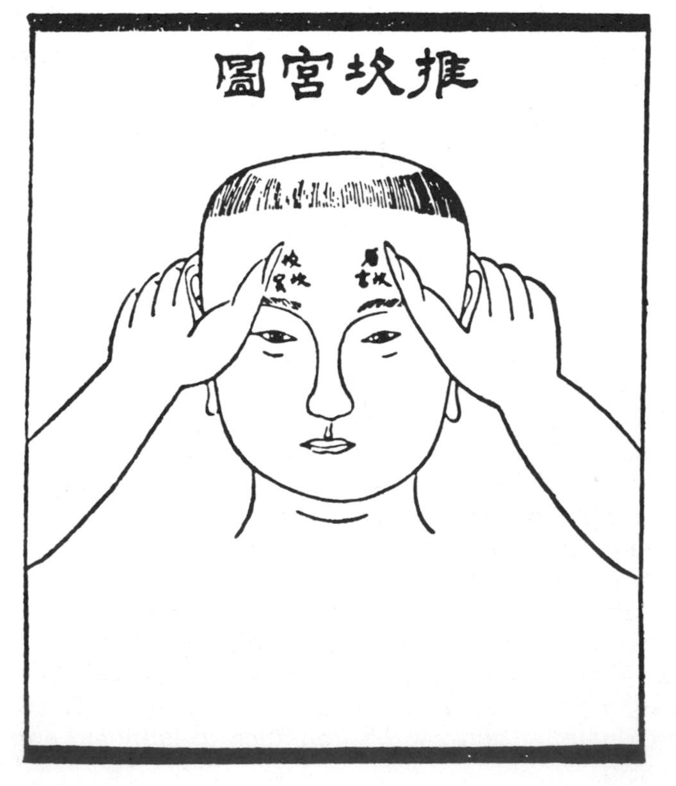


*Massage of the forehead. Illustration from the Chinese work Synopsis of the Technique of Remedial Massage, 1889. Courtesy New York Public Library picture collection.*

### Japanese Tsubu and Shiatsu

The practice of the amma method of massage entered Japan around the sixth century A.D. The points of stimulation remained much the same but were called *tsubo.* These points are pressed to improve circulation and stimulate nerves in a finger pressure technique the Japanese call *shiatsu.* This massage method has become quite popular in recent years. Early records show that a book on massage, *The San-Tsai-Tou-Hoei,* was published by the Japanese in the sixteenth century and listed both passive and active massage procedures.

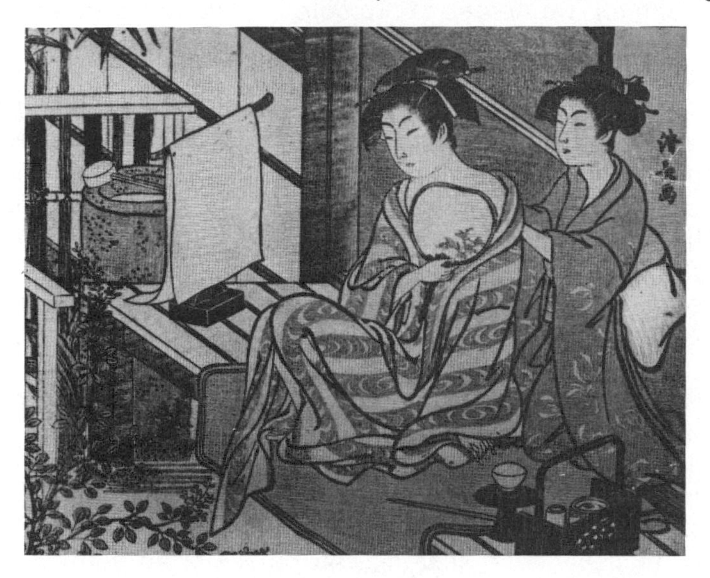

*The art of massage was practiced by the Japanese centuries ago. This illustration shows a woman being given a shoulder and back massage by her servant. Louvre collection. Courtesy New York Public Library picture collection.*

### Arabian, Persian, Egyptian, and Hindu Practices

The Persians and the Egyptians employed various forms of massage as effective health treatment. The *Ayur-Veda (Art of Life),* a sacred book of the Hindus written around 1800 B.C., included massage treatments among its hygenic principles. Avicenna ((980-1037 A.D.), an Arabian physician, gave detailed descriptions of uses and effects of massage in a book titled, *Canon of Medicine.*

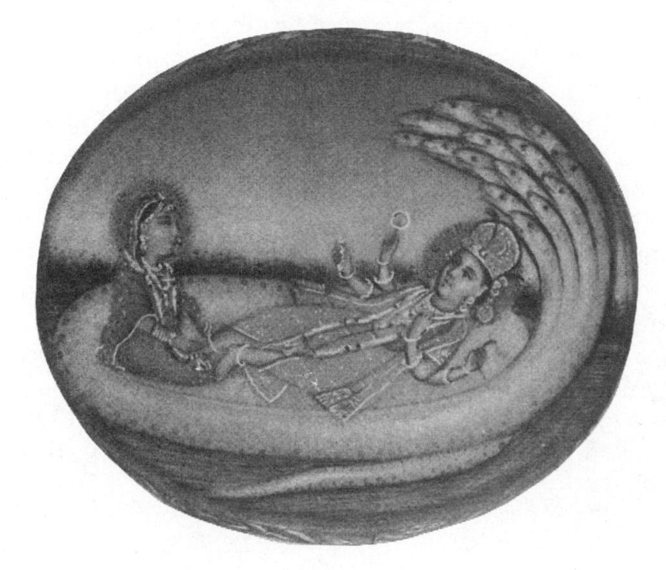

*Massage, rubbing and shampooing were understood and practiced by the Hindus many centuries ago, and they recognized their value in diminishing fatigue, inducing sleep, and in reducing excess fat. Copyright by the Wellcome Historical Medical Museum. Courtesy New York Public Library picture collection.*

## Greek Massage and Gymnastics

From the East, the practice of massage spread to Europe and is believed to have flourished well before 300 B.C. The Greeks made gymnastics and the regular use of massage part of their physical fitness rituals. Asclepiades, a Greek physician of the second century B.C., is said to have recommended therapeutic massage and exercises for athletes and gladiators before contests and as a relief from fatigue or injuries that often followed. Homer, the Greek poet who wrote the *Odyssey* (the story of the Trojan war), spoke of the use of nutritious foods, exercise, and massage for war heroes to promote healing and relaxation.

Greek women also participated in gymnastics and dancing, and used massage as part of their health and beauty regimens. The Greeks referred to exercise as *ascesis,* based on their belief that an *ascete* was a person who exercised his or her body and mind. This was the same principle as today's "holistic" health concept of the cultivation of total health of body and mind.

The Greek physician Herodicus of the fifth century B.C. prolonged the lives of many of his patients by having them massaged with beneficial herbs and oils. Herodotus, the Greek historian of the time, wrote of the benefits of massage. Hippocrates (460-380 B.C.), a pupil of Herodicus, later became known as the father of medicine. His code of ethics for physicians, the Hippocratic oath, is still in use today. This oath, which incorporates a code of ethics for physicians and those about to receive medical degrees, binds them to honor their teachers, do their best to maintain the health of their patients, honor their patients' secrets, and prescribe no harmful treatment or drug. The Hippocratic oath can be found in its entirety in most medical dictionaries.

That Hippocrates understood the effects of massage is revealed in one of his descriptions of massage movements. He said, "Hard rubbing binds, much rubbing causes parts to waste, and moderate rubbing makes them grow." This has been interpreted to mean that rubbing can help to bind a joint that is too loose or loosen a joint that is too tight. Vigorous rubbing can tighten and firm while moderate rubbing tends to build muscle. In his writings, Hippocrates used the word *anatripsis,* which means the art of rubbing a part upward, not downward. He stated that it is necessary to rub the shoulder following reduction of a dislocated shoulder. The advice Hippocrates gave still serves as a valuable guideline for modern practitioners. Hippocrates believed that all physicians should be trained in massage as a method of healing.

## Roman Art of Massage and Therapeutic Bathing

The Romans acquired the practice of therapeutic bathing and massage from the Greeks. The Romans built public baths that were available to rich and poor alike. A brisk rubdown with fragrant oils could be enjoyed following the bath. The art of massage was also highly respected as a treatment for weak and diseased conditions and as an aid in removing stiffness and soreness from muscles.

Romans, as the Greeks before them, used massage as part of their gymnastics. Celsus, who lived during the reign of Emperor Tiberious (about 42 B.C. to 37 A.D.), was considered to be one of the most eminent of Roman physicians. He recommended rubbing the head to relieve headaches and rubbing limbs to strengthen muscles and to combat paralysis. Massage was used to improve sluggish circulation and internal disorders and to reduce edema. Although circulation of the blood was not completely understood, physicians of the time followed the teaching of Hippocrates in rubbing upward as being more effective than rubbing downward.

The Greek physician Claudius Galen (130-200 A.D.), who became physician to the Roman emperor Marcus Aurelius, is said to have discovered that arteries and veins contained blood; however, William Harvey (1578-1657), an English physician is credited with discovering the circulation of the blood in 1628. Galen was a prolific writer, and his medical texts were the principal ones in use for more than a thousand years. As a physician to gladiators, Galen gained great knowledge of anatomy. His books on hygienic health, exercise, and massage stressed specific exercises for various physical disorders. Greek and Roman philosophers, statesmen, and historians such as Cicero, Pliny, Plutarch, and Plato wrote of the benefits of massage and passive and active exercise to the maintenance of a healthy body and mind. Even Julius Gaius Caesar, Roman general and Emperor of Rome (100-44 B.C.), is said to have demanded his daily massage.

**The Decline of Arts and Sciences in the West**

With the decline of the Roman Empire, the popularity of bathing and massage also declined, and the magnificent baths soon became ruins. There is little recorded history of health practices during the Middle Ages (the Dark Ages), which is the period between classical antiquity and the European Renaissance, extending from the downfall of Rome in about 476 to about 1450. The sciences and arts suffered severe setbacks during the Dark Ages. Few historical books were written, and much recorded history was lost. This decline was due in part to wars and to religious superstitions that caused people to fear placing too much importance on the physical self.

**The Renaissance Revives Interest in Health Practices**

The Renaissance (rebirth, 1450-1600) revived interest in the arts and sciences. Once again, the people became interested in the improvement of physical health and appearance. By the second half of the fifteenth century, the printing press had been invented, which led to the publication of many scholarly writings in the arts and sciences. The advancement in the distribution of printed materials also helped to stimulate interest in better health practices.

**The Growth and Acceptance of Massage as a Healing Aid**

By the sixteenth century, medical practitioners began to employ massage as part of their healing treatments. Ambroise Pare (1517-1590), a French barber-surgeon, one of the founders of modern surgery and inventor of the ligation of arteries,

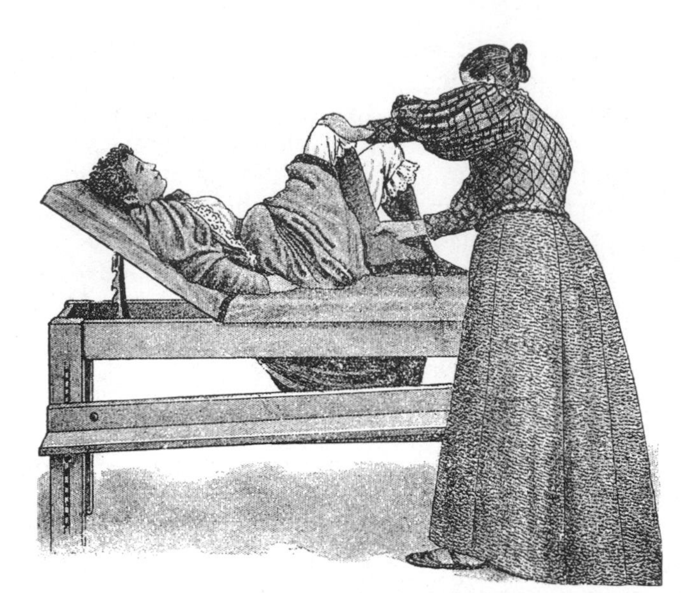

*This illustration from a French manual (1898) shows how massage and flexion of the foot and leg are being used to treat a pulled muscle. Courtesy New York Public Library picture collection.*

described in one of his publications the positive effects of massage in the healing processes. He classified massage movements as gentle, medium, and vigorous. His concepts were passed down to other French physicians who believed in the value of physical therapeutics. During his lifetime, Pare served as personal physician to four of France's kings. He is credited with restoring the health of Mary, Queen of Scots (1542-1587), by use of massage. Mercurialis (1530-1606), a professor of medicine at the University of Padua, Italy, published a book in 1569 on gymnastics and the benefits of massage when integrated into treatments for the body and mind.

## THE DEVELOPMENT OF MODERN MASSAGE TECHNIQUES

Per Henrik Ling (1776-1839) of Smaaland, Sweden, who was a physiologist, and fencing master, systemized and developed movements he found to be beneficial in improving his own physical condition. The Ling (Swedish movement) System consisted of movements classified as passive and active. Ling worked out a series of movements that he called "Swedish Remedial Gymnastics." He based this system on physiology, which was then developing into a science. In 1813 the Swedish government created the Royal Swedish Central Institute of Gymnastics and named Ling president. Ling died in 1839; however, his students published his works posthumously. The Ling System spread throughout the world.

Modern massage therapy is credited to Dr. Johann Mezger (1839-1909) of Holland who established the practice and art of massage as a scientific subject for physicians in the remedial treatment of disease. Through Dr. Mezger's efforts, massage became recognized as fundamental to rehabilitation in physical therapy.

In the early part of the nineteenth century, John Grosvenor (1742-1823), a well-respected English surgeon, stressed to his colleagues the value of massage in the relief of stiff joints, gout, and rheumatism. His efforts helped to further the belief in massage as an aid to healing.

By the early part of the nineteenth century, physicians in medical schools in Germany and Scandinavia were including massage in their teachings as a dignified and beneficial asset in the medical field. In 1900, the distinguished physician Albert J. Hoffa published *Technik Der Massage* in Germany. The publication remains one of the most basic books in the field and contains many of the techniques used in Swedish massage.

Throughout Germany, Denmark, Norway, and Sweden, therapeutic exercises, massage, and baths were recommended by physicians for the restoration and maintenance of health. These physicians believed that massage helped the body rid itself of toxins, relieved such ailments as rheumatism, and promoted the healthy functioning of all body systems.

In England in 1884, a group of women formed The Society of Trained Masseuses. By 1920 this society had grown in members and prestige. Later the society became known as the Chartered Society of Massage and Medical Gymnastics; it was registered in 1964 as the Chartered Society of Physiotherapy.

The introduction of massage in the United States is credited to Dr. S. Weir Mitchell of Philadelphia, Pennsylvania, who in 1870 published a treatise on the value of massage and good nutrition in the treatment of some disorders of the blood and the ill effects of poor nutrition. In 1884, the first book in English on massage was published by Dr. O. Graham of Boston, Massachusetts.

Massage became even more important during and immediately following World War I (1914-1918) when it proved beneficial in the treatment of injuries. Again in World War II (1939-1945), massage was employed on an even larger scale in the hospitals of the Armed Forces. In the years following World War II manual massage played a secondary role in physical therapy as more mechanical means of stimulation and rehabilitation became more generally employed. As a result, the time spent in training physical therapists in "hands on" massage techniques became limited to an average of 75 to 150 hours.

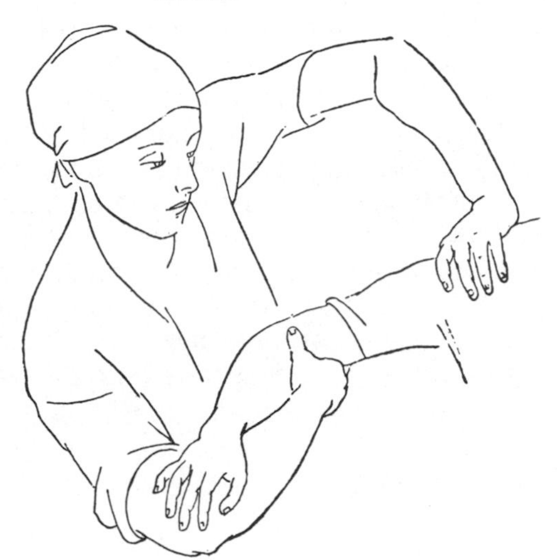

*This illustration from Methuen's book, "What Every Masseuse Should Know," 1917. Reprinted courtesy of the New York Public Library picture collection.*

During the post-war recovery, massage was directed more toward athletes and less toward rehabilitation. Most practitioners were employed in athletic clubs or YMCAs or as trainers for athletic teams. It was during this time that chiropractic began to receive more recognition. Chiropractic developed in the West when Dr. David Palmer began teaching techniques of directed manual pressure against the bony processes to manipulate the vertebrae of the spine and other articulations of the body.

Today, chiropractors use more subtle massage-type techniques and many times employ massage practitioners as assistants.

**Massage Systems**

The methods of massage generally in use today are Swedish, Japanese, French, English, and German systems.

1. The Swedish system employs basic movements that can be slow and gentle, vigorous or bracing, according to the results the practitioner wishes to achieve.
2. The German method combines many of the Swedish movements and emphasizes the use of various kinds of therapeutic baths.
3. The French and English systems also employ many of the Swedish massage movements for body massage. Many excellent facial massage and beauty therapy treatments originated in France and England.
4. The Japanese system, called *shiatsu,* a finger pressure method, is based on the Oriental concept that the body has a series of energy (tsubo) points. When pressure is properly applied to these points, circulation is improved and nerves are stimulated. This system is said to greatly improve body metabolism and to relieve a number of physical disorders.
5. Sports massage refers to a method of massage especially designed to prepare an athlete for an upcoming event and to aid in the body's regenerative and restorative capacities following a rigorous workout or competition. This is achieved through specialized deep tissue manipulations that stimulate circulation of the blood and lymph. Some sports massage movements are designed to break down lesions and adhesions and reduce fatigue. Sports massage generally follows the Swedish system, with variations of movements applied according to the judgment of the practitioner and the results he or she wishes to achieve. Sports teams, especially those in professional baseball, football, basketball, hockey, ice skating, and swimming, often retain a professionally trained massage practitioner. Athletes, dancers, and others who must keep muscles strong and supple are often instructed in automassage (how to massage one's own muscles) and in basic massage on a partner.

6. The physiotherapist or massotherapist is concerned with diseases and injuries for which massage is recommended and supervised by the patient's physician. This requires specialized training and is generally done in hospitals and clinics. Schools of nursing usually include some massage techniques in their training programs. The nurse or nursing assistant gives beneficial massage, particularly back rubs, to relax the patient and to prevent wasted muscles and bed sores as a result of lack of exercise. Gertrude Beard (1887-1971), a physical therapist, is credited with contributing to the acceptance of massage in physical therapy. Today, massage is recognized as an essential part of almost all physical therapy.
7. Acupressure stems from the Chinese medical practice of acupuncture. It employs various methods of stimulating acupuncture points in order to regulate Chi (life force energy). The aim of this method is to achieve therapeutic and pathological changes in the person being treated as well as relieve some pain, discomfort, or other physiological imbalance.
8. Rolfing is a systematic program developed out of the technique of structural integration developed by Dr. Ada Rolf. Rolfing aligns the major body segments through manipulation of the fascia or the connective tissue.

The following are additional systems tnat have gained recognition as beneficial forms of massage.

*Polarity Therapy:* A method developed by Randolph Stone using massage manipulations derived from both Eastern and Western practices. Exercises and thinking practices are included in order to better balance the body both physically and energetically.

*The Trager Method:* Developed by Dr. Milton Trager, this method uses movement exercises called *mentastics* along with massagelike, gentle shaking of different parts of the body to prevent pent-up tensions.

*Reflexology:* This method originated with the Chinese and is based on the idea that stimulation of particular points on the surface of the body has an effect on other areas or organs of the body. Dr. William Fitzgerald is credited with first demonstrating the effects of reflexology, while Eunice Ingham later systemized the technique (popular today) that focuses mainly on the hands and feet.

*Touch For Health:* A simplified form of applied kinesiology (principles of anatomy in relation to human movement) developed by John Thie. This method involves techniques from both Eastern and Western origins. Its purpose is to relieve stress on muscles and internal organs.

Although there are many excellent massage methods, the Swedish system is still the most widely used and is incorporated into other procedures. Whatever method the practitioner prefers, it is essential to be thoroughly knowledgeable in all technical movements and their effects on the various body systems. The objectives of all professional practitioners are generally the same: to provide a service that enhances the client's physical health and sense of well-being.

### Physiological and Psychological Benefits of Massage

Although body massage is not a magic "cure all," it is a safe and beneficial health aid for everyone from infants to elderly people. Just as some active exercise daily is beneficial, passive exercises by way of massage can be included in the daily health regimen, except when there are certain contraindications. When there is doubt on the part of the practitioner as to whether to give massage or to recommend a particular exercise, the client should be asked to first have a physical checkup and to obtain his or her physician's recommendations in writing.

Massage has direct psychological and physiological benefits. Physically, massage increases metabolism, hastens healing, relaxes and refreshes the muscles, and improves the detoxifying functions of the lymphatic system. Massage helps to prevent muscle cramps and spasms, assists the digestive process and assimulation of nutrients, and improves circulation of blood to all body systems. Since blood carries nutrients to the skin, massage is beneficial in keeping the skin functioning in a normal, healthy manner.

Psychologically, massage relieves fatigue, reduces tension, calms the nervous system, and promotes a sense of relaxation and renewed energy.

### Concerns of Educators and Practitioners

Since 1960, there has been a massage renaissance in the United States. Not all of this has been good for the profession. The "massage parlor" boom has associated the word *massage* with such illegal practices as prostitution. This has become a concern for legitimate massage educators and practitioners and is a problem that has not as yet been entirely remedied. Today, there are several professional massage organizations in the United States that are working diligently to legitimize professionalism in massage by standardizing educational requirements and advocating just and equitable laws at state and local levels.

It is important for practitioners to be trained in schools that are licensed and that have credentials meeting the professional standards required by state boards and ethical associations.

## QUESTIONS FOR DISCUSSION AND REVIEW

1. Define the meaning of massage.
2. How do we know that ancient civilizations used therapeutic massage and exercise in their social, personal, or religious practices?
3. Why did the Greeks and Romans place so much emphasis on exercise and massage?
4. Which Greek physician became known as "The Father of Medicine"?
5. Why were the Middle Ages also called the "Dark Ages"?
6. Why was the Renaissance an important turning point for the arts and sciences?

7. How did the invention of the printing press in the fifteenth century help to further the practice of massage and therapeutic exercise?
8. Why did the acceptance of massage and therapeutic exercise increase during the World Wars I and II?
9. Why has there been more interest in health and personal attractiveness in recent years?
10. Why has it become necessary to establish licenses and official guidelines for the practice of therapeutic body massage?
11. What is meant by "holistic" health?
12. Which body systems are said to benefit from regular therapeutic massage and exercise?
13. What are some of the psychological benefits attributed to massage?
14. When should massage be avoided?
15. In what way does improved circulation of the blood benefit the skin?
16. What is the difference between passive and active exercise?
17. Describe the theory upon which the Japanese shiatsu system of massage is based.
18. What part does proper exercise and use of massage play in athletics?
19. Why is it important for nurses and their aides to learn basic massage techniques?
20. How does the job of the physical therapist who works in a hospital differ from that of the massage therapist who works in a salon?
21. Of what benefit is the history of therapeutic massage to the student who wishes to pursue a career in this field?
22. Which massage system is the most widely used in general massage?
23. Why is massage said to be the most natural and instinctive means of relieving pain and discomfort?
24. What did the Chinese call their early massage system?
25. In what way are the Chinese and Japanese systems similar?
26. Why did manual massage become a secondary treatment following World War II?
27. Why is massage used as a treatment in sports or athletic medicine?
28. How are legitimate practitioners helping to stamp out illegal practices that have used massage as a "front"?

**ANSWERS TO QUESTIONS FOR DISCUSSION AND REVIEW**

1. Massage is the manual (use of hands) or mechanical (use of machines or apparatus) manipulation of a part of the body by rubbing, kneading, pressing, rolling, slapping, and like movements for the purpose of improving circulation of the blood, relaxation of muscles, and other benefits to body systems.
2. Various artifacts show evidence that ancient civilizations used massage and exercise in their social, personal, and religious practices.
3. The Greeks and Romans were health and beauty conscious. Both men and women believed that exercise improved the body and the mind. Exercise and massage were utilized in the training and rehabilitation of gladiators. Both Greek and Roman physicians prescribed various kinds of exercise and massage movements as aids to the healing of diseases and wounds.
4. Hippocrates, the Greek physician, became known as the Father of Medicine and originator of the Hippocratic Oath, which is still used as the ethical guide to the medical professions. The Hippocratic oath can be found in its entirety in most modern dictionaries.
5. The Middle Ages were called the "Dark Ages" because the arts and sciences were allowed to deteriorate, leading to the decline of learning.
6. The Renaissance, meaning "rebirth," revived interest in the arts and sciences as well as renewed interest in health and personal hygiene practices.
7. The invention of the printing press in the latter part of the fifteenth century led to the publishing of more writings in the arts and sciences. This improved circulation of educational materials, leading to a better understanding of the value of massage and exercise as therapeutic aids.
8. Because there were more diseases and injuries during wartime, physicians employed therapeutic massage and exercise more often. The good results led to wider acceptance of massage and exercise as aids to healing.
9. Mainly the increase in life expectancy has made most people conscious of their health practices. Because men and women of today look forward to longer, more productive lives, they want to remain healthy and attractive as long as possible. The increase in media coverage has also stimulated awareness of physical and psychological health.
10. The establishment of licenses and official guidelines for the practice of therapeutic massage protects ethical people who uphold the standards of the profession and discourages those who misrepresent the field.
11. The word holistic means wholeness of body and mind; it has been derived from the theory of holism, which says that a living organism has a reality other than the sum of its constituent parts.

12. Massage is beneficial to all body systems including the circulatory, nervous, skeletal, muscular, digestive, glandular, integumentary (skin), respiratory, and excretory systems.
13. The psychological benefits of massage result from the reduction of tension and relief from stress and anxiety. Massage can also promote a sense of renewed energy and well-being.
14. Massage should be avoided when there is a contraindication, such as a physical or mental condition that needs medical attention, and when there is doubt of its benefits.
15. Massage improves the circulation of the blood, which in turn supplies beneficial nutrients to the skin.
16. Passive exercise of muscles incorporates massage and is done by the practitioner on the client. Active exercise of muscles is movement done by the individual, as in sports or gymnastics.
17. The Japanese use a system called shiatsu (shi, fingers; atsu, pressure). It is the finger pressure method based on the Oriental concept that the body has a series of energy points that proper pressure or digital compression can reactivate, thus benefiting all body systems.
18. Athletes often have injuries and sore muscles that can be relieved by massage. Massage and proper exercise also helps to prevent fatigue and contribute to the maintenance of optimum fitness.
19. Nurses and their aides are responsible for the comfort and welfare of patients. They often administer massage (especially back rubs) to help the patient to relax, to prevent sore muscles, and to improve circulation of the blood.
20. The physical therapist is professionally trained to work with the sick and injured as part of the medical team. The massage therapist is professionally trained in the art and science of therapeutic massage and exercise for those who are in good health. The massage therapist does not work with sick or injured people unless such treatment is prescribed by a physician.
21. A person contemplating a career in any important field should have some understanding of problems of the past and the progress that has been made over a period of time. Understanding the past helps us to measure our own progress in the development of the art and practice of therapeutic body massage.
22. The Swedish massage system is still the most widely used and is most frequently incorporated into other systems.
23. Massage is said to be the most effective and most natural means of obtaining relief from pain or discomfort, because a person can use his or her hands to rub, touch, or exercise a part of the body to obtain immediate relief.

24. The Chinese called their massage system amma. This method grew from various pressing and rubbing of parts of the body to produce therapeutic effects.
25. The points of stimulation in Japanese massage (Tsubo) are much the same as points the Chinese use in the method called amma.
26. Manual massage became a secondary treatment following World War II because new mechanical and electrical devices were designed to take over some of the manipulative movements.
27. Sports massage is used in sports medicine as an aid to treating injuries that have occurred during sports activities. It is also used as a means of keeping the athlete's muscles supple and strong.
28. Legitimate practitioners are educating the public about the benefits of massage done by licensed practitioners. The public should be aware of the dangers associated with illegal practices of massage by unlicensed and untrained imposters who use massage as their "front."

# Chapter 2 Requirements for the Practice of Therapeutic Massage

**LEARNING OBJECTIVES**

After you have mastered this chapter you will be able to:

1. Explain why the massage practitioner must be aware of the laws, rules, regulations, restrictions, and obligations governing the practice of therapeutic massage.
2. Explain why it is necessary to obtain a license to practice therapeutic body massage.
3. Explain how the education laws of most states define the practice of body massage.
4. Give 10 reasons a license might be revoked, canceled, or suspended.

**INTRODUCTION**

Therapeutic massage is a personal health service employing the use of various manipulations for the improvement of the client's health and well-being, therefore, the massage practitioner has a responsibility to the public and to individual clients. In addition to being well trained, the practitioner must have an understanding of the laws, rules, regulations, restrictions, and obligations concerning the practice of massage.

**LAWS, REGULATIONS, AND LICENSES**

Laws governing the practice of body massage may differ from one country to another. In the United States, state laws often differ from one state to another. It is not possible in the scope of this text to provide a thorough study of the complete laws and educational requirements pertaining to the practice of massage. However, the following information can serve as a valuable guide. When in doubt about laws pertaining to your profession, check with your own city and state departments of education.

Education laws in most states define body massage as the following: "The applying of a scientific system of activity to the muscular structure of the human body by means of stroking, kneading, rubbing, tapping, and vibrating movements with the hand (manually) or by mechanical apparatus for the purpose of improving muscle tone to promote relaxation, stimulate circulation of the blood and lymph and to produce therapeutic effects on the respiratory and nervous sytems."

Massage when correctly applied, improves the client's sense of physical and psychological well-being. Webster's Dictionary defines massage as: "Rubbing or kneading manipulation of a part of the body, usually with the hands, as to stimulate circulation and to make muscles or joints supple."

The massage practitioner is a person who has completed courses of study in the principles of anatomy, physiology, techniques of body massage (manually or with mechanical or electrical apparatus) safety procedures, hydrotherapy, and other approved, related subjects.

Being licensed in one state does not guarantee that the same license will be valid in another state or another country. A person who has a license and wishes to practice in another state or country should provide proof of ability to meet the requirements and make application as required. Not all states have massage laws. Where they are found, laws may differ because some states have had fewer problems, while others have found it necessary to establish state boards and stringent guidelines for licensing practitioners, schools, and establishments. In recent years, stricter laws have been put into effect in some states to curb unethical practices, misleading advertising, and use of the term *massage* to conceal questionable or unlawful activities such as prostitution.

People who have been educated and trained in another country are required to take a licensing examination by individual states upon presentation of the appropriate credentials.

**EDUCATIONAL REQUIREMENTS**

Licensed physical therapists, physicians, registered nurses, osteopaths, chiropractors, and podiatrists may practice massage as part of their therapeutic treatments when it has been included in their training programs. However, these professionals usually obtain a license specifically for the practice of massage when they wish to be known as massage practitioners.

In some states a student actively enrolled in a qualified school of massage may work as an apprentice under the supervision of a licensed massage practitioner.

Educational requirements to enroll in a program of instruction at a degree-granting institution or a school or institute of massage may differ, but generally a high school diploma or equivalency diploma is required. In most states a practitioner must be at least 18 years of age to be licensed and is expected to be of good moral character and free of any communicable disease.

In most states it is unlawful for any person to engage in the practice of massage or to teach any form of massage without the proper license or licenses. The massage practitioner is not authorized to engage in the practice of medicine; only duly licensed physicians may prescribe drugs or medication.

It is the duty of the massage practitioner to refuse to give treatments to persons who are obviously in need of medical attention and for whom massage treatments have contraindications. It should be remembered that massage techniques included in the training of physicians, nurses, and physical therapists who work with the sick and injured should not be confused with basic nonmedical therapeutic massage.

Massage establishments must abide by certain laws, rules and regulations. They must be licensed and employ only licensed practitioners. Most states require massage practitioners to display their licenses at their place of business.

### HEALTH REQUIREMENTS FOR PRACTITIONERS

Since massage is a "touch" or "hands-on" profession, the massage practitioner is expected to be physically and mentally fit. Some employers request a health certificate or written confirmation from a physician. It is the practitioner's duty to keep himself or herself in top physical condition. Massage is hard work and requires that the practitioner have physical stamina and the ability to concentrate on giving a therapeutic massage.

### REASONS LICENSE MAY BE REVOKED, SUSPENDED, OR CANCELED

Because the practice of massage deals with the health and welfare of the public and specifically that of individual clients, the profession must necessarily be regulated by the issuance of licenses only to people who have met the requirements to practice. The professional massage practitioner must have integrity, the necessary technical skills, and a willingness to comply with rigid health standards.

The following are grounds upon which the practitioner's license may be revoked, canceled, or suspended:

1. Being guilty of fraud or deceit in obtaining a license.
2. Having been convicted of a felony.
3. Being engaged currently or previously in any act of prostitution.
4. Practicing under a false or assumed name.
5. Being addicted to narcotics, alcohol, or like substances that interfere with the performance of duties.
6. Being willfully negligent in the practice of massage so as to endanger the health of a client.
7. Prescribing drugs or medicines (unless you are a licensed physician).
8. Being guilty of fraudulent or deceptive advertising.
9. Being physically or mentally incompetent to practice.
10. Practicing while being knowingly afflicted with a communicable disease.

### QUESTIONS FOR DISCUSSION AND REVIEW

1. Why must the massage practitioner be concerned about the laws, rules, regulations, and obligations pertaining to the practice of therapeutic body massage?
2. How do education laws define massage?
3. Why do laws governing the practice of massage often differ from one state to another?
4. What is the general educational requirement for a license to practice massage?
5. What are the 10 specific grounds upon which the practitioner's license may be revoked, canceled, or suspended?

## ANSWERS TO QUESTIONS FOR DISCUSSION AND REVIEW

1. The practitioner must be concerned about the laws, rules, regulations, and obligations concerning the practice of therapeutic body massage because the practitioner has a responsibility to the public and to individual clients. Massage is a personal, health-related service, and as such, strict rules must be observed.
2. The education law defines massage as, "The applying of a scientific system of activity to the muscular structure of the human body by means of stroking, kneading, rubbing, tapping and vibrating movements by hand (manually) or by means of a mechanical or electrical apparatus for the purpose of improving muscle tone, to promote relaxation, to stimulate the circulation of the blood and to improve the client's sense of physiological and psychological well-being."
3. Laws governing the practice of massage often differ because some states have fewer complaints, or problems, while others have found it necessary to establish state boards and stringent guidelines for licensing practitioners, schools, and establishments. The professional practice of massage is a legitimate profession that requires protection from those who misuse it for unlawful purposes.
4. The general educational requirement for a license to practice massage is a high school or high school equivalency diploma.
5. The grounds upon which the practitioner's license may be revoked, canceled, or suspended are:
   1. Fraud or deceit in obtaining a license.
   2. Convicted of a felony.
   3. Being engaged in any act of prostitution.
   4. Practicing under a false or assumed name.
   5. Addiction to drugs, alcohol, etc.
   6. Being willfully negligent of the health of a client.
   7. Prescribing drugs or medicine.
   8. Being guilty of fraudulent or deceptive advertising.
   9. Being physically or mentally incompetent to practice.
   10. Practicing while being knowingly afflicted with a communicable disease.

# Chapter 3 Professional Ethics for Massage Practitioners

**LEARNING OBJECTIVES**

After you have mastered this chapter, you will be able to:

1. Define the meaning of professional ethics.
2. Explain how the practice of good ethics helps to build a successful massage practice.
3. Discuss the importance of good health habits and professional projection.
4. Discuss the importance of human relations and success attitudes.
5. Discuss ways to build a sound business reputation.

**INTRODUCTION**

Ethics is the study of the standards and philosophy of human conduct and is defined as a system or code of morals of an individual, a group, or a profession. To practice good ethics is to be concerned about the public welfare, the welfare of individual clients, and the reputation of the profession you represent. A professional person is one who is engaged in an avocation or occupation requiring some advanced training to gain education and skills. However, without ethics there can be no true professionalism.

Ethical conduct on the part of the practitioner gives the client confidence in the place of business, the services rendered, and the entire industry. A satisfied client is your best means of advertising because his or her good recommendation helps you to maintain public confidence and build a sound business following. The business establishment that becomes known for its professional ethics will stay in business longer than one that makes extravagant claims and false promises or that is involved in questionable practices.

**BUSINESS ETHICS FOR THE MASSAGE PRACTITIONER**

Successful business managers prefer employees who can help them build their business and keep their customers. The following are points of business ethics you should keep in mind:

1. Treat all clients with the same fairness and courtesy.
2. Set an example of professionalism by your conduct at all times.
3. Live up to your promises and your obligations.
4. Give efficient service, backed by knowledge and skills.
5. Be loyal to clients, co-workers, your employer, and your associates.

6. Know the laws, rules, and regulations of your city, county, and state.
7. Obey all laws, rules, and regulations pertaining to your work.
8. Be fair and honest in all advertising of services.
9. Communicate in a professional manner on the telephone, in personal conversations, and in letters.
10. Refrain from the use of improper language and any form of gossip.
11. Be well organized so that you make the most of your time.
12. Make the most of your appearance so that you are looked upon as a credit to your profession.
13. Continue to learn about new developments in your profession.
14. Keep foremost in your mind that you are a professional person engaged in giving an important and beneficial personal service.
15. Do your utmost to keep your place of business clean, neat, and attractive. Remember that people judge you by first impressions.

## PERSONAL HYGIENE AND HEALTH HABITS

In order to inspire confidence and trust in your clients, you should project a well-groomed, professional appearance at all times. Personal health and good grooming are assets much admired by the client and are essential for your protection and that of the client when you are employed in a personal service business.

Your personal health and grooming habits should include the following:

1. Take a bath or shower daily and use a deodorant as necessary.
2. Keep your teeth and gums healthy. Visit your dentist regularly.
3. Use mouthwash and avoid foods that contribute to offensive breath odor.
4. Keep your hair fresh and clean, and wear an appropriate hairstyle. Hair should be worn in a style so that it is not touched during a massage session.
5. Avoid strong fragrances such as perfumes, colognes, and lotions.
6. Keep your hands free of blemishes and callouses. Use lotion to keep your hands soft and smooth.
7. Keep your nails clean and filed so they do not extend to the tips of the fingers. Sharp nails should never come in contact with the client's skin. Never wear garish nail polish.
8. If you are a woman, wear appropriate makeup in subdued, flattering colors. Be sure makeup is applied neatly.
9. If you are a man, keep beard or mustache neat and well groomed. If you prefer the clean-shaven look, be sure to shave as often as necessary.

10. Avoid gum chewing or smoking in the presence of clients.
11. Keep your face clean and free of blemishes.
12. Practice all rules of sanitation for the client's and for your own protection.
13. Have a complete physical examination by a physician before beginning work as a massage practitioner. Continue to have checkups, follow your physician's advice, and do all that is possible to maintain optimum health.
14. Eat a well-balanced, nutritious diet in order to maintain your physical and mental health.
15. Take time for relaxation and to keep fit. Exercise is important to the massage practioner. You should keep your muscles strong and flexible. A regimen of daily exercise is recommended. This may be accomplished by participation in active sports of your choice (swimming, tennis, etc.), working out at the gym, or by devising a set of beneficial exercises you can do at home.
16. Maintain your normal weight for your height and bone structure. You should not be extremely overweight nor extremely underweight. If you have a weight problem, follow your physician's advice on how to attain your most healthful weight.
17. Be aware of good posture when walking, standing, sitting, and working. Poor posture habits such as slouching contribute to fatigue, foot problems, and strain to your back and neck.
18. Wear the appropriate clothing for your profession. Clothing should be loose enough to allow for optimal movement. It should be free of accessories that might catch on the massage table or touch the client when you are performing the massage, such as a long chain, necklace or tie, a wide belt, or long sleeves.
19. Consider clothing that allows your body heat to escape. Clothing items made of natural fibers such as cotton are good. Clothing made of synthetic fabrics hold the heat of your body and will be uncomfortable for the physical exertion of this profession.

## HUMAN RELATIONSHIPS

In addition to gaining the necessary technical skills as a professional massage practitioner you must be able to understand your client's needs. This is the basis of all good human relations. A pleasant voice, good manners, cheerfulness, patience, tact, loyalty, empathy, and interest in the client's welfare are some of the desirable traits that help to build the client's confidence in you and your place of business.

It is important to be able to interact with people without becoming too familiar. Many times clients will confide their personal feelings and they trust you not to betray their confidence. This is where the art of listening is an invaluable asset. Listen with empathy, change the subject when necessary (tactfully), and never betray the client's confidence in you. This subject will be covered in more detail in another part of this text.

The following rules for good human relations will help you to interact successfully with people from all walks of life:

*Tact:* Tact is your ability to deal with a client who is overly critical, finds fault, and is hard to please. It may be that he or she just wants attention. Tact helps you to deal with this client in an impersonal but understanding manner. To be tactful is to avoid what is offensive or disturbing and to do what is most considerate for all concerned. For example, you might discover that a client needs medical care and you feel you should suggest that he or she see a physician. You must approach the problem with the utmost tact and diplomacy.

*Cheerfulness:* A cheerful attitude and a pleasant facial expression will go a long way toward putting a client at ease.

*Patience:* Patience is the ability to be tolerant under stressful or undesirable conditions. Your patience and understanding will be the best medicine when you deal with people who are ill, handicapped, or in pain. Patience helps you to change negative feelings to more positive ones.

*Honesty:* To be honest does not mean that you must be brutally frank with a client. You can answer questions in a factual but tactful manner. For example, if a client has unrealistic expectations regarding the benefits of a treatment, you can discuss what can or cannot be accomplished in a sincere, conscientious manner.

*Intuition:* Intuition is your ability to have insight into people's feelings. When you genuinely like people, it is easier to show sympathy and understanding for their problems. People will often confide in you when their intuition tells them you are trustworthy. In turn, your own intuition will help you to avoid embarrassing situations and involving yourself in problems you cannot solve. Remember the primary reason your clients come to you is for relaxation. Keep conversations to a minimum to allow the client maximum relaxation.

*Sense of humor:* It is important to have a sense of humor, especially when dealing with difficult people or situations. A good sense of humor helps you to remain optimistic, courteous, and in control.

*Maturity:* Maturity is not so much a matter of how old you are, but what you have gained from your life experience. Maturity is the quality of being reliable, responsible, self-disciplined, and well adjusted.

*Self-esteem:* Self-esteem is projected by your attitudes about yourself and your profession. If you respect yourself and your profession, you will be respected by others.

*Self-motivation:* Self-motivation is your ability to set positive goals and go after what you want. It is having the courage to work a little harder and a lot smarter. It means making sacrifices when necessary to save time and your money in order to put them toward the achievement of your goals.

## BUILDING A PROFESSIONAL IMAGE

If you want to be successful in business, you must prepare for success. Preparation, planning, and performance are the assets that help you do your job in the most professional manner. You should take every opportunity to pursue new avenues of knowledge. Attend professional seminars, read trade papers and other publications relating to your business, and become active in associations where you can exchange ideas with other dedicated people.

Your business image is important and should be built on good service and truth in advertising. The sensational seeking "quick buck" business won't fool the public long. A reliable reputation is particularly important in the personal service business because you are dealing with the health and well-being of individuals. Consistently high standards and good service are the foundations upon which successful businesses are built.

## YOUR BUSINESS NAME

Using appropriate wording in your business name and in advertising will help you to establish a good reputation. You can see how the name "Smitty's Massage Parlour" or "Smith Massage Clinic" can totally change how your business is perceived by potential clients.

Some massage professionals, especially those entering a new community, may feel they need to state in their advertising that only therapeutic and proper massage is given. Keeping regular business hours, rather than late night hours, also improves your reputation.

Another point to remember is that using proper draping techniques to always ensure your client's privacy is very important in building a good reputation. Word of mouth is the massage professional's best advertising. People will spread the message that you work in a professional manner.

## QUESTIONS FOR DISCUSSION AND REVIEW

1. Why is it important to have a code of ethics for your business?
2. Why is a satisfied client your best means of advertising?
3. Why do successful business managers prefer employees who are concerned with personal and professional ethics?
4. Why is it necessary for the massage practitioner to have strict personal hygiene and health habits?
5. What is meant by "professional projection" in attitude and appearance?
6. How do you define human relations as applied to working with or serving others.
7. Why is the practice of human relations so important to the massage practitioner?
8. When building your business (practice) image, how can you be sure the public gets the right message?

## ANSWERS TO QUESTIONS FOR DISCUSSION AND REVIEW

1. It is important to have a code of ethics for your business in order to protect the public and your reputation.
2. A satisfied client is your best means of advertising because he or she will recommend you, your business, and your services.
3. Successful business managers know that employees who practice sound personal and professional ethics will help them to build their business and keep their customers.
4. It is necessary for the massage practitioner to be concerned with personal hygiene and health habits because his or her own good health inspires confidence on the part of clients. Good health is also a form of protection for the practitioner and the client.
5. Professional projection in attitude and appearance means that the practitioner acts, speaks, and dresses to project a professional image.
6. Human relations is defined as the art of being able to work successfully with others and to give excellent service.
7. The practice of good human relations is important because it helps the practitioner interact successfully with different personalities.
8. When building your business image, pay attention to the use of appropriate wording in your business name and in advertising so that potential clients get the right message.

# PART II HUMAN ANATOMY AND PHYSIOLOGY

# Chapter 4 Histology— Cells and Tissues

## LEARNING OBJECTIVES

After you have mastered this chapter you will be able to:

1. Demonstrate knowledge of basic histology, anatomy, and physiology requisites for mastering the practice of therapeutic massage.
2. Explain the basic functions of the cells.
3. Explain the basics of body metabolism.
4. Describe the various types of tissues and their functions.
5. Explain the importance of the study of cells and tissues to the practice of body massage.

## INTRODUCTION

An elementary knowledge of histology, anatomy, and physiology is a necessary requisite in mastering the theory and practice of therapeutic massage. The massage practitioner should study the structures and functions of the human body in order to know when, where, and how to apply massage movements for the most beneficial results. This knowledge enables the practitioner to adjust the massage treatment to the needs of the individual and to control results.

## HISTOLOGY DEFINED

*Histology* is a form of microscopic anatomy. It is the branch of biology concerned with the microscopic structure of tissues of a living organism. All living structures are composed of cells and intercellular materials that are organized from the various systems of the body. Massage has a beneficial effect on the body when it promotes or stimulates cellular activity.

*Anatomy* is defined as the gross structure of the body or the study of an organism and the interrelations of its parts. For example, when we describe the skeleton or other anatomic parts of the body, naming the parts and how they relate to one another, we are describing anatomy.

*Physiology* is the science and study of the vital processes, mechanisms, and functions of an organ or system of organs. When we describe how the organs or parts of the body function, we are speaking of physiology. Histology, anatomy, and physiology are interrelated in that the structures are associated with their functions. Structure and function are dependent on the interaction of the organism's parts, and each part has a role in the operation of the whole.

## LEVELS OF COMPLEXITY OF LIVING MATTER

All materials are composed of chemical substances. These substances are made up of subatomic particles called *molecules.* Within the human organism the basic unit of structure and function is the *cell.* Cells are organized into layers or groups called *tissues.* Groups of various tissues form complex structures which perform certain functions. These structures are called *organs* and are arranged in *organ systems.* Organ systems are arranged together to form an organism. The human body is the organism we study in relation to body massage.

### Cells

Cells are the basic units of all living matter of animals, plants, and bacteria. Living cells differ from one another in size, shape, structure, and function. In the human body cells are highly specialized and perform such vital functions as movement, digestion, and reproduction. The principal parts of a cell are the *cytoplasm, centrosome, nucleus,* and *cell membrane.* Cells are composed of *protoplasm,* a colorless, jellylike substance in which food elements, such as protein, fats, carbohydrates, mineral salts, and water, are present. A thin cell membrane or wall permits soluble substances to enter and leave the protoplasm. Near the center of the cell is a nucleus (dense protoplasm). Outside the nucleus are the cytoplasm (less dense protoplasm) and a centrosome.

#### *Structure of the Cell*

The protoplasm of the cell contains the following structures:

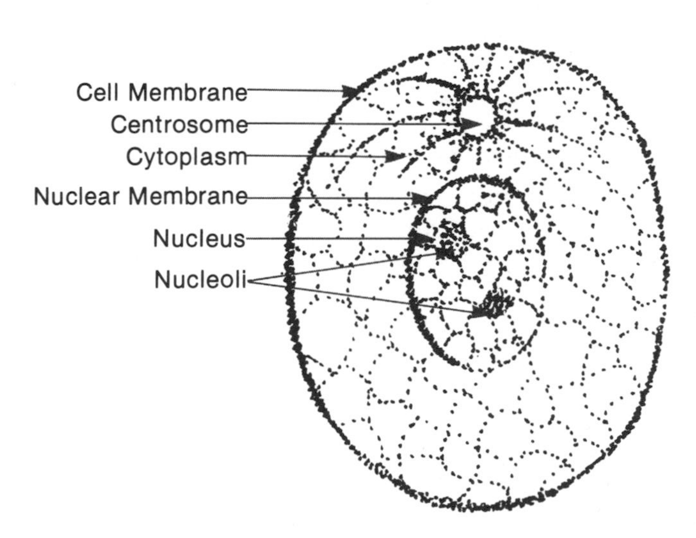


Nucleus (***NOO** klee us*)—dense protoplasm found in the center, which plays an important part in the reproduction of the cell.

Cytoplasm (***SI** to plaz um*)—less dense protoplasm found outside of the nucleus and contains food materials necessary for the growth, reproduction and self-repair of the cell.

Centrosome (***SEN** tro sohm*)—a small, round body in the cytoplasm, which also affects the reproduction of the cell.

Cell membrane—encloses the protoplasm. It permits soluble substances to enter and leave the cell.

The cytoplasm contains a network of various membranes that mark off several distinct parts called *cytoplasmic organelles* that perform specific functions necessary for cell survival.

The centrosome and nucleus control cell reproduction. As long as the cell receives an adequate supply of food, oxygen, and water, eliminates waste products, and is surrounded by a favorable environment (proper temperature, and the absence of waste products, toxins, and pressure), it will continue to grow and prosper. When these requirements are not filled, the cell will stop growing and will eventually die.

**Chart of Structure and Function of Cellular Organelles**

An organelle is a discreet structure within a cell, having specialized functions, identifying molecular structures, and a distinctive chemical composition.

| ORGANELLE | STRUCTURE | FUNCTION |
|---|---|---|
| Cell membrane | A thin covering of the outer surface of the cytoplasm composed of protein and lipid molecules. | Transports materials between the outside and inside of the cell. Helps to control cell activity and contains cellular material. |
| Centrosome | A nonmembranous structure near the nucleus—two rod-shaped centrioles. | Divides into two parts during mitosis and moves to the opposite poles of the dividing cell. |
| Chromatin | Network of fibers composed of protein and DNA that form the chromosomes. | Contains the genes by which hereditary characteristics are transmitted and determined. |
| Endoplasmic reticulum | Network of sacs and canals. | There are two varieties: a smooth type that produces lipid and a rough type that produces protein. Synthesizes protein for cell utilization and transport. |
| Fibrils and microtubules | Minute rods and tubules | Support the cytoplasm and contribute to movement of substances within the cytoplasm. |
| Golgi apparatus | Composed of flattened membranes and small vesicles. | Collects the products of cell synthesis, synthesizes carbohydrates, holds protein molecules for secretion. |
| Lysosome | Membraneous structure containing hydrolytic enzymes. | Digests foreign substances. |
| Mitochrondria | Shape varies according to function, but all exhibit a double membrane with the inner membrane lifted into folds. | Contains enzymes for releasing energy and converting it to useful forms for cell operation. |
| Nuclear membrane | The covering structure of the nucleus that separates the nucleus and the cytoplasm. | Controls passage of substances between the nucleus and the cytoplasm. |
| Nucleolus | A dense body composed mainly of protein with some RNA molecules, and found in the nucleus of most cells. | Forms ribosomes. |
| Nucleus | Protein-coated hereditary material (DNA) containing chromosomes that transmit heredity. | Supervises all cell activity. |
| Ribisome | Minute particle or granule composed of RNA and protein molecules. | Synthesizes proteins. |
| Vacuole | Membrane-lined containers. | Involved in rapid ejection of fluids or introduction of substances. |

## Cell Mitosis

As a cell matures and is nourished; it grows in size and eventually divides into two smaller daughter (like) cells. This series of changes, from the time the cell forms until it reproduces, is the life cycle of a cell.

The human body is composed of more than 100 trillion cells, which develop from a single cell, the fertilized ovum (egg). The repeated division of the ovum results in many specialized cells that differ from one another in composition and function. This process is termed *differentiation.* The basic structure of the cells is common to all.

In the human body, some cells reproduce continually, some occasionally, and some not at all. For example skin and intestinal lining cells reproduce continually throughout life.

Bone and nerve cells stop growing at maturity. Most body cells are capable of growth and self-repair during their life cycle. However, delicate nerve cells are incapable of self-repair after injury or destruction and disease. In the human body, when a cell reaches maturity, reproduction takes place by indirect division. This is a process called *mitosis,* in which a series of changes occur in the nucleus before the entire cell divides in half. In mitosis, two daughter cells are produced that are identical to the parent type, or one may become a special cell while the other remains the same as the parent cell. Mitosis is accomplished in five stages. These phases are called: interphase, prophase, metaphase, anaphase and telophase.

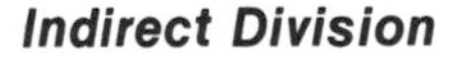

### *Indirect Division*

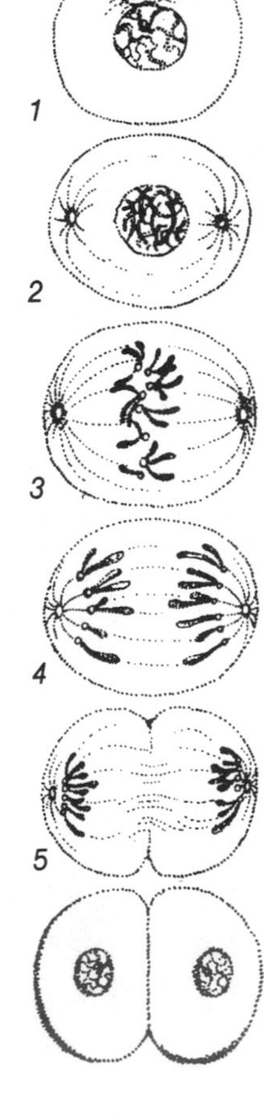


1. *Interphase:* This is a normal state of the cell or the resting phase during which most of the cellular work and growth are done. During interphase, chromosomes exist in thin threads. It is during mitosis that the chromosomes assume the twin helical (rodlike) structure.
2. *Prophase:* Prophase occurs when the chromosomes, composed of DNA (deoxyribonucleic acid), which houses the genes, become larger. They can be seen within the cell duplicated in two coiled strands called chromatids. During the last part of the prophase, the nucleus disappears.
3. *Metaphase:* During metaphase, the chromosomes arrange themselves in a plane called the equatorial plane. The nuclear membrane and the nucleolus are absent.
4. *Anaphase:* During anaphase, the chromatids are separated and are again called chromosomes.
5. *Telophase:* This is the stage when the chromosomes reach the centroles (small bodies) and begin to uncoil. The cytoplasm divides into two parts or two cells.

Direct division of a cell, *amitosis,* is the method of reproduction in which the nucleus and cytoplasm divide by simple construction without the splitting of chromosomes.

*Mitosis is the indirect and complex division of the human cell. This is a process whereby a series of changes occur in the nucleus before the cell divides in half. In this procedure the centrosome plays an important role in maintaining the characteristics of the original cell. This method of reproduction occurs in human tissues, including hair and skin.*

## Muscle Cells

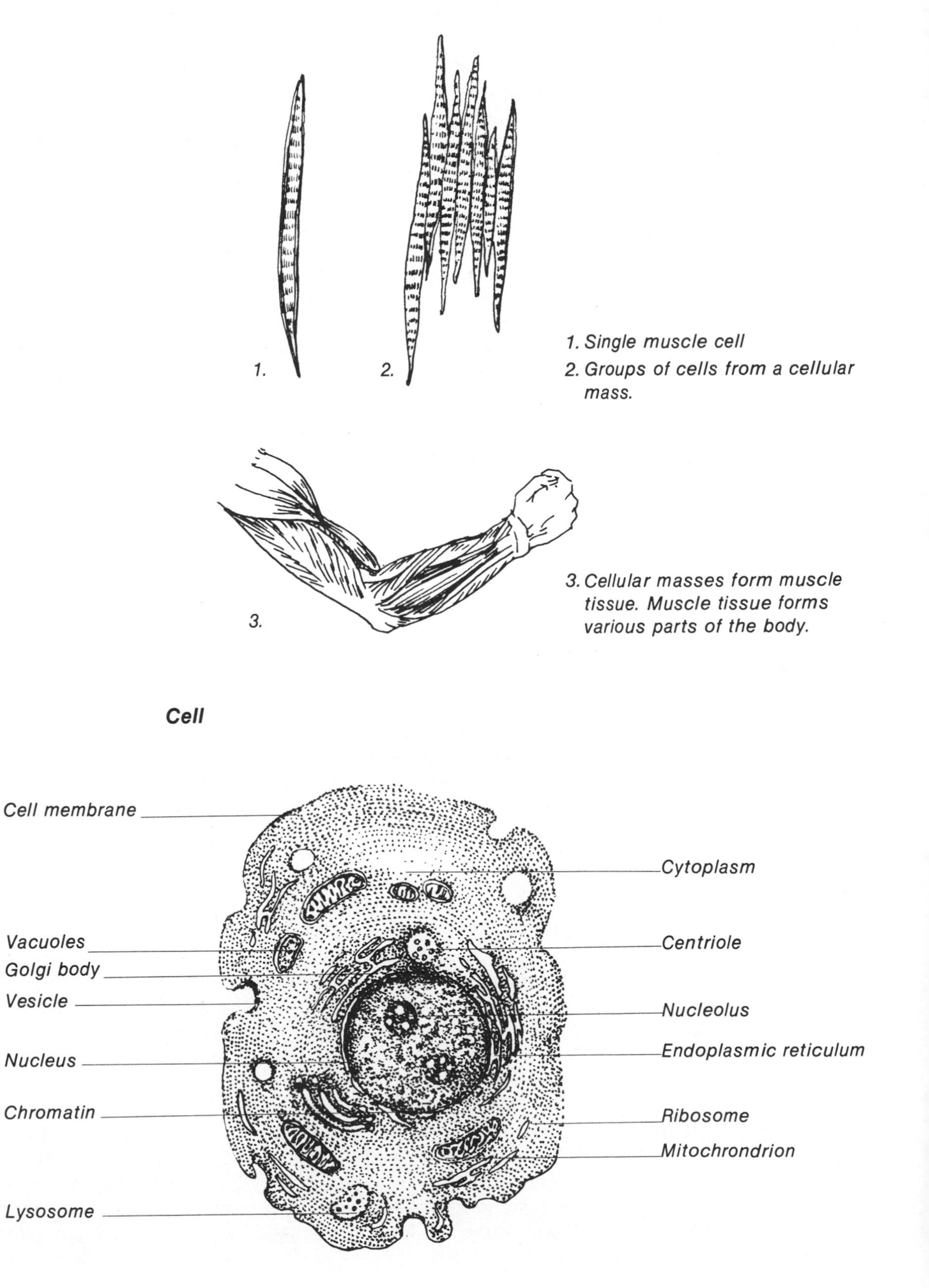


1. Single muscle cell
2. Groups of cells from a cellular mass.
3. Cellular masses form muscle tissue. Muscle tissue forms various parts of the body.

## Cellular Activity

The activity of cells may be divided into three categories: vegetative, growth and reproduction, and specialized.

1. *Vegetative:* Vegetative activities include maintenance of the cell such as absorption, assimilation, and excretion of waste products.
2. *Growth and reproduction:* Growth involves the development of additional structural materials. Reproduction is the process of mitosis or indirect division of cells. The centriole and nucleus play important roles in this process.
3. *Specialized activities:* This refers to cell differentiation, which means that some cells are more prominent than others, and different cells perform different functions. For example, muscle cells exhibit contractility. Epithelial cells secrete and absorb. Nerve cells are involved in transmission of impulses. The cell is usually in the vegetative state, then as time passes it undergoes regression (atrophy) and finally dies.

## Metabolism

As the basic units of life, cells perform individually much like a small factory. All chemical reactions within a cell that transforms food for cell growth and operation are broadly termed *cellular metabolism.* Metabolism is a complex chemical and physical process that takes place in living organisms whereby the cells are nourished and carry out their various activities. *Intermediate metabolism* includes all chemical reactions taking place from the moment a nutrient is ingested until the chemical products are returned to the environment. Different kinds of cells perform specialized metabolic processes; however, all cells perform basic reactions that include the building up or breaking down of proteins, carbohydrates, fats, and other nutrients. There are two phases of metabolism: anabolism and catabolism. *Anabolism* is the process of building up of larger molecules from smaller ones. This process requires energy because it is the constructive phase of the cellular metabolism during which time substances needed for cell growth and repair are manufactured. *Catabolism* is the breaking down of larger substances or molecules into smaller ones. This process releases energy that may be stored by special molecules to be used for other reactions, such as muscle contraction or heat production. Digestion is an example of catabolism.

Anabolism and catabolism are carried out simultaneously and continuously in the cells. Their activities are closely regulated so that the breaking-down or energy-releasing reactions are balanced with building-up or energy-using reactions. Therefore, homeostasis (the maintenance of normal, internal stability in an organism) is maintained.

## ENZYMES

*Enzymes* are protein substances formed in the cells that act as organic catalysts to initiate or accelerate specific chemical reactions in the metabolic process, while they themselves remain unchanged. The reaction promoted by a particular enzyme is very specific. Therefore, because cellular metabolism includes hundreds of different chemical reactions, there are hundreds of different kinds of enzymes.

Enzymes are involved in the process of releasing energy from nutrients, principally from carbohydrates, fats, and proteins. Energy is the capacity to produce change in matter or to do work. Carbohydrates are broken down into simple sugars (glucose), fats are split into fatty acids, and proteins are converted into amino acids. As these materials are broken down into simpler compounds, energy is released. Some of this energy is in the form of heat, while some is used to carry on the various cellular functions or to promote further cellular metabolism. Some energy may be stored in a special molecule called *adenosine triphosphats (ATP).* ATP is involved in the release of energy for muscular and other cellular activity.

**TISSUES**

The basic unit of tissue is the cell. Tissues are collections of similar cells that carry out specific functions of the body. Tissues comprise all body organs and are subdivided into five main categories:

1. Epithelial Tissue.
2. Connective tissue.
3. Muscular tissue.
4. Nervous tissue.
5. Liquid tissue.

The human body develops from a single cell, and by the second week of growth of a human fetus (the embryonic stage), there is development of distinct layers of cells. The innermost layer of cells is called the *endoderm,* the middle layer is the *mesoderm,* and the outermost layer is called the *ectoderm.* Together these layers form the primary germ layer from which all body tissues and organs are formed.

The endodermal (inner layer) cells produce the epithelial linings of the respiratory and digestive tracts as well as linings of the urethra and urinary bladder. The mesodermal (middle layer) cells develop into all types of muscle, bone, blood, blood vessel tissues, various connective tissues, lymph, and the linings of all body cavities as well as the kidneys and the reproductive organs. The ecodermal (outer layer) cells form the glands of the skin, linings of the mouth, the anal canal, the epidermis, hair, nails, and the nervous system.

*Epithelial tissue* is a thin protective layer or covering that functions in the process of absorption, excretion, secretion, and protection. There are various classifications of epithelial tissue named according to shape or number of layers of cells. Epithelial cells are classified by shape as *squamous* (flat), *cuboidal* (small cube shape), and *columnar* (tall or rectangular). These cells are also classified according to arrangement. For example, a simple squamous arrangement is one cell thick, the stratified squamous arrangement is several cells thick and the transitional squamous is an arrangement of several layers of cells that are flat and closely packed.

Epithelial tissue covers all the surfaces of the body both inside and out. It forms the skin, the covering of the organs, and the inner lining of all the hollow organs. It also makes up the major tissue of the glands. Because epithelial tissue acts as a surface covering or a lining, it always has a free surface that is exposed to outside influences, whereas the other surface is well anchored in the connective tissue from which it derives nourishment.

**Types of Epithelial Tissue**

*Simple squamous*

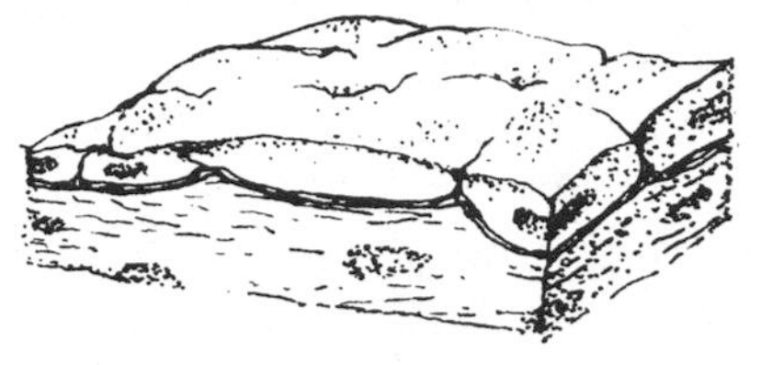

1. *Simple squamous:* found in protective layers of tissue.

*Stratified squamous*

2. *Stratified squamous:* Found in vocal chords, intestines, and like organs.

*Simple columnar*

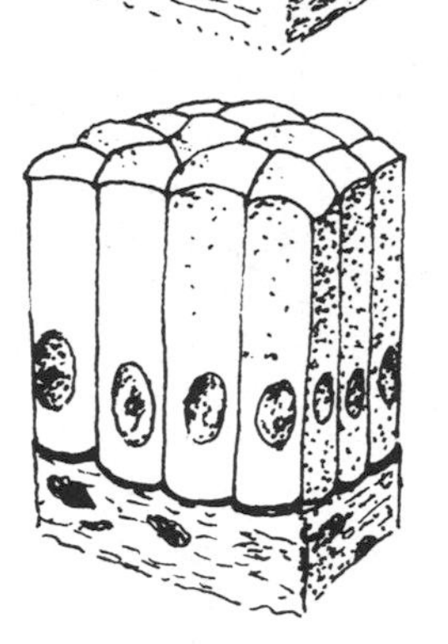

3. *Simple columnar:* Found in the stomach and bowels.

*Cuboidal*

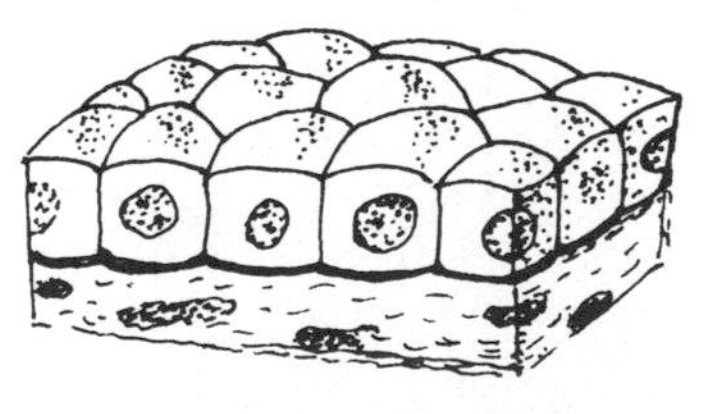

4. *Cuboidal:* Found in lining of ducts and pigmented layer of the retina of the eye.

*Transitional squamous*

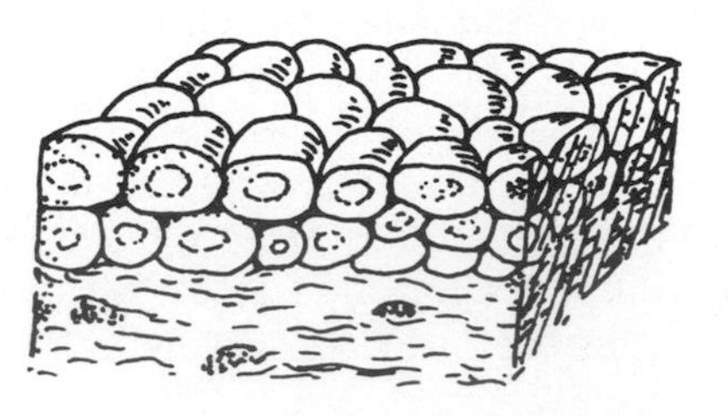

5. *Transitional squamous:* Found in the lining of the urinary bladder and kidney.

**Membranes**

Membranes are structures closely associated with epithelial tissue. There are two main categories of membranes: epithelial membranes and fibrous connective tissue membranes. *Epithelial membranes* have their outer surface faced with epithelium. They are further divided into two main subgroups: mucuous membranes and serous membranes. *Mucuous membranes* produce a thick, sticky substance that acts as a protectant and lubricant. *Serous membranes* produce a more watery substance that also acts as a lubricant. In some instances their secretions contain a high number of enzymes that perform specific actions, such as digestion. Serous membranes line the body cavities and sometimes form the outermost surface of the organs contained in those cavities. The covering of the serous membranes in the body cavities is a special epethelial tissue called the mesothelium. This is a smooth covering that allows the movements of the organs to take place with little or no friction. Three major serous membranes are the pleura that encase the lungs, the peracardium around the heart and peritoneum, that lines the abdominal cavity.

The second category of membranes is known as the *connective tissue membranes.* These include the *fascial membranes,* which serve to anchor and support the organs and the skeletal membranes that cover bones and cartilage. *Superficial fascia* refers to the connecting layer between the skin and those structures underlying the skin. *Fascia* is the fibrous tissue between muscle bundles or forming the sheath around muscles or other deep (deep fascia) structures that support nerves and blood vessels. *Deep fascia* refers to tissues, containing little or no fat, that penetrate deep into the body. Deep fascia may also cover and protect muscles. Blood vessels, nerves, and the spinal cord are also covered by fascia.

*Skeletal membrane* covers bones and cartilage. The membrane covering bone is termed *periosteum.* The membrane covering cartilage is called *perichondrium.* Cavities and capsules in and around joints are lined with connective tissue called *synovial membrane,* which secretes synovium, or synovial fluid, an agent that acts as lubricant between the ends of bones and in spaces of great activity and friction. There are many other membranes in the body, and all of them can be classified as either epithelial or connective.

**Connective Tissue**

Connective tissue binds structures together, provides support and protection, and serves as a framework. There is an abundance of intercellular substance (matrix) in connective tissue, consisting of fibers or thick, gel-like fluid.

The loose connective tissue, or *areolar* tissue, binds the skin to the underlying tissues and fills the spaces between the muscles. This is the tissue that lies beneath most layers of epithelium. It is rich in blood vessels and provides nourishment to the epithelial tissues. *Adipose* tissue is areolar tissue that has an abundance of fat-containing cells. Adipose tissue acts as a protection against heat loss and stores energy in the form of fat molecules. It is found in abundance in certain abdominal membranes, around the surface of the heart, between the muscles, around the kidneys, and just beneath the skin.

*Reticular tissue* resembles fine fibers, when viewed under a microscope. These fibers form the framework of the liver and lymphoid organs. *Fibrous connective tissue* is composed of collagen (albuminoid substance) and elastic fibers that are closely arranged to form tendons and ligaments. *Tendons* or sinews are white, glistening cords or bands that serve to attach muscle to bone and are found wherever great strength with a certain amount of rigidity is required. Ligaments are tough, fibrous bands that connect bones or support viscera. Bone is tissue consisting of inorganic salts, cells, and fibers.

*Dentine* is the hard, calcareous tissue forming the body of a tooth beneath the enamel. Unlike bone, dentine contains no cells or vessels.

***Cartilage***

*Fibrous cartilage* is found between the vertebrae and where minimal-range movement is required. In dense fibrous connective tissue, repair to damaged tissue is slower due to poor blood supply.

*Hyaline* is a type of cartilage that contains little fibrous tissue and is made up of cells embedded in a somewhat translucent matrix, as found in the nose and trachea and on the end of bones and in many joints.

*Elastic cartilage* is the most resilient of cartilages and is found in the external ear, the larynx, and like structures.

***Bone Tissue***

*Bone* or osseous (bonelike) tissue is connective tissue in which the intercellular substance is rendered hard by being impregnated with mineral salts, chiefly calcium phosphate and calcium carbonate. Compact, dense material forms the dense, outer layer of a long bone, while cancellous (porous) material forms the bone's inner tissue. Dentine, the substance beneath the enamel of the teeth, closely resembles bone but is harder and denser.

**Muscle Tissue**

The main function of muscle tissue fibers is to contract their elongated cells, which pulls attached ends closer together, causing a body part to move. The three types of muscle tissue are: skeletal muscle tissue, smooth muscle tissue, and cardiac muscle tissue.

*Skeletal muscles* are usually attached to bone or other muscle by way of tendons and can be controlled by conscious effort. These are called *voluntary muscles.* Skeletal muscles are responsible for moving the limbs of the body, facial expression, speaking, and other voluntary movements. Voluntary muscle cells appear long and threadlike under a microscope and have alternating light and dark cross-markings called *striations.* Muscles containing striations are called *striated muscles.*

*Smooth muscle tissue* lacks striations (nonstriated) and cannot usually be stimulated to contract by conscious effort. Muscle contractions generally result from involuntary nerve or gland activity. Smooth muscle tissue is found in the hollow organs of the stomach, small intestine, colon, bladder, and the blood vessels. Nonstriated muscle is responsible for the movement of food through the digestive tract, the constriction of blood vessels, and the emptying of the bladder.

***Cardiac Muscle Tissue***

*Cardiac muscle tissue* occurs only in the heart. It is controlled involuntarily and can continue to function without being directly stimulated by nerve impulses. Cardiac tissue is responsible for pumping blood through the heart into the blood vessels.

**Nervous Tissue**

*Nervous* or *nerve tissue* is composed of neurons (nerve cells) enclosed in connective tissue. Nerves act as channels for the transmission of messages to and from the various parts of the body, such as sensory nerves in the skin and organs of hearing, taste, smell, and sight.

*Nervous tissue proper* (fundamental cellular units of nervous tissue) initiates, controls, and coordinates the body's adaptation to its surroundings. Neurons (nerve cells) are linked together to form pathways.

Connective and supportive tissues in the central nervous system are called neuroglia.

**Liquid Tissue**

*Liquid tissue* is represented by blood and lymph. Bone marrow is an example of hematopiotic (blood forming) tissue. Blood is a fluid tissue that circulates throughout the body and from which the body cells obtain nutrients and by which waste products are removed. According to some sources, liquid tissue is considered to be connective tissue. Lymphoid tissue is found in the lymph nodes (small compact, knotlike structures) and in the adenoids, thymus, tonsils, and spleen. Lymphoid tissue is important in the production of antibodies.

**TISSUE**

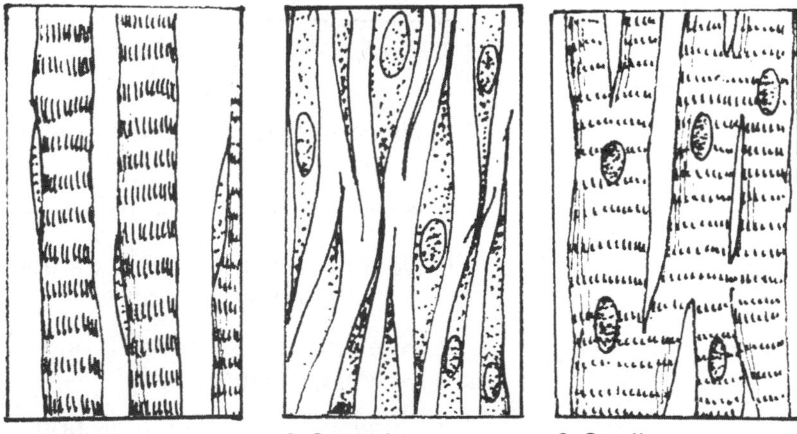

*1. Striated* *2. Smooth* *3. Cardiac*

**Types of Tissue**

1. *Striated:* Cylindrical fibers in voluntary muscles.
2. *Smooth:* Smooth fibers without striations found in involuntary muscles.
3. *Cardiac (striated):* Cardiac muscles found exclusively in the heart.

**Types of Tissue**
*(continued)*

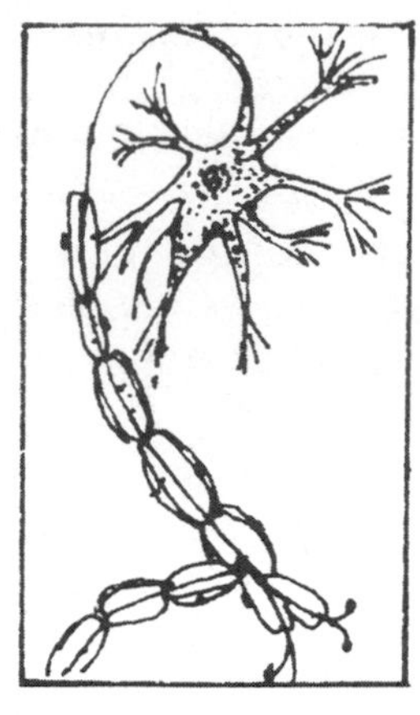

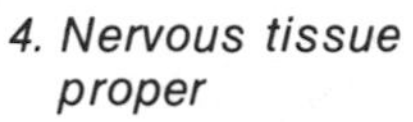

*4. Nervous tissue proper*

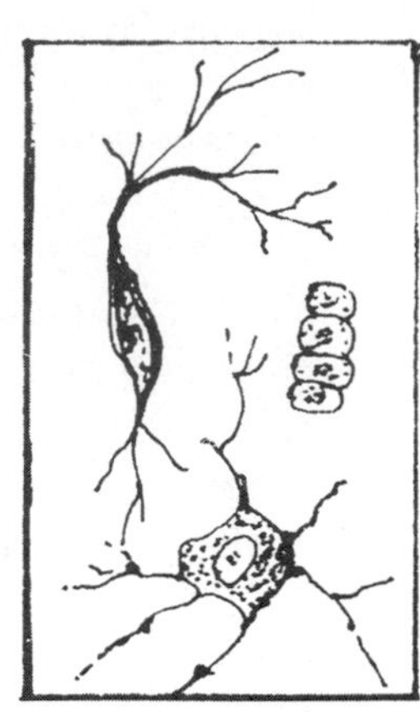

*5. Neuroglia*

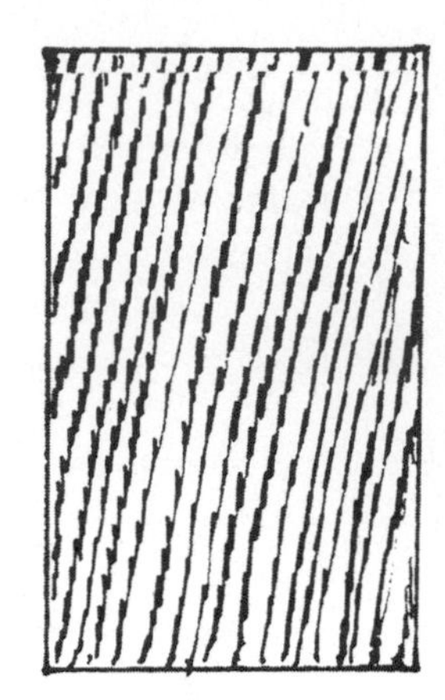

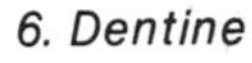

*6. Dentine*

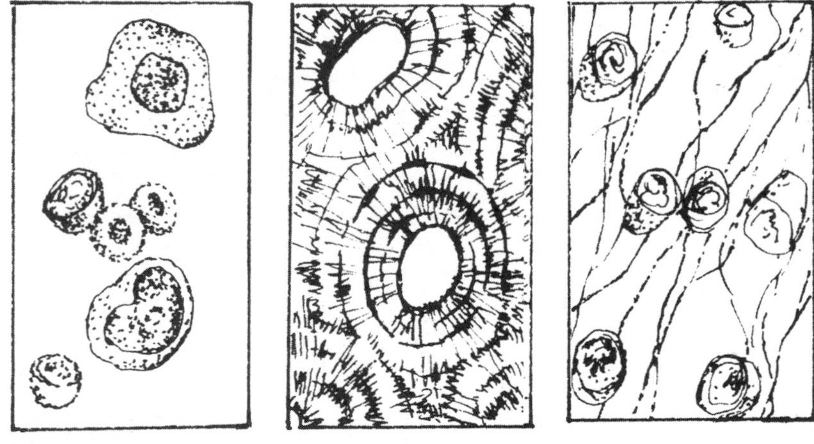

*7. Hemopoietic* *8. Bone* *9. Lymphoid*

4. *Nervous tissue proper:* Neurons consisting of the body and nerve fibers.
5. *Neuroglia:* Supportive tissue of the central nervous system.
6. *Dentine:* Hard, dense, calcareous tissue forming the body of a tooth beneath the enamel.
7. *Hemopoietic:* Tissue found in bone, marrow and the vascular system.
8. *Bone:* Tissue found in all bones of the skeleton.
9. *Lymphoid:* Tissue found in lymph nodes and other compact structures such as the tonsils and adenoids.

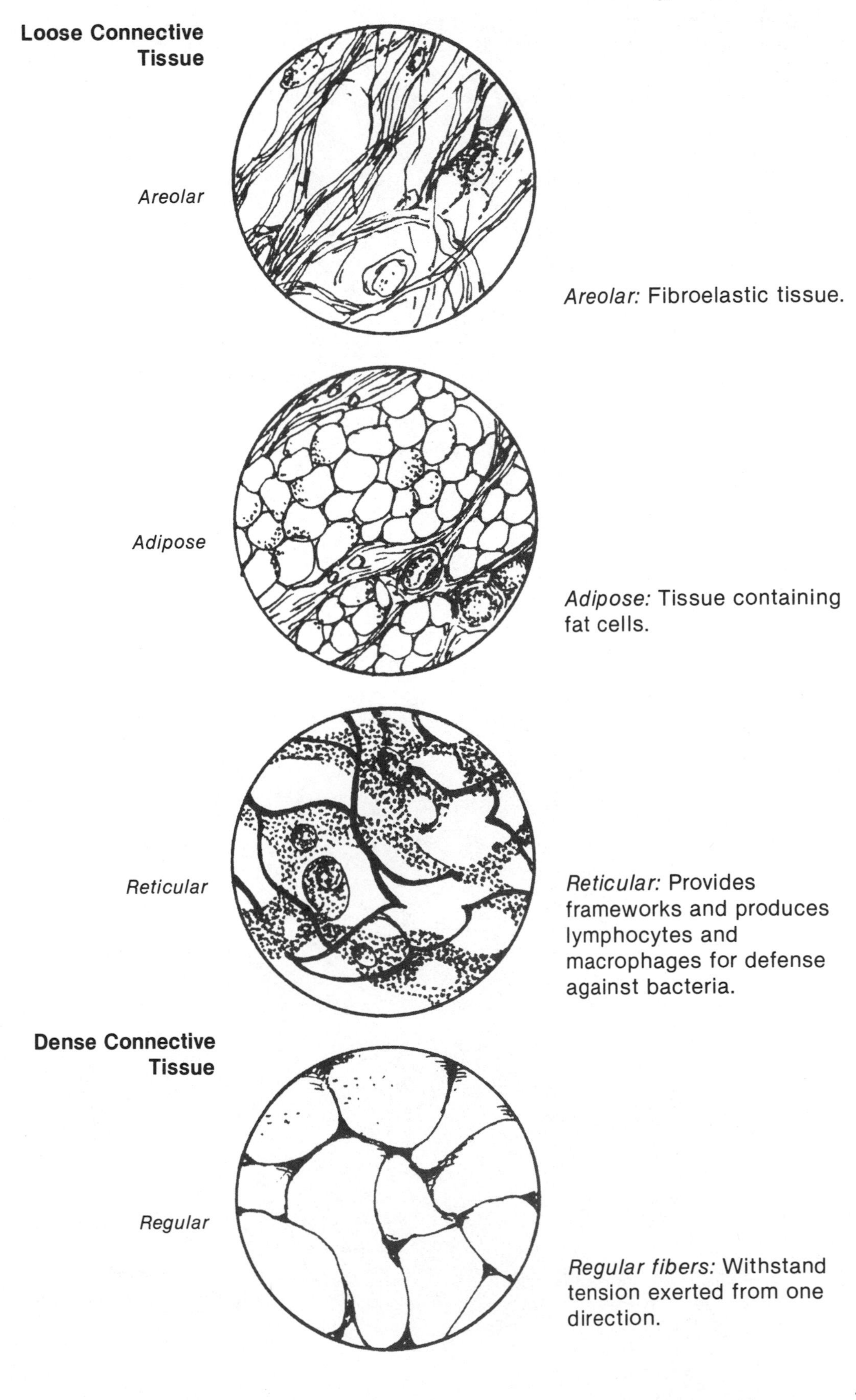


*Areolar:* Fibroelastic tissue.

*Adipose:* Tissue containing fat cells.

*Reticular:* Provides frameworks and produces lymphocytes and macrophages for defense against bacteria.

*Regular fibers:* Withstand tension exerted from one direction.

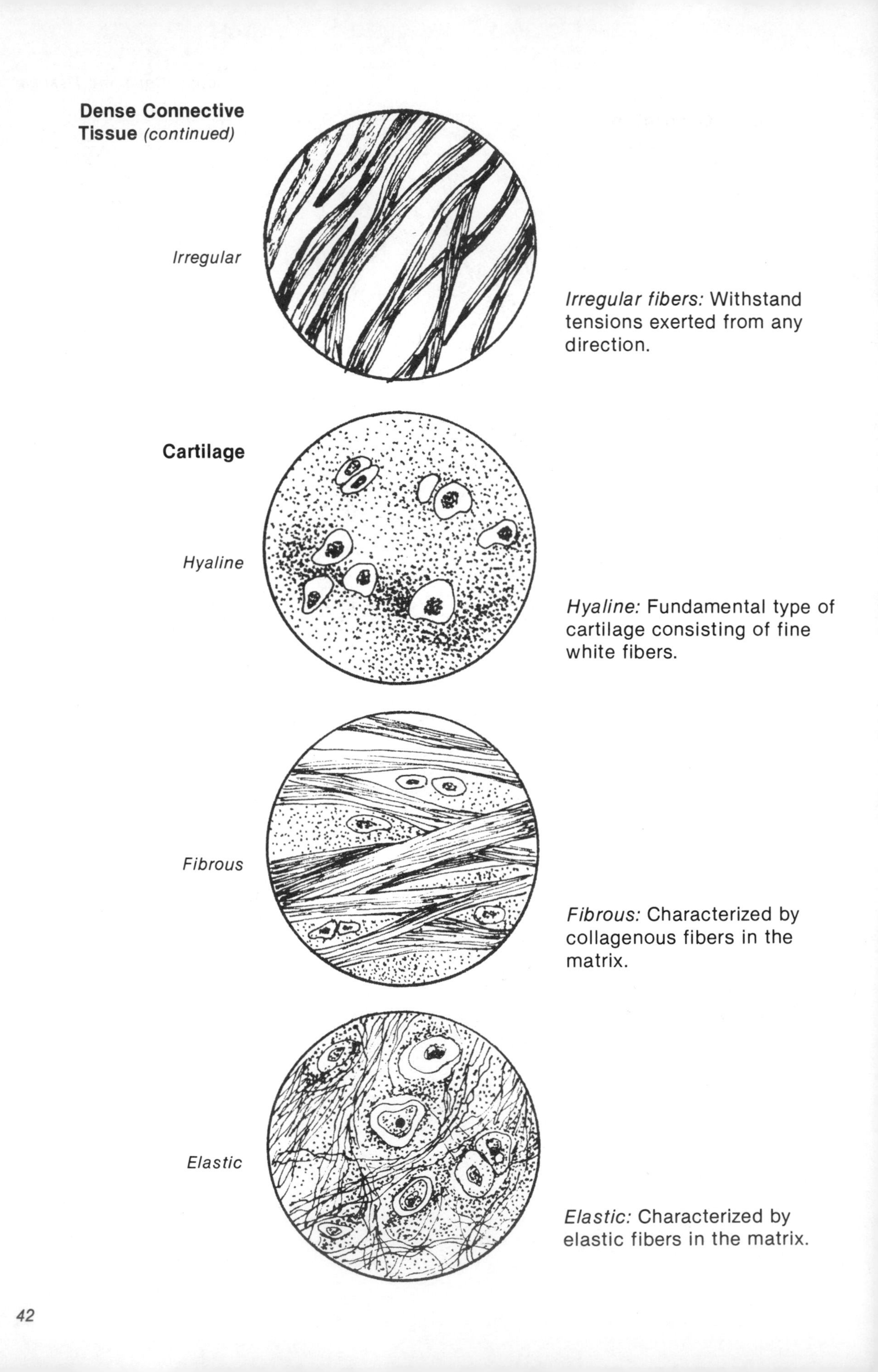
Dense Connective Tissue (continued)
Irregular
Irregular fibers: Withstand tensions exerted from any direction.
Cartilage
Hyaline
Hyaline: Fundamental type of cartilage consisting of fine white fibers.
Fibrous
Fibrous: Characterized by collagenous fibers in the matrix.
Elastic
Elastic: Characterized by elastic fibers in the matrix.

**QUESTIONS FOR DISCUSSION AND REVIEW**

1. Why is the cell called the basic unit of all living matter?
2. Name the four principle parts of a cell.
3. Which parts of the cell control reproduction?
4. How does cell reproduction occur in human tissue?
5. Name the five phases of cell mitosis.
6. Name the two phases of metabolism.
7. Explain the process of anabolism.
8. Explain the process of catabolism.
9. Of what substances are tissues composed?
10. Name the five main categories of tissues.
11. What parts of the body do epithelial tissues cover?
12. Name the two main types of membranes.
13. What is the main function of connective tissue?
14. What is the main function of areolar (loose) tissue?
15. What is adipose tissue?
16. Name the three types of cartilage.
17. What makes bone tissue hard?
18. Name the three types of muscle tissue.
19. What is the difference between striated and smooth muscle tissue?
20. Where is liquid tissue found?
21. In what part of the body is cardiac muscle tissue found?
22. What is the main function of nervous tissue proper?
23. What is dentine?
24. Name an example of blood-forming or hematopoietic tissue.

**ANSWERS TO QUESTIONS FOR DISCUSSION AND REVIEW**

1. All living matter consists of various cells.
2. Nucleus, centrosome, cytoplasm, and the cell membrane or wall.
3. The nucleus and the centrosome.
4. By the process called mitosis, the indirect division of cells.
5. The five phases of mitosis are: interphase, prophase, metaphase, anaphase, and telephase.
6. Catabolism and anabolism.
7. Anabolism is the process of building up of larger molecules from smaller ones.
8. Catabolism is the process of breaking down of larger molecules into smaller ones.
9. All tissues are composed of specialized cells.
10. The five main categories of tissues are: epithelial, connective, muscular, nervous, and liquid tissue.
11. Epithelial tissues cover all surfaces of the body, both inside and out.
12. Epithelial and connective.
13. To bind structures together, to create a frame work, and to provide support.

14. To bind the skin to underlying tissues and to fill spaces between the muscles.
15. Adipose tissue is areolar tissue with an abundance of fat-containing cells.
16. Three types of cartilage are: fibrous, hyaline, and elastic.
17. Bone tissue is made hard by mineral salts, calcium phosphate, and calcium carbonate.
18. Three types of muscle tissue are: skeletal, smooth, and cardiac tissue.
19. Striated muscle tissue is made of cylindrical fibers and is found in voluntary muscles. Smooth muscle tissue fibers are not striated and are found in involuntary muscles.
20. Liquid tissue is found in blood and lymph.
21. Cardiac muscle tissue is found only in the heart.
22. The main function of nervous tissue proper is to initiate, control, and coordinate the body's adaptions to its surroundings and environment.
23. Dentine is the hard, dense, calcareous tissue that forms the body of a tooth beneath the enamel.
24. Bone marrow is an example of blood forming or hematopoietic tissue.

# Chapter 5 Human Anatomy and Physiology

**LEARNING OBJECTIVES**

After you have mastered this chapter, you will be able to:

1. Demonstrate knowledge of basic human anatomy and physiology as a requisite in mastering the theory and practice of therapeutic body massage.
2. Name the anatomical parts of the body.
3. Name the 10 most important body systems.
4. Explain the structures and functions of the various body systems.
5. Explain the various planes, regions, and cavities of the body.
6. Know the planes and regions of the body.

**INTRODUCTION**

An elementary knowledge of anatomy and physiology is a necessary requisite in mastering the theory and practice of therapeutic body massage. To obtain the most beneficial results, the practitioner who knows the principles of anatomy and physiology is better able to adjust the massage treatment to the needs of the client, and to control results.

Anatomy is the science of morphology or structure of an organism or body. Physiology concerns the normal functions performed by the various systems of the body.

**THE ANATOMICAL POSITION OF THE BODY**

When studying anatomy, it is essential to know the terms that have been devised to designate specific regions in the body. These terms refer to the body as seen in the anatomic position, which shows a figure standing upright with the palms of the hands facing forward. Anatomists have divided the body by three imaginary planes called the sagittal (vertical), the coronal (frontal), and the transverse (horizontal) planes.

1. The sagittal plane divides the body into left and right halves by an imaginery line running vertically down the center of the body. Midsagittal refers to the plane that divides the body or an organ into right and left halves.
2. The coronal plane is an imaginary line that divides the body into the anterior (front) or vertical half of the body and the posterior (back) or dorsal half of the body.
3. The transverse plane is an imaginary line that divides the body at about midsection into an upper and lower portion. A transverse section cuts through the body perpendicular to the long axis of the body part.

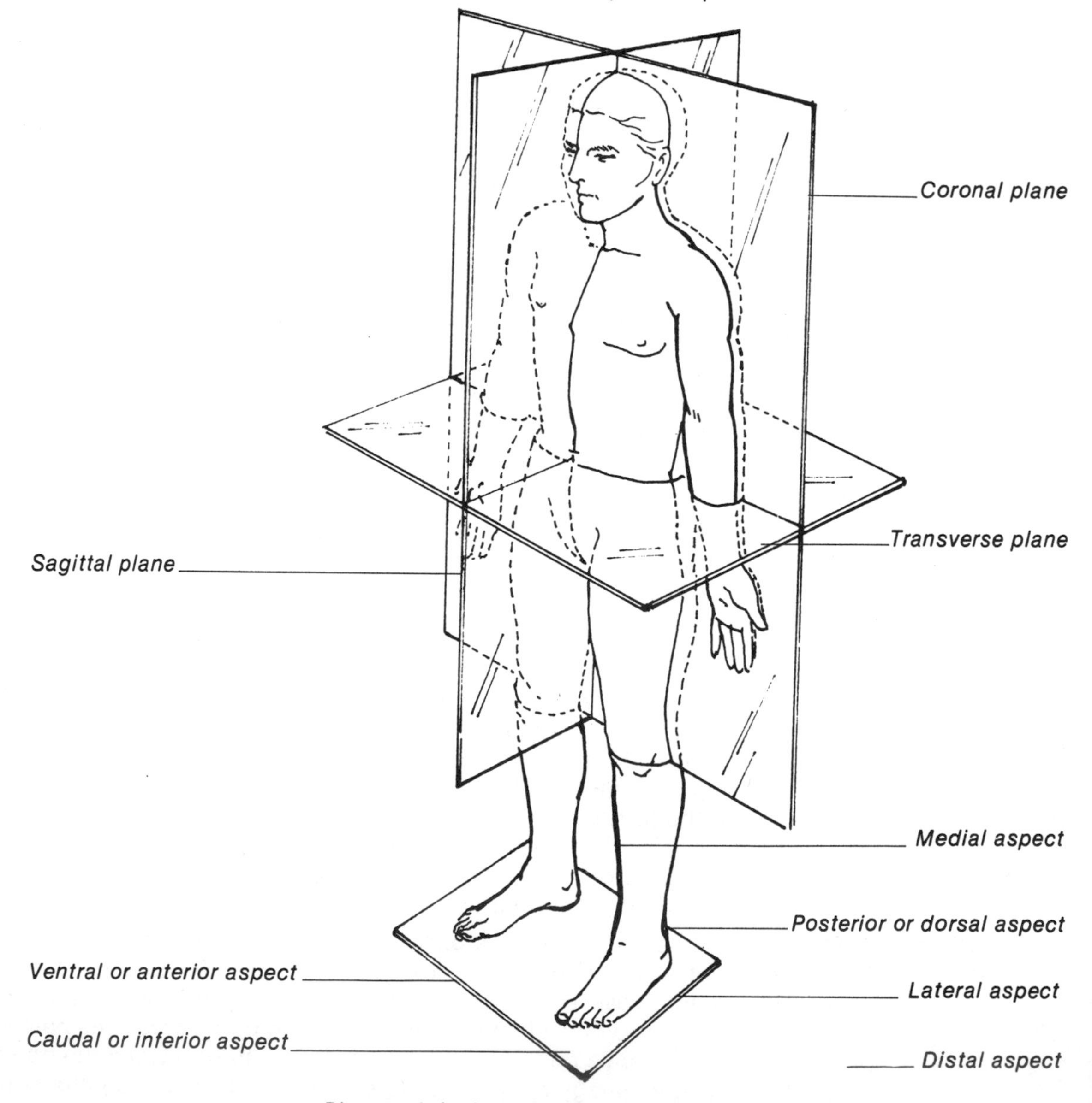


*Planes of the body and terms of location and position.*

## Anatomical Terms and Meanings

| TERM | MEANING |
|---|---|
| 1. Cranial or superior aspect | Situated higher, toward the crown of the head. |
| 2. Caudal or inferior aspect | Situated lower, farther from the crown of the head. |
| 3. Anterior or ventral aspect | Situated before or in front of. |
| 4. Posterior or dorsal aspect | Situated behind or in back of. |
| 5. Transverse plane | Division of the body at the mid-section into an upper and lower half. Transverse section refers to a plane through the body perpendicular to the axis, which is the vertical center line around which the body parts are arranged. |
| 6. Sagittal plane | Vertical plane or section dividing the body into right and left halves, in front to back direction, and mid-sagittal divides the body into equal left and right halves. |
| 7. Coronal plane | Pertaining to the corona or crown of the skull, the frontal plane or section passes through the long axis of the body, dividing it into front and back halves. |
| 8. Medial aspect | Pertaining to the middle or center, nearer to the midline. |
| 9. Lateral aspect | On the side, farther from the midline or center. |
| 10. Distal aspect | Farthest point from the origin of a structure or point of attachment. |

**Additional Words *(Not shown in illustration)***

| | |
|---|---|
| Proximal | Nearest the origin of a structure or point of attachment. |
| Anguli | At an angle. |
| Levator | That which lifts or raises. |
| Dilator | That which expands or enlarges. |
| Erector | That which draws upward. |
| Vertical | Long axis, in erect position. |
| Afferent | Bearing or conducting inward. |

## BODY CAVITIES AND ORGANS

Once you know the body planes, it is easier to remember where body cavities and organs are located. There are two groups of body cavities: the dorsal or posterior cavities and the ventral or anterior cavities. The dorsal cavities contain the brain and spinal cord, with the skull forming the cranial cavity and the vertebrae forming the vertebral cavity. The ventral cavities are the thoracic cavity and abdominal cavities. The thoracic is subdivided into the pericardial cavity, which contains the heart, and the pleural cavity, which contains the lungs. The lesser or true pelvis cavity contains the bladder, rectum, and some of the reproductive organs.

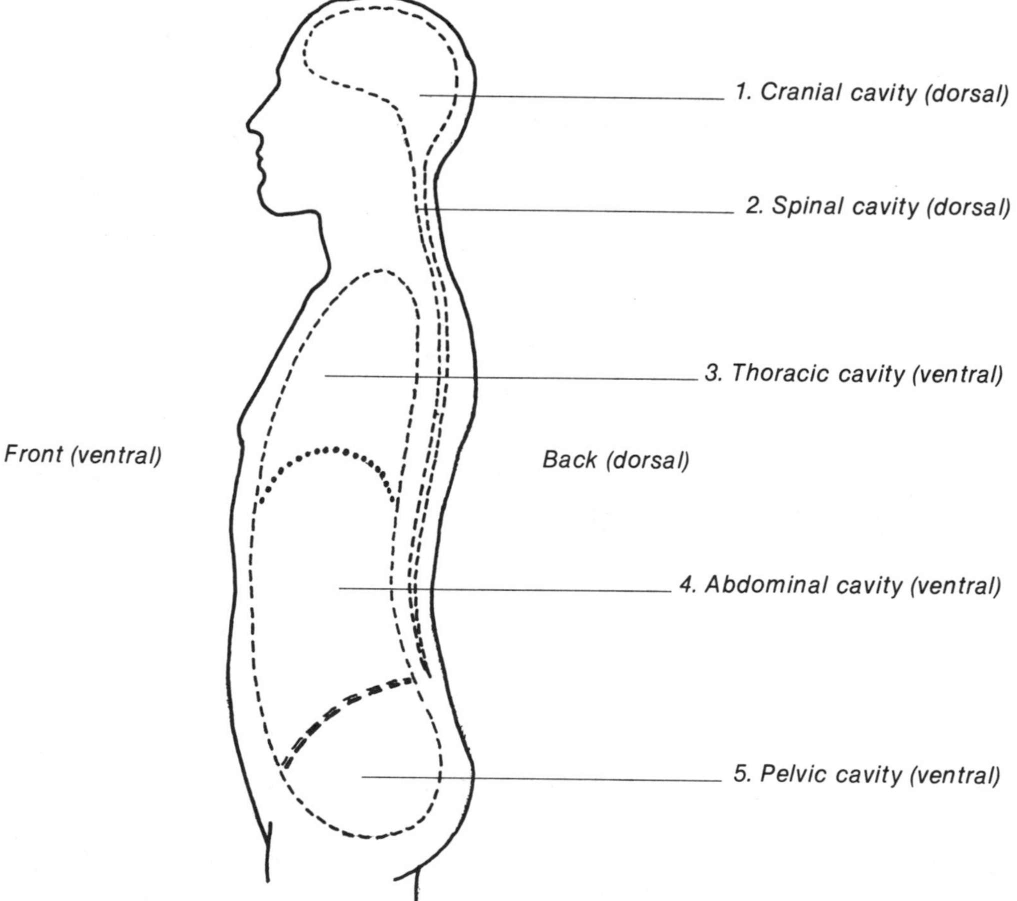


**Body Cavities**

1. Cranial cavity (dorsal).
2. Spinal cavity (dorsal).
3. Thoracic cavity (ventral).
4. Abdominal cavity (ventral).
5. Pelvic cavity (ventral).

## THE REGIONS OF THE HUMAN BODY

Knowing the regions of the body helps us to pinpoint a particular area of the body. For example, the pectoral muscle is located in the pectoral or chest region. The brachial nerve is located in the brachial region. If a client complains of pain in the lower back, you will remember that the lower back is the lumbar region. Study the illustrations of regions of the body until you can locate each region and name the parts of the body associated with each region.

### Anterior View of the Human Body Regions

1. *Frontal:* Region of the head.
2. *Temporal:* Region of the temples.
3. *Cervical:* Region of the neck.
4. *Deltoid:* Region of the shoulder joint and deltoid muscle.
5. *Axillary:* Region of the armpit.
6. *Brachial:* Region between the elbow and shoulder.
7. *Hypochrondriac:* Region of the abdomen lateral to the epigastric region.
8. *Umbilical:* Region of the navel (umbilicus). The middle of the three median abdominal regions, below the epigastric region and above the pubic region.
9. *Hypogastric:* Region under the stomach and inferior to the umbilical region.
10. *Patella:* Region of the knees and kneecap.
11. *Femoral:* Region of the femur or thigh.
12. *Inguinal:* Region of the groin.
13. *Lumbar:* Region of the lower back.
14. *Epigastric:* Region of the abdomen.
15. *Pectoral:* Region of the breast and chest.

*Illustration of Posterior View of the Human Body Regions appears on the following page.)*

## Posterior View of Regions of the Body

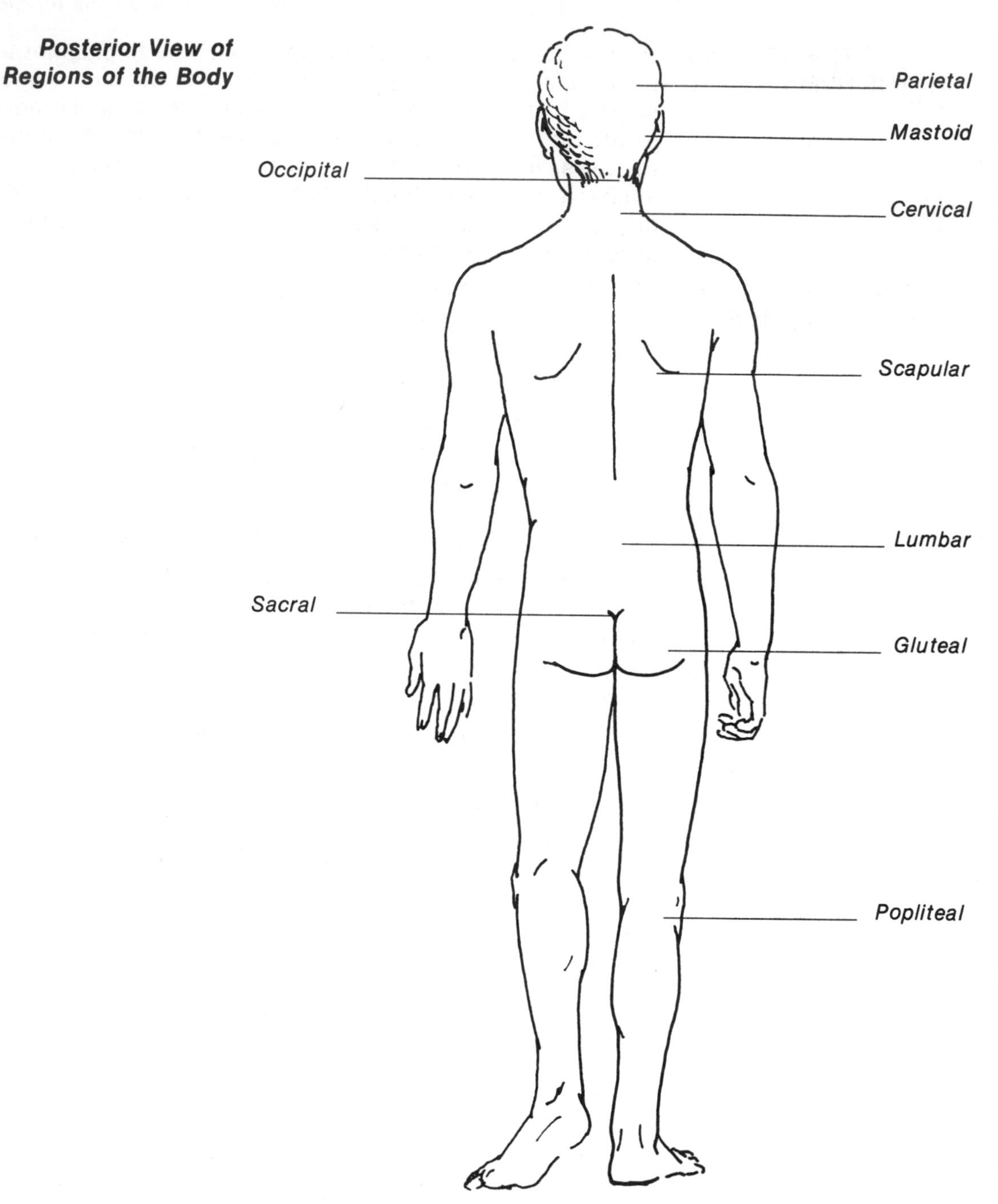


*Posterior view of the regions of the body.*

**Posterior View of the Human Body Regions**

1. *Parietal:* Region of the head, posterior to the frontal region and anterior to the occipital region.
2. *Mastoid:* Region of the temporal bone behind the ear.
3. *Cervical:* Region of the neck.
4. *Scapula:* Region of the back of the shoulder or shoulder blade.
5. *Lumbar:* Region of the back lying lateral to the lumbar.
6. *Gluteal:* Region of muscles of the buttocks.
7. *Popliteal:* A diamond-shaped area behind the knee joint.

**Anterior View of the Regions of the Body**

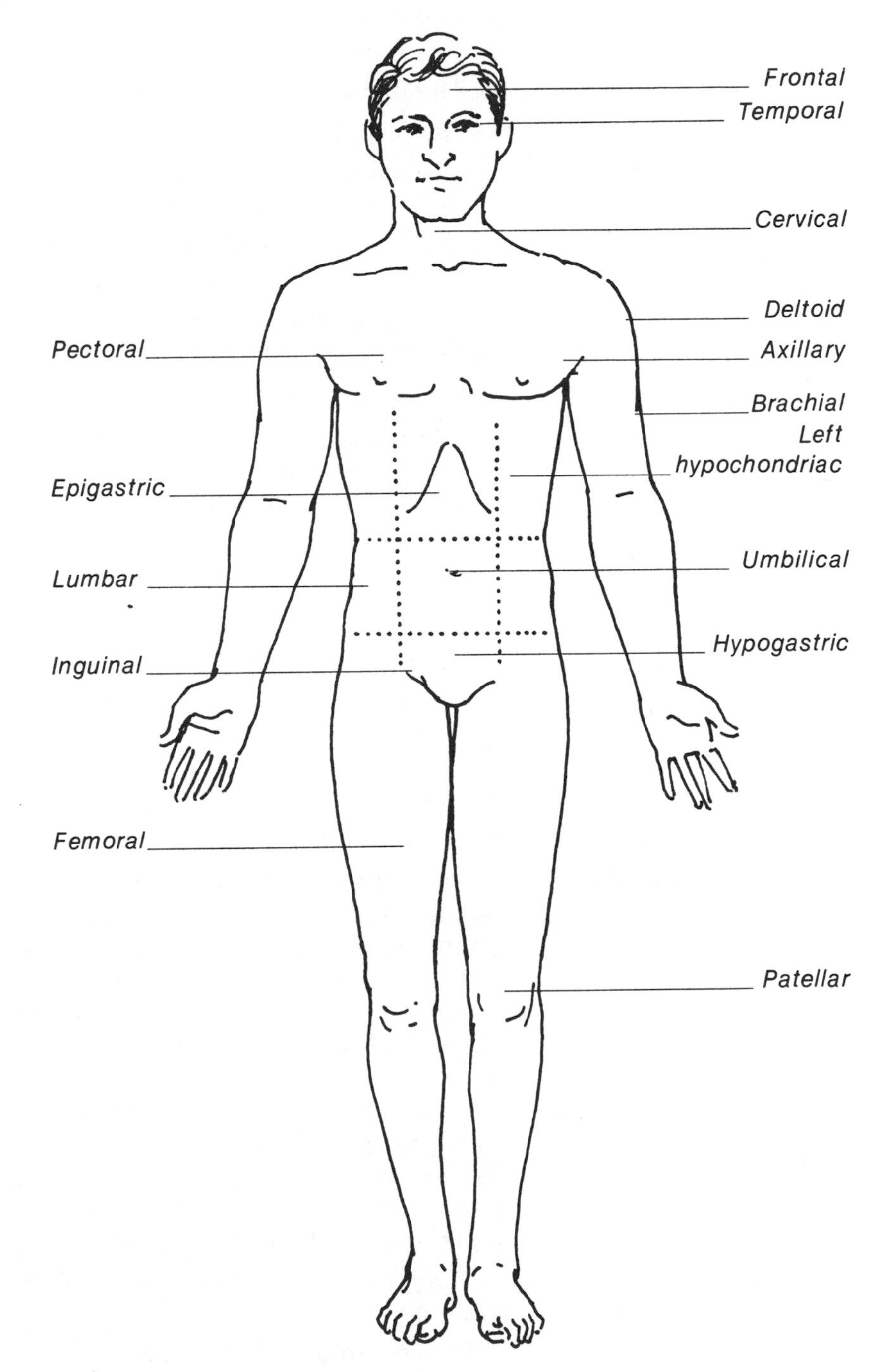


*Anterior view of the body in the anatomical position showing the regions. Sometimes the regions of the abdomen are designated as the right and left upper quadrants and the right and left lower quadrants.*

## THE STRUCTURE OF THE HUMAN BODY

The main anatomical parts of the body are:

1. The head.
2. The spine.
3. The trunk.
4. The extremities.

The head is subdivided into:

1. *The cranium:* The front and lower part of the skull including the eyes, nose, and mouth.
2. *The face:* The front and lower part of the skull including the eyes, nose, and mouth.

The spine is a column of bones that supports the head and trunk of the body and protects the spinal cord.

The trunk is subdivided into:

1. *The thorax or chest:* The upper part of the trunk containing the lungs, heart, esophagus (food tube), and part of the trachea or windpipe.
2. *The abdomen:* Situated below the diaphram and including the stomach, intestines, liver, and kidneys. The diaphram is the partition of muscles and tendons located between the chest cavity and the abdominal cavity or the main muscle associated with breathing. Located below the abdomen and containing the bladder, reproductive organs, lower bowel, and rectum.

The extremities include:

1. *The upper limbs:* The shoulder, forearm, wrist, and hand.
2. *The lower limbs:* the hip, thigh, leg, ankle, and foot.

### Body Organs

Body organs are structures containing two or more different tissues that are combined to accomplish a definite function. Each organ is so constructed that in a state of health it will perform its function with ease and efficiency. Among the important organs of the body are the brain, heart, lungs, kidneys, liver, sense organs, organs of digestion, organs of reproduction, and the skin.

### Body Systems

When a number of bodily organs work together to perform a bodily function, they are called a system. All systems cooperate for a common purpose, namely the maintenance of the entire body or function of the organism. Systems are not independent units, but are dependent upon one another.

The human body is composed of the following 10 important systems.

1. Integumentary system (skin).
2. Skeletal system.
3. Muscular system.
4. Nervous system.
5. Endocrine system.
6. Circulatory system (blood vascular and lymph vascular).
7. Digestive system.
8. Excretory system (including urinary system).
9. Respiratory system.
10. Reproductive system.

***The Integumentary System***

The skin is the largest organ of the body. It is often referred to as the outer covering or the integumentary system, because it is the organ involved in the protection, heat regulation, secretion and excretion, sensation, absorption, and respiration of the body.

***The Skeletal System***

The skeletal system is the structure and hard framework upon which the other body systems depend for support and protection. The skeletal system is the physical foundation of the body. It is composed of differently shaped bones united by movable and immovable joints. The main function of the skeletal system is to serve as a means of protection, support, and attachment for muscles of locomotion.

***The Muscular System***

The muscular system is made up of voluntary and involuntary muscles that are necessary for movement of the parts of the body. The muscular system covers and shapes the skeleton. Practically every contraction and movement of the body is due to the action of the muscles. The obvious movements of the arms and hands, the contraction of the heart and stomach, and the changes in facial expression are the direct result of muscular activity.

***The Nervous System***

The nervous or neurological system controls and coordinates all the body systems, helping them to work efficiently and harmoniously. The neurological system includes all the nerves of the body, spinal cord, and the brain. It is a highly developed and sensitive organization of nerve tissues. Through the nervous system the individual is made aware of his or her existence and relationship to the outside world. Nerves, branching out from the brain and spinal cord, coordinate all voluntary and involuntary functions of the body.

***The Endocrine System***

The endocrine system represents a group of specialized organs or glands capable of manufacturing secretions called *hormones* that affect (beneficially or adversely) many functions of the body including its growth, reproduction, and health. The endocrine glands, such as the pituitary and thyroid, secrete hormones in the blood and regulate the processes of growth and metabolism. Reproduction is made possible by the sex glands and their secretions.

***The Circulatory System (Blood Vascular and Lymph Vascular)***

The circulatory (vascular) system controls the circulation of blood throughout the body. It consists of two divisions: the blood vascular system and the lymph vascular system. The blood vascular system includes the heart and blood vessels (arteries, veins, and capillaries). The pumping action of the heart distributes the vital fluids, being blood and lymph, through the blood vessels to all parts of the body. The blood acts as a two-way carrier of supplies, bringing oxygen and food materials to the cells and taking away waste products and secretions from the tissues.

The lymph (a clear, yellow fluid) bathes all cells and assists in the exchange of supplies required by the cells and carries waste and impurities away from the environment of the cells. The lymph vascular system consists of lymph glands, nodes, and lymph vessels (lymphatics) through which the lymph circulates. The lymph system also includes the spleen, thymus, tonsils, and adnoids.

***The Digestive System***

The digestive system consists of all the structures involved in the process of digestion including the mouth, stomach, intestines, salivary and gastric glands. The intestines are part of a continuous tube about 30 feet in length. The function of digestion is to break down complex food substances into simple materials fit to be absorbed and used by the body cells. Various digestive glands including the salivary glands, pancreas, and liver, along with glands in the stomach and small intestine, form and discharge enzymes that act on food in the process of digestion.

***The Excretory System***

The excretory system includes the skin, kidneys, bladder, liver, lungs, and large intestines, which are engaged in the process of eliminating waste products from the body. The skin (integumentary system) gives off perspiration. The lungs exhale carbon dioxide gas, the kidneys excrete urine, and the large intestines discharge refuse from the body. The liver produces bile, which contains certain waste products.

***The Respiratory System***

The respiratory system includes the lungs, air passages, nose, mouth, pharynx, trachea, and bronchial tubes, which leads to the lungs. The blood, as it passes through the lungs is purified by the removal of carbon dioxide and the intake of oxygen.

***The Reproductive System***

The reproductive system is the system whose function it is to ensure continuance of the species by the reproduction of other human beings. In the female, the ovaries discharge an ovum or egg cell that appears prior to menstruation. The testes in the male manufacture sperm cells. The union of the ovum with sperm results in fertilization and conception.

**QUESTIONS FOR DISCUSSION AND REVIEW**

1. What is anatomy?
2. Why should the massage practitioner study anatomy?
3. Why is it important to know the anatomical position and the planes and regions of the human body?
4. What are the four main anatomical parts of the body?
5. Name the 10 important systems of the body.

**ANSWERS TO QUESTIONS FOR DISCUSSION AND REVIEW**

1. Anatomy is the science of morphology or structure of an organism or body.
2. The massage practitioner should study anatomy to understand why certain parts of the body are benefited by therapeutic massage, and how to apply appropriate massage movements.
3. When studying anatomy, it is important to know the anatomical position and the regions and planes of the human body in order to describe the position of a structure or to locate one structure in relation to another. Once you know the body planes you will understand the location of body cavities and which organs are located in a particular cavity.
4. The four main anatomic parts of the body are: the head, spine, trunk, and extremities.
5. The 10 most important systems of the body are: the integumentary (skin), skeletal, muscular, nervous, endrocine, circulatory (blood and lymph vascular), digestive, excretory, respiratory, and reproductive systems.

## SYSTEM ONE THE INTEGUMENTARY SYSTEM — THE SKIN

The word *integument* means covering or skin. The skin is the largest organ of the body and serves as interface with the environment and protection for the body.

The principle functions of the skin are:

1. *Protection:* The skin protects the body from injury and bacterial invasion.
2. *Heat regulation:* The healthy body maintains a constant internal temperature of about 98.6 degrees Fahrenheit (37°C). As changes occur in the outside temperature, the blood and sweat glands of the skin make the necessary adjustments in their functions.
3. *Secretion and excretion:* By means of its sweat (sudoriferous) and oil (sebaceous) glands, the skin acts both as a secretory and an excretory organ. The sudoriferous (sweat) glands excrete (eliminate) perspiration which is waste matter. The sebaceous (oil) glands secrete (produce and release) sebum which is a lubricant.
4. *Sensation:* The papillary layer of the dermis provides the body with a sense of touch. Nerves supplying the skin register basic types of sensations, such as heat, cold, pain, pressure, and touch. Nerve endings are most abundant in the fingertips. Complex sensations, such as the feelings of vibration, seem to depend on a combination of these nerve endings.
5. *Absorption:* The skin has limited powers of absorption through its pores. Some cosmetics, chemicals, and drugs can be absorbed in small amounts. The skin is about 50 to 70 percent moisture. Sebum (oil) coats the surface of the skin and helps to maintain its moisture level. The sebum level slows down evaporation of moisture and keeps excess water from penetrating the skin.
6. *Respiration:* The skin breathes through its pores much as the body breathes through its lungs, but on a much smaller scale. Oxygen is taken in and carbon dioxide is discharged.

### The Structure of The Skin

The structure of the skin contains two clearly defined divisions: the *epidermis* (cuticle or scarf), which is the outermost layer, and the *dermis* (corium or true skin), which is the deeper layer that extends to form the subcutaneous tissue.

Although the epidermis comprises almost a solid sheet of cells, the dermis is a more semisolid mixture of fibers, water, and a gel called "ground" substance. There are three kinds of fibers that make up the cells of the dermis: collagen, reticulum, and elastin. Collagen makes up about 70 percent of the dry weight of the skin and gives it strength, form, and flexibility. Reticulum fibers form a fine branching pattern in connective tissue that helps to link the bundles of collagen fibers. Collagen contains a protein called elastin that has elastic properties and helps to give the skin its resiliency. The dermis contains an elastic network of cells through which are distributed nerves, blood and lymph vessels, and sweat and oil glands.

## The Integumentary System *(showing the skin and hair)*

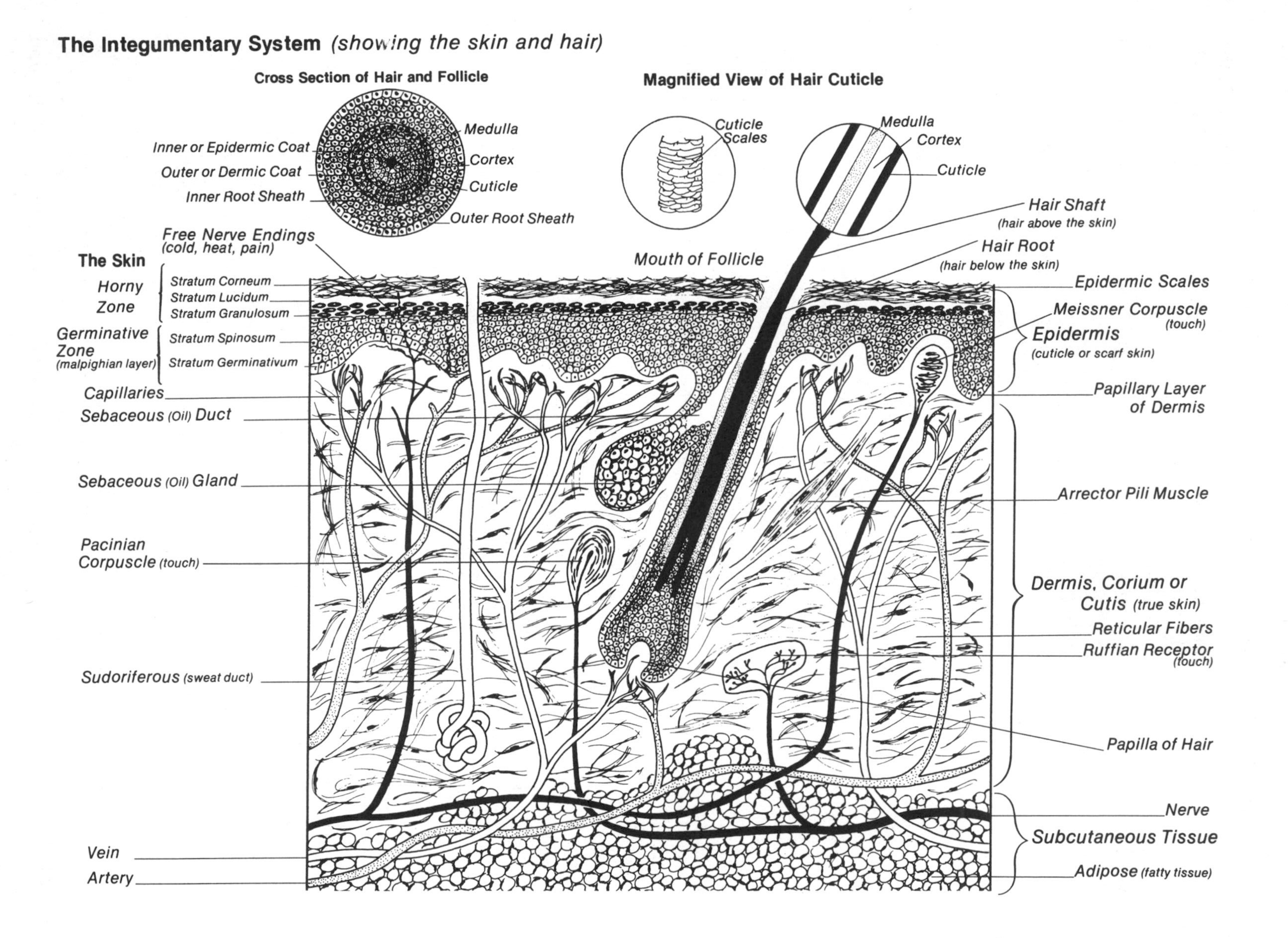

**Structures in the Skin**

*1 Square Inch (6.452 Sq. cm) of Skin Contains*

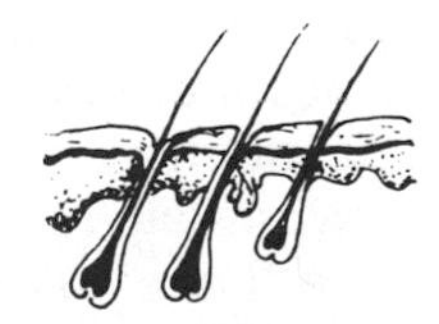

*65 hairs*

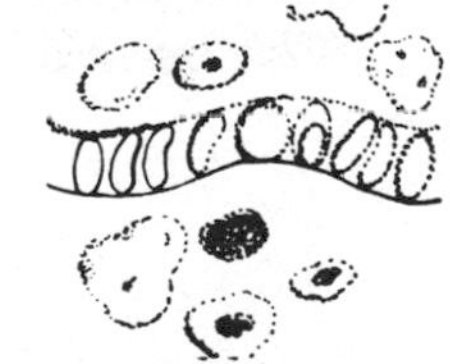

*9,500,000 cells*

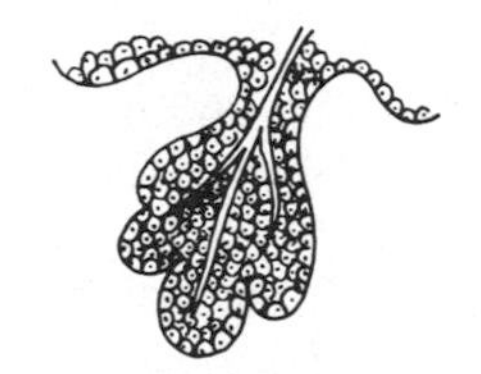

*95-100 sebaceous glands*

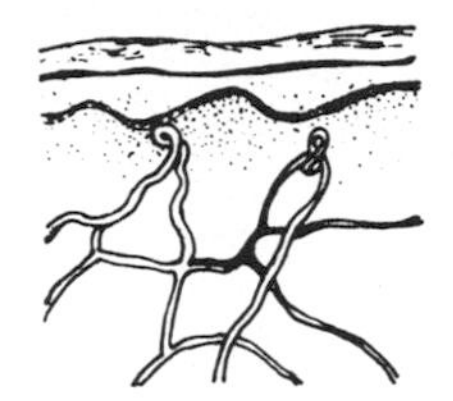

*19 yards (17 meters) of blood vessels*

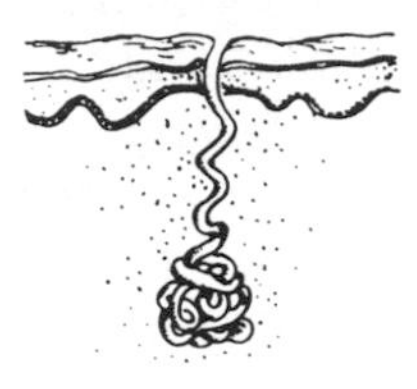

*650 sweat glands*

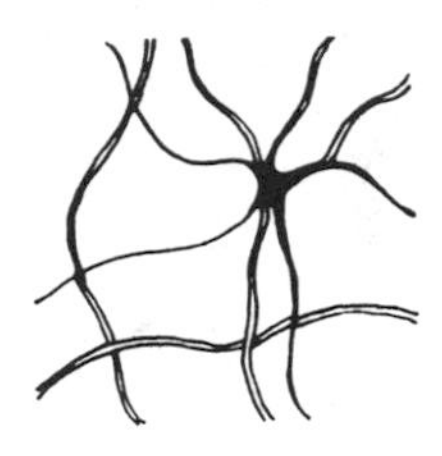

*78 yards (70 meters) of nerves*

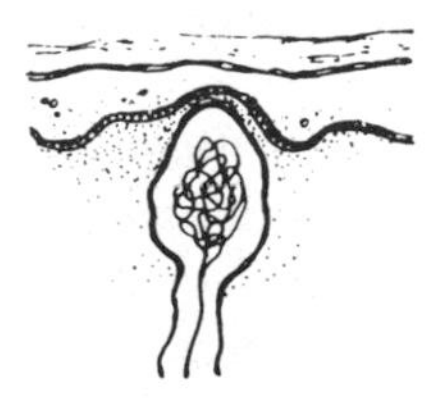

*78 sensory apparatuses for heat*

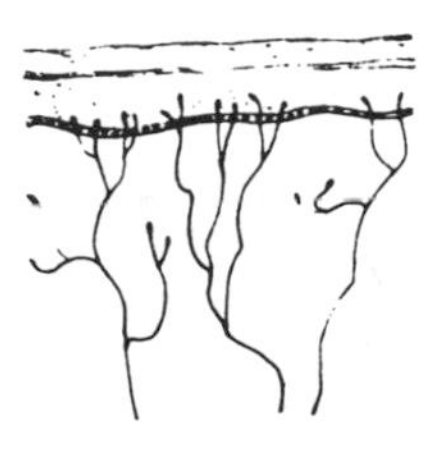

*19,500 sensory cells at the ends of nerve fibers*

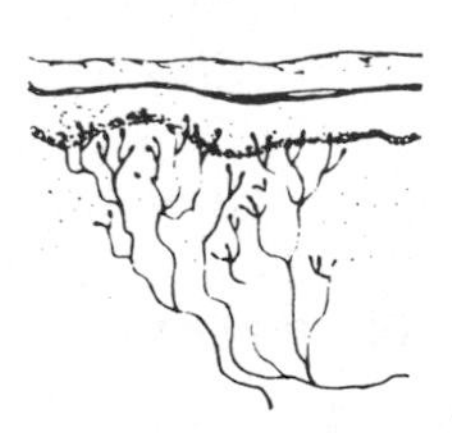

*1,3000 nerve endings to record pain*

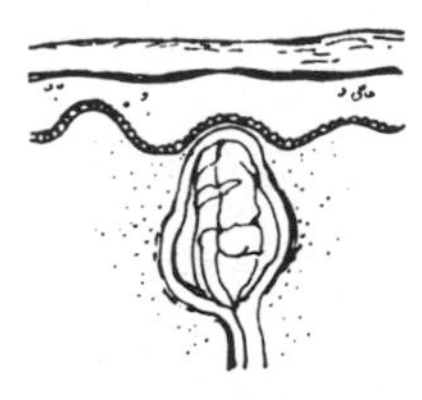

*160-165 pressure apparatuses for the perception of tactile stimuli*

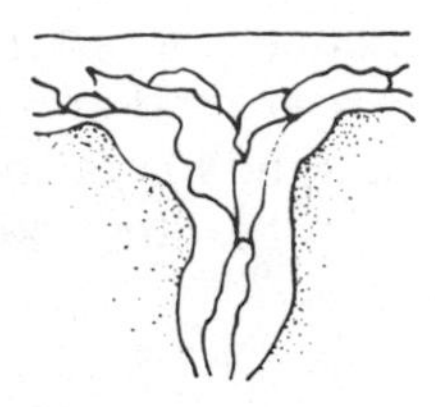

*13 sensory apparatuses for cold*

**The Dermis**

The papillary layer of the skin (directly beneath the epidermis) contains the papillae, the conelike projections, made of fine strands of elastic tissue that extend upward into the epidermis. Some of the papillae contain looped capillaries; others contain terminations of nerve fibers called *tactile corpuscles.*

*The reticular layer* of the skin contains fat cells, blood and lymph vessels, sweat and oil glands, hair follicles, and nerve endings.

The subcutaneous tissue (subcutis) is regarded as a continuation of the dermis. It varies in thickness according to the age, sex, and general health of the individual. Fatty (adipose) tissue gives smoothness and contour to the body, provides a reservoir for fuel and energy, and serves as a protective cushion for the upper skin layers.

**The Epidermis**

The *stratum granulosum* (granular layer of the skin) consists of cells that look like granules. These cells are almost dead and undergo a change into a horny substance called keratin.

The *stratum* or *malpighian* layer (also called stratum mucosum) consists of cells containing melanin (coloring matter) of the skin. Melanin also helps to protect the sensitive cells from the action of strong light rays.

The *stratum germinativum* is the deepest layer of the epidermis comprising a single layer of cells that are well nourished by the dermis. These cells undergo mitosis, pushing other cells closer to the body surface. This layer also contains melanocytes that produce the pigment melanin.

The skin varies in thickness, being thinnest on the eyelids and thickest on the palms of the hands and soles of the feet. Continued pressure over any part of the skin will cause it to thicken and may produce a callus.

## NUTRITION AND THE SKIN

Blood and lymph supply nutrients to the skin. About one-half to two-thirds of the total blood supply of the body is distributed to the skin. Blood and lymph, as they circulate through the skin, contribute certain materials for growth, nourishment, and repair of skin, hair, and nails. In the subcutaneous tissue are found networks of arteries and lymphatics, which send their smaller branches to hair papillae, hair follicles, and the glands of the skin. Capillaries are quite numerous in the skin.

**Aging Skin**

As people age, the collagen network of the skin tends to lose its elasticity causing the skin to become less firm and supple. With age, the deeper or dermal layer of the skin undergoes changes. The skin may become thinner, dryer and more prone to growths. It may become lined and crepey. Swelling (edema) of tissues may appear around and under the eyes. Pliability of the skin depends on elasticity of the fibers of the dermis. For example, after expansion healthy skin will regain its former shape almost immediately.

## STRUCTURAL CHANGES OF THE SKIN

Because the skin is the covering of the entire body, its condition must be taken into consideration before massage treatment is given. The skin may be sensitive to touch or it may show signs of damage due to disease or injury. The massage practitioner must be aware of any skin condition that may require the attention of the client's physician. Freckles, birthmarks (port-wine stains), and the like, present no problem; however, a lesion or any discontinuity of tissue should be examined by a physician before massage.

Healthy skin is slightly moist, soft, flexible, and possesses a slightly acid reaction. The texture of skin revealed by feel and appearance should be smooth and fine grained. The color of the skin depends partly on the blood supply but more on the coloring matter melanin. Skin pigment varies in different people and is determined by genetics. Regardless of native pigmentation, healthy skin is of good color. An overly pale, ashy, reddish, or yellow cast to the skin may indicate health problems.

Massage benefits the skin by improving circulation of the blood, which carries nutrients to the cells.

## THE APPENDAGES ASSOCIATED WITH THE SKIN

### Glands of the Skin

The skin contains two types of duct glands that extract materials from the blood to form new substances. These are the *sudoriferous* (sweat) glands and *sebaceous* (oil) glands. Sweat glands are under the control of the autonomic nervous system and are located in the dermis. They (tubular type) consist of a coiled base or fundas and a tubelike duct that terminates at the surface of the skin to form a sweat pore. Practically all parts of the body are supplied with sweat glands, but more abundant from the armpits, soles of the feet, palms of the hands, and forehead. The activity of the sweat glands is greatly increased by heat, exercise, and mental excitement. The two types of sweat glands are the *epocrine* and the *eccrine glands.* The epocrine glands respond to emotional stimuli, and their secretions generally produce odor. These are located primarily in the armpits and groin and are usually connected with hair follicles.

***Hair Follicle***

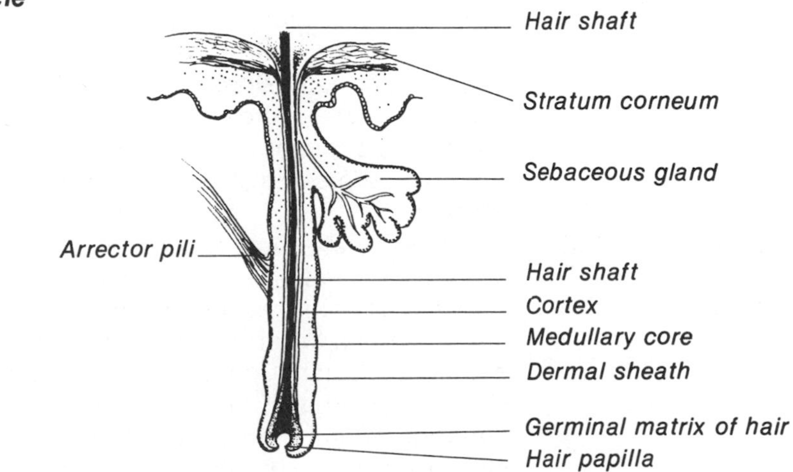

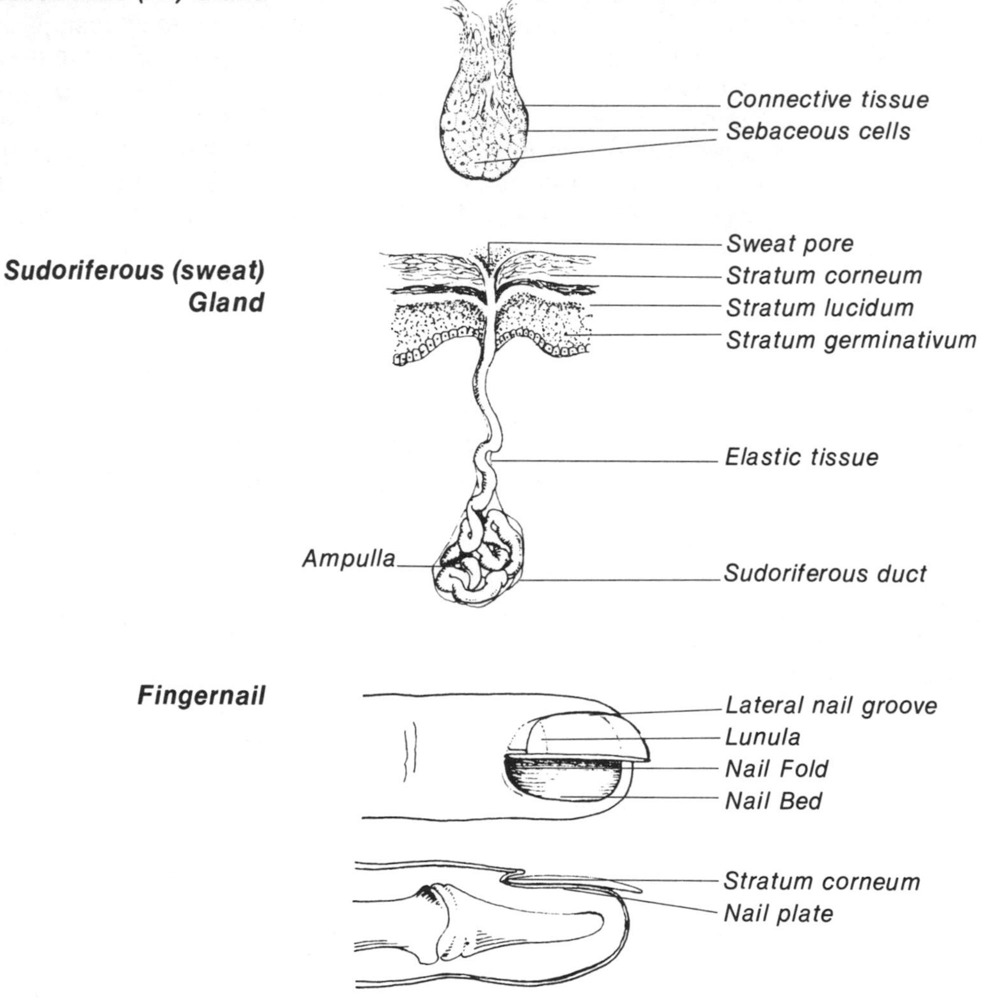


The eccrine glands respond to elevated body temperatures resulting from environmental conditions or physical activity. The tubular extensions of these glands open at the body surface as a pore. Fluid secreted by the eccrine glands is mostly water and contains some bodily wastes, such as urea and uric acid. Therefore, the skin acts in some degree as an organ of excretion.

**The Hair and Nails**

Hair and nails are appendages of the skin. They are composed of hard keratin, a protein which in its soft form is found in skin. Hard keratin, as found in hair, has a sulfur content of 4 to 8 percent and a lower moisture and fat content than soft keratin and is particularly tough, elastic material. It forms continuous sheets (fingernails) or long endless fibers (hair). Soft keratin contains about 2 percent sulfur, 50 percent moisture, and a small percentage of fats. In the epidermis keratin occurs as flattened cells or dry scales.

### *Hair*

Hair grows over the entire body, with the exception of the palms of the hands, soles of the feet, some areas of the genitalia, the mucous membranes of the lips, the nipples, the navel, and the eyelids. The heavier concentration of hair is on the head, under the armpits, on and around the genitals, and on the arms and legs. An individual's genes strongly influence the distribution of hair, its thickness, quality, color, and rate of growth, and whether it is curly or straight.

Each hair develops from a tubelike depression (hair follicle) that extends through the epidermis, into and often through the dermis, and into the subcutaneous layer. As epidermal cells at the base of the follicle are nourished by the blood supply, they divide and push up through the hair follicle, die, and keratinize, becoming a shaft of hair.

Associated with hair follicles are sebaceous (oil) glands, specialized sweat (apocrine) glands, and arrector pili muscles. The arrector pili muscles are fanlike muscles connected with the base of the follicle and positioned in such a way that they contract in reaction to cold or emotional stimuli. This reaction often results in a condition called *goose bumps* because the skin appears bumpy, like that of a plucked goose.

## LESIONS OF THE SKIN

A lesion is a structural change in the tissues caused by injury or disease. There are three types: primary, secondary and tertiary. The massage practitioner is concerned with primary and secondary lesions only. Knowing how to identify the principal skin lesions helps the practitioner to avoid affected areas. The client should be advised to seek medical attention.

### Definitions Pertaining to Primary Lesions

*Bulla:* A blister containing a watery fluid, similar to a vesicle, but larger.

*Macule:* A small, discolored spot or patch on the surface of the skin, neither raised nor sunken, as freckles.

*Papule:* A small, elevated pimple in the skin, containing fluid, but which may develop pus.

*Pustule:* An elevation of the skin having an inflamed base, containing pus.

*Tubercle:* A solid lump larger than a papule. It projects above the surface or lies within or under the skin. It varies in size from a pea to a hickory nut.

*Tumor:* An external swelling, varying in size, shape, and color.

*Vesicle:* A blister with clear fluid in it, vesicles lie within or just beneath the epidermis. (Example: Poison ivy produces small vesicles.)

*Wheal:* An itchy, swollen lesion that lasts only a few hours. (Examples: hives, or the bite of an insect, such as a mosquito.)

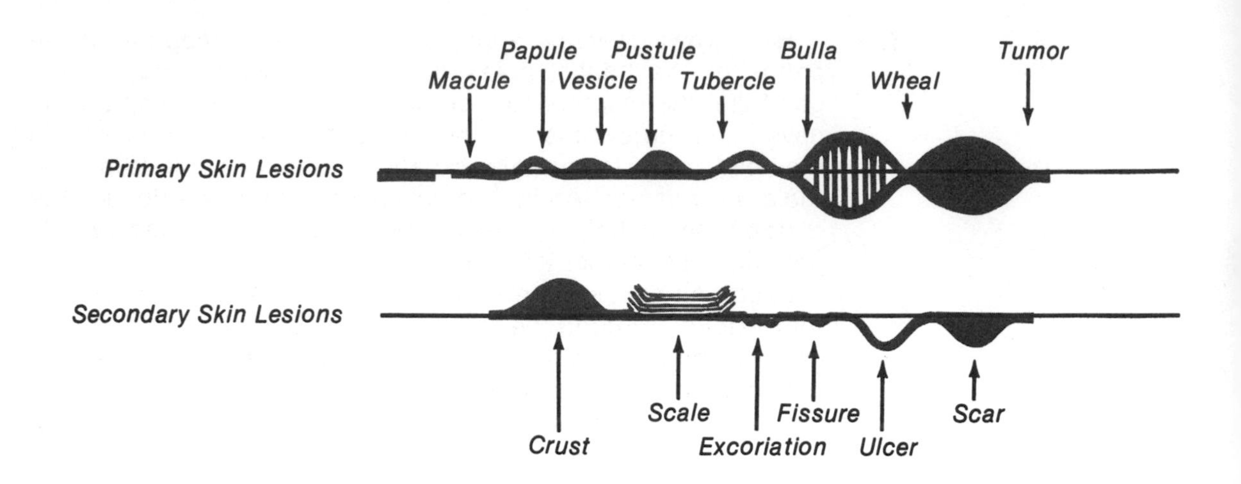


**Definitions Pertaining to Secondary Lesions**

The secondary skin lesions are those in the skin that develop in the later stages of disease. These are:

*Crust:* An accumulation of serum and pus, mixed perhaps with epidermal material. (Example: the scab on a sore.)

*Excoriation:* A skin sore or abrasion produced by scratching or scraping. (Example: a raw surface due to the loss of the superficial skin after an injury.)

*Fissure:* A crack in the skin penetrating into the derma, as in the case of chapped hands or lips.

*Scale:* An accumulation of epidermal flakes, dry or greasy. (Example: abnormal or excessive dandruff.)

*Scar:* (cicatrix) Likely to form after the healing of an injury or skin condition that has penetrated the dermal layer.

*Stain:* An abnormal discoloration remaining after the disappearance of moles, freckles, or liver spots, sometimes apparent after certain diseases.

*Ulcer:* An open lesion on the skin or mucous membrane of the body, accompanied by pus and loss of skin depth.

## DISORDERS OF THE SKIN

**Problem Blemished Skin**

The massage practitioner need not be concerned about diagnosis or treatment of skin disorders, but he or she should be able to recognize some of the more common conditions in order to explain to the client why massage should or should not be given. The practitioner can suggest or recommend that the client see a dermatologist for skin conditions that are contraindications for massage.

*Blackheads (comedones)* are small masses of hardened, discolored sebum that appear most frequently on the face, shoulders, chest, and back. Blackheads are often accompanied by pimples during adolescence and are primarily due to overstimulated sebaceous glands. Proper cleansing of the skin will help to reduce the skin's oiliness. Any case of excessive pimples or blackheads should be treated by a dermatologist.

Massage should not be given over areas where these skin conditions are more severe. However, stimulation of blood circulation is beneficial and massage, exercise, and proper diet will, in most cases, help to improve these conditions.

*Dermatitis* is an inflammatory condition of the skin. The lesions come in various forms, such as vesicles or papules.

*Eczema,* an inflammation of the skin, either acute or chronic in nature, can appear in many forms of dry or moist lesions. The term *eczema* is applied to any number of surface lesions. It is usually a red, blistered, oozing area that itches painfully. Eczema may be the result of some type of allergy or internal disorder and should be referred to a physician for treatment.

*Psoriasis* is a common chronic, inflammatory skin disease whose cause is unknown. It is usually found on the scalp, elbows, knees, chest and lower back, but rarely on the face. The lesions are round dry patches covered with course, silvery scales. If irritated, bleeding points occur. Although not contagious, it can be spread by irritation. Massage over such a condition should be avoided.

Occupational disorders refer to abnormal conditions resulting from contact with chemicals. Some individuals may develop allergies to ingredients in some substances with which they work. An example is often seen when a cosmetologist is allergic to hair tints.

A client may have a condition of the skin known as *staphylodermatitis,* an inflamation caused by staphylococci, bacteria that are generally found in milk and other dairy products. Massage should not be given when the skin is inflamed. The client should have the condition diagnosed by a physician.

A *bruise* is a superficial injury (contusion) generally caused by a blow or impact with some object; while not breaking the skin, it causes a reddish blue or purple discoloration. Severe bruises should be avoided during massage.

*Acne* is a chronic inflammatory disorder of the skin, usually related to hormonal changes and overactive sebaceous glands during adolescence. Common acne is also known as *acne simplex* or *acne vulgaris.* Although acne generally starts at the onset of puberty, it also afflicts adult men and women.

Modern studies show that acne is often due to heredity, but the condition can be aggravated by emotional stress and environmental factors. A well-balanced diet, drinking plenty of water, and developing healthful personal hygiene are recommended. Acne may be present on the back, chest, and shoulders. Acne may be accompanied by blackheads, pustules, and pimples that are red, swollen, and containing pus. In more advanced cases of acne, cysts (which are red, swollen lumps beneath the surface of the skin) may appear. Massage should be avoided when acne is present.

*Seborrhea* is a skin condition caused by overactivity and excessive secretion of the sebaceous glands. An oily or shiny condition of the nose, forehead, or scalp indicates the presence of seborrhea. It is readily detected on the scalp by the unusual amount of oil on the hair. Seborrhea is often the basis of an acne condition. Massage should not be given over infected areas.

*Rosacea* is associated with excessive oiliness of the skin and a chronic inflammatory condition of the cheeks and nose. It is characterized by redness owing to dilation of blood vessels and the formation of papules and pustules. The skin becomes coarse, and the pores enlarged. Rosacea is usualy caused by an inability to digest certain foods and intolerance to strong beverages. It may also be caused by overexposure to extreme climate, faulty elimination, and hyperacidity. Massage is not given over affected areas.

A *steatoma* or *sebaceous cyst* is a subcutaneous tumor of the sebaceous glands that contains sebum. It usually appears as a small growth on the scalp, neck, or back. A steatoma is sometimes called a *wen.* Massage is not given over the affected area.

*Asteatosis* is a condition of dry, scaly skin, characterized by absolute or partial deficiency of sebum, usually due to aging or bodily disorders. In local conditions, such as scaling of the hands, it may be caused by alkalies in soaps and similar products. When the skin is unbroken, a mild lubricant may be massaged into the skin.

A *furuncle,* or boil, is caused by bacteria that enter the skin through the hair follicles. It is a subcutaneous abscess that fills with pus. A boil can be painful if neglected and should be treated by a physician.

## SERIOUS SKIN CONDITIONS

The massage practitioner should not attempt to diagnose any kind of bump, lesion, ulceration, or discoloration as skin cancer but should be able to recognize serious skin disorders and suggest that the client seek medical attention without delay.

### Skin Cancer

There are three kinds of skin cancer. The least malignant and most common is called *basal cell carcinoma.* This type of cancer is characterized by light or pearly nodules and visible blood vessels.

*Squamous cell carcinoma* is different in appearance from the basal type; it consists of scaly, red papules. Blood vessels are not visible. This cancer is more serious than the basal cell carcinoma.

The most serious skin cancer is the *malignant melanoma.* This cancer is characterized by dark (brown, black, or discolored) patches on the skin.

A *tumor* is an abnormal growth of swollen tissue that can be located on any part of the body. Some tumors are benign (mild in character) and are not likely to recur after removal, which means they are not harmful. Some tumors are malignant and are more serious, as they can recur after removal. Tumors are removed by surgery, X-ray, or chemical treatments.

**Venereal Diseases**

Venereal diseases are those diseases associated with the sexual organs and are characterized by sores and rashes on the skin. Venereal diseases can become latent and appear at a later time. This can be dangerous because the affected person may not seek treatment. Venereal diseases can also affect unborn children.

*Syphilis* is a serious disease that is transmitted by sexual contact with an infected person. When a sore first appears, especially one that is hard and ulcerated (with a hole in the center), a physician should be consulted. Without treatment the sore may go away only to appear later in the form of a rash. This is called *secondary syphilis* which can cause degeneration of various parts of the body, ultimately causing death.

*Gonorrhea* is a more common disease than syphilis and is characterized by a discharge and burning sensation when urinating. Women may show no symptoms. If left untreated, harmful bacteria can enter the bloodstream.

**Herpes**

*Herpes* generally affects the mouth, skin, and other parts of the face (commonly called *cold sores* and *fever blisters*). Herpes virus can cause a variety of diseases known for their persistence in a latent state and re-occurance at regular intervals. The virus usually enters the body through the mucous membranes. *Herpes simplex* is generally defined as a recurrent spreading cutaneous infection. Examples are *herpes facialia* (herpes simplex), a type of herpes that affects the lips, mouth, pharynx, or parts of the face. *Herpes progenitalis* is a type of herpes simplex in which vesicles occur on the genitalia.

**AIDS**

Just a few years ago AIDS (acquired immune deficiency syndrome) was unheard of, but the disease has spread at an alarming rate since the early 1980s. The World Health Organization has reported that AIDS has become an international concern. AIDS is caused by a virus that is linked to the viral family that causes leukemia (a cancer of the blood). The virus breaks down the body's immune system, which produces anitbodies and cells that destroy harmful bacteria. When the body loses its natural resistance, it is unable to combat various infections.

There is a great deal of controversy about how AIDS is spread, but intensive research has revealed that it is not spread by casual contact such as being in the same room with an AIDS patient or by just touching a person. The disease is most often transmitted by sexual activity, by blood transfusions, and by the use of contaminated needles, and it can be transmitted to an unborn child through the placenta.

Progress is being made in the prevention and treatment of AIDS by screening tests and by educating the public about the seriousness of the disease.

**Allergies**

An *allergy* is a sensitivity that certain persons develop to normally harmless substances. Contact with certain types of cosmetics, medicines, and hair preparations or consumption of certain foods may bring about an itching skin eruption, accompanied by redness, swelling, blisters, oozing, and scaling. Many allergies are accompanied by headaches, congestion, or emotional inconsistency.

Millions of people suffer from various forms of allergies. *Allergic dermititis* (eczema), one of the more common allergies, can be caused by a number of different factors: food, substances in the air, or materials the victim uses. Many objects, including necklaces, rings, hairpins, and bracelets, contain metals (such as nickel) that cause dermatitis. Hair dyes, makeup, and chemicals are a few of the substances to which some people are allergic.

**Pigmentations of the Skin**

Changes in skin color may be observed in various skin disorders and in many systemic disorders. Certain drugs taken internally can affect pigmentation. Foods eaten in excess can affect the skin. The carotene in carrots is an example. A suntan is an example of external changes in the pigmentation of the skin. The fairer the skin, the easier it is to sunburn and the more difficult it may be to acquire an even suntan.

Generally, a skin that tans easily will not be sensitive to massage. However, when skin has been overexposed, it may become sensitive. When there is sunburn or peeling due to sunburn, massage may be painful.

*Lentigines,* or freckles, are small yellowish to brownish color spots on parts exposed to sunlight and air.

*Stains* are abnormal brown skin patches, having circular and irregular shape. Their permanent color is due to the presence of blood pigment. They occur during aging, after certain diseases, and after the disappearance of moles, freckles, and liver spots. The cause of these stains is unknown.

*Chloasma* is characterized by increased deposits of pigment in the skin. It is found mainly on the forehead, nose, and cheeks. Chloasma is also called *moth patches* or *liver spots.*

*A naevus* is commonly known as a birthmark. It is a small or large discoloration of the skin due to pigmentation or dilated capillaries and is present on the skin at birth. Generally, such colored spots or areas are not affected by massage.

*Leucoderma* are abnormal light patches of skin, due to congenital defective pigmentations. *Vitiligo* is an acquired condition of leucoderma that affects skin or hair.

*Albinism* is a congenital absence of melanin pigment in the body that affects the color of the skin, hair, and eyes. In albinos the hair is silky and white, and the skin is pinkish white and will not tan.

A *kertoma,* or callus, is a superficial, thickened patch of epidermis caused by friction on the hands and feet. This condition is usually treated by a chiropodist.

Color changes of the skin, such as a crack on the skin, a type of thickening, or any discoloration ranging from shades of red to brown and purple to almost black, may be danger signals and should be examined by a dermatologist.

**QUESTIONS FOR DISCUSSION AND REVIEW**

1. Define skin as the integumentary system
2. Name the major functions of the skin
3. Name the two main layers of the skin.
4. Name the layers of the epidermis.
5. Name two forms of keratin and where they are found in most abundance.
6. What is subcutaneous tissue?
7. How does the skin receive its color?
8. Name the layers of the dermis.
9. What is a gland?
10. Name the two major glands found in the skin and give the function of each.
11. Define the following: sebum, pore, duct.
12. Name the appendages of the skin.
13. What is a lesion?
14. What kind of skin condition is called an occupational disorder?
15. Why is it important for the massage practitioner to observe a client's skin condition?

**ANSWERS TO QUESTIONS FOR DISCUSSION AND REVIEW**

1. The skin (integumentary system) is the external covering and largest organ of the body.
2. The skin protects the parts of the body situated beneath its surface, regulates body temperature, and functions as an organ of secretion and excretion, absorption, and respiration.
3. The two main layers of the skin are the epidermis and the dermis.
4. The layers of the epidermis are the stratum corneum, lucidum, granulosum, and mucosum.
5. Keratin is both hard and soft. Soft keratin is found in the skin, and hard keratin is found in hair and nails.
6. Subcutaneous tissue is a layer of fatty tissue found below the dermis. It contains a network of arteries and a superficial and deep layer of lymphatics.
7. The color of the skin depends partly upon the blood supply but more upon melanin, the pigment or coloring matter deposited in the deepest layer of the epidermis and the superficial layer of the dermis.
8. The layers of the dermis are the papillary and the reticular layers.
9. A gland is an organ of either excretion of secretion, taking materials from the blood and forming new substances.
10. The two major glands in the skin are the sudoriferous glands, which excrete sweat, and the sebaceous glands, which secrete sebum.

11. Sebum is an oily substance of the sebaceous glands. A pore is a minute opening of the sweat glands on the surface of the skin and is also referred to as a follicle. A duct is a passage or canal for fluids.
12. Appendages of the skin include hair and nails. Also the oil and sweat glands are appendages.
13. A lesion is a structural change in tissues caused by injury or disease.
14. An occupational disorder is a skin condition or reaction caused by some substance a worker uses in his or her occupation.
15. The massage practitioner should observe the client's skin condition because the skin often gives clues as to whether massage would be beneficial or potentially harmful.

## SYSTEM TWO THE SKELETAL SYSTEM

The skeletal system is the framework of the body that supports and protects the other body systems. It is composed of bones, cartilage, and ligaments.

### THE SKELETON AS A WHOLE

The skeleton is divided into two main parts, the *appendicular skeleton* and the *axial skeleton.* The appendicular skeleton is made up of bones of the shoulder, upper extremeties, hips and lower extremities. The name *appendicular* identifies these parts as appendages or extensions of the axis or axial skeleton. The bones of the skull, thorax, and vertebral column comprise the axial skeleton.

In the human adult, the skeleton consists of 206 bones, which are distributed as follows:

HEAD
- Cranium (8)
- Face (14)
- Ear (6)
- Hyoid bone (1)

THORAX
- Ribs and sternum (25)

SPINE
- Vertebrae (26)

EXTREMITIES
- Upper extremities (64)
- Lower extremities (62)

In all massage manipulations, the form or outline of the bones must be carefully followed, and strenuous massage movements must be avoided. Knowing the names of bones serves as a guide in recalling the names of related structures connected with the part being massaged.

#### Composition

Other than dentine, the dense hard tissue covering the teeth, bone is the hardest structure of the body. Bone is composed of about one-third animal matter and two-thirds mineral or earthy matter. The animal (organic) matter consists of bone cells, blood vessels, connective tissues, and marrow. The mineral (inorganic) matter consists mainly of calcium phosphate and calcium carbonate.

*Marrow* is the connective tissue filling the cavities of bones. Its function is largely concerned with the formation of red and white blood cells. There are two types of bone marrow: *red* and *yellow* marrow. Red bone marrow functions in the production of red and white blood cells and platelets. It occupies nearly all the bone cavities of the newborn; however, in the adult it is found in the bone spaces of the skull, ribs, sternum, vertebrae, and pelvis. Yellow marrow is the result of inactive blood producing cells filling with fatty material.

There are two types of bone tissue: *cancellous* (spongy) and *dense* (compact). Cancellous tissue forms the interior of bones, the end of the bone shaft and very thin bones. It consists of a meshwork of bony arches through which blood vessels and nerves pass. The two ends of the long bone are called epiphyses, the shaft of the bone, or diaphysis, is compact bone covered with periosteum. Compact tissue forms the hard bone found in the shafts of long bones along the outside of flat bones. *Channels,* called *Haversian canals,* are where branches of blood vessels penetrate to nourish the bone. Canals are made up of clusters of bone cells that run longitudinal in compact bone tissue.

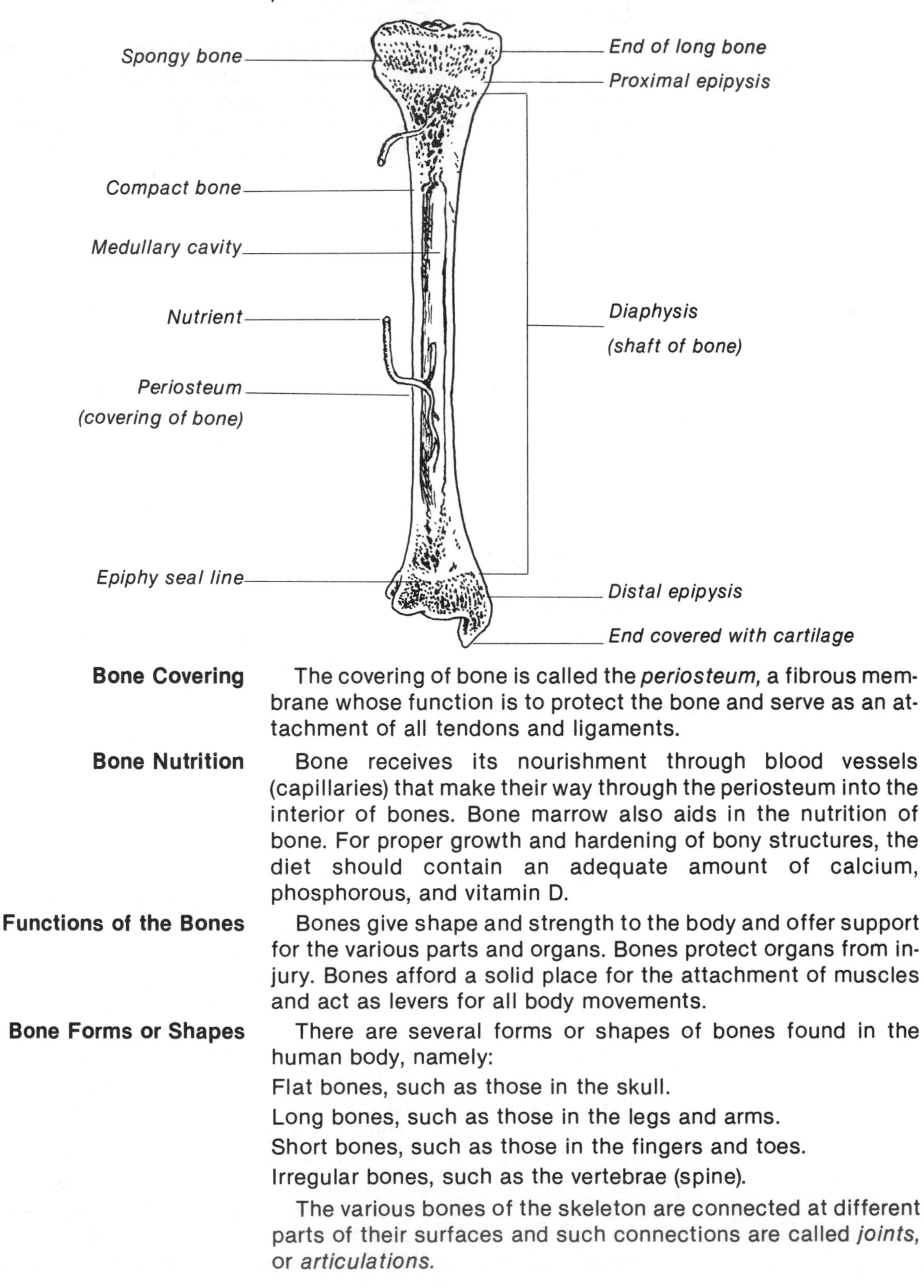


**Bone Covering**

The covering of bone is called the *periosteum,* a fibrous membrane whose function is to protect the bone and serve as an attachment of all tendons and ligaments.

**Bone Nutrition**

Bone receives its nourishment through blood vessels (capillaries) that make their way through the periosteum into the interior of bones. Bone marrow also aids in the nutrition of bone. For proper growth and hardening of bony structures, the diet should contain an adequate amount of calcium, phosphorous, and vitamin D.

**Functions of the Bones**

Bones give shape and strength to the body and offer support for the various parts and organs. Bones protect organs from injury. Bones afford a solid place for the attachment of muscles and act as levers for all body movements.

**Bone Forms or Shapes**

There are several forms or shapes of bones found in the human body, namely:

Flat bones, such as those in the skull.

Long bones, such as those in the legs and arms.

Short bones, such as those in the fingers and toes.

Irregular bones, such as the vertebrae (spine).

The various bones of the skeleton are connected at different parts of their surfaces and such connections are called *joints,* or *articulations.*

**Joints**

The various kinds of joints come under the following classifications:

Movable, as in fingers.
Immovable, as in the skull.

Slightly movable, as in the spine.

The various types of joints found in the human body are classified as:

Pivot, as in the neck.

Hinge, as in the elbow and knees.

Ball and socket, as in the hips and shoulders.

Gliding, as in the spine or hand.

Saddle, as in the wrist and thumb.

**Cartilage and Ligaments**

*Cartilage* (also called *gristle*) is a firm and tough, elastic substance, similar to bone but without its mineral content. It serves the following purposes:

To cushion the bones at the joints.

To prevent jarring between bones in motion, as in walking.

To give shape to external features, such as the nose and ears.

*Ligaments* are bands or sheets of fibruous tissue that help to support the bones at the joints, as in wrist and ankle. The *synovial fluid* is the lubricating fluid whose function is to prevent friction at the joints.

**Vertebral Column**

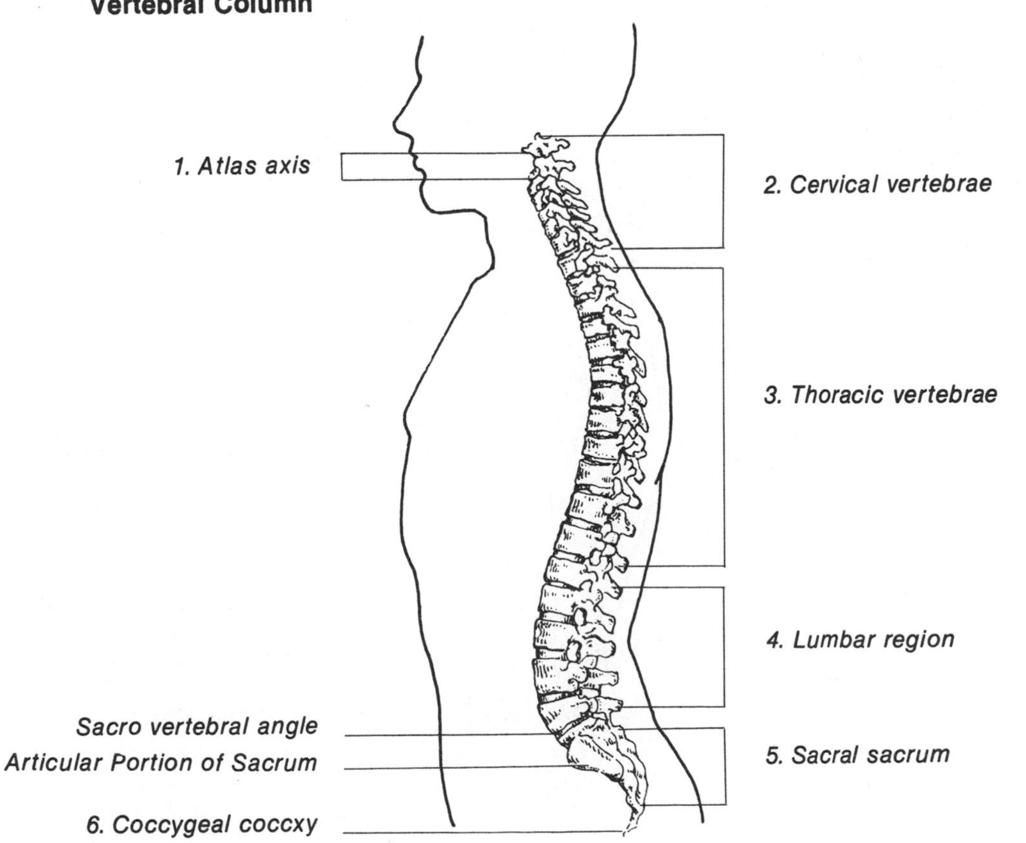

## The Skeletal System — Anterior View

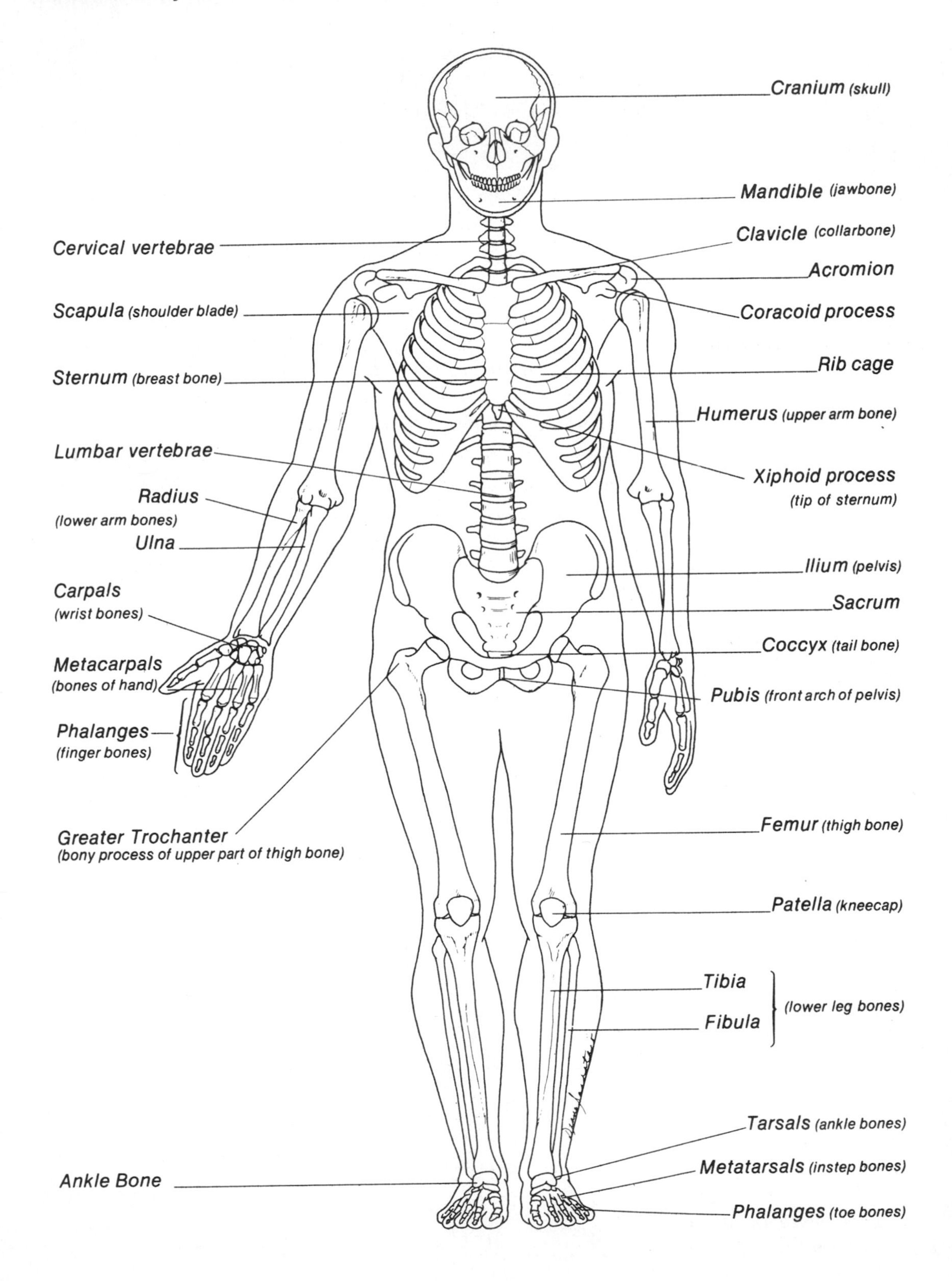

## The Skeletal System — Posterior View

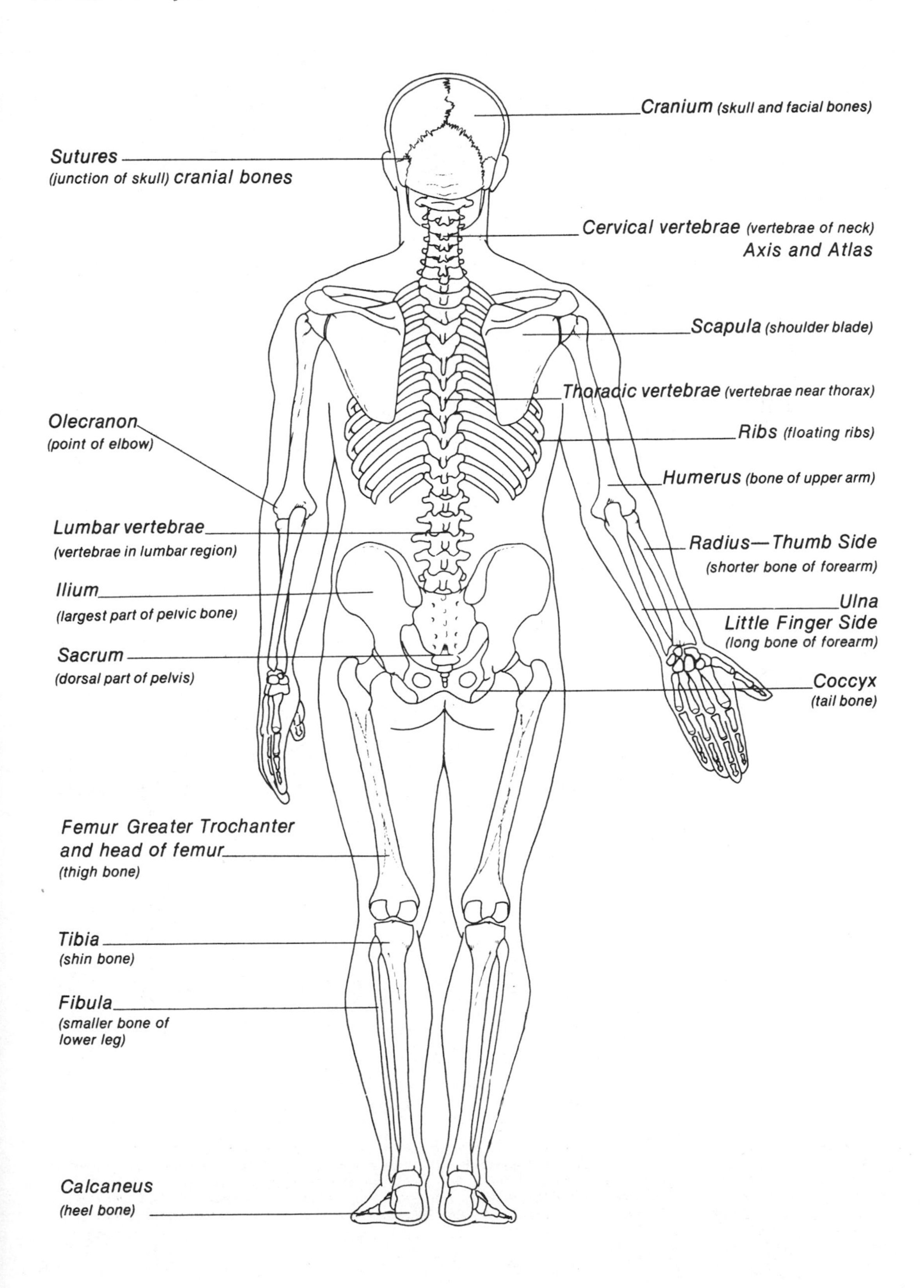

## Cranium, Face and Neck Bones

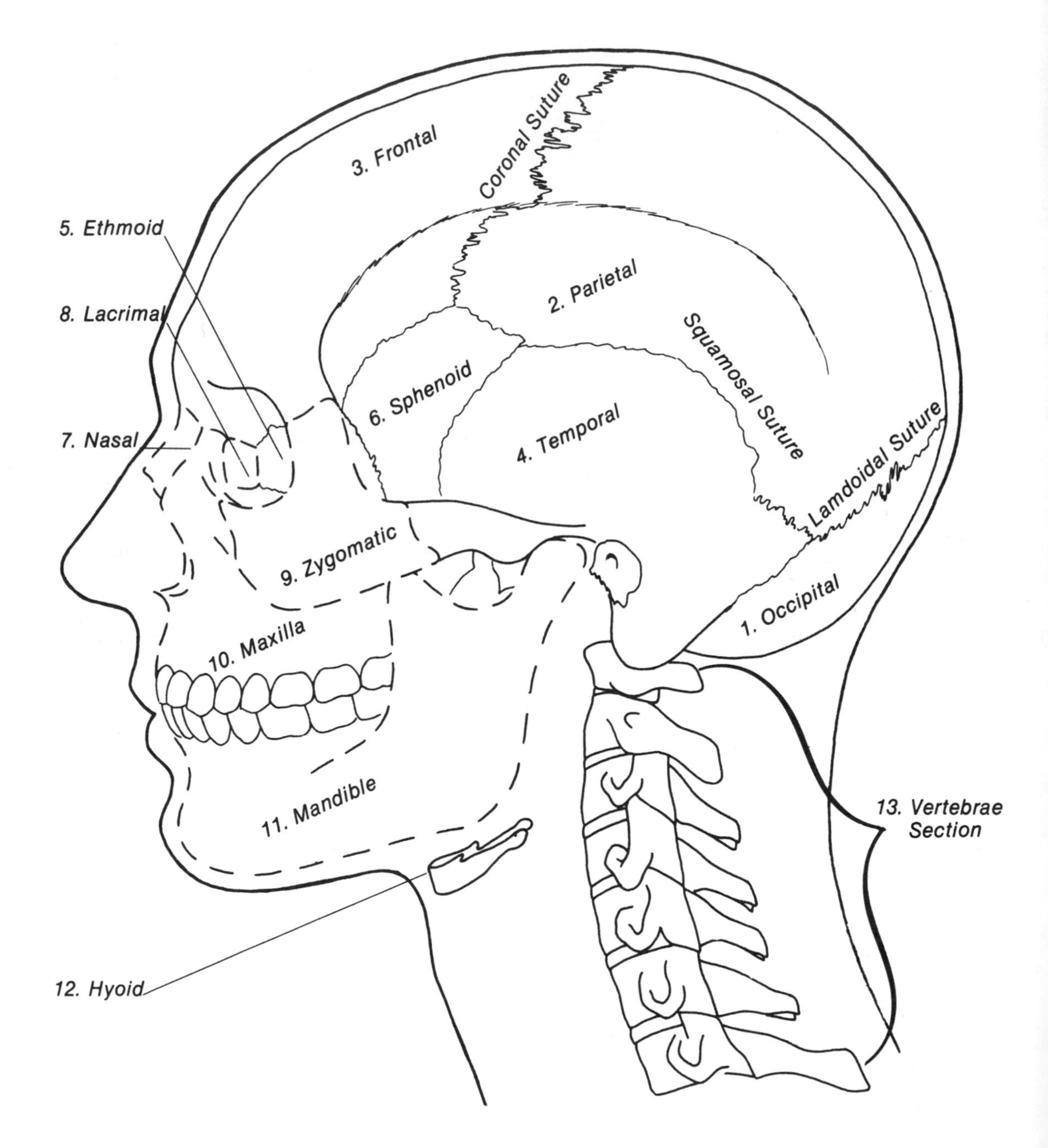


**1.** Base of skull. **2.** Large part of upper and side walls of cranium. **3.** Forms forehead, nasal cavity and orbits. **4.** Forms sides and base of cranium. **5.** Supports nasal cavity and helps to form orbits. **6.** Forms anterior part of base of cranium. **7.** A pair of bones forming the bridge of the nose. **8.** A pair of bones making up part of the orbit at the inner angle of the eye. **9.** Bone which helps to form the cheek. **10.** Bone of the upper jaw. **11.** Bone forming the lower jaw. **12.** Bone located between the mandible and the larynx. **13.** Smallest vertebrae of the spinal column; forming the framework of the neck.

**Important Bones of the Body**

| NUMBER OF BONES | FUNCTION |
|---|---|
| **Head** | |
| 8 cranial bones | Form a protective structure for the brain. |
| 14 facial bones | Form the structure of the eyes, nose, cheeks, mouth and jaws. |
| 6 ear bones | Form the structure of the ears. |
| 1 hyoid bone | Supports the base of the tongue. |
| **Spine** | |
| 26 vertebrae | Form the spinal column which supports the head and trunk, provides attachment for the ribs, and also protects the spinal cord. |
| **Thorax or Chest** | |
| 1 sternum (breast bone) | Serves as an attachment for the ribs at the front of the chest. |
| 24 ribs | Form a protective cage for the lungs and heart. |
| **Upper Extremities** | |
| *(The following bones are for one side of the body)* | |
| 1 clavicle (collar bone)<br>1 scapula (shoulder blade) | Both clavicle and scapula form the shoulder girdle to which the upper limbs are attached. |
| 1 humerus | Forms the upper part of the arm. |
| 1 ulna | Forms the bone at the finger side of the forearm. |
| 1 radius | Forms the bone at the thumb side of the forearm. |
| 8 carpus | Form the wrist bones. |
| 5 metacarpus | Form the bones in the palm of the hand. |
| 14 phalanges | Form the bones of the fingers. |
| **Lower Extremities** | |
| *(The following bones are for one side of the body)* | |
| 1 pelvis (hip bone) | Serves as an attachment for the lower limb. |
| 1 femur | Forms the upper part of the leg. |
| 1 patella (kneecap) | Forms the front of the knee joint. |
| 1 tibia (shin bone) | Forms the inner side of the leg. |
| 1 fibula (calf bone) | Forms the outer side of the leg. |
| 7 tarsus | Form the ankle bones. |
| 5 metatarsus | Form the bones between the ankle and toes. |
| 14 phalanges | Form the bones of the toes. |

**Words That Describe Bone Markings**

| | |
|---|---|
| Process | a bone prominence or projection |
| Condyle (***KON*** *dil*) | a rounded knuckle-like prominence usually at a point of articulation |
| Head | a rounded articulating process at the end of a bone |
| Spine | a sharp slender projection |
| Tubercle (*tu* ***BER****-kl*) | a small rounded process |
| Tuberosity (*tu-****BER*** *os i tee*) | a large rounded process |
| Trochanter (***TRO****-kan tur*) | a large process for muscle attachment |
| Fossa (***FOS*** *uh*) | a depression or hollow |
| Foramen (***FO****-ray mun*) | a hole |
| Crest | a ridge |
| Line | a less prominent ridge of a bone than a crest |
| Meatus (***ME****-ay tus*) | a tubelike passage |
| Sinus or antrum | a cavity within a bone |

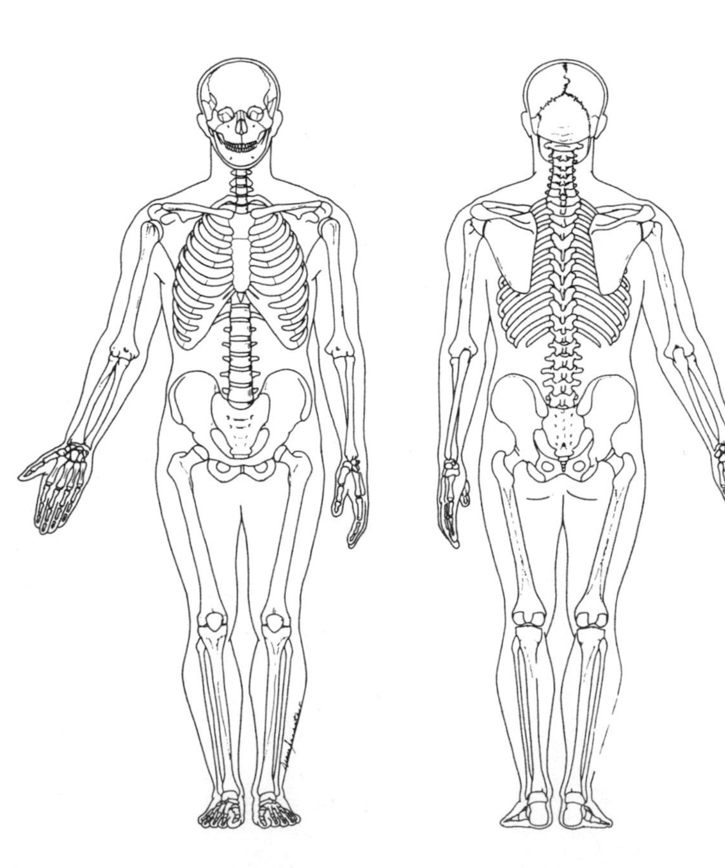

**Review** IMPORTANT BONES OF THE BODY

### Matching Test

*Match the following definitions. Insert the proper term in front of each definition.*

| | | |
|---|---|---|
| 1. .............. | Upper arm. | Fibula |
| 2. .............. | Wrist bones. | Tarsus |
| 3. .............. | Ankle bones. | Scapula |
| 4. .............. | Toe or finger bones | Tibia |
| 5. .............. | Palm bones. | Phalanges |
| 6. .............. | Spinal column. | Vertebrae |
| 7. .............. | Collar bone. | Carpus |
| 8. .............. | Shoulder blade. | Metacarpus |
| 9. .............. | Calf bone. | Humerus |
| 10. .............. | Shin bone. | Clavicle |

### True or False Test

*Carefully read each statement and decide if it is True or False by drawing a circle around the letter T or F.*

| | | | |
|---|---|---|---|
| 1. | T | F | The hyoid bone supports the base of the ear. |
| 2. | T | F | The metatarsus and metacarpus are different bones. |
| 3. | T | F | The patella forms the front of the knee joint. |
| 4. | T | F | The upper limbs are attached to the pelvis. |
| 5. | T | F | The clavicle and scapula serve as an attachment for the lower limbs. |
| 6. | T | F | The femur forms the upper part of the leg. |
| 7. | T | F | The ulna and radius are found in the forearm. |
| 8. | T | F | The lungs and heart are found in the thorax. |
| 9. | T | F | The vertebrae provide an attachment for the ribs. |
| 10. | T | F | The pelvis is known as the kneecap. |

### Answers

Matching Test

| | |
|---|---|
| 1—Humerus. | 6—Vertebrae. |
| 2—Carpus. | 7—Clavicle. |
| 3—Tarsus. | 8—Scapula. |
| 4—Phalanges. | 9—Fibula. |
| 5—Metacarpus. | 10—Tibia. |

True or False Test

| | |
|---|---|
| 1—F | 6—T |
| 2—T | 7—T |
| 3—T | 8—T |
| 4—F | 9—T |
| 5—F | 10—F |

**QUESTIONS FOR DISCUSSION AND REVIEW**

1. Why should every massage practitioner study the skeletal system?
2. In what manner is massage applied over the bones?
3. Name the organic and inorganic matter found in bones.
4. Name two types of bone tissue.
5. Which covering protects the bone?
6. How are the bones nourished?
7. Name the various shapes of bones found in the body. Give an example of each.
8. What are joints?
9. Which structure cushions the bones at the joints?
10. Which structure supports the bones at the joints?
11. Which fluid lubricates the joints?
12. About how many bones are found in the human body?

**ANSWERS TO QUESTIONS FOR DISCUSSION AND REVIEW**

1. The massage practitioner studies the skeletal system because bones form the framework of the body and protect other body systems.
2. The form of the bones must be carefully followed, and strenuous movements must be avoided.
3. Organic matter consists of bone cells, blood vessels, connective tissue and marrow. Inorganic matter consists of calcium phosphate and calcium carbonate.
4. Two types of bone tissue are cancellous (spongy) tissue and dense (compact) tissue.
5. The periosteum covers and protects bone.
6. Bones receive their nourishment through blood vessels that enter through the periosteum into the interior of the bone. Bone marrow also aids in the nutrition of the bone.
7. Flat bones, such as the skull; long bones, such as the legs; short bones, such as the fingers; and irregular bones, such as the vertebrae of the spine.
8. Joints are the connections between the surfaces of bones.
9. Cartilage or gristle cushion bony joints.
10. Ligaments support the bones at their joints.
11. Synovial fluid lubricates the joints.
12. The body comprises 206 bones.

## SYSTEM THREE THE MUSCULAR SYSTEM

The muscular system covers, shapes, and supports the skeleton. Its function is to produce all movements of the body. The muscular system relies upon the skeletal and nervous systems for its activities.

The muscular system consists of over 600 muscles, large and small. In the human body it comprises approximately 40 to 50 percent of the total body weight of an adult.

Deep massage has a profound effect not only on the development of muscles but also on the activity of the blood, lymph, and nerves associated with the muscles of the body.

### Muscle

*Muscle* is a contractile fibrous tissue by which movements of every part of the body are affected. Muscles do not cover and surround the body in continuous sheets, but consist of separate bundles made up of elastic fibers varying in size and length, according to the function of each.

Muscles are attached to bones, cartilage, ligaments, tendons, skin, and sometimes to each other. Usually muscles are not directly connected to bones, but are joined by means of glistening cords, called *tendons,* sometimes called *sinews.* Where one muscle connects with another, each muscle ends in an expanded tendon or fibrous sheet, called an *aponeurosis.* The *origin of a muscle* is the more fixed attachments of that muscle and is generally located more proximally, or the center of the body. The *insertion of muscle* is the term applied to the more movable attachments such as muscle attached to skin or movable and generally more distal aspect of the appendage. Each muscle has a vast network of blood vessels, nerves, and lymphatics from which it receives nourishment.

### *Types of Muscles*

There are three kinds of muscular tissue:

1. Voluntary or striated or skeletal muscles, which are controlled by the will.
2. Involuntary or nonstriated muscles, which function without the action of the will.
3. Heart or cardiac muscle, found only in the heart, and is not duplicated anywhere else in the body.

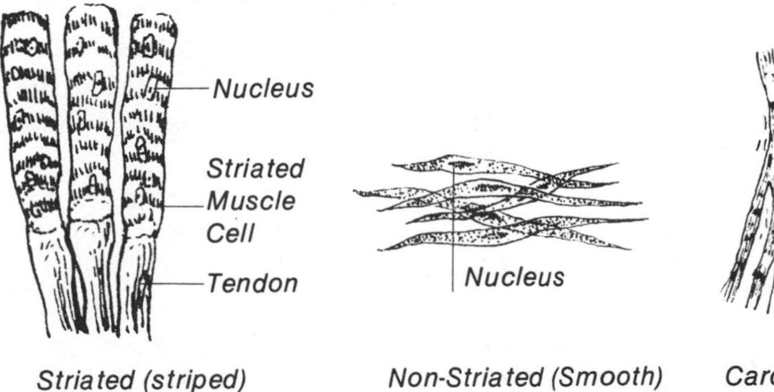


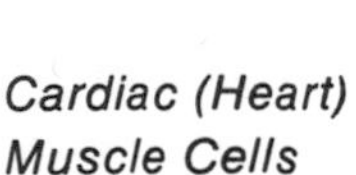

*Striated (striped) Muscle Cells*

*Non-Striated (Smooth) Muscle Cells*

*Cardiac (Heart) Muscle Cells*

*Voluntary* (striated) muscles are put into action by will. They are governed by the cerebrospinal system and appear striated or striped under the microscope. They are attached to the skeleton and are in turn fastened to the bones, skin, and other muscles by tendons.

*Involuntary* (nonstriated) muscles function without the action of the will. They are controlled by the sympathetic nervous system. Involuntary muscles consist of spindle-shaped cells that overlap at the ends, often forming fibrous bands, such as those found in the walls of the stomach, intestines, and blood vessels where they contract and expand.

*Cardiac* (heart) *muscles* are found in the heart. They are composed of cells that are as distinctly striated as the cells of skeletal muscle. Cardiac muscle cells are quadrangular in shape, joined end to end, and grouped in bundles supported by a framework of connective tissue.

***Characteristics of Muscles***

The characteristics that enable muscles to perform their functions of contraction and movement are: irritability,contractility, and elasticity. *Irritability* or excitability is the power of muscles to receive and react to stimuli, whether mechanical (massage), electrical (currents), thermal (heat), chemical (acid or salt), or impulses of nervous origin.

Muscle also has *contractility,* which is the ability to exert force. A muscle possesses tone if it is firm and responds promptly to stimulation under normal conditions. Lack of tone is evidenced by a condition of flabbiness. Exercise and massage help to improve muscular tone. Muscle has *elasticity,* which is the ability to return to its original shape after being stretched. *Extensibility* is the ability of the muscle to stretch.

Muscular activity brings about a chemical change in which glucose, a simple sugar, is consumed by oxidation. As a result, heat and energy are liberated, and various waste products are formed. The blood supplies food and oxygen and also removes the waste products from the active muscles. Rapid or prolonged contractions fatigue the muscles, either because the blood cannot keep pace with the demand for nutritive materials or because the waste products accumulate faster than they can be removed.

**Definitions**

A *spincter muscle* is a muscle that closes an orifice.

An *aponeurosis* is a fibrous sheet or expanded tendon that serves to connect one muscle to another.

A *tendon* is a white glistening bundle of fibrous tissue that attaches muscle to bone.

A *fascia band* is a delicate membrane of connective tissue covering muscles and separating their several layers or groups of layers.

*Skeletal muscles* are those having their attachments to the bones.

*Muscle tone* is the normal degree of muscle tension.

**Terms to Remember**

A review of the following words will be helpful in understanding the meaning of technical terms when studying the muscular system.

*Anterior:* Before, or in front of.

*Posterior:* Behind, or in back of.

*Superior:* Situated above.

*Inferior:* Situated lower.

*Anguli:* At an angle.

*Levator:* That which lifts.

*Dorsal:* Behind, or in back of.

*Medial:* Pertaining to the middle or center.

*Dilator:* That which expands or enlarges.

*Depressor:* That which presses or draws down.

*Proximal:* Nearest from the center or medial line.

*Distal:* Farthest from the center or medial line.

**Muscle Movement and Energy Source**

The energy from muscle contraction comes from the breakdown of *adenosine triphosphate (ATP)*, a high-energy compound of the cell. It is the immediate source of energy for muscular contractions. When a muscle is stimulated, an enzyme causes one of the phosphates to split, releasing energy and forming *adenosine diphosphates (ADP)*. ADP is found in all living cells and is vital to the energy processes of life.

During the oxidation of carbohydrates, ADP is converted to ATP, and the resulting energy is stored in the ATP molecules. ATP is converted back to ADP when energy is released, as in muscular contraction. Each muscle cell, when stimulated gives a total response, or it does not contract at all. The strength of the contraction of the entire muscle depends on the number of cells stimulated and the condition of the entire muscle. Both chemical and electrical changes take place during muscle contraction.

**Muscle Tone**

*Muscle tone* is a type of muscle contraction that is present in healthy muscles. Exercise and massage help to retain muscle tone.

**Muscle Cells or Fibers**

Muscles contain bundles of muscle *cells* or *fibers.* A single fiber is composed of fibrils that contain *actin* and *myosin* filaments. During contraction, the actin and myosin filaments move closer together, shortening the muscle.

## PRIME MOVERS AND ANTAGONISTS

The massage practitioner is concerned with helping the client to relax tense muscles. Consequently, it is important to understand the contraction and relaxation of muscles. When a prime mover contracts, its antagonist must relax. The antagonist does the opposite of the prime mover. For example, when the elbow is flexed, the biceps is the prime mover and the triceps, the antagonist, must relax. To extend the elbow, the triceps becomes the prime mover, the biceps relaxes. Muscles that assist a prime mover are called *synergists.*

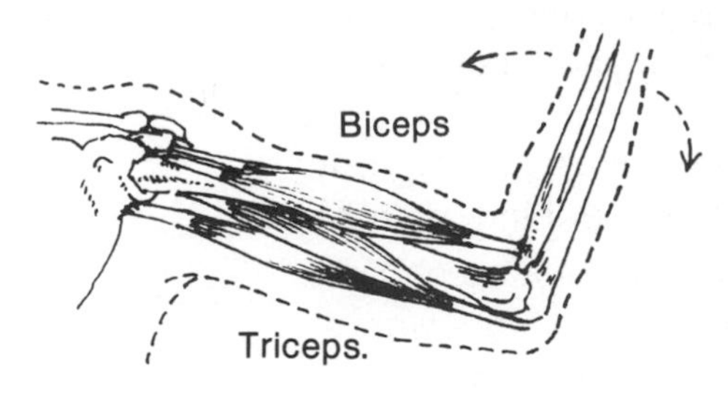


Antagonist muscles. During elbow flexion, the triceps relax while the biceps contract. For extension, the biceps relax while the triceps contract.

**Muscle Interaction**

Skeletal muscles function in groups rather than each muscle functioning alone. When a person wishes to move a muscle, a group of muscles respond. For example, if you wish to lift your arm, the deltoid muscle is the prime mover (contracting), while related muscles (synergists) assist the action. Other muscles act as antagonists. Muscles at movable joints produce movement in different planes and directions.

**Articulations of Joints**

Joints are classified according to the amount of motion they permit. *Diarthrotic joints* are freely movable. The articulating ends of the bones that meet at these joints are covered with hyaline cartilage. A strong fibrous capsule surrounds the joint and is firmly attached to both bones. The lining of the capsule consists of synovial membrane, which secretes a fluid for lubrication. Diarthrotic joints are capable of several kinds of movements: pivot movement, as in turning head; saddle movement, as in the wrist and thumb; ball and socket movement, as in the hip; and hinge movement as in the knees.

DIARTHROSES
Joints are classified according to the degree of movement.

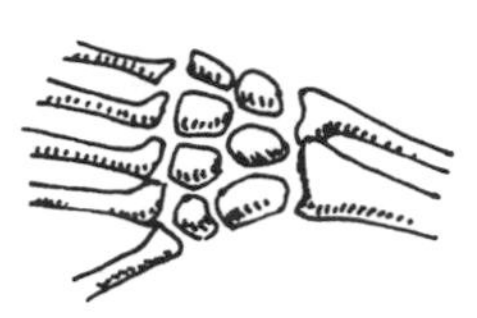

*1. Gliding*

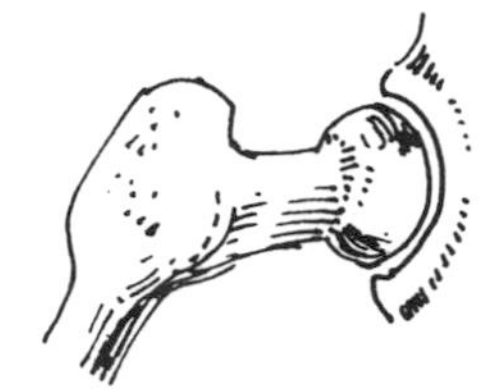

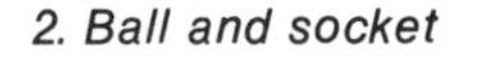

*2. Ball and socket*

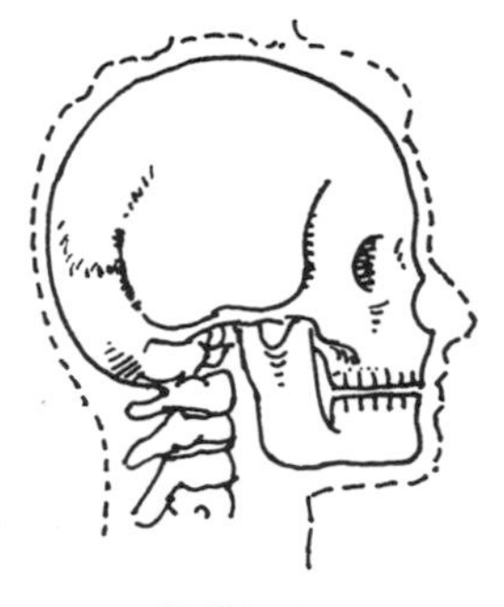

*3. Pivot*

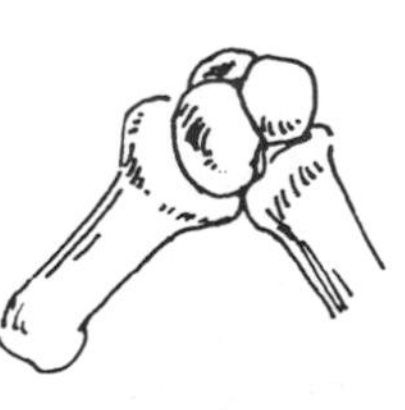

*4. Saddle*

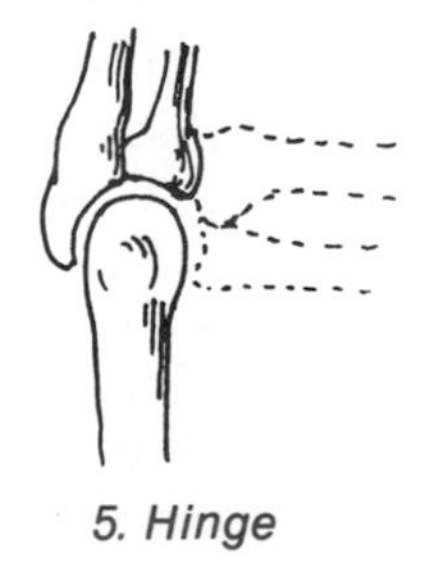

*5. Hinge*

*Amphiarthrotic joints* have limited motion. Examples are the symphysis pubic and vertebral joints.

*Synarthrotic joints* such as those in the skull, are immovable.

*Bursae,* little sacks lined with synovial membrane and lubricated with synovial fluid, are important to movement. The purpose of bursae is to function as a slippery cushion in areas where pressure is exerted, such as between bones and overlying muscle, tendons, or skin. Injury to bursae can cause inflammation and swelling and is called *bursitis.*

AMPHIARTHROSIS

Pelvis.

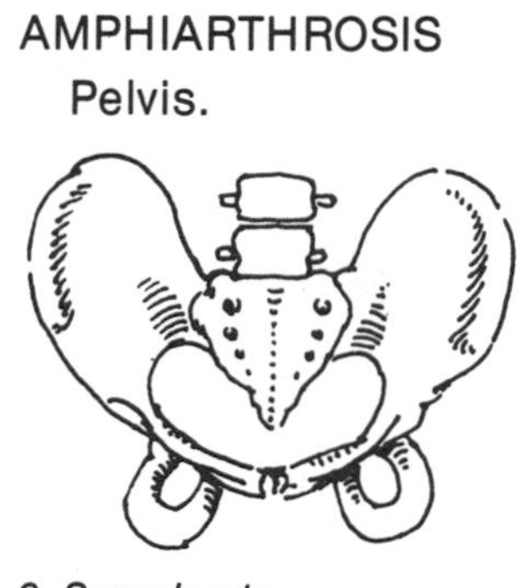

*6. Symphysis*

SYNARTHROSES

Skull

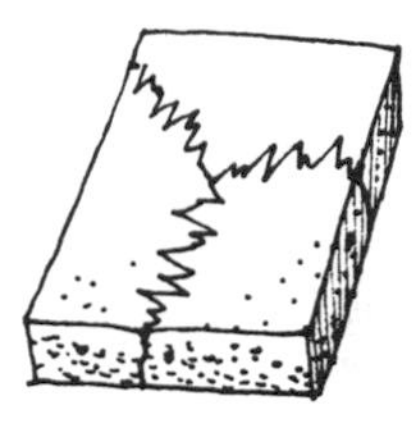

*7. Suture*

### *Motion in Diarthrotic Joints*

| ACTION | MOVEMENT |
| --- | --- |
| *Hyperextension* | Increase the angle beyond the anatomical position. |
| *External rotation* | To move laterally or away from midline (as shown here by the feet). |
| *Internal Rotation* | To move medially or toward the midline. |

***Motion in Diarthrotic Joints*** *(continued)*

| ACTION | MOVEMENT |
|---|---|
| *Rotation* | 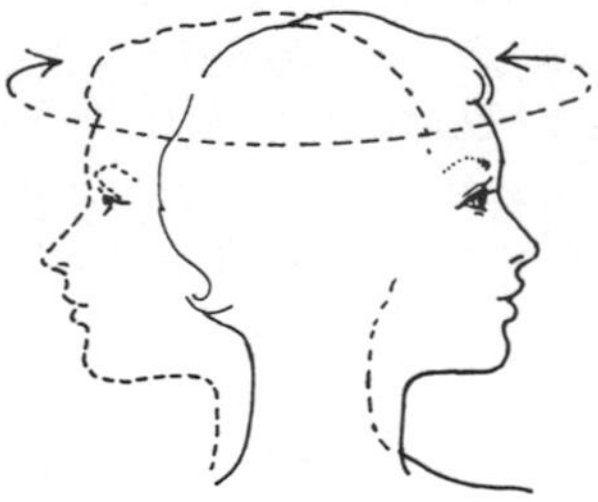 To revolve a part about the longitudinal axis. |
| *Dorsiflexion* | 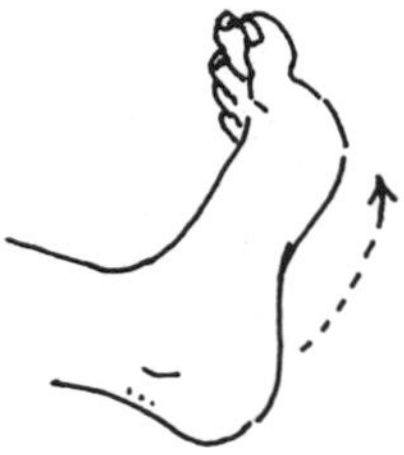 To move the foot upward. |
| *Eversion* | 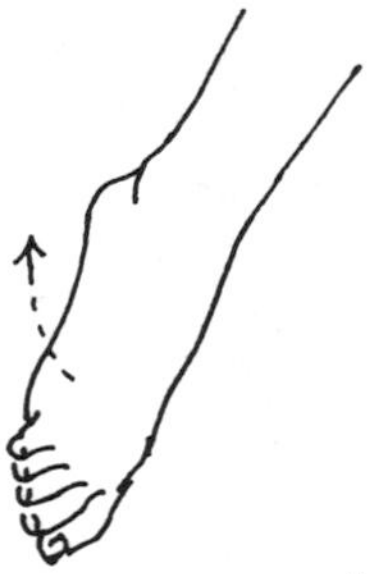 To turn the plantar surface away from the midline. |
| *Inversion* | 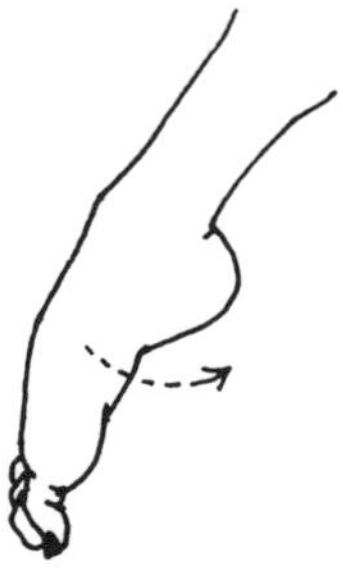 To turn the plantar surface toward the midline. |
| *Plantar flexion* | 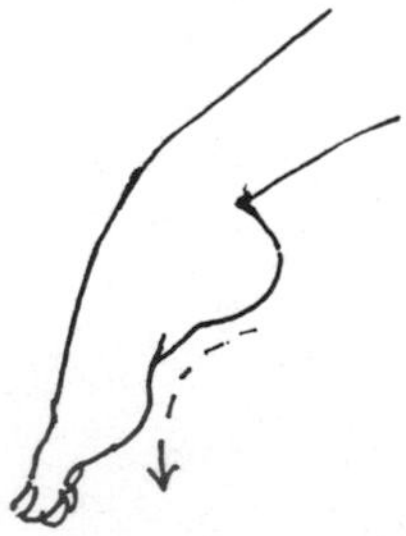 To move the foot downward (extension). |

***Motion in Diarthrotic Joints*** *(continued)*

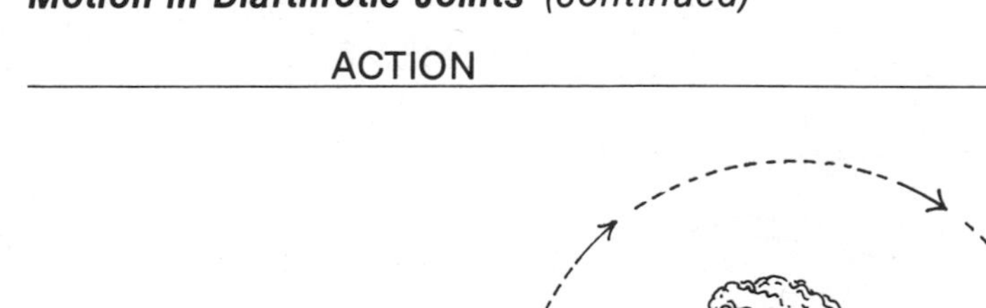

| ACTION | MOVEMENT |
|---|---|
| *Circumduction* | To move the distal end of an extremity in a circle while the proximal end remains fixed. |
| *Adduction* | To move a part toward the midline. |
| *Abduction* | To move a body part away from the midline. |
| *Flexion* | To decrease the angle at a joint. |
| *and* | |
| *Extension* | To increase the angle at a joint. |

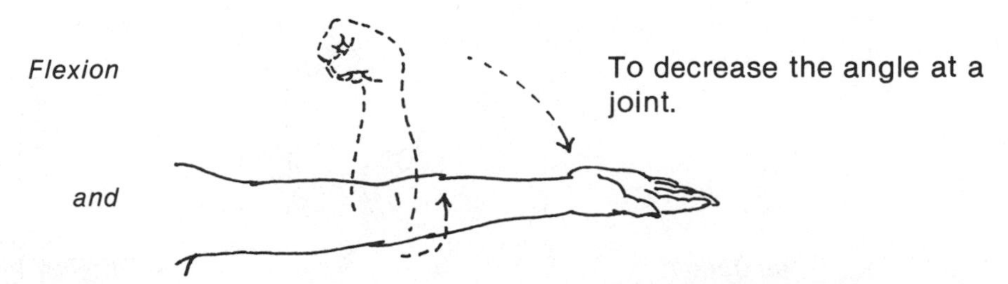

**Motion in Diarthrotic Joints** *(continued)*

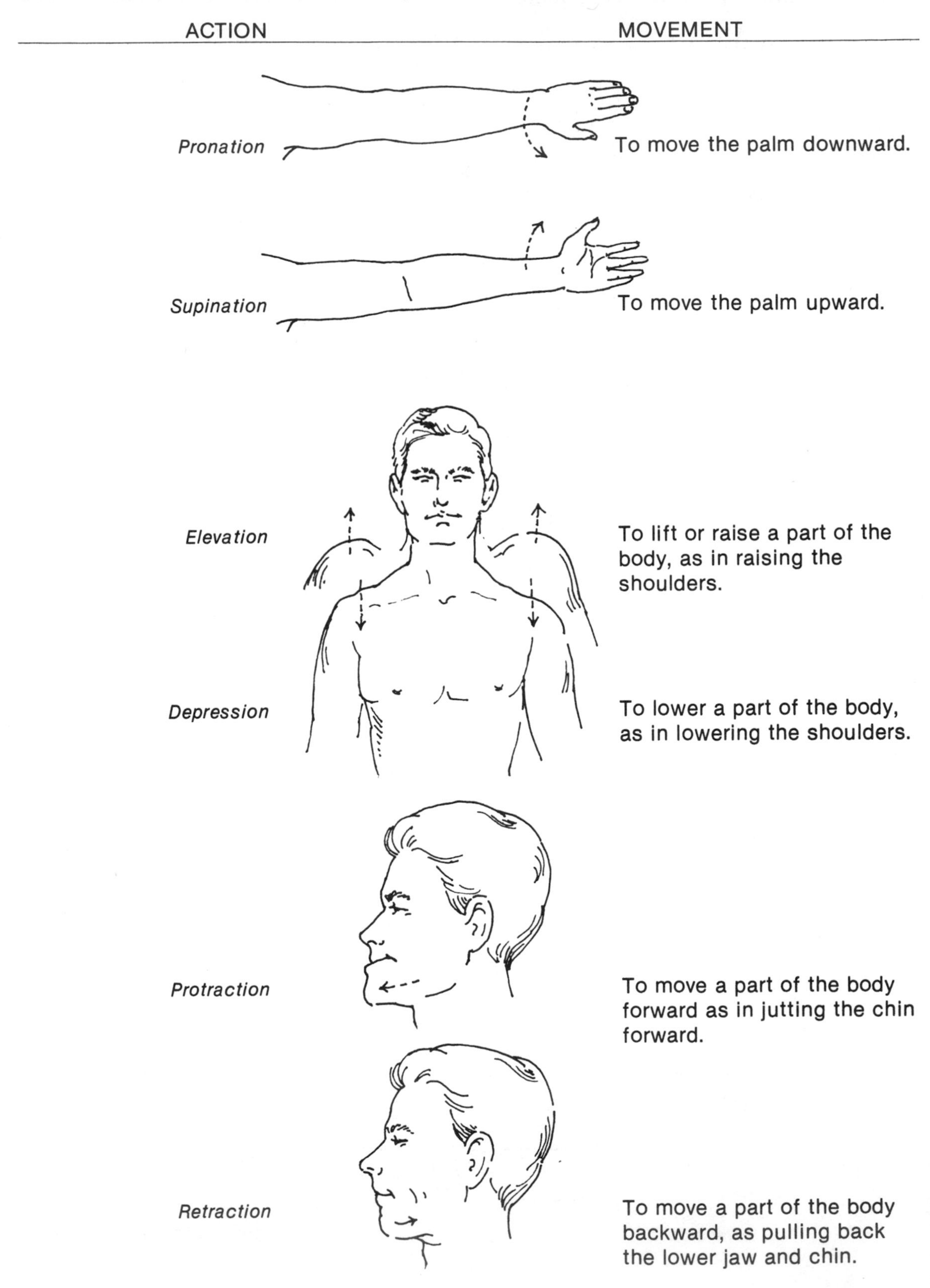

## The Muscular System-Anterior View

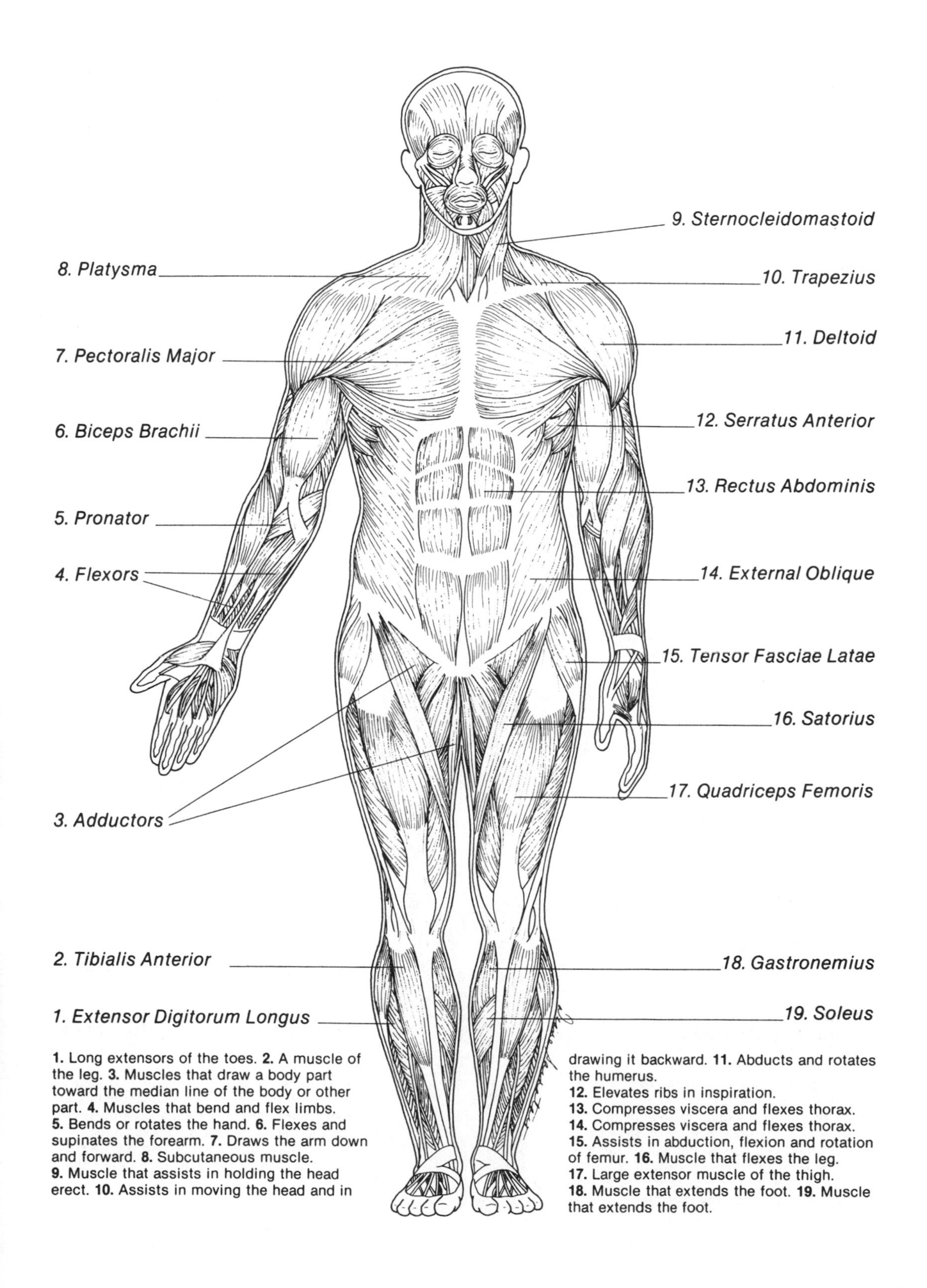


**1.** Long extensors of the toes. **2.** A muscle of the leg. **3.** Muscles that draw a body part toward the median line of the body or other part. **4.** Muscles that bend and flex limbs.
**5.** Bends or rotates the hand. **6.** Flexes and supinates the forearm. **7.** Draws the arm down and forward. **8.** Subcutaneous muscle.
**9.** Muscle that assists in holding the head erect. **10.** Assists in moving the head and in drawing it backward. **11.** Abducts and rotates the humerus.
**12.** Elevates ribs in inspiration.
**13.** Compresses viscera and flexes thorax.
**14.** Compresses viscera and flexes thorax.
**15.** Assists in abduction, flexion and rotation of femur. **16.** Muscle that flexes the leg.
**17.** Large extensor muscle of the thigh.
**18.** Muscle that extends the foot. **19.** Muscle that extends the foot.

## The Muscular System-Posterior View

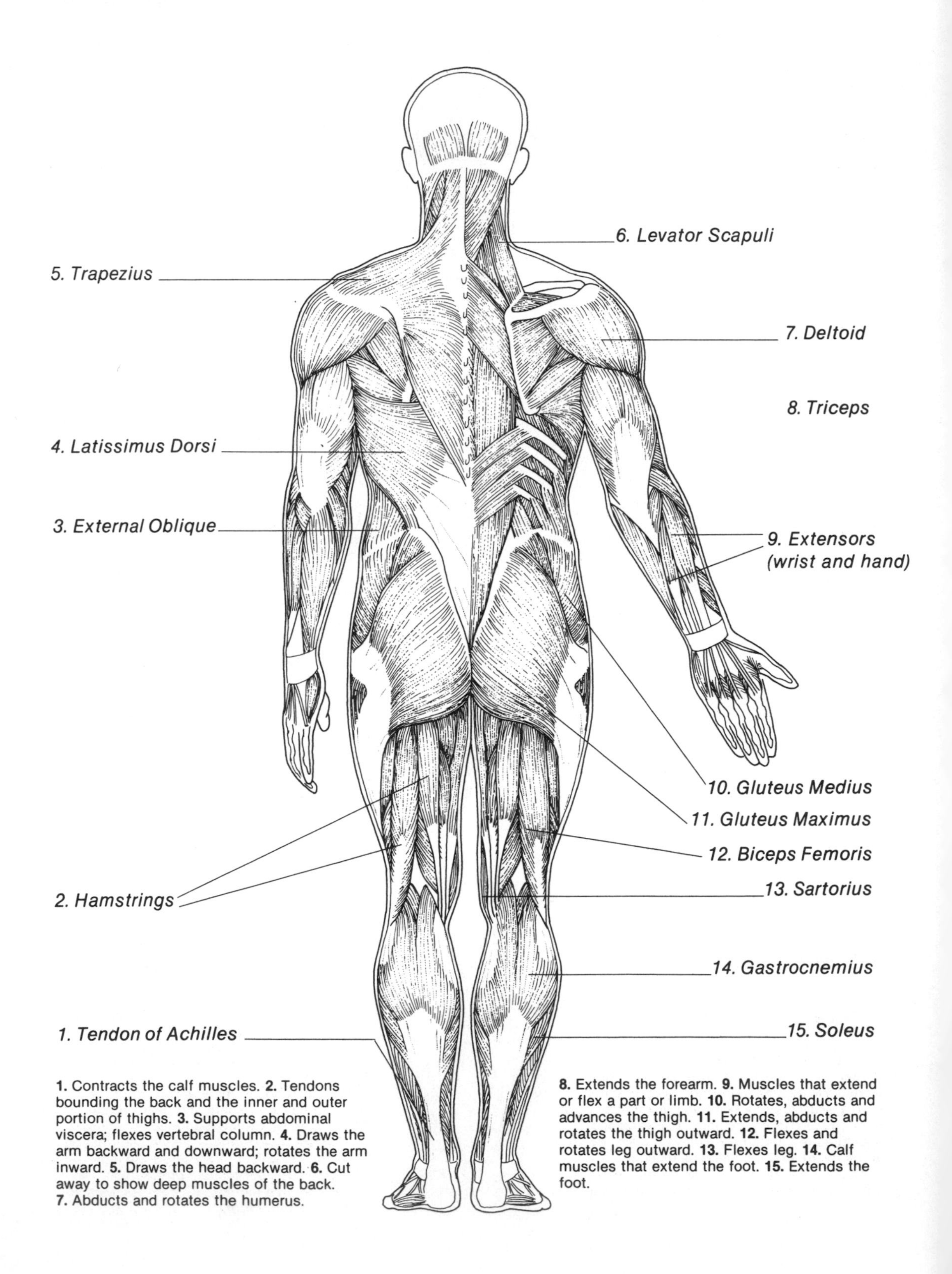


**1.** Contracts the calf muscles. **2.** Tendons bounding the back and the inner and outer portion of thighs. **3.** Supports abdominal viscera; flexes vertebral column. **4.** Draws the arm backward and downward; rotates the arm inward. **5.** Draws the head backward. **6.** Cut away to show deep muscles of the back. **7.** Abducts and rotates the humerus.

**8.** Extends the forearm. **9.** Muscles that extend or flex a part or limb. **10.** Rotates, abducts and advances the thigh. **11.** Extends, abducts and rotates the thigh outward. **12.** Flexes and rotates leg outward. **13.** Flexes leg. **14.** Calf muscles that extend the foot. **15.** Extends the foot.

## Muscles of the Head, Face and Neck

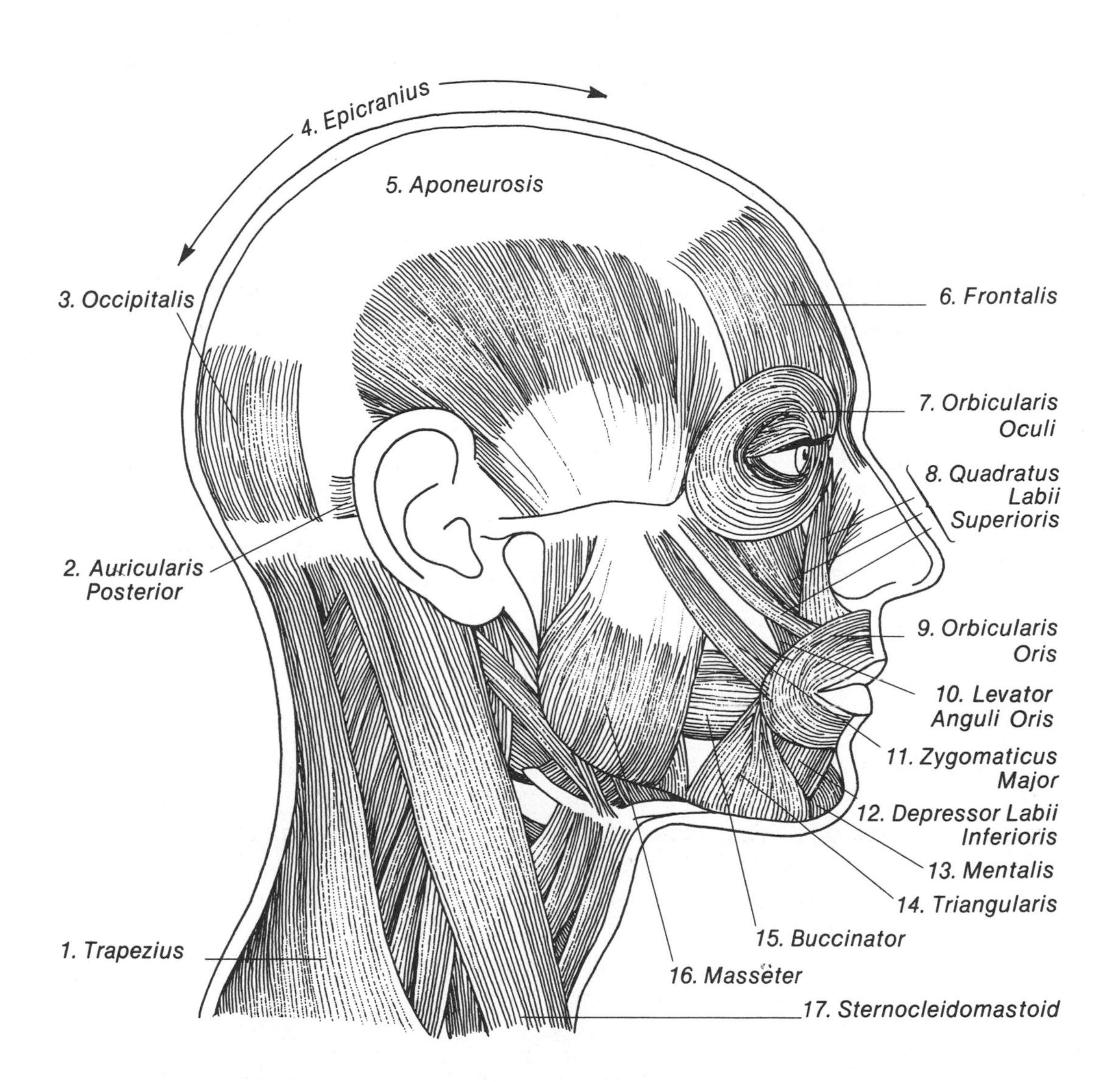


**1.** Allows movement of shoulders. **2.** Moves auricle, the external part of the ear. **3.** Posterior part of the epicranius muscle. **4.** Draws scalp backward. **5.** Fibrous or membranous sheet to which flat muscles are attached at origin of insertion. **6.** Elevates eyebrows and wrinkles skin of forehead. **7.** The ring muscle of the eye. **8.** A muscle of facial expression with insertion in skin of upper lip. **9.** Muscle of expression, especially smile; opens and closes lips; ring muscle of the mouth. **10.** Muscle of facial expression at the angle of the mouth. **11.** Muscle which pulls the mouth upward and back when laughing. **12.** Muscle of facial expression; everts and draws the lower lip downward. **13.** Muscle which raises and protrudes lower lip. **14.** Muscle of facial expression at angle of mouth. **15.** Largest muscle of facial expression; purses the lips. **16.** Muscle which closes the jaw. **17.** Muscle which helps to hold the head erect.

**Muscles of the Head and Face**

| NAME | FUNCTION | NERVE SUPPLY |
|---|---|---|
| Epicranius (occipito-frontalis) | Moves scalp and raises eyebrows. | Posterior auricular, small occipital and facial. |
| Temporalis | Raises lower jaw and presses it against upper jaw. | Inferior maxillary. |
| Masseter | Raises lower jaw and presses it against upper jaw. | Inferior maxillary. |
| Pterygoideus externus (2) internus (2) | Draw lower jaw forward and sideways. | Inferior maxillary. |
| Buccinator | Used in blowing and whistling. | Facial. |
| Zygomaticus | Draws corners of mouth upward and backward. | Facial. |
| Orbicularis oris | Presses lips together and pushes them outward. | Facial. |
| Recti muscles (4) Obliquus superior Obliquus inferior | Rotate eyeball in various directions | Oculomotor, abducent, and trochlear. |
| Levator palpebrae superioris | Opens the eye. | Oculomotor. |
| Orbicularis oculi | Closes the eye. | Facial. |
| Corrugator | Draws eyebrows downward and inward. | Facial. |
| Nasalis | Compresses nostril. | Facial. |
| Quadratus labii superioris | Raises lip and dilates nostril. | Facial. |
| Quadratus labii inferioris | Depresses lower lip. | Facial. |
| Triangularis | Pulls down corners of mouth. | Facial. |
| Risorius | Draws corners of mouth back. | Facial. |
| Auricularis (3) | Raise and move ears. | Facial. |
| Caninus | Raises and draws in angle of mouth. | Facial. |
| Procerus | Draws down inner angle of eyebrows. | Facial. |
| Mentalis | Raises chin and pushes up lower lip. | Facial. |
| Depressor septi | Closes opening of nostrils. | Facial. |
| Dilatator naris posterior and interior | Expand opening of nostrils. | Facial. |

**Muscles of the Neck**

| NAME | FUNCTION | NERVE SUPPLY |
|---|---|---|
| Platysma | Draws down corners of the mouth, and flexes the head. | Facial. |
| Sterno-cleido-mastoideus | Bends head forward and to one side. | Spinal accessory. |
| Digastric | Depresses jaw and raises hyoid bone. | Facial and inferior dental. |
| Stylo-hyoid | Depresses jaw and raises hyoid bone. | Facial. |
| Mylo-hyoid | Depresses jaw and raises hyoid bone. | Inferior dental. |
| Genio-hyoid | Depresses jaw and raises hyoid bone. | Hypoglossal. |
| Omo-hyoid | Depresses and draws back hyoid bone. | Hypoglossal. |
| Scaleni (3) | Bends head sideways and forward. | Cervical. |
| Rectus capitis anterior minor | Rotates and bends head forward. | Suboccipital. |
| Rectus capitis lateralis | Bends the head. | First cervical. |
| Longus colli (3) | Bends and rotates cervical portion of spine. | Lower cervical. |
| Obliquus capitais superior | Draws head backward. | Occipital. |
| Rectus capitis posterior minor | Draws head backward. | Suboccipital. |
| Rectus capitis posterior major | Rotates cranium. | Occipital. |
| Obliquus capitis inferior | Rotates cranium. | Occipital. |

**Muscles of the Chest**

| NAME | FUNCTION | NERVE SUPPLY |
|---|---|---|
| Pectoralis major | Draws arm downward and forward. | External anterior thoracic. |
| Pectoralis minor | Depresses point of shoulder. | Internal anterior thoracic. |
| Serratus anterior | Raises ribs in breathing and draws shoulder blade forward. | Posterior thoracic. |
| Intercostales externi (11)<br>Intercostales interni (11) | Stretch the chest during breathing. | Intercostal. |
| Levatores costarum (12) | Raise ribs in breathing. | Intercostal. |
| Diaphragm | Chief muscle of respiration. | Phrenic. |

**Muscles of the Abdomen**

| NAME | FUNCTION | NERVE SUPPLY |
|---|---|---|
| Obliquus externus abdominis | Compresses abdomen and bends chest. | Intercostal. Ilio-hypogastric. Ilio-inguinal. |
| Obliquus internus abdominis | Compresses abdomen and bends chest. | Intercostal. Ilio-hypogastric. Ilio-inguinal. |
| Transversus abdominis | Compresses abdomen and bends chest. | Intercostal. Ilio-hypogastric. Ilio-inguinal. |
| Rectus abdominis | Compresses abdomen and bends chest. | Intercostal. Ilio-hypogastric. Ilio-inguinal. |
| Quadratus lumborum | Aids in breathing and bends trunk. | Branches of lower dorsal and upper lumbar. |
| Psoas major | Bends thigh on trunk or trunk on thigh. | Second and third lumbar. |

**Muscles of the Back**

| NAME | FUNCTION | NERVE SUPPLY |
|---|---|---|
| Trapezius | Draws head sideward and backward. | Spinal accessory. |
| Latissimus dorsi | Draws arm backward, downward and rotates it inward | Subscapular. |
| Rhomboid | Draws shoulder blade backward and upward. | Fifth cervical. |
| Infra-spinatus | Rotates arm outwardly. | Suprascapular. |
| Supra-spinatus | Aids to raise arm sideward. | Suprascapular |
| Sacrospinalis (7) | Keep spine erect. | Cervical, dorsal, lumbar and sacral. |
| Multifidus | Keeps spine erect and rotates spinal column | Cervical, dorsal, lumbar and sacral. |
| Obliquus externus abdominis | Compresses abdomen and bends chest. | Intercostal. Ilio-hypogastric. Ilio-inguinal. |
| Glutaeus medius | Rotates and bends thigh inwardly. | Superior gluteal. |
| Glutaeus maximus | Extends hip joint. | Inferior gluteal. |

**Muscles of the Arms and Hands**

| NAME | FUNCTION | NERVE SUPPLY |
|---|---|---|
| Deltoid | Bends and extends arm. | Circumflex. |
| Teres minor | Rotates humerus outward. | Circumflex. |
| Teres major | Helps to draw humerus downward and backward | Subscapular. |
| Subscapularis | Rotates humerus inward. | Subscapular. |
| Biceps brachii | Bends forearm and draws palm upward. | Musculo-cutaneous. |
| Brachialis | Bends forearm. | Musculo-cutaneous. |
| Brachioradialis | Bends forearm and draws palm upward. | Musculo-spiral. |
| Extensor carpi radialis longus | Extends hand and bends elbow. | Musculo-spiral. |
| Pronator teres | Turns palm of hand downward. | Median. |
| Flexor digitorum sublimis | Bends fingers, elbow and wrist. | Median. |
| Flexor carpi radialis | Bends hand sideways. | Median. |
| Palmaris longus | Helps to bend hand. | Median. |
| Abductor pollicis | Draws thumb from fingers. | Median. |
| Opponens pollicis | Draws thumb across palm. | Median. |
| Flexor pollicis brevis | Bends and separates thumb. | Median and ulnar. |
| Adductor pollicis | Draws thumb to fingers. | Ulnar. |
| Flexor carpi ulnaris | Bends hand and draws it to ulnar side. | Ulnar. |
| Palmaris brevis | Wrinkles skin of palm. | Ulnar. |
| Abductor digiti quinti | Separates little finger. | Ulnar. |
| Flexor digiti quinti brevis | Bends little finger. | Ulnar. |
| Lumbricales (4) | Assists in quick, short movements of fingers. | Ulnar. |
| Interossel (7) | Separates fingers from each other. | Ulnar. |
| Flexor digitorum profundus | Bends fingers and wrist. | Ulnar and anterior interosseous. |
| Flexor pollicis longus | Bends thumb. | Anterior interosseous. |
| Triceps brachialis | Extends forearm. | Radial. |
| Extensor carpi ulnaris | Extends hand and wrist. | Dorsal interosseous. |
| Extensor carpi radialis brevis | Extends hand and bends elbow. | Dorsal interosseous. |
| Extensor digitorum communis | Extends fingers. | Dorsal interosseous. |
| Extensor indicis propius | Extends index finger. | Dorsal interosseous. |
| Extensor pollicis brevis | Extends thumb. | Dorsal interosseous. |
| Extensor pollicis longus | Extends thumb. | Dorsal interosseous. |

**Muscles of the Legs and Feet**

| NAME | FUNCTION | NERVE SUPPLY |
|---|---|---|
| Rectus femoris<br>Vastus lateralis<br>Vastus medialis | Extends leg. | Anterior crural. |
| Sartorius | Bends thigh and leg, rotates thigh outward and leg inward. | Anterior crural. |
| Pectineus | Bends thigh. | Anterior crural and obturator. |
| Adductor longus | Bends thigh. | Obturator. |
| Gracilis | Bends thigh and leg. | Obturator. |
| Tibialis anterior | Extends foot. | Common peroneal. |
| Extensor digitorum longus | Extends toes. | Anterior tibial. |
| Extensor hallucis longus | Extends big toe. | Anterior tibial. |
| Extensor digitorum brevis | Extends four inner toes. | Anterior tibial. |
| Interossei (7) | Draw toes to and from middle line. | External plantar. |
| Peronaeus longus<br>Peronaeus brevis | Extend foot and raise outer border. | Musculo-cutaneous. |
| Semi-membranosus<br>Semitendinosus<br>Biceps femoris | Bend leg. | Sciatic. |
| Gastrocnemius Soleus | Extend foot. | Tibial. |
| Flexor digitorum<br>Flexor hallucis | Bend toes. | Tibial. |

## Review MUSCLES OF THE HEAD AND FACE

### Matching Test

*Match the following definitions. Insert the proper term in front of each definition.*

| | Definition | Term |
|---|---|---|
| 1. ............... | Move ears. | Orbicularis oculi |
| 2. ............... | Move scalp. | Orbicularis oris |
| 3. ............... | Opens eye. | Auricularis |
| 4. ............... | Presses lips together. | Masseter |
| 5. ............... | Raises lower jaw. | Epicranius |

### True or False Test

*Carefully read each statement and decide if it is True or False by drawing a circle around the letter T or F.*

1. T F Obliquus inferior and superior muscles do not rotate the eyeball.
2. T F Only the temporalis muscle moves the lower jaw.
3. T F The levator palpebrae superioris muscle opens the eye.
4. T F The epicranius is also known as the occipito-frontalis muscle.
5. T F The corrugator muscle controls the movement of the mouth.

### Answers

| Matching Test | True or False Test |
|---|---|
| 1—Auricularis. | 1—F |
| 2—Epicranius. | 2—F |
| 3—Orbicularis oculi. | 3—T |
| 4—Orbicularis oris. | 4—T |
| 5—Masseter. | 5—F |

## Review MUSCLES OF THE NECK AND CHEST

### Matching Test

*Match the following definitions. Insert the proper term in front of each definition.*

| | | |
|---|---|---|
| 1. .............. | Rotates cranium. | Serratus anterior |
| 2. .............. | Draws head backward. | Longus colli |
| 3. .............. | Rotates spine. | Obliquus capitis inferior |
| 4. .............. | Muscle of respiration. | Obliquus capitis superior |
| 5. .............. | Raises ribs in breathing. | Diaphragm |

### True or False Test

*Carefully read each statement and decide if it is True or False by drawing a circle around the letter T or F.*

| | | | |
|---|---|---|---|
| 1. | T | F | Several muscles depress the jaw and raise the hyoid bone. |
| 2. | T | F | The sterno-cleido-mastoideus is the only muscle which bends the head forward and sideways. |
| 3. | T | F | The platysma muscle does not draw down the corners of the mouth. |
| 4. | T | F | The pectoralis major and minor muscles control the movement of the arm and shoulder. |
| 5. | T | F | Several groups of muscles raise the ribs in breathing. |

### Answers

| Matching Test | True or False Test |
|---|---|
| 1—Obliquus capitis inferior. | 1—T |
| 2—Obliquus capitis superior. | 2—F |
| 3—Longus colli. | 3—F |
| 4—Diaphragm. | 4—T |
| 5—Serratus anterior. | 5—T |

## Review MUSCLES OF THE ABDOMEN AND BACK

### Matching Test

*Match the following definitions. Insert the proper term in front of each definition.*

| | | |
|---|---|---|
| 1. .............. | Bends trunk. | Rectus abdominis |
| 2. .............. | Keeps spine erect. | Quadratus lumborum |
| 3. .............. | Draws head backward. | Sacrospinalis |
| 4. .............. | Draws arm backward. | Trapezius |
| 5. .............. | Compresses abdomen. | Latissimus dorsi |

### True or False Test

*Carefully read each statement and decide if it is True or False by drawing a circle around the letter T or F.*

1. T F The obliquus externus abdominis is an external muscle of the abdomen and back.
2. T F Only one muscle compresses the abdomen and bends the chest.
3. T F The infra-spinatus and supra-spinatus muscles control the movement of the arm.
4. T F The glutaeus medius muscle extends the hip joint.
5. T F The spine is kept erect with the aid of the sacrospinalis and multifidus muscles.

### Answers

| Matching Test | True or False Test |
|---|---|
| 1—Quadratus lumborum. | 1—T |
| 2—Sacrospinalis. | 2—F |
| 3—Trapezius. | 3—T |
| 4—Latissimus dorsi. | 4—F |
| 5—Rectus abdominis. | 5—T |

**Review** MUSCLES OF THE ARMS AND HANDS

## Matching Test

*Match the following definitions. Insert the proper term in front of each definition.*

| | | |
|---|---|---|
| 1. .............. | Bends hand. | Brachialis |
| 2. .............. | Bends forearm. | Triceps brachialis |
| 3. .............. | Bends arm. | Interossei |
| 4. .............. | Separates fingers. | Deltoid |
| 5. .............. | Extends forearm. | Palmaris longus |

## True or False Test

*Carefully read each statement and decide if it is True or False by drawing a circle around the letter T or F.*

| | | | |
|---|---|---|---|
| 1. | T | F | The movement of the thumb is controll-ed by one muscle. |
| 2. | T | F | The biceps brachii muscle draws the palm downward. |
| 3. | T | F | The brachioradialis muscle draws the palm upward. |
| 4. | T | F | Quick, short movements of the fingers are produced by the lumbricales muscles. |
| 5. | T | F | The subscapularis muscle rotates the humerus inward. |

## Answers

| Matching Test | True or False Test |
|---|---|
| 1—Palmarus longus. | 1—F |
| 2—Brachialis. | 2—F |
| 3—Deltoid. | 3—T |
| 4—Interossei. | 4—T |
| 5—Triceps brachialis. | 5—T |

**Review** MUSCLES OF THE LEGS AND FEET

### Matching Test

*Match the following definitions. Insert the proper term in front of each definition.*

| | | |
|---|---|---|
| 1. . . . . . . . . . . . . . . | Bends leg. | Flexor digitorum |
| 2. . . . . . . . . . . . . . . | Extends leg. | Biceps femoris |
| 3. . . . . . . . . . . . . . . | Bends thigh. | Rectus femoris |
| 4. . . . . . . . . . . . . . . | Extends foot. | Pectineus |
| 5. . . . . . . . . . . . . . . | Bends toes. | Soleus |

### True or False Test

*Carefully read each statement and decide if it is True or False by drawing a circle around the letter T or F.*

1. T F The sartorius muscle bends the thigh and leg.
2. T F The movement of the big toe is controlled by the extensor hallucis longus muscle.
3. T F The extensor digitorum brevis muscle does not extend the four inner toes.
4. T F The soleus and gastrocnemius muscles both extend the foot.
5. T F The gracilis adducts femur and flexes knee joint.

### Answers

| Matching Test | True or False Test |
|---|---|
| 1—Biceps femoris. | 1—T |
| 2—Rectus femoris. | 2—T |
| 3—Pectineus. | 3—F |
| 4—Soleus. | 4—T |
| 5—Flexor digitorum. | 5—F |

## QUESTIONS FOR DISCUSSION AND REVIEW

1. What is the structure and function of muscles?
2. To which structures are muscles attached?
3. What are skeletal muscles?
4. What is the origin of a muscle? Give an example.
5. What is the insertion of a muscle? Give an example.
6. Which structure attaches the muscle to the bone?
7. What is fascia?
8. Name three types of muscular tissue.
9. What is the difference between voluntary and involuntary muscles?

10. Which characteristics enable muscles to produce movements?
11. When does a muscle have tone?
12. When does a muscle lack tone?
13. Why is it important for the massage practitioner to understand how muscles contract and relax?
14. What is meant by extensibility of muscle?
15. When flexing the elbow would the triceps become the prime mover or the antagonist?
16. Do diarthrotic joints remain motionless or are they capable of free movement?
17. What joints have limited motion?
18. Are synarthrotic joints movable or immovable?

## ANSWERS TO QUESTIONS FOR DISCUSSION AND REVIEW

1. Muscles are contractile fibrous tissue that produce various movements of the body.
2. Muscles are attached to bones, cartilage, ligaments, tendons, skin, and sometimes to each other.
3. Skeletal muscles are striated muscles attached to the bones of the skeleton.
4. Origin of a muscle refers to the more fixed attachments, such as muscles attached to bones that act as anchors for movements.
5. Insertion of a muscle refers to the more movable attachments, such as muscles attached to skin, or movable muscles or the more distal and movable attachment.
6. Tendon or sinew attaches muscles to the bone.
7. Fascia is a delicate membrane of connective tissue covering muscles and separating their several layers or groups of layers.
8. Voluntary (striated) muscle; involuntary (nonstriated) muscle; heart (cardiac) muscle.
9. Voluntary muscles are controlled by the will; involuntary muscles are not controlled by the will.
10. Irritability, contractility, and elasticity.
11. A muscle has tone if it is firm and responds readily to stimulation.
12. A muscle lacks tone if it is flabby.
13. The massage practitioner is concerned with helping the client to relax tense muscles.
14. Extensibility is the ability of a muscle to stretch.
15. When flexing the elbow the triceps become the antagonist.
16. Diarthrotic joints are freely movable.
17. Amphiarthrotic joints have limited motion.
18. Synarthrotic joints, as in the skull, are immovable.

## SYSTEM FOUR THE NERVOUS SYTEM

The nervous system is one of the most important systems of the body because it controls and coordinates the functions of other systems so that they work harmoniously and efficiently.

The nervous system is comprised of the brain, spinal cord, cranial nerves, and spinal nerves.

The functions of the nervous system are:

1. To rule the body by controlling all visible and invisible activities.
2. To control human thought and conduct.
3. To govern all internal and external movements of the body.
4. To give the power to see, hear, move, talk, feel, think, and remember.

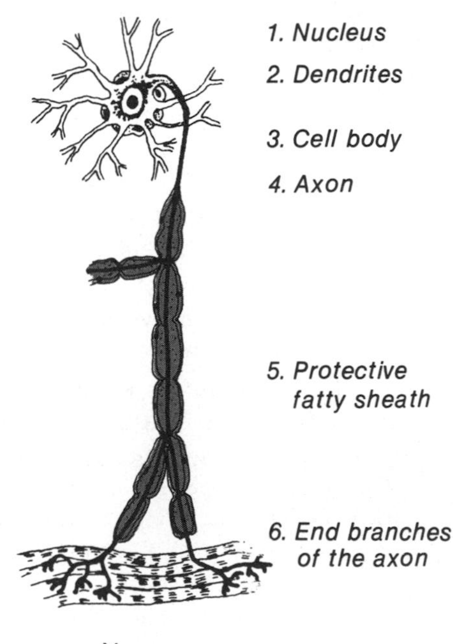


Neuron

1. *Nucleus:* Nerve cells.
2. *Dendrites:* The branched part of a nerve cell that carries impulses toward the cell body.
3. *Cell body:* A nerve cell.
4. *Axon:* The central core that forms the essential conducting part of a nerve fiber.
5. *Protective fatty sheath:* A thin covering of fat.
6. The branched end of the axon.

A *neuron* is the structural unit of the nervous system. It is comprised of a *nerve cell* (cell body) and its outgrowth of long and short fibers, called *cell processes.* The nerve cell stores energy and nutrients for the cell processes that convey the nerve impulses throughout the body. Practically all the nerve cells are contained in the brain and spinal cord.

Nerves are long white cords consisting of fibers (cell processes) from nerve cells. They have their origin in the brain and spinal cord and distribute branches to all parts of the body.

Nerves furnish both sensation and motion. *Sensory nerves,* termed *afferent nerves,* carry impulses or messages from sense organs to the brain where sensations of touch, cold, heat, sight, hearing, taste, and pain are experienced.

*Motor nerves,* termed *efferent nerves,* carry impulses from the brain to the muscles, where the transmitted impulses cause movement.

The nervous system is divided into two main divisions: the cerebrospinal nervous system and the autonomic nervous system.

**Cerebrospinal Nervous System**

The *cerebrospinal nervous system,* which consists of the brain and spinal cord as well as the spinal nerves, the peripheral nerves, and cranial nerves, controls speech, taste, sight, touch, and smell. It likewise governs the voluntary muscles. Comprising this large system are the central peripheral system that supply nerves throughout the body.

The central nervous system consists of the *brain* and *spinal cord.* The brain, the principal nerve center, is the body's largest and most complex nerve tissue. It controls sensations, voluntary muscles, and the power to think and feel. The central nervous system comprises:

1. The cerebrum, the large frontal of the brain, which presides over such mental activities as memory, reasoning, will, and emotions.
2. The cerebellum, the smaller, lower part of the brain which keeps the body balanced, coordinates voluntary muscles, and makes muscular movement smooth and graceful.
3. The medulla oblongata, which connects the brain with the spinal cord and regulates movements of the heart as well as the organs of digestion and respiration.
4. Twelve pairs of cranial nerves, originating in the brain, which serve various parts of the head, face, and neck.

The peripheral system consists of peripheral nerves that connect the central nervous system to the rest of the body parts and is located in the skin, muscles, and sense organs. Peripheral nerves send sensory impulses to the brain and spinal cord and transmit motor impulses from the brain to the muscles.

***Cranial Nerves***

There are 12 pairs of cranial nerves, all connected to some part of the brain surface and pass through openings on the sides and base of the cranium. They are classified as *motor, sensory,* and *motor-sensory* nerves, which contain both motor and sensory fibers.

The cranial nerves are named numerically according to the order in which they arise from the brain, and also by names that describe their type, function, or location.

**Nerves of the Head, Face and Neck**

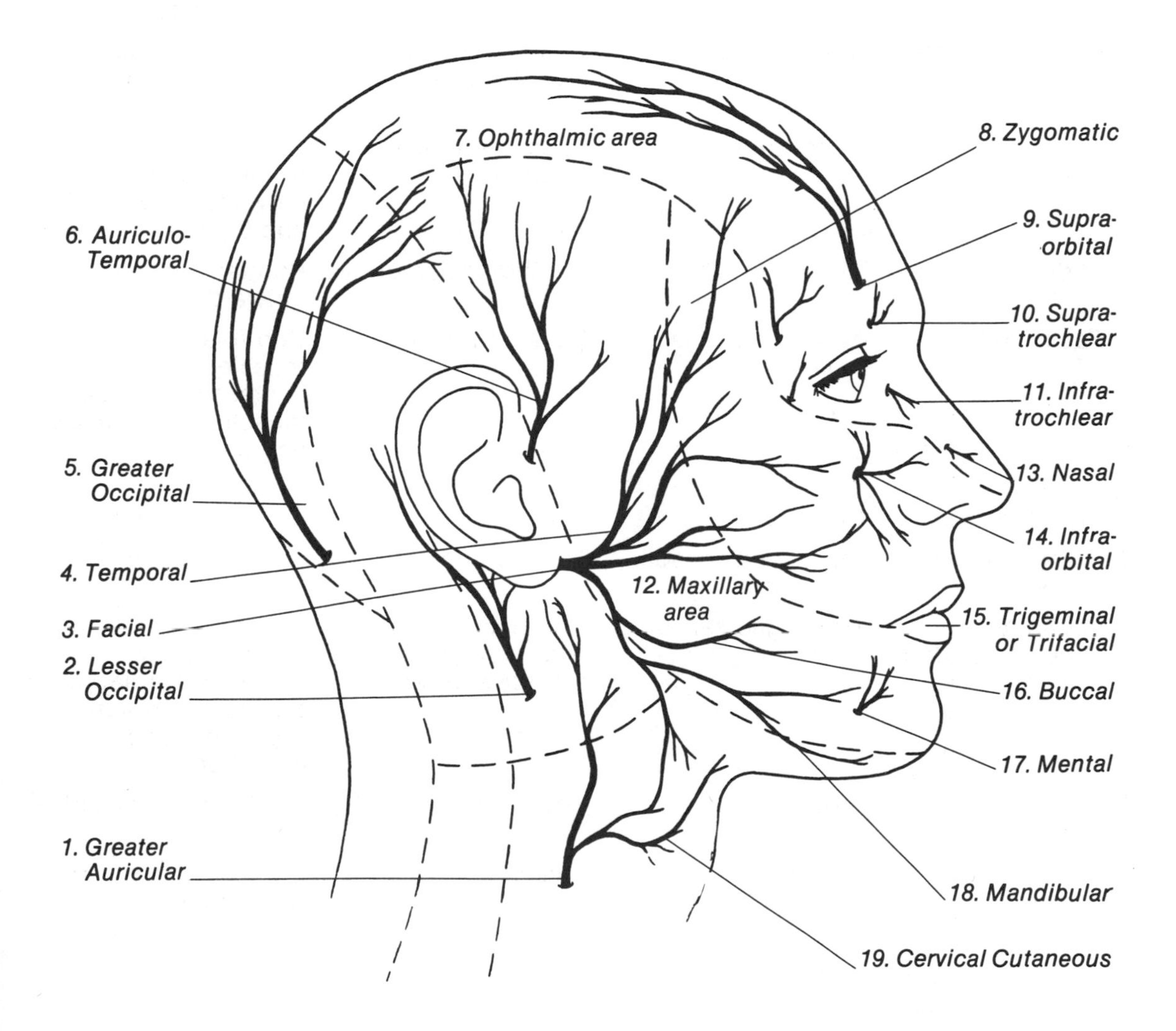


**1.** Nerves of the side of the neck and ear. **2.** Nerves of skin behind the ear and back of scalp. **3.** Nerves of muscles of expression. **4.** Nerves of the temporal muscle. **5.** Nerves of skin over back part of the head. **6.** Nerves of the side of the scalp. **7.** Nerves of tear glands, eye membrane, skin of forehead and nose. **8.** Zygomatic sensory nerve, a branch of the maxillary nerve which innervates the skin in the temple area, side of forehead and upper part of cheek. **9.** Nerves of the skin of the forehead. **10.** Nerves of the skin of upper eyelids and root of the nose. **11.** Nerves of skin of lower eyelids and sides of nose. **12.** Nerves of the nasal pharynx, teeth of the upper jaw and skin of the cheek. **13.** Nerves of skin and mucous membrane of the nose. **14.** Nerves of the skin of the cheek and lower eyelid. **15.** Nerves of skin of face, tongue, teeth and muscles of mastication. **16.** Nerves of buccinator and orbicularis oris. **17.** Nerves of lower lip and chin. **18.** Nerves of teeth and lower jaws and cheek area. **19.** Nerves which supply the skin of the jaw back of ear, lateral and anterior sides of neck and skin of upper anterior thorax.

**Classification of Cranial Nerves**

| CRANIAL NERVES | TYPE OF NERVE | LOCATION | FUNCTION |
|---|---|---|---|
| 1. Olfactory nerve. | Sensory nerve. | Nose. | Sense of smell. |
| 2. Optic nerve. | Sensory nerve. | Retina of eye. | Sense of sight. |
| 3. Oculomotor nerve. | Motor nerve. | Muscles of eye. | Controls eye movements. |
| 4. Trochlear nerve. | Motor nerve. | Obliquus superioris muscle of eye. | Rotates eyeball downward and outward. |
| 5. Trigeminal or trifacial nerve. | Motor and sensory nerve. | Face, teeth, and tongue. | Controls sensations of the face and movements of the jaw and tongue. |
| 6. Abducent nerve. | Motor nerve. | Recti muscles of eye. | Rotates eyeball outward. |
| 7. Facial nerve. | Motor and sensory nerve. | Face and neck. | Controls facial muscles of expression and some muscles of the neck and ear. |
| 8. Acoustic or auditory nerve. | Sensory nerve. | Ear. | Sense of hearing. |
| 9. Glossopharyngeal nerve. | Motor and sensory nerve. | Tongue and pharynx. | Sense of taste. |
| 10. Vagus or pneumogastric nerve. | Motor and sensory nerve. | Pharynx, larynx, heart, lungs, and digestive organs. | Controls sensations and muscular movements relating to talking, heart action, breathing, and digestion. |
| 11. Spinal accessory nerve. | Motor nerve. | Shoulder. | Controls movement of neck muscles |
| 12. Hypoglossal nerve. | Motor nerve. | Tongue and neck. | Controls movement of the tongue. |

**The Nervous System:**
**The Brain, Spinal Cord and Main Nerves of the Body**

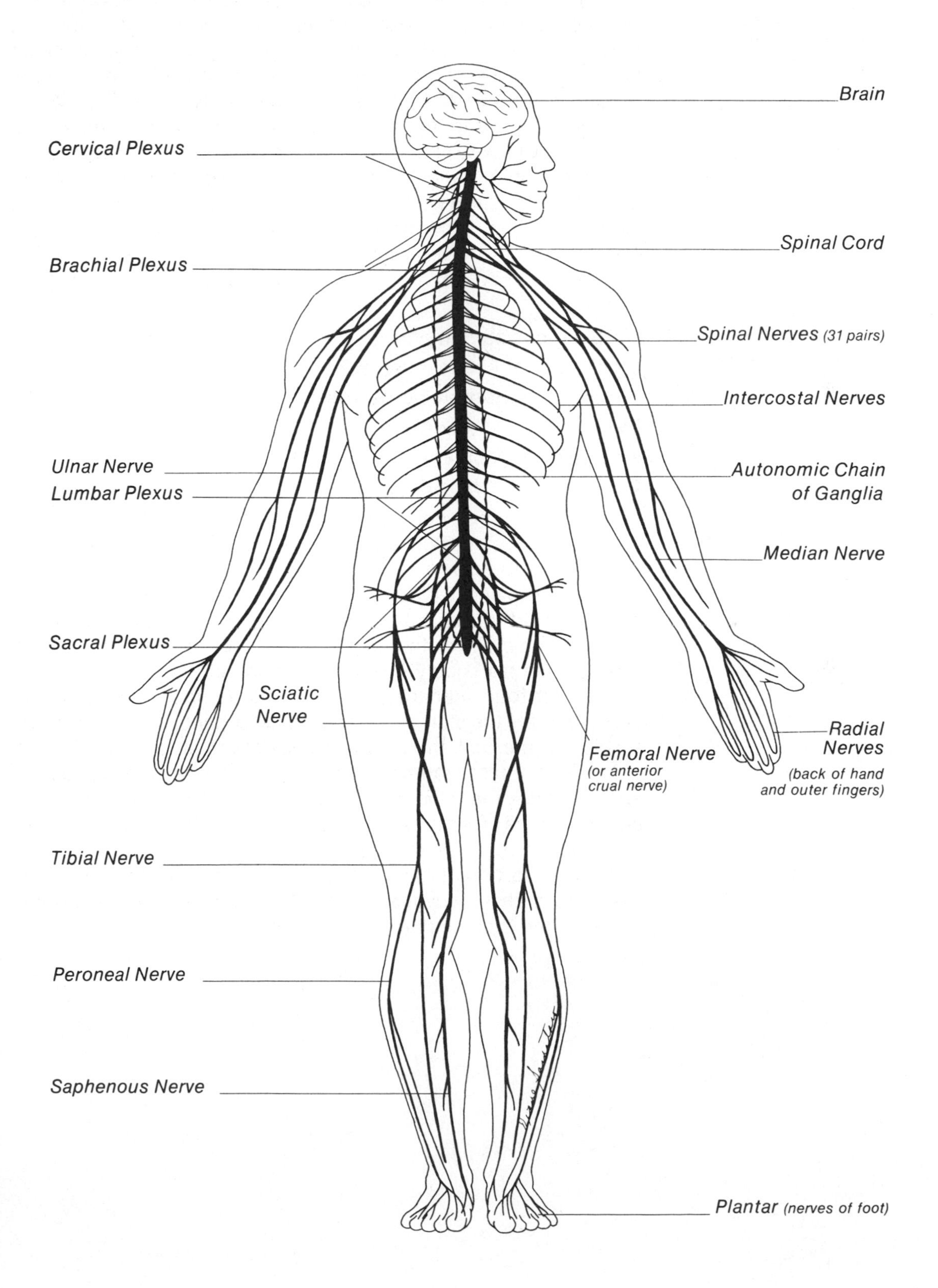

### *The Sympathetic Nervous System*

The *sympathetic nervous system* consists of a double chain of small *ganglia* (masses of neurons), extending along the spinal column from the base of the brain to the coccyx. These ganglia are connected with each other by nerves and with the cerebrospinal system by fibers. The sympathetic nervous system supplies the glands, involuntary muscles of internal organs, and walls of blood vessels with nerves.

Important sympathetic nerves are the *splanchnics* and *vasomotor nerves.* The cervical splanchnics control the circulation of the heart, lungs, and stomach. A second group of splanchnics controls the vascular area of the intestines; while a third set of splanchnics controls blood circulation to the sex glands. The vasomotor nerves regulate the supply of blood to various parts of the body by causing the arterial walls to contract or dilate.

### Classification of Spinal Nerves

Spinal nerves number:

Eight pairs of cervical nerves.

Twelve pairs of thoracic nerves.

Five pairs of lumbar nerves.

Five pairs of sacral nerves.

One pair of coccygeal nerves.

The four upper cervical nerves form the *cervical plexus,* which supplies the skin and controls the movement of the head, neck, and shoulders.

The four lower cervical nerves and the first pair of thoracic nerves form the *brachial plexus,* which controls the movement of the arm by way of the median and ulnar nerves. The next 11 thoracic nerves supply the organs in the chest.

The first four lumbar nerves form the *lumbar plexus,* whose nerves supply the skin of the abdominal organs, hip, thigh, knee, and leg. The crural and sciatic nerves reach all parts of the leg.

The fifth or last lumbar nerves, the first sacral nerves, second sacral nerves, the third sacral nerves, and a portion of the fourth sacral nerves form the *sacral plexus,* which controls the movements of the flexor muscles of the leg.

Another portion of the fourth sacral nerves and the fifth sacral nerves form the *coccygeal plexus.* The coccygeal nerves supply the skin and muscles around the coccyx.

**The Autonomic Nervous System**

*Autonomic* means self-governing. The *autonomic nervous system* regulates action of glands, smooth muscles, and the heart. The motor neurons of the autonomic nervous system originate in the central system. Its divisions are:

1. The *sympathetic nervous system,* which originates in the thoracolumbar (thoracic and lumbar portions of the spine).
2. The *parasympathetic nervous system,* which balances action of the sympathetic system. The sympathetic division mainly expands energy. Stimulation can bring about rapid responses, such as increased respiration, dilated pupils, and increased heart rate and cardiac output. Muscles dilate, the skin constricts, and the liver increases conversion of glycogen to glucose for more energy. There is increased mental activity and production of adrenal hormones. All these activities prepare us to meet emergencies. The general function of the parasympathetic division is to calm and to conserve energy and to reverse action of the sympathetic division.

**Reflex Action**

*Reflex action,* the simplest form of nervous activity, is an involuntary response to a stimulus. A simple reflex, such as a knee jerk, involves at least two neurons (sensory and motor) that pass into and out of the spinal cord without influencing any other nerve centers. The more complex reflexes resulting from massage may affect parts of the body distant from the point of stimulation.

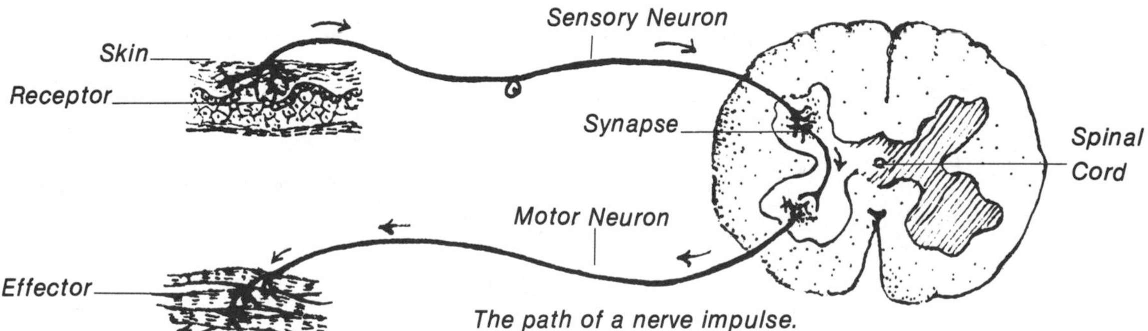

*The path of a nerve impulse.*

The areas of the body that are particularly sensitive to reflex influences are:

1. The skin of the back between the shoulders.
2. The side of the chest between the fourth and sixth ribs.
3. The skin at the upper and inner portion of the thigh.
4. The skin overlying the gluteal muscles.
5. The sole of the foot.

***Motor Points***

Motor points are sensitive spots that readily respond to stimulation. Every muscle and nerve has a motor point. Proper stimulation of muscles, whether by massage or electrical apparatus, can be obtained by contracting each nerve at its motor point. The contraction of healthy muscles can be obtained not only by direct stimulation through their motor points but also indirectly through stimulation of their nerve trunks.

## Motor Nerve Points of the Face and Neck

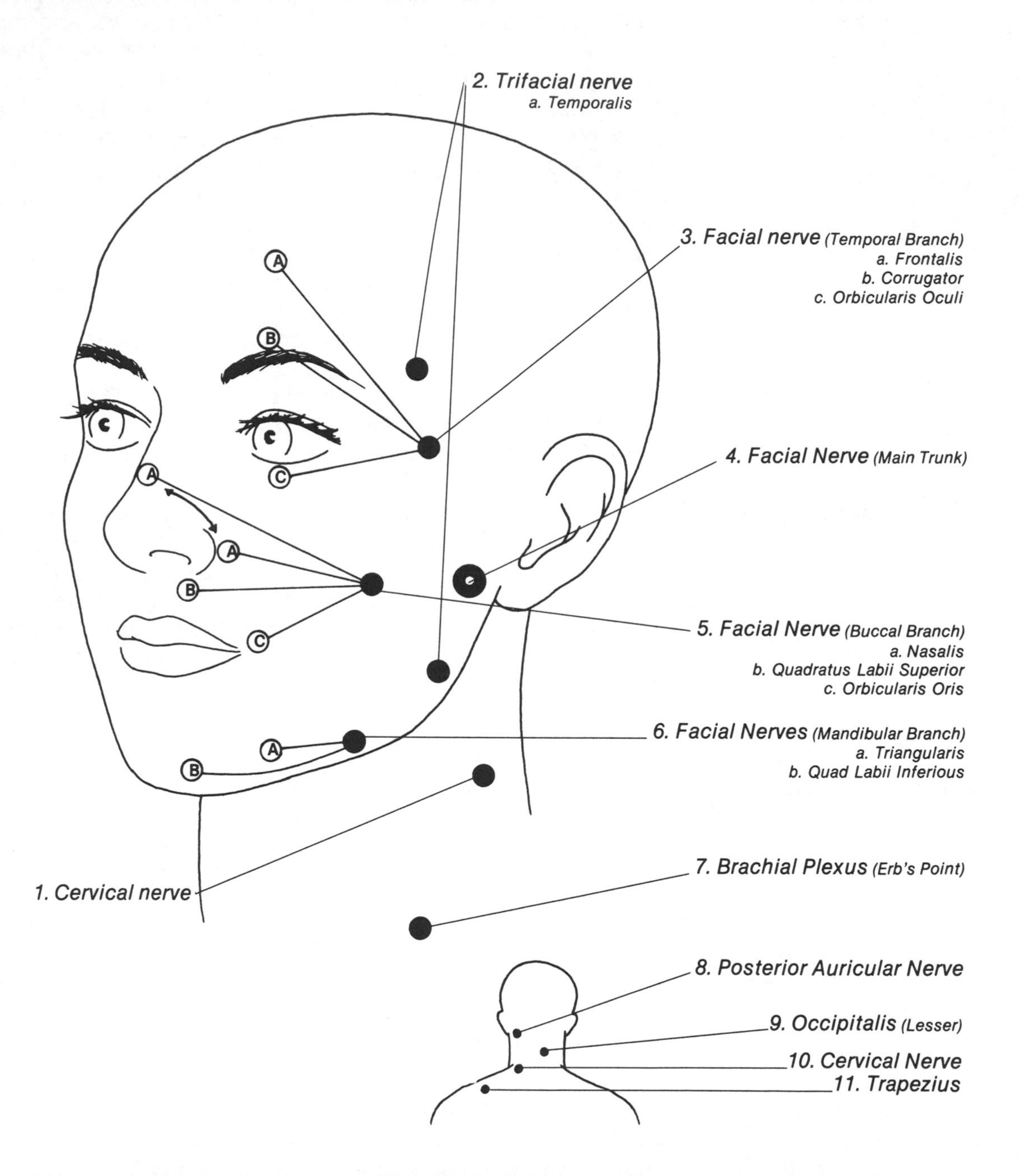


**1.** Nerve serving the skin of jaw, back of ear, lateral and posterior sides of the neck, and skin of upper anterior thorax. **2.** Nerves of skin of face, tongue, teeth and muscles of mastication. **2a.** Nerves of the temporal muscle. **3a.** Nerve serving skin of forehead. **3b.** Nerve serving the muscle that draws eyebrows downward and inward. **3c.** Nerves of muscle surrounding the orbit. **4.** Controls facial muscles of expression. **5a.** Serves skin and mucous membrane of the nose. **5b.** Nerves that raise lip and dilate nostrils. **5c.** Muscles ringing the mouth that function in pursing of the lips. **6a.** Nerves serving the triangularis muscle. **6b.** Nerves of the lower lip. **7.** Nerves located in the neck and axilla. **8.** Nerve of epicranius and auricular muscle. **9.** Nerve of skin behind the ear and on back of scalp. **10.** Nerve serving the skin of back of neck. **11.** Nerve serving the trapezius muscles that draw the head sideward and backward.

**Nerves of the Head and Face**

| NAME | FUNCTION | DISTRIBUTION |
|---|---|---|
| Auriculo-temporal | Sensation. | Side of scalp. |
| Auditory | Sensory nerve of hearing. | Ear. |
| Abducent | Motion. | Obliquus externus muscle of eye. |
| Trochlear | Motion. | Obliquus superior muscle of eye. |
| Auricular, anterior | Sensation. | Skin of external ear. |
| Auricular, great | Sensation. | Side of neck and ear. |
| Auricular, inferior | Sensation. | Ear lobe. |
| Auricular, posterior | Motion | Epicranius and auricularis posterior muscle. |
| Buccal | Motion. | Buccinator and orbicularis oris muscles. |
| Dental, inferior | Sensation-Motion. | Teeth of lower jaw and skin of chin. |
| Facial | Sensation-Motion. | Muscles of expression. |
| Frontal | Sensation. | Skin of forehead. |
| Glossopharyngeal | Sensation-Motion. | Muscles and mucous membranes of pharynx and back of tongue. |
| Infra-orbital | Sensation. | Skin of cheek and lower eyelid. |
| Infra-trochlear | Sensation. | Skin of lower eyelid and side of nose. |
| Mandibular | Sensation-Motion. | Teeth and skin of lower jaw and cheeks. |
| Masseteric | Motion. | Masseter muscle. |
| Maxillary | Sensation. | Nasal pharynx, teeth of upper jaw and skin of cheek. |
| Mental | Sensation. | Skin of lower lip and chin. |
| Nasal | Sensation. | Skin and mucous membrane of nose. |
| Occipital, greater | Sensation-Motor | Skin over back part of head. |
| Occipital, lesser | Sensation. | Skin behind ear and on back of scalp. |
| Oculomotor | Motion. | Levator palpebrae superioris, recti muscles and obliquus inferior muscle of eye. |
| Olfactory | Sensory nerve of smell. | Nose. |
| Ophthalmic | Sensation. | Tear glands, eye membrane, skin of forehead and nose. |
| Optic nerve | Sensory nerve of sight. | Retina of eye. |
| Orbital | Sensation. | Skin of temple. |
| Supra-orbital | Sensation. | Skin of forehead. |
| Pterygoid, external | Motion. | External pterygoid muscle. |
| Pterygoid, internal | Motion. | Internal pterygoid muscle. |
| Trigeminal or trifacial | Sensation-Motion. | Skin of face, tongue, teeth and muscles of mastication. |
| Supratrochlear | Sensation. | Skin of upper eyelid and root of nose. |
| Pneumogastric | Sensation-Motion. | Pharynx. |
| Temporal | Motion. | Temporal muscle. |

### Nerves of the Neck

| NAME | FUNCTION | DISTRIBUTION |
|---|---|---|
| Auricular, great | Sensation. | Skin of neck. |
| Colli, superficial | Sensation. | Skin of neck and throat. |
| Dental, inferior | Sensation-Motion. | Mylo-hyoid muscle. |
| Digastric | Motion. | Stylo-hyoid and posterior portion of digastric muscle. |
| Hypoglossal | Motion. | Genio-hyoid and omo-hyoid muscles. |
| Mylo-hyoid | Motion. | Mylo-hyoid and anterior part of digastric muscle. |
| Spinal accessory | Motion. | Neck muscles. |
| Stylo-hyoid | Motion. | Stylo-hyoid and posterior part of digastric muscle. |
| Suboccipital | Motion. | Muscles of back and neck. |
| Cervical, superficial | Sensation. | Skin of front of neck. |
| Occipital, greater | Sensation-Motion. | Muscles of back of neck. |
| Pneumogastric | Sensation-Motion. | Larynx or voice-box. |

### Nerves of the Chest

| NAME | FUNCTION | DISTRIBUTION |
|---|---|---|
| Pneumogastric | Sensation-Motion. | Heart and lungs. |
| Phrenic | Motion. | Diaphragm. |
| Suprasternal | Sensation. | Skin over top of breast bone. |
| Thoracic, external anterior | Motion. | Pectoralis major. |
| Thoracic, internal anterior | Motion. | Pectoralis major and minor. |
| Thoracic, external posterior | Motion. | Serratus anterior. |
| Thoracic, spinal | Sensation-Motion. | Muscles and skin of chest. |
| Cervical (8) | Sensation-Motion. | Trunk and upper extremities. |
| Dorsal (12) | Sensation-Motion. | Muscles and skin of chest and trunk. |

### Nerves of the Abdomen

| NAME | FUNCTION | DISTRIBUTION |
|---|---|---|
| Hypogastric | Sensation-Motion. | Muscles and skin of abdominal wall. |
| Ilio-hypogastric | Sensation-Motion. | Muscles and skin of lower abdomen. |
| Ilio-inguinal | Sensation-Motion. | Obliquus internus abdominis muscle and skin of groin. |
| Intercostal | Sensation-Motion. | Muscles and skin of upper abdomen. |
| Lumbar (5) | Sensation-Motion. | Front of lower abdomen. |
| Pneumogastric | Sensation-Motion. | Stomach. |

**Nerves of the Back**

| NAME | FUNCTION | DISTRIBUTION |
|---|---|---|
| Coccygeal | Sensation-Motion. | Coccygeus muscle and skin over coccyx of spine. |
| Gluteal, inferior | Motion. | Glutaeus maximus muscle. |
| Gluteal, superior | Motion. | Glutaeus medius muscle. |
| Intercostal | Sensation-Motion. | Muscles and skin of back. |
| Subscapular | Motion. | Latissimus dorsi muscle. |
| Suprascapular | Motion. | Supra-spinatus and infra-spinatus muscles. |
| Spinal accessory | Motion. | Trapezius muscle. |
| Supraacromial | Sensation. | Skin over shoulder. |
| Iliac | Sensation. | Skin of gluteal region. |
| Sacral (5) | Sensation-Motion. | Multifidus muscles of spine and gluteal region. |

**Nerves of the Arms and Hands**

| NAME | FUNCTION | DISTRIBUTION |
|---|---|---|
| Cervical (8) | Sensation-Motion. | Upper extremities. |
| Circumflex | Sensation-Motion. | Deltoid, teres minor, shoulder joint and overlying skin. |
| Cutaneous, internal | Sensation. | Skin of inner part of forearm. |
| Interosseous, anterior | Motion. | Deep flexor and pronator muscles of forearm. |
| Interosseous, posterior | Sensation-Motion. | Muscles and skin of back of forearm and wrist. |
| Median | Sensation-Motion. | Pronator and flexor muscles of forearm, external lumbricales, and skin of fingers. |
| Musculo-cutaneous | Sensation-motion. | Flexors of upper arm and skin of external part of forearm. |
| Musculo-spiral | Sensation-Motion. | Extensor muscles of entire arm and hand, and skin of back of forearm. |
| Radial | Sensation. | Back of hand and outer fingers. |
| Subscapular | Motion. | Teres major and subscapularis muscles. |
| Ulnar | Sensation-Motion. | Flexor carpi ulnaris and flexor digitorum profundus muscles, elbow and wrist joints and skin of fingers. |

**Nerves of the Legs and Feet**

| NAME | FUNCTION | DISTRIBUTION |
|---|---|---|
| Crural | Sensation. | Skin of upper thigh. |
| Musculo-cutaneous of leg | Sensation-Motion. | Peroneal muscles and skin of external part of lower leg and foot. |
| Obturator | Sensation-Motion. | Adductor muscles of thigh, hip and knee joints, and skin of inner portion of thigh. |
| Pectineal | Motion. | Pectineus muscle. |
| Popliteal, external Peroneal, common | Sensation-Motion. | Extensor muscles of lower leg and foot and overlying skin. |
| Popliteal, internal | Sensation-Motion. | Flexor muscles of lower leg and foot and overlying skin. |
| Sacral | Sensation-Motion. | Muscles and skin of lower extremities. |
| Saphenous, external | Sensation. | Skin of foot and toe. |
| Saphenous, internal | Sensation. | Skin of inner part of knee, leg, ankle, and dorsum of foot. |
| Sciatic, great | Sensation-Motion. | Flexor muscles of thigh, leg, foot, and skin of calf and sole. |
| Sciatic, small | Sensation. | Skin of back of thigh. |
| Tibial, anterior Peroneal, deep | Sensation-Motion. | Extensor muscles of foot and toes and skin of dorsum of foot. |
| Tibial, posterior | Sensation-Motion. | Flexor muscles of foot and toes, and skin of sole. |
| Cutaneous, dorsal | Sensation. | Top of foot. |
| Plantar | Sensation-Motion. | Sole of foot, deep muscles of foot and toes. |

**Review** NERVES OF THE HEAD AND FACE

**Matching Test**

*Match the following definitions. Insert the proper term in front of each definition.*

| | | |
|---|---|---|
| 1. ............... | Sense of hearing. | Facial nerve |
| 2. ............... | Sense of smell. | Trifacial nerve |
| 3. ............... | Sense of sight. | Auditory nerve |
| 4. ............... | Supplies skin of face. | Olfactory nerve |
| 5. ............... | Supplies muscles of expression. | Optic Nerve |

**True or False Test**

*Carefully read each statement and decide if it is True or False by drawing a circle around the letter T or F.*

| | | | |
|---|---|---|---|
| 1. | T | F | The great auricular nerve supplies the epicranius muscle. |
| 2. | T | F | The frontal and supra-orbital nerves supply the skin of the forehead. |
| 3. | T | F | The abducent nerve supplies the obliquus superior muscle of the eye. |
| 4. | T | F | The trigeminal nerve supplies the muscles of mastication. |
| 5. | T | F | The auriculo-temporal nerve supplies the side of the scalp. |

**Answers**

| Matching Test | True or False Test |
|---|---|
| 1—Auditory nerve. | 1—F |
| 2—Olfactory nerve. | 2—T |
| 3—Optic nerve. | 3—F |
| 4—Trifacial nerve. | 4—T |
| 5—Facial nerve. | 5—T |

## Review NERVES OF THE NECK AND CHEST

### Matching Test

*Match the following definitions. Insert the proper term in front of each definition.*

| | | |
|---|---|---|
| 1. .............. | Supplies neck muscles. | Greater occipital nerve |
| 2. .............. | Supplies front of neck. | Phrenic nerve |
| 3. .............. | Supplies back of neck. | Pneumogastric nerve |
| 4. .............. | Supplies heart and lungs. | Superficial cervical nerve |
| 5. .............. | Supplies diaphragm. | Spinal accessory nerve |

### True or False Test

*Carefully read each statement and decide if it is True or False by drawing a circle around the letter T or F.*

| | | | |
|---|---|---|---|
| 1. | T | F | The cervical nerves supply the trunk and the lower extremities. |
| 2. | T | F | The suboccipital nerve supplies the backof the neck. |
| 3. | T | F | The dorsal and spinal thoracic nerves supply the muscles and skin of the chest. |
| 4. | T | F | The pneumogastric nerve supplies the heart and lungs but not the larynx. |
| 5. | T | F | Branches of the thoracic nerve supply the pectoralis major, pectoralis minor and serratus anterior muscles. |

### Answers

| Matching Test | True or False Test |
|---|---|
| 1—Spinal accessory nerve. | 1—F |
| 2—Superficial cervical nerve. | 2—T |
| 3—Greater occipital nerve. | 3—T |
| 4—Pneumogastric nerve. | 4—F |
| 5—Phrenic nerve. | 5—T |

**Review** NERVES OF THE ABDOMEN AND BACK

**Matching Test**

*Match the following definitions. Insert the proper term in front of each definition.*

| | | |
|---|---|---|
| 1. .............. | Supplies lower abdomen. | Supraacromial nerve |
| 2. .............. | Supplies upper abdomen. | Ilio-hypogastric nerve |
| 3. .............. | Supplies shoulders. | Pneumogastric nerve |
| 4. .............. | Supplies stomach. | Spinal accessory nerve |
| 5. .............. | Supplies trapezius muscle. | Intercostal nerve |

**True or False Test**

*Carefully read each statement and decide if it is True or False by drawing a circle around the letter T or F.*

| | | | |
|---|---|---|---|
| 1. | T | F | The sacral, coccygeal, and suprascapular nerves supply various muscles of the spine. |
| 2. | T | F | The subscapular and suprascapular nerves supply the same muscles of the back. |
| 3. | T | F | The lumbar nerves supply the upper part of the abdomen. |
| 4. | T | F | Superior gluteal nerve supplies the glutaeus medius muscle. |
| 5. | T | F | Subscapular nerve supplies latissimus dorsi muscle of back. |

**Answers**

| Matching Test | True or False Test |
|---|---|
| 1—Ilio-hypogastric nerve. | 1—T |
| 2—Intercostal nerve. | 2—F |
| 3—Supraacromial nerve. | 3—F |
| 4—Pneumogastric nerve. | 4—T |
| 5—Spinal accessory nerve. | 5—T |

## Review NERVES OF THE ARMS AND HANDS

### Matching Test

*Match the following definitions. Insert the proper term in front of each definition.*

| | | |
|---|---|---|
| 1. .............. | Supplies elbow joint. | Median Nerve |
| 2. .............. | Supplies shoulder joint. | Ulnar nerve |
| 3. .............. | Supplies wrist joint. | Circumflex nerve |
| 4. .............. | Supplies deltoid muscle. | Radial nerve |
| 5. .............. | Supplies muscles of forearm. | Subscapular nerve |

### True or False Test

*Carefully read each statement and decide if it is True or False by drawing a circle around the letter T or F.*

| | | | |
|---|---|---|---|
| 1. | T | F | The subscapular nerve supplies the teres minor muscle. |
| 2. | T | F | The cervical nerves supply the upper extremities. |
| 3. | T | F | The musculo-spiral nerve supplies the extensor muscles of the entire arm and hand. |
| 4. | T | F | The musculo-cutaneous nerve supplies the pronator muscles of the upper arm. |
| 5. | T | F | The ulnar nerve supplies the skin of the fingers. |

### Answers

| Matching Test | True or False Test |
|---|---|
| 1—Ulnar nerve. | 1—F |
| 2—Circumflex nerve. | 2—T |
| 3—Ulnar nerve. | 3—T |
| 4—Circumflex nerve. | 4—F |
| 5—Median nerve. | 5—T |

**Review** NERVES OF THE LEGS AND FEET

**Matching Test**

*Match the following definitions. Insert the proper term in front of each definition.*

| | | |
|---|---|---|
| 1. .............. | Supplies soles of foot. | Small sciatic nerve |
| 2. .............. | Supplies upper thigh. | Obturator nerve |
| 3. .............. | Supplies inner portion of thigh. | Crural nerve |
| 4. .............. | Supplies back of thigh. | External saphenous nerve |
| 5. .............. | Supplies foot and toe. | Plantar nerve |

**True or False Test**

*Carefully read each statement and decide if it is True or False by drawing a circle around the letter T or F.*

1. T F The obturator nerve supplies the hip and knee joints.
2. T F The internal popliteal nerve supplies the extensor muscles of the lower leg and foot.
3. T F The sacral nerve supplies the muscles and skin of the lower extremities.
4. T F The anterior tibial nerve supplies the flexor muscles of the foot and toes.
5. T F The dorsal cutaneous nerve supplies the top of the foot.

**Answers**

| Matching Test | True or False Test |
|---|---|
| 1—Plantar nerve. | 1—T |
| 2—Crural nerve. | 2—F |
| 3—Obturator nerve. | 3—T |
| 4—Small sciatic nerve. | 4—F |
| 5—External saphenous nerve. | 5—T |

## QUESTIONS FOR DISCUSSION AND REVIEW

1. Why should the massage practitioner understand how the nervous system functions?
2. What are the two divisions of the autonomic nervous system?
3. Which division of the nervous system expands energy?
4. What is a motor point?
5. Why should the massage practitioner be aware of motor points?
6. Where is the peripheral system located?
7. How many pairs of cranial nerves branch out from the brain?
8. How many pairs of spinal nerves branch out from the spinal cord?
9. Name the important groups of spinal nerves.
10. Give the name and number of spinal nerves that supply the head, neck, and shoulders.
11. Give the name and number of spinal nerves that supply the arms.
12. Give the name and number of spinal nerves that supply the chest.
13. Give the name and number of spinal nerves that supply the abdomen and legs.
14. Which organs are supplied by the sympathetic nervous system?
15. What is a reflex action?
16. Which areas of the body are sensitive to reflex influences?
17. Name the 12 cranial nerves.
18. Which cranial nerves are important in facial massage?
19. Name the important nerve motor points of the head, face, and neck.
20. Name the important nerve motor points of the trunk and extremities.

## ANSWERS TO QUESTIONS FOR DISCUSSION AND REVIEW

1. Massage affects the nervous system. The nervous system is one of the most important systems of the body because it controls and coordinates the functions of the other systems to make them work harmoniously and efficiently.
2. The parasympathetic and sympathetic are the two divisions of the autonomic nervous system.
3. The sympathetic division expands energy.
4. A motor point is a sensitive spot on the body that responds readily to stimulation.
5. Motor points are important when giving facial or body massage. Every muscle and nerve has a motor point and can be stimulated by appropriate massage techniques.
6. The peripheral system is located in the skin, muscles, and sense organs.
7. There are 12 pairs of cranial nerves.
8. There are 31 pairs of spinal nerves.

9. The important groups of spinal nerves consist of the cervical nerves, thoracic nerves, lumbar nerves, sacral nerves, and coccygeal nerves.
10. The four upper cervical nerves supply the head, neck, and shoulders.
11. The four lower cervical nerves and first pair of thoracic nerves supply the arms.
12. Eleven pairs of thoracic nerves supply the chest.
13. Five pairs of lumbar nerves, four pairs of sacral nerves, and a portion of the fifth pair of sacral nerves supply the abdomen and legs.
14. The involuntary muscles, heart, lungs, stomach, intestines, and blood vessels are supplied by the sympathetic nervous system.
15. Reflex action is the involuntary response of a muscle to a stimulus.
16. The back between the shoulders, side of chest, upper and inner portion of the thigh, gluteal muscles, and sole of the foot are sensitive to reflex influences.
17. The 12 cranial nerves are the olfactory nerve, optic nerve, oculomotor nerve, trochlear nerve, trigeminal or trifacial nerve, abducent nerve, facial nerve, acoustic or auditory nerve, glossopharyngeal nerve, vagus or pneumogastric nerve, accessory nerve, and hypoglossal nerve.
18. The trifacial and facial nerves are important to facial massage.
19. The posterior auricular nerve, facial nerve and its branches, spinal accessory nerve, and hypoglossal nerve are important nerve motor points of the head, face and neck.
20. Important motor points of the trunk and extremities are the: circumflex nerve, anterior thoracic nerve, spinal accessory nerve, brachial plexus, ulnar nerve, median nerve, radial nerve, sciatic nerve, and tibial nerve.

## SYSTEM FIVE THE ENDOCRINE SYSTEM

The endocrine system comprises a group of specialized glands that may beneficially or adversely affect the growth, reproduction, and health of the body, depending on the quality and quantity of their secretions.

The major functions of the endocrine system is to assist the nervous system in regulating body processes.

### Glands of the Body

The glands are specialized organs that vary in size and function. The blood and nerves are intimately connected with the glands, with the nervous system controlling the glands' functional activities. The glands act as chemical factories, having the ability to remove certain constituents from the blood and to convert them into new compounds. The secretions manufactured by the endocrine glands are known as *hormones.*

There are two main sets of glands. One group is called the *exocrine* or *duct glands* (possessing canals leading from a gland to a particular part of the body). Certain skin and intestinal glands belong to this group. The other group, known as *ductless* or *endocrine glands,* throws its secretions directly into the bloodstream, which in turn influences the welfare of the entire body.

The endocrine glands operate as a unit. If there is an under- or over-functioning of any duct gland, it will upset the delicate balance of the entire chain of the endocrine glands. Some of the endocrine glands exert a regulatory and restraining influence over the other glands.

Among the important endocrine glands are the pituitary gland, thyroid gland, adrenal gland, sex gland (gonad), and pancreas. The *pituitary gland* is the main gland and is often called the *master gland* because it controls the ductless glands.

#### *The Pituitary Gland*

The pituitary gland is a small gland about the size of a cherry that produces a number of hormones that regulate many body processes. The pituitary gland is located in a depression just behind the point of the optic nerve crossing, in the brain. It has an interior and posterior lobe, each of which produces different hormones. The production of hormones can be affected by both emotional and physical conditions. The anterior lobe of the pituitary gland produces hormones that stimulate other glands. The following are the main hormones:

*Somatorropic or growth hormone.* This hormone stimulates growth of bones, muscles, and organs. A deficiency of this hormone will inhibit growth.

*Thyrotropic hormone.* This hormone stimulates the thyroid gland. Thyroid hormones regulate metabolism for the production of heat and energy in body tissues. The proper manufacture of these hormones requires adequate iodine in the blood. Proper diet assures adequate iodine, which helps to prevent goiter (enlarged thyroid).

## The Endocrine System

*(Both male and female glands are shown)*

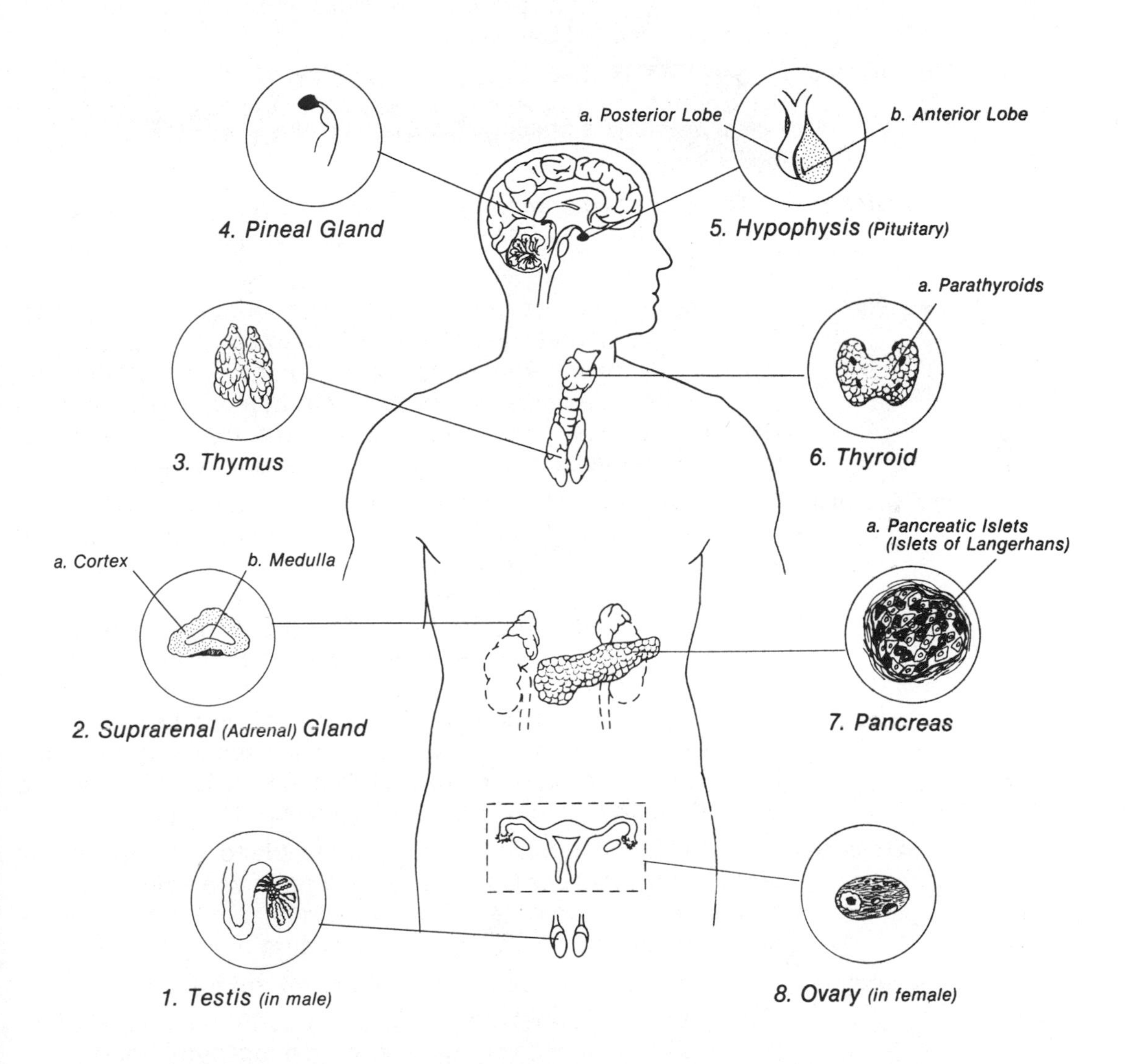


**1.** Two glandular male reproductive organs which produce testosterone, the hormone which controls sex characteristics in males. **2.** Two small glands located above the upper end of each kidney.
**2a.** External tissue. **2b.** Chromaphil tissue. **3.** The thymus is part of the lymphatic system located in the upper chest cavity along the trachea. Necessary in early life for development and maturation of immunological functions. **4.** A gland attached to the roof of the third ventricle of the brain. Function is stimulation of adrenal cortex.
**5.** Called the master or dominating gland. Controls skeletal growth, thyroid secretion and other metabolic processes. **5a.** Affects blood pressure, heartbeat, constriction and contraction of some muscles.
**5b.** Affects thyroid secretions. **6.** Gland that influences growth and development. Located in front of trachea below thyroid cartilage. **6a.** Four glands arranged in pairs that play a part in maintaining the normal calcium level of the blood, regulate phosphorus metabolism and play a part in the functioning of the nervous system and muscles. **7.** Located between the first and second lumbar vertebrae behind the stomach. Aids in the synthesis of sugar to glycogen, storage of glycogen, and conversion of glycogen to glucose in the liver.
**7a.** A special group of cells that secrete insulin, which is essential for normal glucose metabolism.
**8.** Two almond shaped bodies located on each side of the uterus that produce estrogen and progesterone and are essential in the development of female characteristics.

***The Thyroid Gland***

The thyroid gland, situated on either side of the trachea, produces the hormone *thyroxin,* which controls the weight and the metabolic rate of the body. The parathyroid glands, situated behind the thyroid, produce *parathoromone,* which regulates the blood level of calcium.

***The Thymus***

The thymus, located inferior to the thyroid, has endocrine and lymphatic functions and is active until puberty at which time it diminishes. The main purpose of the thymus is to produce lymphocytes.

***The Adrenal Glands***

There are two adrenal glands, each situated above a kidney. Adrenal glands play an important role in regulating blood circulation.

***The Sex Glands***

The sex glands (gonads) are both duct and ductless glands. The male and female sex glands manufacture the reproductive cells and sex hormones that are required for fertility and reproduction. *Testosterone* is the male hormone (a potent androgen). *Estrogen* and *progesterone* are the two essential ovarian hormones of the female reproductive system.

***The Pancreas***

The pancreas is located behind the stomach and is made up of small groups of specialized cells called *islets (Islands of Langerhands).* The pancreas has both endocrine and exocrine functions. It produces digestive enzymes that are excreted into the small intestine through the pancreatic duct. This is an exocrine function. Certain cells in the pancreas produce the hormone *insulin,* which favors the storage and metabolism of sugars in the body. When insulin is lacking, there is not enough glucose for proper cell metabolism, which results in abnormal breakdown of proteins and fats. Diabetes is a condition caused by faulty functioning of the pancreatic islets.

***Obesity***

Faulty functioning of the endocrine glands may be partly responsible for obesity. Many reducing remedies contain thyroid extract or other glandular products. Such products should be used only under the supervision of a physician.

**Overview**

Glands are made of cells that secrete different fluids.

Duct glands (exocrine) are the sweat (sudoriferous) glands, tear glands (lacrimal), salivary glands, oil (sebaceous) glands, and milk glands.

The ductless glands (endocrine) manufacture hormones and pass their secretions directly into the bloodstream. The glands of internal secretion are the pituitary, thyroid, parathyroids, thymus, adrenals, and islet cells of the pancreas and gonads.

**QUESTIONS FOR DISCUSSION AND REVIEW**

1. What is the composition and function of the endocrine system?
2. How are the glands connected with other parts of the body?
3. Why are the glands dependent upon an adequate nerve and blood supply?
4. What is the function of the duct glands?
5. Are sebaceous (oil) glands classified as duct or ductless glands?
6. What is the function of a ductless or endocrine gland?
7. What is an important difference between a duct and ductless gland?
8. Which glands function as both duct and ductless glands?
9. Which glands produce hormones?
10. Why are hormones important to the body?
11. Why is the pituitary gland called the master gland?
12. Why is the functioning of the adrenal cortex so important to life?

**ANSWERS TO QUESTIONS FOR DISCUSSION AND REVIEW**

1. The endocrine system is composed of a group of glands whose functions are vital to the maintenance of health. Each gland is an organ capable of producing a secretion or hormone.
2. Each gland is linked with other parts of the body by means of nerves and the bloodstream.
3. The blood supplies the raw materials that glands utilize to produce secretions. The nerves control the functional activities of the glands.
4. Duct glands manufacture substances that are carried away through canals to particular parts of the body.
5. Sebaceous glands are duct glands that provide sebum (oil) to lubricate the skin.
6. A ductless or endocrine gland has no duct, but delivers its secretion directly into the blood or lymph streams, causing actions remote from the regions of their formation.
7. A duct gland possesses a duct or canal, whereas a ductless gland has no duct.
8. The pancreas and sex glands (gonads) function as both duct and ductless glands.
9. The ductless or endocrine glands produce hormones.
10. Hormones in the bloodstream have a profound influence on external appearance and body processes. An absence or deficiency of certain hormones in the blood is the cause of various diseases.
11. The pituitary gland controls the ductless glands.
12. The functioning of the adrenal cortex allows the body to adapt to its environment.

## SYSTEM SIX THE CIRCULATORY SYSTEM (Blood Vascular)

The vascular or circulatory system controls the circulation of the blood and lymph through the body in a steady stream, by means of the heart and blood vessels, whose function it is to supply body cells with nutrient materials and carry away waste products.

There are two divisions to the vascular system:

1. The *blood-vascular system,* which comprises the heart and blood vessels (arteries, capillaries, and veins) for the circulation of the blood.
2. The *lymph-vascular system,* or lymphatic system, consisting of lymph glands and lymphatics through which the lymph circulates.

These two systems are intimately linked with each other. Lymph is derived from the blood and is gradually shifted back into the blood stream.

The heart is an efficient pump that keeps the blood moving in a steady stream through a closed system of arteries, capillaries, and veins.

### The Blood-Vascular System

#### *The Heart*

The heart is a muscular, conical-shaped organ, about the size of a closed fist, located in the chest cavity, and enclosed in a membrane, the pericardium. Two sets of nerves, the *vagus* and *sympathetic,* regulate the heart beat. In a normal adult, the heart beats about 72 to 80 times a minute.

The interior of the heart contains four chambers and four valves. The upper thin-walled cavities are the right and left atrium or auricle. The lower thick-walled chambers are the right and left ventricle. Valves allow the blood flow in only one direction, either upward or downward. With each contraction and relaxation of the heart, the blood flows in, travels from the auricles to the ventricles, and is then driven out to be distributed all over the body.

#### *The Blood Vessels*

The *arteries, capillaries,* and *veins* transport blood to and from the heart and the various tissues of the body. The main artery of the body is the *aorta,* which arches up from the left ventricle of the heart, extending over and down along the vertebral column, and subdividing into smaller arteries.

Arteries are thick-walled muscular and elastic vessels that carry oxygenated blood from the heart to the capillaries. They vary in size from the aorta, which is about an inch in diameter, to capillaries whose walls are just a single cell in thickness and are only large enough to pass one blood cell at a time.

The muscular tissue, which controls the movements of the arterial walls, is chiefly supplied with nerves from the sympathetic system. These vasomotor nerves are of two kinds:

1. *Vasoconstrictor nerves,* which contract blood vessels, thereby decreasing the flow of blood to a particular area and raising blood pressure.
2. *Vasodilator nerves,* which expand the blood vessel, thereby increasing the flow of the blood to a particular area.

**_Capillaries_**

Capillaries are microscopic, thin-walled blood vessels whose networks connect the smaller arteries with the veins. Through their walls, the tissues receive nourishment and eliminate waste products.

**_Veins_**

Veins are thin-walled inelastic blood vessels containing cuplike valves to prevent backflow and carry impure blood from the various capillaries back to the heart.

**_Arteries_**

Arteries are usually located deeper into the tissues, whereas the veins are usually located nearer to the surface of the body.

**The Circulation of the Blood**

The blood is in constant circulation from the moment it leaves until it returns to the heart. There are two systems involved in circulation: pulmonary and systemic.

*Pulmonary circulation* is the blood circulation from the heart to the lungs and back again to the heart. During the pulmonary circulation, the blood is pumped from the right side of the heart to the lungs where carbon dioxide is replaced by oxygen. With each respiration, an exchange of gases takes place. The exchange is continuous. Breathing is the process whereby oxygen is made available and carbon dioxide is carried out of the body.

*General* or *systemic circulation* is the blood circulation from the left side of the heart throughout the body and back again to the heart. The course that blood travels is as follows:

1. The right atrium or auricle receives impure blood from a large vein, the vena cava.
2. From the right atrium or auricle, the venous blood passes through a valve into the right ventricle.
3. From the right ventricle, the venous blood is carried through the pulmonary artery up to the lungs to be oxygenated or purified.
4. The left atrium or auricle receives the oxygenated blood through the pulmonary vein.
5. From the left atrium or auricle, the purified blood passes through a valve into the left ventricle.
6. From the left ventricle, the aorta sends the arterial blood to all parts of the body, except the lungs.
7. This cycle is repeated when the venous blood is brought back again to the right atrium or auricle.

**The Blood**

Blood is the nutritive fluid circulating throughout the blood-vascular system. It is salty and sticky, has an alkaline reaction, and maintains a normal temperature of 98.6° Fahrenheit (37° Celsius). About 8 to 15 pints of blood fill the blood vessels of an adult and constitute about one-sixteenth to one-twentieth of the body's weight. The skin holds about one-half to two-thirds of all the blood in the body.

**_The Color of Blood_**

The blood itself is bright red in color in the arteries (except in the pulmonary artery) and dark red in the veins (except in the pulmonary vein). This change in color is due to the gain or loss of oxygen as the blood passes through the lungs and other tissues of the body.

**Composition of Blood**

The blood is a liquid tissue consisting of blood plasma, red corpuscles, white corpuscles, and blood platelets. Plasma constitutes about two-thirds of the blood and other bodies about one-third.

**Plasma**

*Plasma* is the fluid part of the blood, strawlike in color, in which the red corpuscles, white corpuscles, and blood platelets flow. About nine-tenths of plasma is water. It is derived from the food and water taken into the body.

**Red Corpuscles**

*Red corpuscles* (red blood cells) or erythrocytes are double concave disklike-shaped cells colored with a substance called *hemoglobin.* The function of the red corpuscles is to carry oxygen from the lungs to the body cells and transport carbon dioxide from the cells to the lungs. The red blood cells are formed in the red bone marrow. They are far more numerous than the white blood cells.

**White Corpuscles**

*White corpuscles* (white blood cells) or leucocytes differ from red blood cells in many respects. They are larger in size, colorless, and can change their form by movements. White corpuscles are produced in the spleen, lymph glands, and the red marrow of the long bones. The most important function of these cells is to protect the body against disease by fighting harmful bacteria and their poisons.

**Blood Platelets**

*Blood platelets* or *thrombocytes* are colorless, irregular bodies, much smaller than the red corpuscles. They are formed in the red bone marrow. These bodies play an important role in the clotting of the blood over a wound.

**Clotting**

When the blood leaves the body and comes in contact with the air, it hardens and clots. This clotting is due to the hardening of the fibrin in the blood, and the clot thus prevents the further flow of the blood.

**Diseases of the Blood**

*Hemophilia* is characterized by extremely slow clotting of blood and excessive bleeding from even very slight cuts. This disease is hereditary, but men are the chief sufferers. Women may, however, transmit this blood condition to their sons.

*Anemia* is a condition in which there are two few red blood cells (corpuscles) and too little hemoglobin, or both, resulting in a lack of body strength and paleness of the complexion. A diet rich in iron, which is found in green vegetables, such as spinach, and organ meats, such as liver, will help to alleviate this condition. A physician should be consulted.

**Chief Functions of the Blood**

1. The blood carries water, oxygen, food, and secretions to all areas of the body.
2. It carries away carbon dioxide and waste products to be eliminated through the excretory channels.
3. It helps to equalize the body temperature, thus protecting the body from extreme heat and cold.
4. It aids in protecting the body from harmful bacteria and infections through the action of the white blood cells.
5. It coagulates (clots) thereby closing injured blood vessels and preventing the loss of blood through hemorrhage.

## The Circulatory System

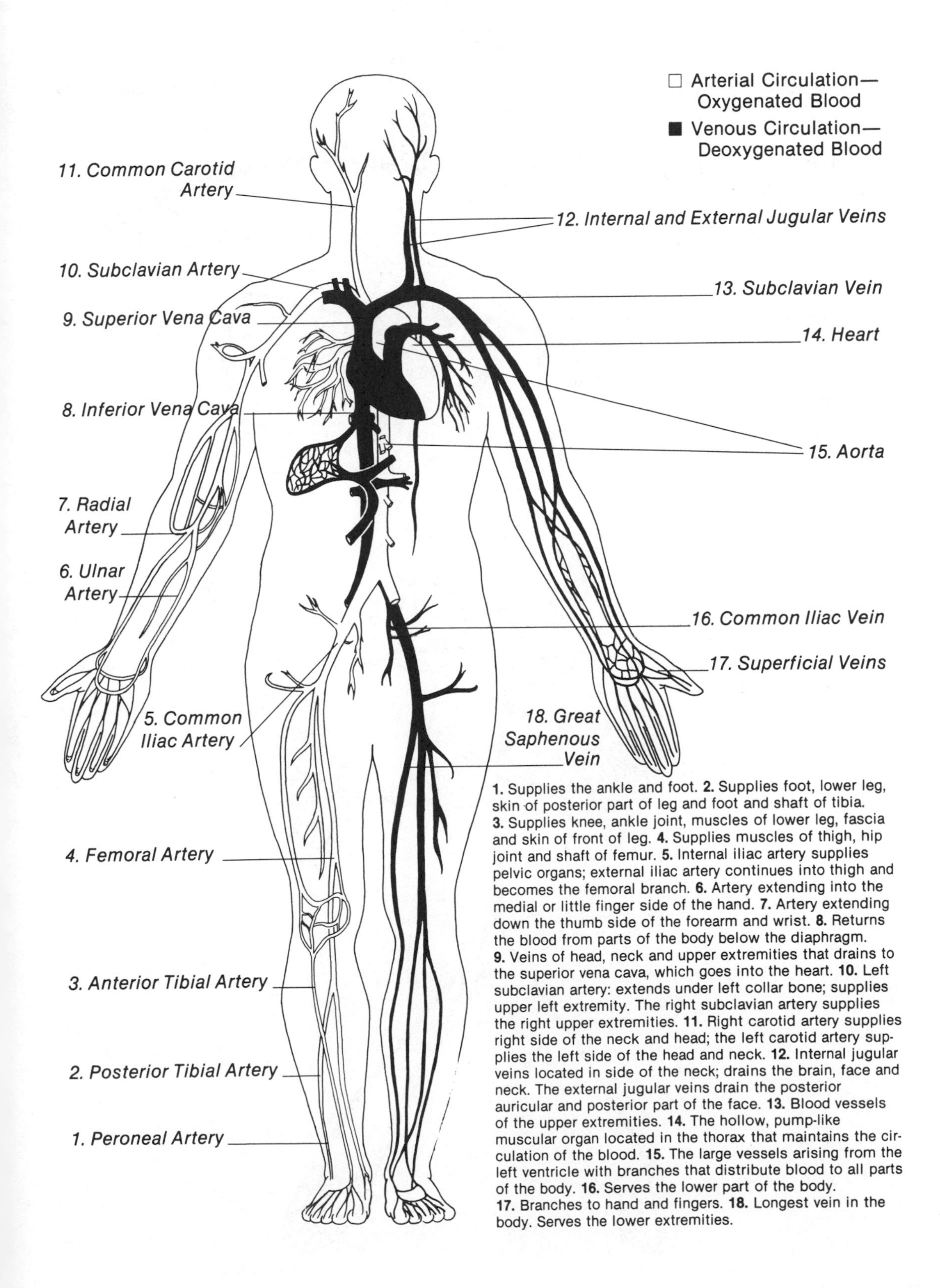


**1.** Supplies the ankle and foot. **2.** Supplies foot, lower leg, skin of posterior part of leg and foot and shaft of tibia. **3.** Supplies knee, ankle joint, muscles of lower leg, fascia and skin of front of leg. **4.** Supplies muscles of thigh, hip joint and shaft of femur. **5.** Internal iliac artery supplies pelvic organs; external iliac artery continues into thigh and becomes the femoral branch. **6.** Artery extending into the medial or little finger side of the hand. **7.** Artery extending down the thumb side of the forearm and wrist. **8.** Returns the blood from parts of the body below the diaphragm. **9.** Veins of head, neck and upper extremities that drains to the superior vena cava, which goes into the heart. **10.** Left subclavian artery: extends under left collar bone; supplies upper left extremity. The right subclavian artery supplies the right upper extremities. **11.** Right carotid artery supplies right side of the neck and head; the left carotid artery supplies the left side of the head and neck. **12.** Internal jugular veins located in side of the neck; drains the brain, face and neck. The external jugular veins drain the posterior auricular and posterior part of the face. **13.** Blood vessels of the upper extremities. **14.** The hollow, pump-like muscular organ located in the thorax that maintains the circulation of the blood. **15.** The large vessels arising from the left ventricle with branches that distribute blood to all parts of the body. **16.** Serves the lower part of the body. **17.** Branches to hand and fingers. **18.** Longest vein in the body. Serves the lower extremities.

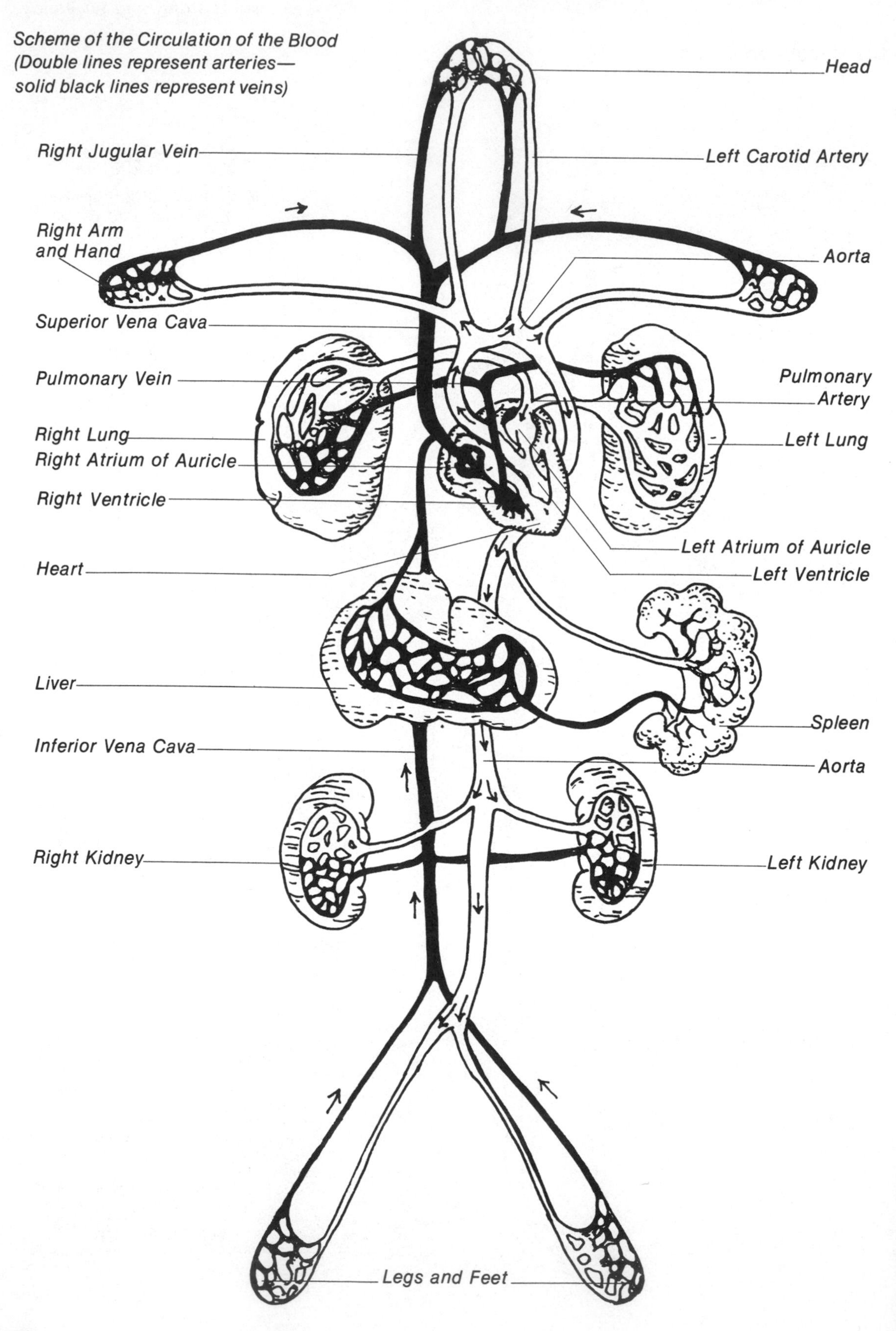
Scheme of the Circulation of the Blood
(Double lines represent arteries—
solid black lines represent veins)
Head
Right Jugular Vein
Left Carotid Artery
Right Arm
and Hand
Aorta
Superior Vena Cava
Pulmonary Vein
Pulmonary
Artery
Right Lung
Left Lung
Right Atrium of Auricle
Right Ventricle
Left Atrium of Auricle
Heart
Left Ventricle
Liver
Spleen
Inferior Vena Cava
Aorta
Right Kidney
Left Kidney
Legs and Feet

**Arteries of the Head, Face, and Neck**

The common carotid arteries are the main sources of blood supply to the head, face, and neck. They are located on either side of the neck, and each artery divides into an internal and external branch. The internal branch of the common carotid artery supplies the cranial cavity, whereas the external branch supplies the superficial parts of the head, face, and neck. The arteries, like the muscles and nerves, are named in accordance with the parts of the body that they serve.

**Arteries of the Head, Face and Neck**

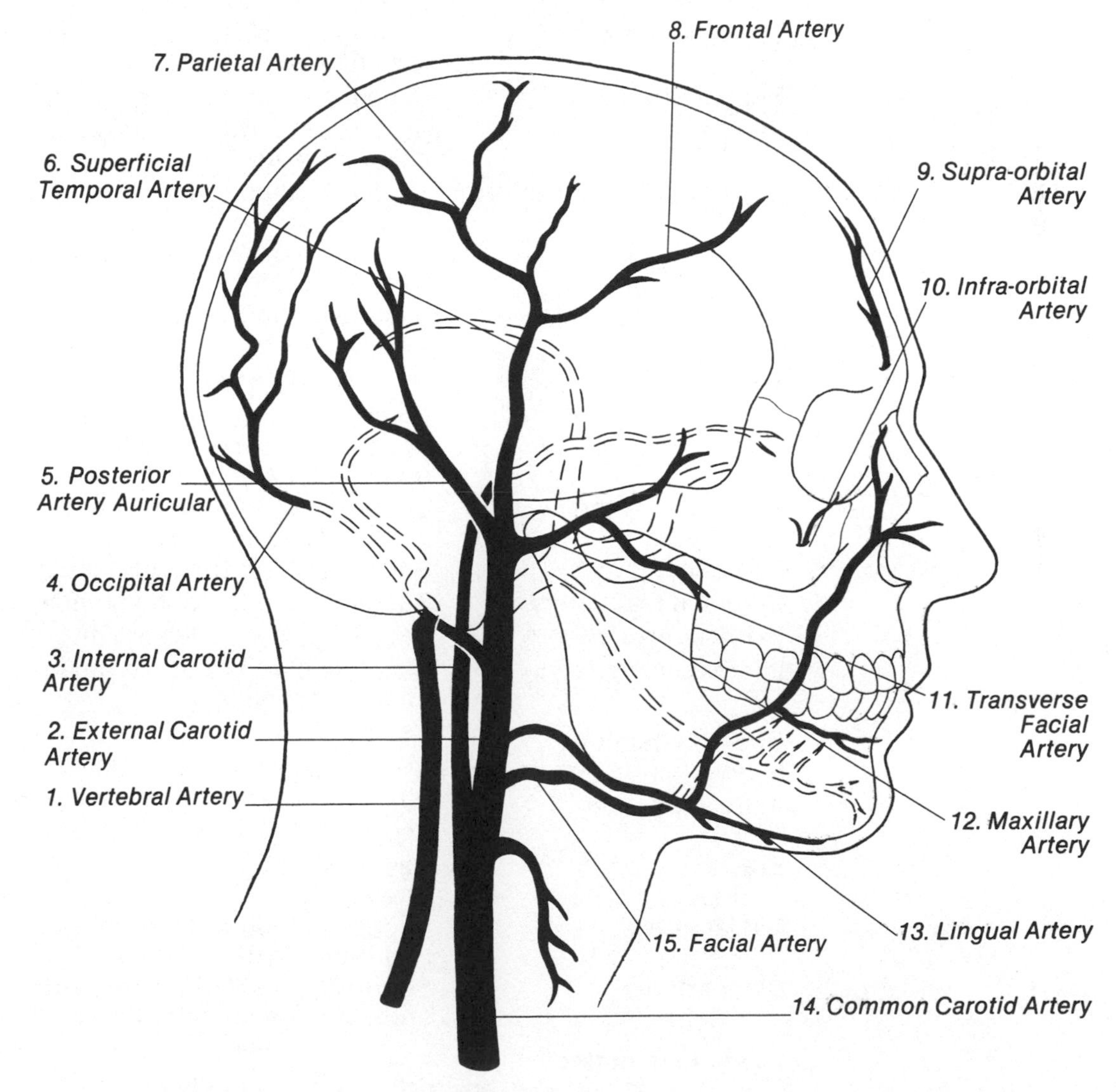


**1.** Supplies muscles of neck, posterior fossa of skull. **2.** Supplies face, tonsils, root of tongue and submandibular gland. **3.** Supplies brain, sinuses, parts of the head. **4.** Supplies muscles of neck, ear area and scalp. **5.** Supplies area of ear, scalp and parotid gland. **6.** Supplies the masseter muscle. **7.** Located in the parietal bone of the skull. **8.** Supplies frontal bone, upper eyelid. **9.** Supplies root of orbit, frontal bone, upper eyelid. **10.** Supplies muscle of eye and upper lip. **11.** Supplies masseter muscle, parotid gland, skin of face. **12.** Supplies jaws, ear and deep structure of face.
**13.** Supplies membrane of tongue and mouth, gums, tonsils, soft palate, epiglottis. **14.** Right side supplies right side of head and face, left side supplies the left side of the head and face. **15.** Supplies face, root of tongue, submandibular gland.

**Important Arteries of the Body**

| NAME | FUNCTION |
|---|---|
| **Head and Neck** | |
| Facial Artery | Supplies blood to face and pharynx. |
| Temporal Artery | Supplies blood to forehead, masseter muscle and ear. |
| Common Carotid Arteries: | |
| Internal branch | Supplies blood to cranial cavity. |
| External branch | Supplies blood to surface of head, face and neck. |
| **Branches of External Carotid Artery** | |
| Ophthalmic artery | Supplies blood to the eyes. |
| Supra-orbital artery | Supplies blood to the eye-socket, forehead and side of nose. |
| Frontal artery | Supplies blood to the forehead. |
| Parietal artery | Supplies blood to the crown and sides of head. |
| Posterior auricular artery | Supplies blood to the scalp and back of ear. |
| Submental artery | Supplies blood to chin and lower lip. |
| Superior labial | Supplies blood to upper lip and center of nose. |
| **Trunk** | |
| Aorta | Forms main trunk of arterial system and subdivides to form large and small branches. |
| Subclavian artery | Supplies blood to neck, chest, and upper part of back. |
| Coronary artery | Supplies blood to heart muscles. |
| Common iliac artery | Supplies blood to abdominal wall. |
| External iliac artery | Supplies blood to lower limb. |
| Internal iliac artery | Supplies blood to pelvic organs and inner thigh. |
| **Upper Extremities** | |
| *(The following arteries are for one side of the body* | |
| Axillary artery | Supplies blood to shoulder, chest, and arm. |
| Brachial artery | Supplies blood to the arm and forearm. |
| Radial artery | Supplies blood to forearm, wrist, and thumb side of hand. |
| Ulnar artery | Supplies blood to forearm, wrist, and small finger side of hand. |
| **Lower Extremities** | |
| *(The following arteries are for one side of the body)* | |
| Femoral artery | Supplies blood to lower part of abdominal wall, pelvic organs and upper thigh. |
| Popliteal artery | Supplies blood to knee and leg. |
| Anterior tibial artery | Supplies blood to leg. |
| Posterior tibial artery | Supplies blood to leg, heel, and foot. |
| Dorsalis pedis artery | Supplies blood to foot. |

## Anatomy of the Heart

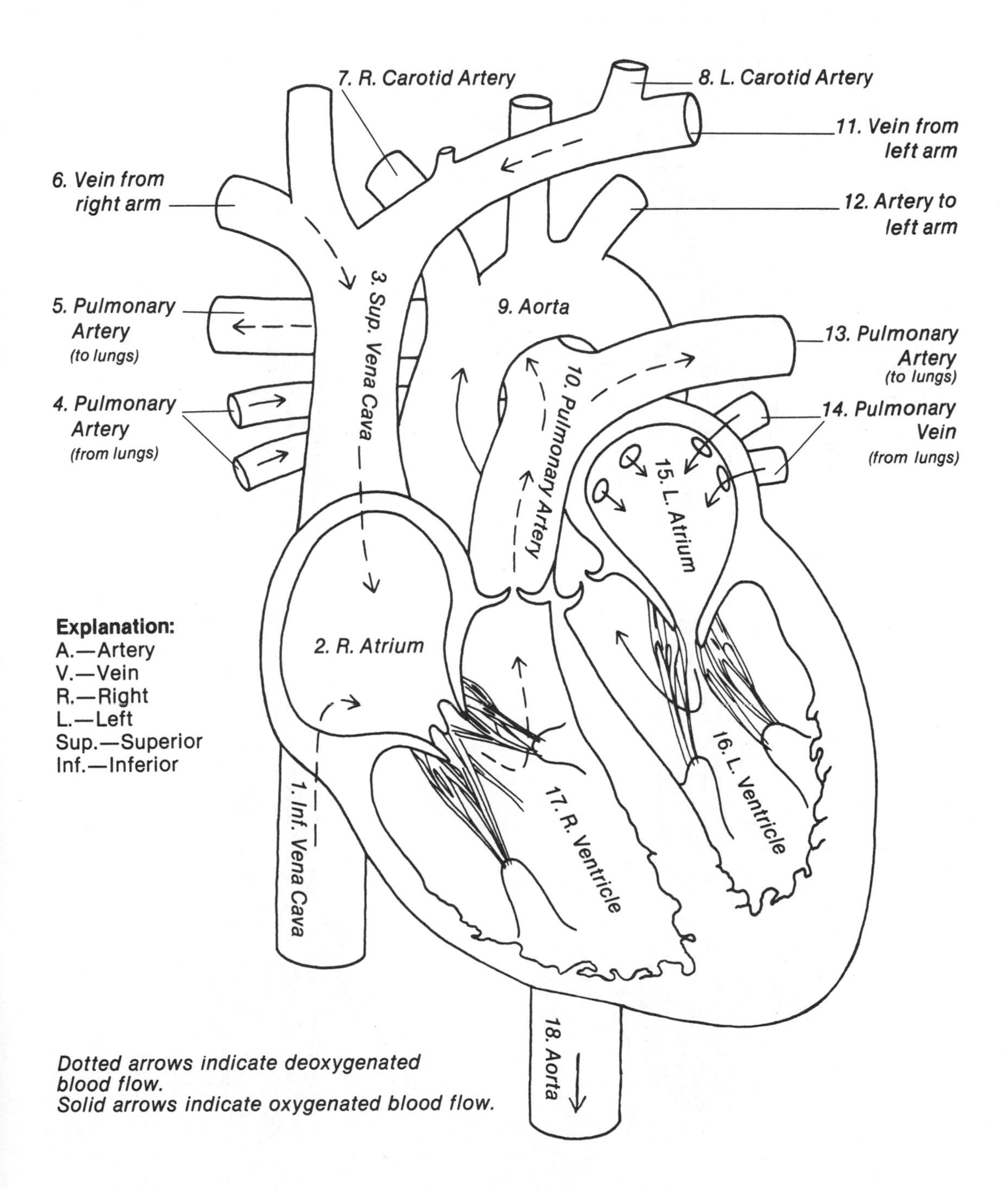


**1.** Veins of abdomen, pelvis and lower extremities empty into this vein. **2.** Receives impure blood from the vena cava. **3.** Veins of the head, neck, thorax and upper extremities empty into this vein. **4.** Conveys oxygenated blood from the lungs to the left atrium. **5.** Conveys venous blood from the right ventricle to the lungs. **7.** The principal large artery on the right side of the neck. **8.** The principal large artery on the left side of the neck. **9.** Main artery of the body; carries blood from the left ventricle to all arteries of the body. **10.** Divides into left and right branches and takes blood into the lungs. **15.** Receives purified blood through the pulmonary vein. **16.** From the left ventricle the aorta sends blood to all parts of the body except the lungs. **17.** Venous blood is carried through the pulmonary artery up to the lungs to be oxygenated and purified. **18.** A large vessel arising from the left ventricle which, by way of its branches, distributes arterial blood to all parts of the body.

## Blood Supply for the Arm and Hand

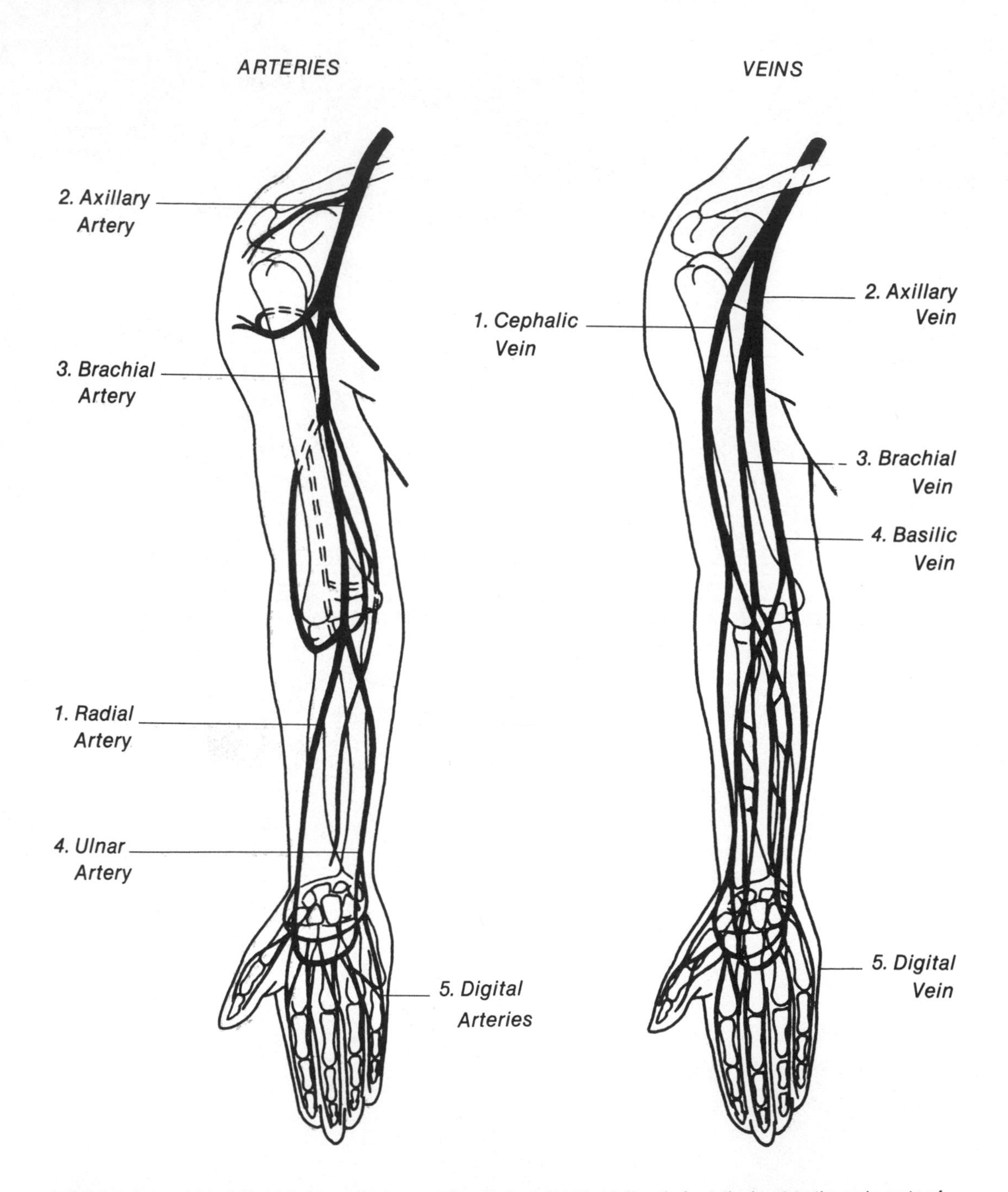


**I.** Arteries: Large thick-walled tubes comprising a system that carries blood directly from the heart to the main parts of the body. **1.** Principal artery of thumb and deep palmar arch. **2.** A continuation of the subclavian extending from the outer border of the first rib to the tendon of the teres major muscle where it becomes the brachial. **3.** Distributes blood to various muscles of the arm, the humerus, elbow joint, forearm and hand. **4.** Artery which supplies muscles of the forearm, shafts of radius and ulna, ulnal half of the hand and skin of these areas. **5.** Arteries serving the dorsal areas of the fingers.

**II.** Veins: Blood vessels that carry blood from parts of the body back toward the heart. **1.** The superficial vein rising from the radial side of the arm which supplies the biceps and deltoid muscles. **2.** A continuation of the basilic ending in the outer border of the first rib in the subclavian vein. **3.** Deep veins of the forearm and arm. **4.** Veins beginning in the ulnar part of the dorsal network and extending to join the accessory cephalic vein. **5.** Veins of the fingers.

## Veins of the Head, Face and Neck

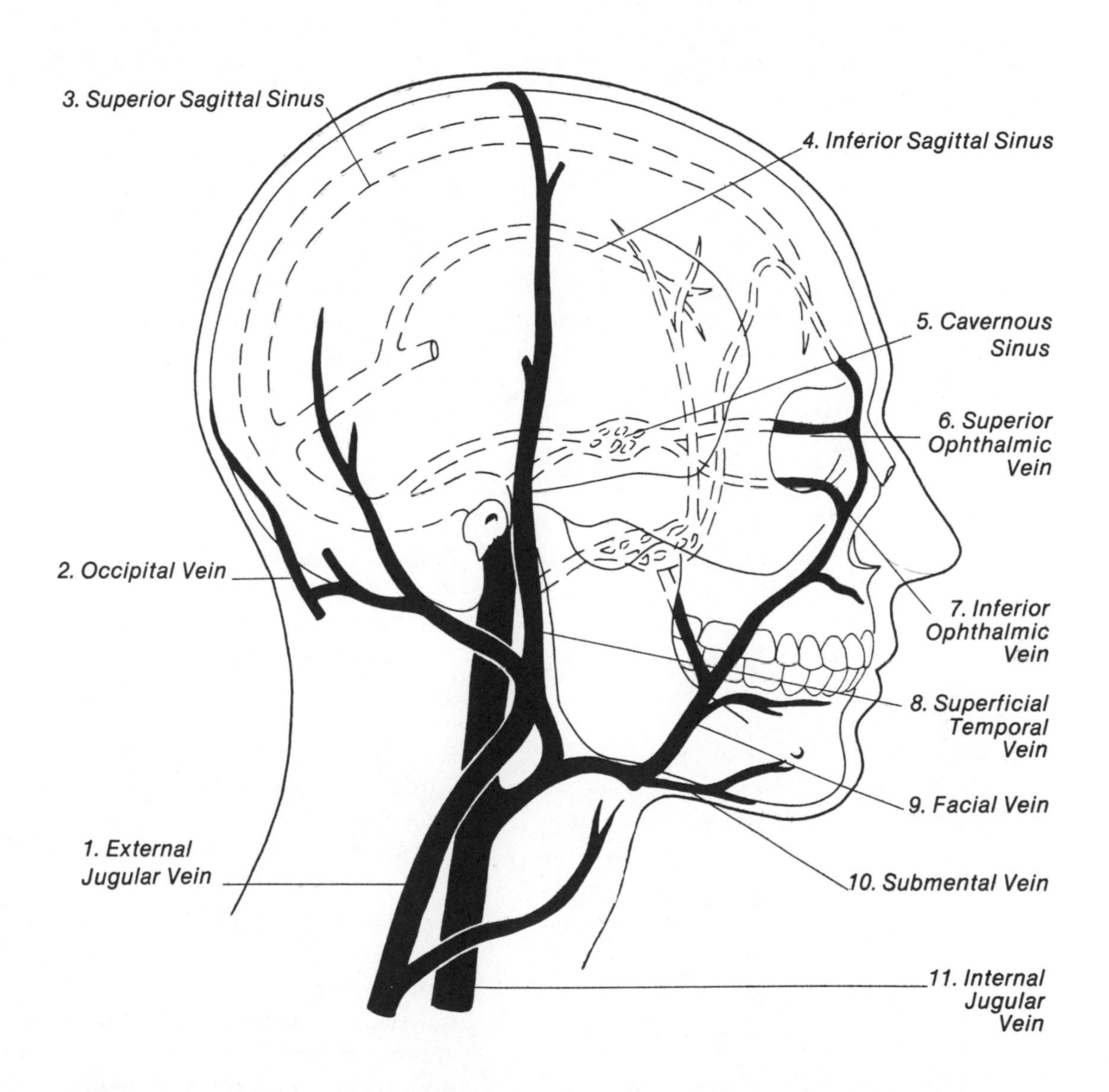


**1.** Vein located in side of the neck that drains the posterior part of the face area supplied by carotid arteries.
**2.** Drains into confluence of sinuses. **3.** A single long space located in midline above the brain. Ends in an enlargement called the confluence of sinuses. **4.** A small venous sinus of the dura mater, situated in the posterior half of the lower concave border of the cerebral falx. **5.** Situated behind the eyeball and drains the ophthalmic veins of the eye.
**6.** Drains veins of the eye. **7.** Veins supplying the eye area. **8.** Vein serving the temple region of the head on either side.
**9.** Vein supplying the anterior side of the face. **10.** A vein situated below the chin that follows the submental artery and opens into the facial vein. **11.** Vein located in side of the neck and drains the brain, face, neck and transverse sinus.

**Important Veins of the Body**

| NAME | FUNCTION |
|---|---|
| **Head and Neck** | |
| Facial vein | Receives blood from face and empties into internal jugular vein. |
| Internal jugular vein | Receives blood from cranial cavity and from surface of face and neck. |
| External jugular vein | Receives blood from deep parts of face and from the surface of cranium. |
| Temporal veins | Receives blood from the tempero-maxillary region of the head. |
| Maxillary anterior vein | Receives blood from the anterior portion of the face. |
| Ophthalmic vein | Receives blood from the eyes. |
| Supra-orbital vein | Receives blood from the forehead and eyebrow. |
| Frontal vein | Receives blood from the anterior portion of the scalp. |
| Superior and inferior labial veins | Receive blood from the upper and lower lips. |
| **Trunk** | |
| Innominate veins | Receive blood from internal jugular and subclavian veins. |
| Coronary veins | Receive blood from heart muscles. |
| Common iliac vein | Receives blood from external and internal iliac veins and empties into inferior vena cava. |
| Inferior vena cava | Receives blood from abdomen, pelvis and lower limbs. |
| Superior vena cava | Receives blood from head, neck, thorax, and upper limbs. |
| **Upper Extremities** | |
| *(The following veins are for one side of the body)* | |
| Cephalic vein | Receives blood from radial side (front) of arm. |
| Basilic vein | Receives blood from ulnar side (outside) of arm. |
| Axillary vein | Returns blood from arm to heart. |
| **Lower Extremities** | |
| *(The following veins are for one side of the body)* | |
| Great saphenous veins | Receive blood from the inner side of front leg. |
| Small saphenous vein | Receive blood from back of leg. |
| Popliteal vein | Receives blood from anterior and posterior tibial veins. |
| Femoral vein | Receives blood from feet, legs, and thigh. |

**Review** IMPORTANT VEINS OF THE BODY

### Matching Test

*Match the following definitions. Insert the proper term in front of each definition.*

| | | |
|---|---|---|
| 1. ............... | Receives blood from eyes. | Femoral vein |
| 2. ............... | Receives blood from heart. | Ophthalmic vein |
| 3. ............... | Receives blood from face. | Coronary veins |
| 4. ............... | Receives blood from outer arm. | Facial vein |
| 5. ............... | Receives blood from legs. | Basilic vein |

### True or False Test

*Carefully read each statement and decide if it is True or False by drawing a circle around the letter T or F.*

1. T F Both the internal and external jugular veins return blood from the head, face and neck to the heart.
2. T F The inferior vena cava receives blood from the abdomen and upper limbs.
3. T F The popliteal vein is located in the lower extremities.
4. T F The innominate veins are found in the upper extremities.
5. T F The superior vena cava receives blood from the head, neck, thorax and upper limbs.

### Answers

| Matching Test | True or False Test |
|---|---|
| 1—Ophthalmic vein. | 1—T |
| 2—Coronary veins. | 2—F |
| 3—Facial vein. | 3—T |
| 4—Basilic vein. | 4—F |
| 5—Femoral vein. | 5—T |

**Review** IMPORTANT ARTERIES OF THE BODY

**Matching Test**

*Match the following definitions. Insert the proper term in front of each definition.*

| | | |
|---|---|---|
| 1. .............. | Supplies blood to heart. | Ophthalmic artery |
| 2. .............. | Supplies blood to eyes. | Subclavian artery |
| 3. .............. | Supplies blood to face. | Frontal artery |
| 4. .............. | Supplies blood to forehead | Coronary artery |
| 5. .............. | Supplies blood to chest. | Facial artery |

**True or False Test**

*Carefully read each statement and decide if it is True or False by drawing a circle around the letter T or F.*

1. T F The posterior auricular artery supplies blood to the scalp.
2. T F The aorta does not form large and small branches.
3. T F The axillary artery supplies blood to the shoulder, chest and arm.
4. T F The external branch of the common carotid artery supplies blood to the cranial cavity.
5. T F The external iliac artery supplies blood to the upper limb.

**Answers**

| Matching Test | True or False Test |
|---|---|
| 1—Coronary artery. | 1—T |
| 2—Ophthalmic artery. | 2—F |
| 3—Facial artery. | 3—T |
| 4—Frontal artery. | 4—F |
| 5—Subclavian artery. | 5—F |

**QUESTIONS FOR DISCUSSION AND REVIEW**

1. Name the important parts comprising the blood-vascular system.
2. Which nerves regulate the heart beat?
3. What is the function of the heart?
4. What is the function of the arteries?
5. Which nerves control the movements of the arterial walls?
6. What is the function of the capillaries?
7. What is the function of the veins?
8. Name the main artery of the body.
9. What controls blood circulation of the body?
10. Which constituents are found in the blood?
11. Which substances are carried by the blood to the body cells?
12. Which substances does the blood remove from the body cells?
13. In what ways does the blood protect the body?
14. What is the normal temperature of the blood?

**ANSWERS TO QUESTIONS FOR DISCUSSION AND REVIEW**

1. The heart and blood vessels (arteries, veins, and capillaries) are the main parts of the blood-vascular system.
2. Two sets of nerves: the vagus and sympathetic nerves regulate the heart beat.
3. The heart is an efficient pump that keeps the blood moving in a steady stream through a closed system of blood vessels.
4. The arteries carry pure blood from the heart to the capillaries.
5. Movements of the arterial walls are controlled by vasomotor nerves consisting of the vasoconstrictor nerves and the vasodilator nerves.
6. The capillaries connect the smaller arteries with the veins, thereby bringing nourishment to the cells and removing waste products.
7. The veins carry impure blood from the various capillaries back to the heart.
8. The main artery is the aorta.
9. Blood flow is controlled by pulmonary circulation and general circulation.
10. Blood consists of plasma, red corpuscles, white corpuscles, and platelets.
11. Blood carries water, oxygen, food, and secretions to the body cells.
12. Blood removes carbon dioxide gas and waste products from the body cells.
13. The blood protects the body against extreme heat or cold, harmful bacteria, and the excessive loss of blood by forming an external clot.
14. Normal body temperature is 98.6 degrees Fahrenheit (37° C).

## THE CIRCULATORY SYSTEM (Lymph-Vascular)

The lymphatic system acts as an aid to, and is interlinked with the blood-vascular system. The lymphatic vessels lie in close proximity to the larger veins and have valves that prevent backflow in much the same way as the valves of the veins. The lymph-vascular system includes the lymph spaces, lymphatics, lymph ducts, lymph nodes, glands, and lacteals.

The *lacteals* are any of the lymphatic vessels that carry chyle (a milky emulsion of lymph and fat) from the intestine to the thoracic duct. Lymph originates as blood plasma and is circulated to all parts of the body not reached by blood. It is a yellowish, alkaline fluid that is formed by the filtering of some of the blood plasma through the capillary walls. By bathing all cells, tissue fluid acts as a medium of exchange, trading to the cells its nutritive materials and receiving in return the waste products of metabolism.

The return supply of lymph to the blood happens when tissue fluid enters the lymph capillaries, travels through lymph vessels and nodes, then connects with the venous blood supply at the bracocephalic vein. This movement depends on the contractions of muscles, pulsation of arteries and the actions of the diaphram in respiration.

*Lymph spaces* or *intercellular spaces* are channels found between the walls of the capillaries and the cells. *Lymphatics* are vessels that transport lymph from the lymph spaces of the body back toward the venous blood system. The structure and arrangement of lymphatics resemble those of the veins except that the lymphatic capillaries are closed, whereas the veins are a continuation from the arteries and capillary beds.

**Collecting Vessels**

The collecting vessels that receive lymph from capillaries empty into one of two terminal ducts: The *thoracic duct* serves the upper left side and all the lower parts of the body and ends in the left subclavian vein. The right *lymphatic duct* drains the rest of the body and empties into the right subclavian vein. The spleen, tonsils, and thymus are also a part of the lymphatic system. Basically, the functions of the lymph are:

1. To reach parts of the body not reached by the blood and to carry on an interchange with the blood.
2. To carry nourishment from the blood to the body cells.
3. To act as a body defense against invading bacteria and toxins.
4. To remove waste material from the body cells to the blood.

The body is made up of approximately two-thirds liquid, and all tissues are bathed in lymph to nourish the cells. The lymphatic system is also the system that fights infections by ridding the body of toxic wastes. It filters and returns tissue fluid to the bloodstream. In general, lymph carries on a constant interchange with the blood. Lymph nodes when inflamed can be felt beneath the skin. Correct massage can increase lymphatic circulation and clear the lymph spaces as well as drain sluggish lymph nodes.

**Lymph Glands or Nodes**

Lymph glands or nodes are made of *lymphoid tissue,* oval or rounded masses from the size of a pin head to an inch in length and resemble the shape of a bean. Lymph nodes are usually massed in groups of two or more. An indented area called the *hilus* serves as the exit for lymph vessels carrying lymph out of nodes. Lymph nodes are placed along the course of the lymphatics. They serve to filter and to neutralize harmful bacteria and toxic matter from the lymph, thereby preventing the spread of infection to other parts of the body.

Lymph nodes are found in the following regions of the body:

1. Back of the head, draining the scalp.
2. Around the neck muscles, draining the back of the tongue, pharynx, nasal cavities, and the roof of the mouth.
3. Under the floor of the jaw, draining the floor of the mouth.
4. Upper extremities, in the bend of elbow, under the armpit, and under the pectoral muscle.
5. Abdomen and pelvis, along the blood vessels in these regions.
6. Lower extremities, in back of the knee and the groin.

Regional lymph nodes are named according to where they are located in the body:

| NODE | LOCATION |
|---|---|
| Submandibular | Beneath the mandible |
| Occipital | Base of the skull |
| Axillary | Armpit |
| Inguinals | Groin |
| Supratrochlear | Elbow |
| Popliteal | Behind the knee |
| Mammary | Breast |
| Femoral | Thigh |
| Tibial | Leg |
| Cervical | Neck |

It is believed that healthy cells are dependent upon lymph circulation and that lymph stagnation causes degeneration of cells. The purpose of lymph drainage is to cleanse and regenerate the tissues and organs of the body. Massage activates the formation of lymphocytes that produce antibodies and increase the body's resistance to infection.

## The Lymphatic System and Lymphatic Ducts

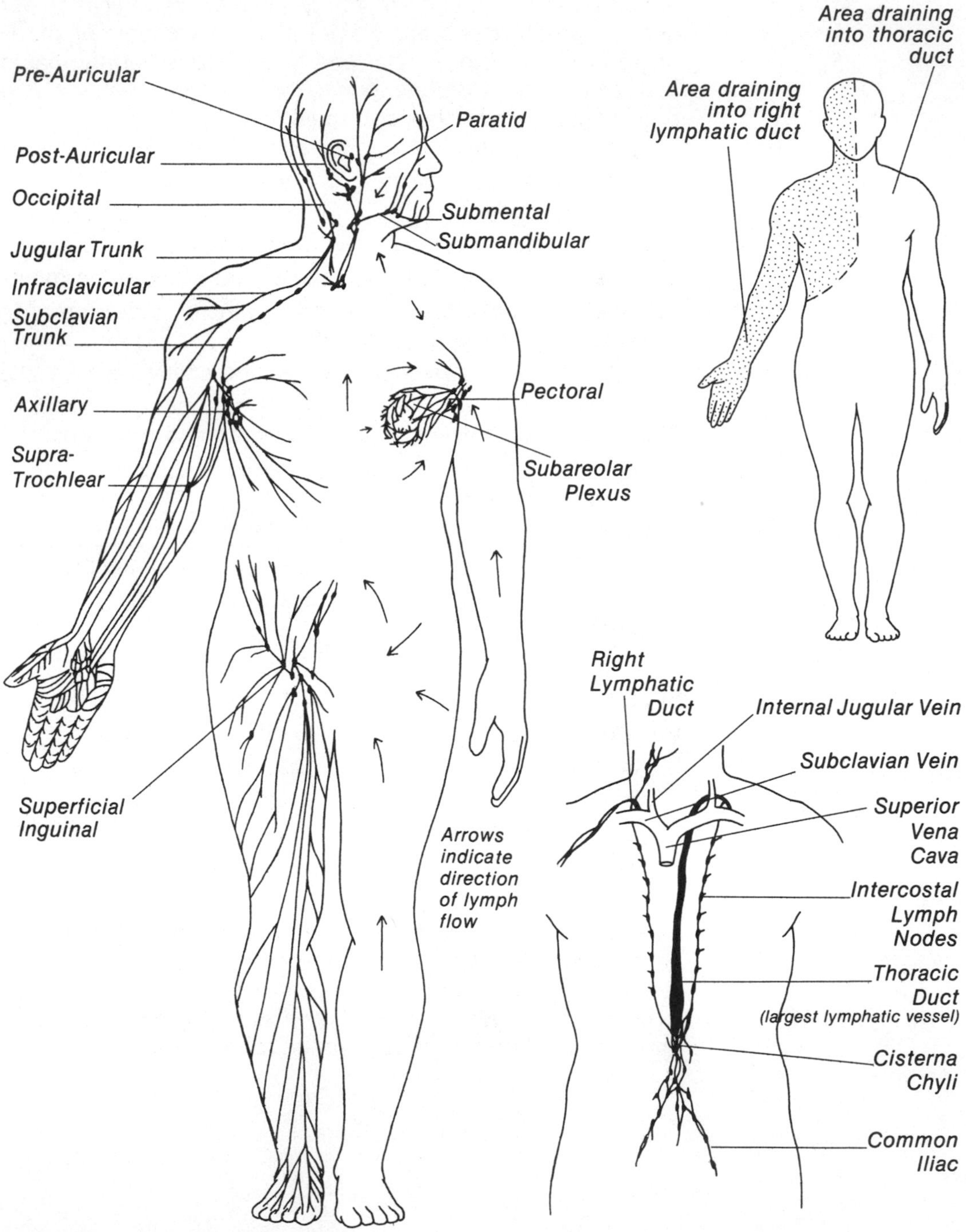

Pre-Auricular
Post-Auricular
Occipital
Jugular Trunk
Infraclavicular
Subclavian Trunk
Axillary
Supra-Trochlear
Superficial Inguinal
Paratid
Submental
Submandibular
Pectoral
Subareolar Plexus
Arrows indicate direction of lymph flow

Area draining into thoracic duct
Area draining into right lymphatic duct

Right Lymphatic Duct
Internal Jugular Vein
Subclavian Vein
Superior Vena Cava
Intercostal Lymph Nodes
Thoracic Duct (largest lymphatic vessel)
Cisterna Chyli
Common Iliac

- *Major locations of lymph nodes*
- *Lymphatic vessels are named according to their location*

**QUESTIONS FOR DISCUSSION AND REVIEW**

1. What is the major function of the lymph-vascular system?
2. What is the major function of the lymph glands or nodes?
3. Which regions of the body contain lymph nodes?
4. Name the important parts of the lymph-vascular system.
5. From what source is lymph derived?
6. Into which blood does the lymph return?
7. What is meant by lymph drainage?
8. What are lacteals?
9. Of what value is massage to the health of the lymphatic system?
10. What determines names of lymphatics?

**ANSWERS TO QUESTIONS FOR DISCUSSION AND REVIEW**

1. The function of the lymph vascular system is to reach parts of the body not reached by blood and to carry on an interchange with the blood.
2. The lymph glands filter harmful bacteria and toxic matter from the lymph.
3. The parts of the body containing lymph nodes are the back of the head, around the neck muscles, under the armpit, under pectoral muscles, along the blood vessels of the abdomen and pelvis, the back of the knees and the groin.
4. Lymph spaces, lymphatics, lymph glands, and lacteals are the main parts of the lymph-vascular system.
5. Lymph is derived from blood plasma.
6. Lymph returns to venous blood.
7. Lymph drainage is draining of lymph fluids from various areas of the body.
8. The lacteals are lymphatic vessels that carry chyle from the small intestine to the thoracic duct.
9. Massage increases flow of lymph and prevents stagnation.
10. Lymphatics are named according to their location in the body.

## SYSTEM SEVEN THE DIGESTIVE SYSTEM

Food undergoes many changes before it is finally digested, absorbed into the blood, and carried to the cells for nourishment.

The process of digestion changes the food into a fluid capable of being absorbed into the blood. Digestion is accomplished through physical and chemical means. The physical means are the teeth and involuntary muscles, which mix the food with digestive juices and propel it through the intestinal canal.

The mouth, called the *oral cavity,* prepares the food for entrance into the stomach. In the mouth the food is masticated by the teeth and mixed by the tongue with the salivary secretion. Saliva contains enzymes that digest starches to the sugar stage through the process of mastication (chewing) and deglutition (swallowing). After food enters the stomach, it is churned with gastric juices, containing an acid and protein-digesting enzyme. From the stomach the food passes into the small intestines by contractions of the intestinal walls. This is called *peristaltic action.*

The small intestine consists of three united parts: the *duodenum, jejunum,* and *ileum.* Various enzymes secreted by the liver, pancreas, and small intestine complete this part of the process. The blood vessels and the lacteals absorb the end products of digestion, which pass through the intestinal wall and are carried by the blood to the liver before entering the systemic circulation. The small intestine (duodenum) is the longest part of the alimentary canal. It is about 20 feet long and is lined with small fingerlike projections within the walls called *villi,* to move the contents along and to greatly increase the surface area available for absorption.

The chemical agents, *enzymes,* are contained in the digestive secretions and can break down complex food substances into simpler materials fit to be used by the body.

Once the digestive processes have been completed in the small intestine, the waste (unusable) materials (water and solids) moves through the iliocecal valve into a small pouchlike part of the large intestine called the *cecum.* Then they pass into the large intestine, the *colon.* The colon ascends into the abdominal cavity and forms the *transverse colon.* It continues downward to become the *descending colon.* This part of the intestine forms an S shape to form the *sigmoid colon,* which empties into the rectum. The *rectum* is a temporary storage area for waste. The distal part of the large intestine is the anal canal, which ends with the anus from which fecal matter is expelled.

## The Digestive System

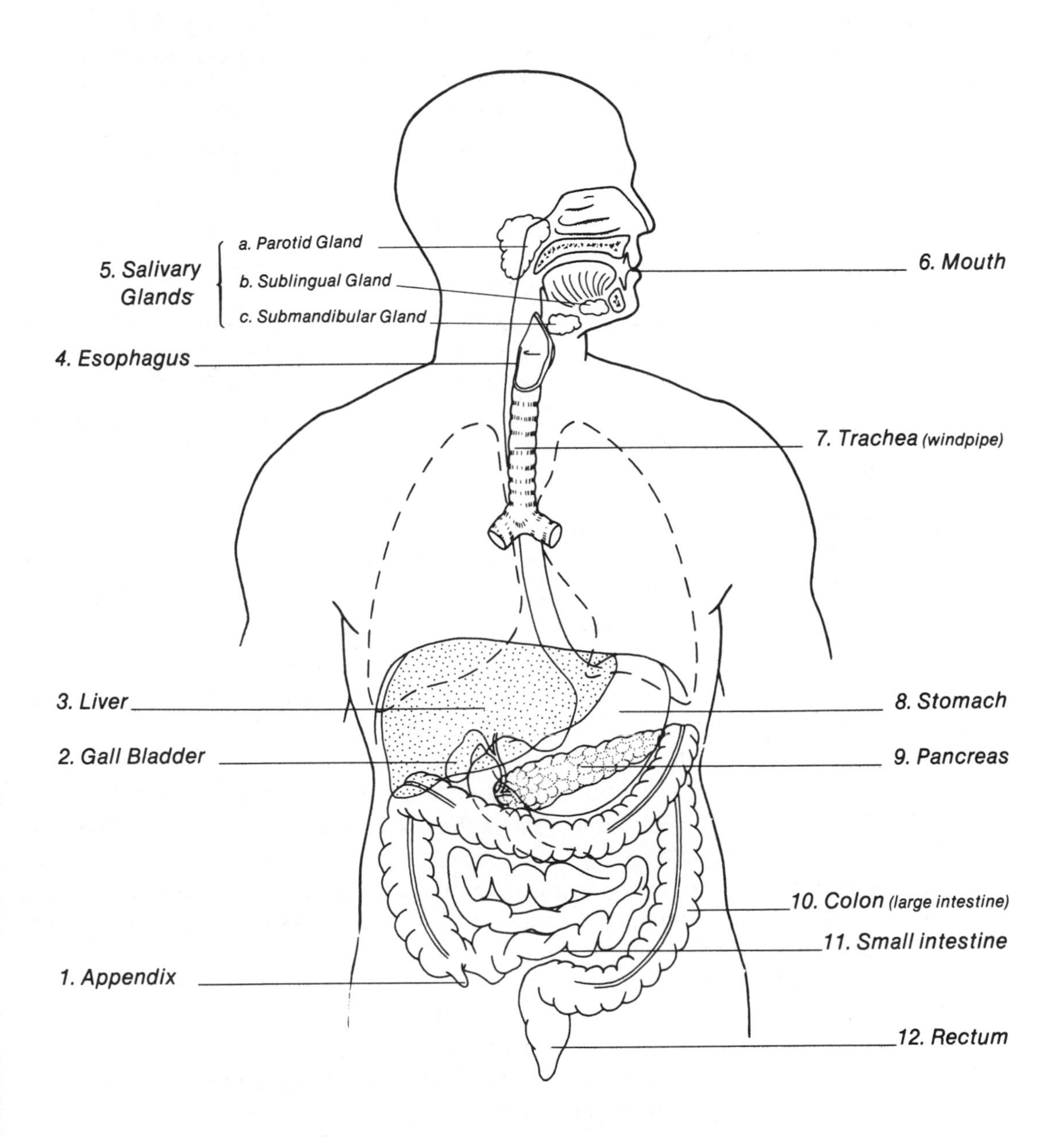


**1.** A narrow tube attached to the cecum, a part of the colon. **2.** The gal! bladder is located on the underside of the liver. It receives bile from liver and expels the bile (as needed) into the duodenum. **3.** Produces bile, which acts as fat solvent. The largest gland of the body, the liver functions to maintain and regulate homeostasis of body fluids and help to control body processes. **4.** Moves food to the stomach.
**5.** Buccal glands. **5a.** Located under and in front of ear. **5b.** Located below the jaw and under the tongue. **5c.** Located in floor of mouth beneath the tongue. **6.** Principal functions of mouth and salivary glands are mastication and changing starch to sugar. **7.** Windpipe (respiratory tract). **8.** Serves as a receptacle for food; manufactures gastric juice during digestion. **9.** Lies behind the stomach and produces enzymes which act on fat, proteins, starch and carbohydrates to complete the digestive process. Aids in regulation of glucose metabolism.
**10.** Responsible for absorption and elimination of foodstuffs. **11.** Serves in the absorption and elimination of foodstuffs.
**12.** Serves to eliminate waste.

**Glands, Digestive Juices, and Enzymes**

| GLANDS AND JUICE | LOCATION | ENZYMES | CHANGES IN FOOD |
|---|---|---|---|
| Saliva (3)<br>Salivary gland | Mouth | Salivary<br>Amalase<br>(ptyalin) | Begins digestion of starch into simple sugars |
| Gastric juice<br>Stomach | Stomach wall | Pepsin | Begins digestion of protein into amino acids |
| Pancreatic juice<br>Pancreas | Small intestine | Amalase<br>Trypsin<br>Lipase | Starches, proteins, fats |
| Juice from small intestine | Small intestine | Lactase<br>Maltase<br>Sucrase | Breaks down complex carbohydrates to simple sugars |
| Bile from liver | Small intestine | No enzymes | Breaks down fats into fatty acids |

**QUESTIONS FOR DISCUSSION AND REVIEW**

1. Which structures are involved in digestion?
2. What is the function of digestion?
3. Which chemical agents in the digestive juices aid digestion?
4. What digestive changes occur in the mouth?
5. What digestive changes occur in the stomach?
6. Which glands supply digestive secretions to the small intestine?
7. What digestive changes occur in the small intestine?
8. Which structures absorb the end products of digestion?
9. From which organ is the undigested food eliminated from the body?

**ANSWERS TO QUESTIONS FOR DISCUSSION AND REVIEW**

1. Digestion involves the mouth, tongue, teeth, salivary glands, stomach, gastric glands, small intestine, liver, gallbladder, and pancreas.
2. Digestion changes food into a fluid capable of being absorbed into the blood.
3. Enzymes aid digestion.
4. Food is chewed and mixed with saliva. Starches are digested to the sugar stage.
5. Food is mixed with gastric juice. Protein foods are digested.
6. Liver, pancreas, and glands in the small intestine.
7. Food is completely digested.
8. The blood vessels and lacteals in villi in the walls of the small intestine.
9. The rectum of the large intestine.

## SYSTEM EIGHT THE RESPIRATORY SYSTEM

To carry on the vital processes of cells, the body requires a continual supply of oxygen and the removal of carbon dioxide from the blood. The needs of the body in these respects are fulfilled by the respiratory system.

The respiratory system includes the air passages, nose, mouth, pharynx, trachea, and bronchial tubes, which lead to the lungs. The lungs are composed of spongy tissue and microscopic air sacs. A network of very fine capillaries bring the blood in close contact with thin walls of air sacs.

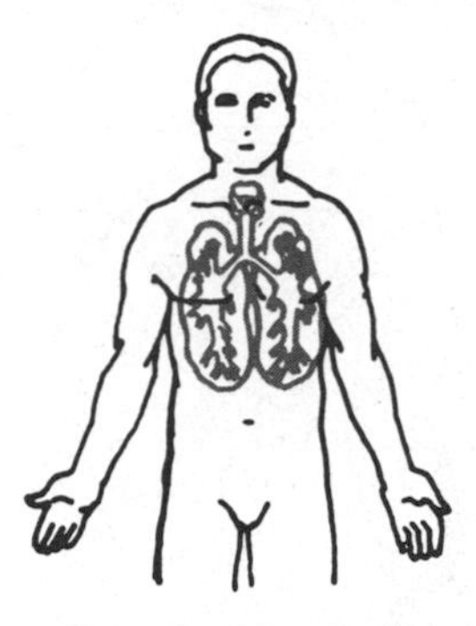

*The Respiratory System*

*Respiration* is the act of inhaling and exhaling air, resulting in an exchange of gases between the blood and air sacs. With each inhalation, the chest expands and the diaphragm is pulled down, causing the lungs to draw in air. During exhalation, the chest contracts and the diaphragm is drawn up, forcing the air out of the lungs. The maximum intake of oxygen and expulsion of carbon doxide is accomplished during deep breathing, which involves movements of both the ribs and diaphragm.

Depending on the individual's lung capacity, the natural rate of breathing for an adult is between 14 and 18 times a minute. The rate of breathing is increased by muscular activity.

From the nose, air passes in the nasal pharynx, which has three parts: *nasal, oral,* and *laryngeal.* The *eustachian* (auditory) tube extends from the pharynx to the middle ear and helps to equalize the pressure in the ear with the pressure of the atmosphere.

The *pharyngeal tonsil* is located in the posterior part of the masopharynx and helps to protect the body from infection. The *larynx* or voice box forms the laryngeal prominance, commonly called the *Adam's apple.* The *epiglottis* is a leaf-shaped cartilage that covers the entrance to the larynx during swallowing.

A healthy respiratory system is maintained by avoidance of air pollution, working with chemicals, and smoking. Deep breathing, regular exercise, and a healthy diet all help to keep the respiratory system functioning normally. Should the massage practitioner notice that a client has trouble breathing normally, it is wise to suggest that the client see a physician. There is a great deal more to the respiratory system than has been covered in this brief overview. Study the illustration of the respiratory system to be sure you understand the location of major parts.

## The Respiratory System

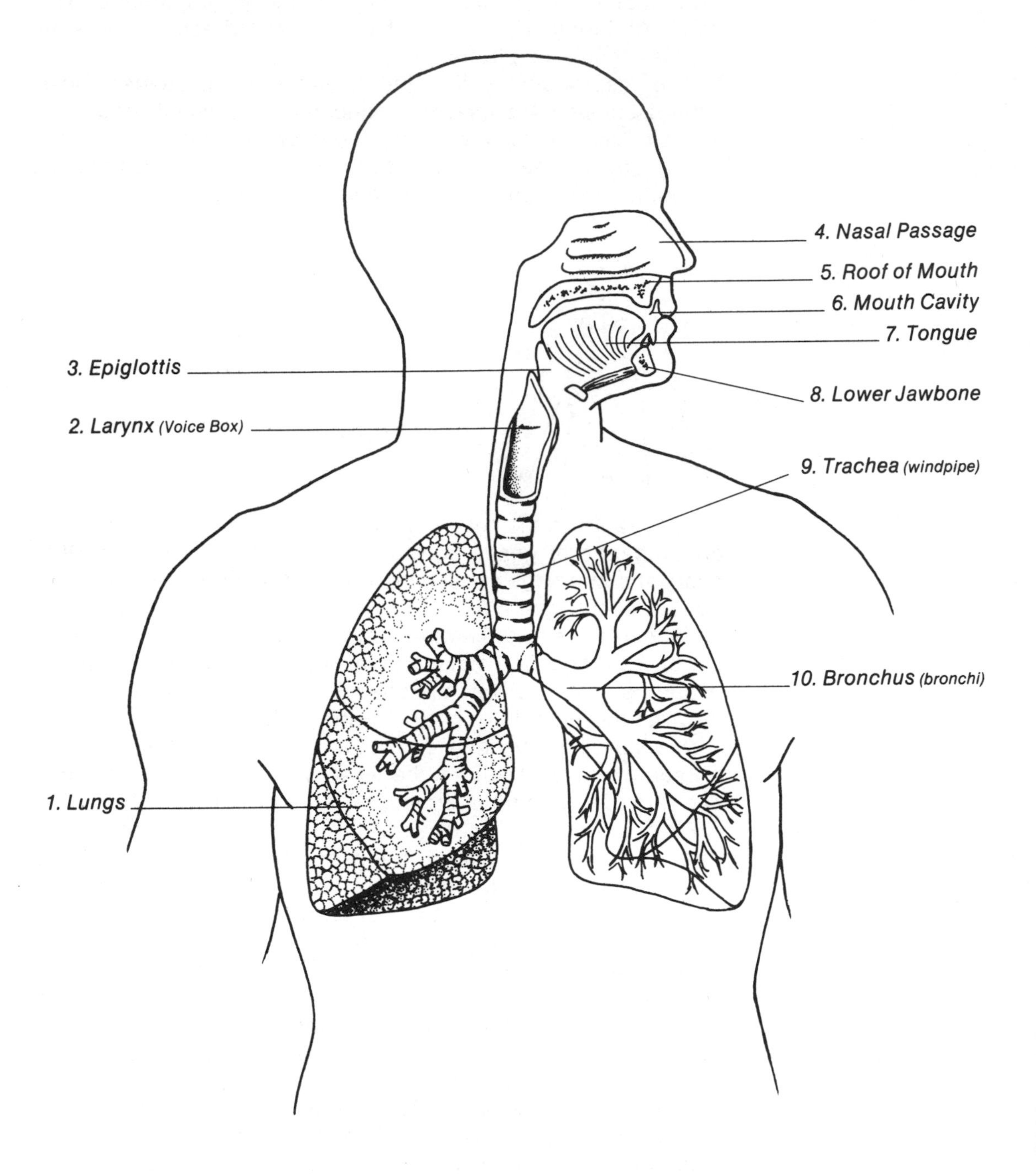


**1.** Organs of external respiration located in lateral chambers of the thoracic cavity and consisting of three right and two left lobes. **2.** Situated between the tongue and trachea. Functions in production of vocal sounds. **3.** Forms part of larynx and assists in swallowing. **4.**Air passage extending from nostrils to pharynx. **9.** Located in front of esophagus. **10.** Air tubes entering the lungs.

**QUESTIONS FOR DISCUSSION AND REVIEW**

1. What are the major organs of the respiratory system?
2. What are the functions of the respiratory system?
3. What is the physical appearance of the lungs?
4. What is the natural rate of breathing for an adult?
5. What is the diaphragm, and what function does it perform?

**ANSWERS TO QUESTIONS FOR DISCUSSION AND REVIEW**

1. The major respiratory organs are mouth and nose, trachea or windpipe, bronchial tubes and the lungs
2. During breathing, oxygen (gas) is inhaled and carbon dioxide (gas) is exhaled.
3. The lungs are two spongy sacs composed of microscopic cells into which the inhaled air penetrates.
4. The natural rate of breathing is 14 to 18 times a minute.
5. The diaphragm is a muscular sheet separating the thorax from the abdominal cavity. This helps to expand and to contract the lungs.

## SYSTEM NINE THE EXCRETORY SYSTEM

The excretory system (including the urinary system) includes the kidneys, liver, skin, intestines, and lungs. Its main function is to remove certain waste products from the blood and eliminate them from the body.

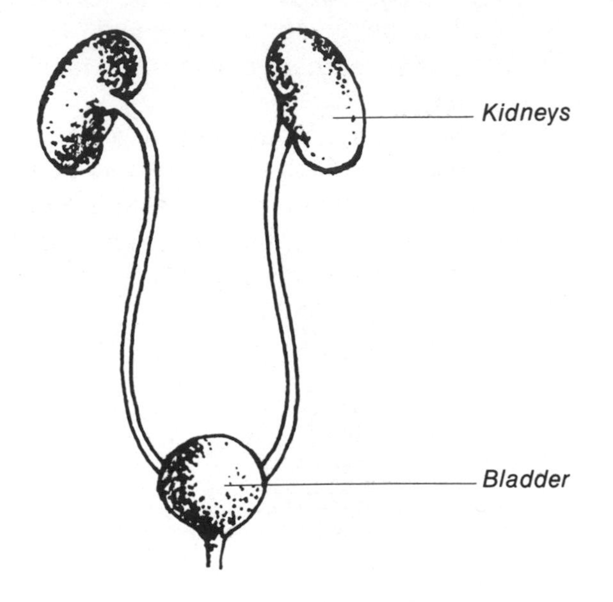


The excretory system adjusts the fluid balance of the body and helps to adjust the blood pH as follows:

1. The kidneys excrete uric acid, urea, electrolytes, and water.
2. The liver discharges bile pigments.
3. The skin eliminates perspiration and heat.
4. The large intestine discharges food wastes.
5. The lungs exhale carbon dioxide.

Cellular metabolism yields various toxic substances that if retained would have a tendency to poison the body.

**Urinary System**

The important organs of the urinary system are the kidneys and the bladder. The *kidneys* are two bean-shaped glands located between the tenth thoracic and third lumbar vertebra and kept in place by fibrous connective and fatty tissues. The *ureters* are tubes that carry urine from the kidneys to the *bladder* where the urine is stored. The emptying of the bladder is accomplished by the passage of the urine through the *urethra*. As the blood circulates through the kidneys, it gives up a certain amount of water and rejects the various end products of metabolism, such as urea, uric acid, and excess electrolytes.

A *urinalysis* is the examination of the urine and part of the routine examination given by most physicians. Normal, healthy urine is a clear yellowish fluid. A change in the color of the urine, such as a reddish or brownish color, may indicate infection or other problems.

**The Liver**

With the exception of the skin, the liver is the largest organ in the body and is situated on the upper right side of the abdomen, immediately below and in contact with the diaphragm. The liver neutralizes or detoxifies toxic substances that may have been absorbed from the intestines such as alcohol, food additives, and drugs. The liver is also the site for the destruction of red blood cells whose pigments are eliminated in the bile. Two other functions of the liver is the production of bile, which aids the digestion of fats, and the storage of glycogen, which is a reserve form of energy to be mobilized when the body needs it.

The liver functions in a great number of other metabolic processes that include changing glucose to glycogen, changing of lactic acid to glucose, production of glucose from noncarbohydrates, changing carbohydrates and protein to fats for storage, production of cholesterol lioproteins, the breaking down and reform of damaged red blood cells and other foreign substances. The liver stores vitamins A, B, and $B^{12}$ and changes potentially toxic substances into inert forms. It forms urea, which is put back into the blood stream to be excreted by the kidneys. The liver also produces and excretes bile through the intestines. *Bile* is a bitter, alkaline, yellowish-brown fluid secreted from the liver into the duodenum and contains water, bile salts, mucin, cholesterol, lechithin, and fat pigments. Bile aids in the emulsification, digestion, and absorption of fats and the alkalinization of the intestines.

**QUESTIONS FOR DISCUSSION AND REVIEW**

1. Name the five important organs of the excretory system.
2. What happens if waste products are retained within the body instead of being eliminated?
3. What is the function of the excretory system?
4. Which organ of the excretory system is the largest?
5. Why do most physicians include urinalysis as a part of a routine physical checkup?
6. Which organ of the body secretes bile?
7. Of what benefit is bile?
8. What colors of urine indicate a problem that needs checking by a physician?

**ANSWERS TO QUESTIONS FOR DISCUSSION AND REVIEW**

1. The lungs, kidneys, skin, liver, and large intestine are the five important organs of the excretory system.
2. The body will become poisoned by its own waste products.
3. The excretory system eliminates waste products that have been formed in the body.
4. The liver is the largest organ in the excretory system.
5. The color and composition of urine can indicate some existing health problem.
6. The liver secretes bile.
7. Bile aids in the emulsification, digestion, and absorption of fats and aids in alkalination of the intestines.
8. Healthy urine has a clear yellowish color. A reddish or brownish color may indicate bleeding and should be checked by a physician.

## SYSTEM TEN THE HUMAN REPRODUCTIVE SYSTEM

The reproductive system is the generative apparatus necessary for organisms to reproduce organisms of the same kind.

The reproductive system in males include the penis, testes, vans deferens, prostate gland and seminal vesicles, bulbourethal glands (Cowper's glands), and the urethra, the canal through which urine is discharged. The reproductive system in females includes the ovaries, uterine tubes (oviducts), uterus, vagina, and labia.

It is not within the scope of this book to describe in detail the entire process of human reproduction. The following is a brief summary.

Lower forms of life such as one-celled organisms do not need a partner to reproduce. They do so by nonsexual means, which is known as *asexual reproduction.*

In humans (and most animals), reproduction is sexual and requires a male and female, each having specialized sex cells. In the male these cells are called *spermatoza* and in females, *ova.*

*Gamete* is the term used to describe a reproductive cell that can unite with another gamete to form the cell (zygote) that develops into a new individual. A *zygote* is the fertilized ovum, the cell formed by the union of a spermatozoon with an ovum. A *gonad* is a sex gland; the ovary in the female and the testes in the male. *Ovulation* is the discharge of a mature ovum from the follicle of the ovary.

### The Male Reproductive System

The glands of the male reproductive system produce a secretion called semen. The secretion contains the spermatoza, the mature male germ cells. The male gonads (two testes) are located in the scrotum, a pouch supporting the testes.

The hormone testosterone is secreted by the testes and helps to maintain the reproductive structure as well as the development of the spermatoza. Spermatoza are tiny detached cells, egg shaped with a tail that enables them to swim until one unites with the ovum (egg) and accomplishes fertilization. Of the millions of spermatozoa that are ejected during copulation, only one will fertilize the reproductive cell (egg) produced by the female. The others die within a short period of time. Testosterone also aids in the development of secondary sexual characteristics in the male (body structure, hair growth). The male reproductive system also includes the following: The duct system, tubes beginning inside the testes that carry spermatoza. The epididymis, located in the scrotum that serves as the storage place for spermatoza. This tube extends upward to become two vans deferens (ductus deferens) and continues through a small canal behind the abdominal wall and behind the urinary bladder. The vans deferens join with the ducts of the seminal vesicles to form the ejaculatory ducts. These two ducts enter the prostate gland where they empty into the urethra.

***The Seminal Vesicles***

Seminal vesicles are two branched, secular, glandular diverticula of each ductus deferens. Each duct unites to form the ejaculatory duct. The seminal fluid forms most of the semen when it is expelled.

***The Prostate Glands***

The prostate gland lies below the urinary bladder. Ducts from the prostate enter the ejaculatory ducts. The prostate gland is supplied with muscular tissue that is involved in the expulsion of the semen.

***The Cowper's or Bulbourethral Glands***

The Cowper's (Bulbourethral) glands are two pea sized glands located beneath the prostate gland. They are the largest of the mucus producing glands and serve to lubricate the urethra.

***Urethra***

The urethra serves to convey urine from the bladder and to carry reproductive cells and secretions to the outside.

***Penis***

The penis is the male organ of copulation consisting of erectile tissue.

**The Female Reproductive System**

The vulva forms the external part of the female reproductive system. It includes the outer lips called the labia majora and the inner, smaller lips called the labia minora. Within the vulva is a fold of connective tissue, the hymen, that partially covers the external orifice of the vagina. The word vagina means sheath. This is a muscular tube or canal leading from the vulva opening to the cervix, and is the lower part of the birth canal. Near the vestibule of the vagina are mucus producing glands called Bartholen's glands. The clitoris is a small sensitive body of erective tissue located beneath the mons pubis.

***The Female Internal Organs***

The ovaries (female gonads) are a pair of glandular organs located within the pelvic area. The ovum is the egg cell capable of being fertilized by a spermatoza and developing into a new life. The ovaducts, also called uterine or fallopian tubes are the egg carrying tubes of the female reproductive system. They extend from near the ovaries to the uterus. Ova are carried into the ovaducts by the action of fibril, which produce a current in the peritoneal fluid. The uterus is a pear-shaped, muscular organ consisting of an upper portion, the body, the cervix or neck.

During each menstrual cycle (the periodically recurring series of changes that take place in the ovaries, uterus, and related structures in the female), a follicle develops in the ovary and produces estrogen (female hormone) as the ovum (egg) matures. Meanwhile the uterus is being prepared by thickening of the lining for possible pregnancy. A hormone from the pituitary gland, called luteinzing hormone, transforms the follicle linto the corpus luteum. This is a yellowish endocrine body formed in the ovary which produces estrogen and progesterone. The ovum travels down the ovaduct to the uterus. If the ovum (egg) is fertilized, pregnancy results. If the ovum is not fertilized, the lining that has been built up sloughs off, and is expelled along with the menstrual blood and secretions.

Menstruation is the cyclic, physiologic uterine bleeding which normally occurs at about four week intervals (except during pregnancy) during the reproductive period of the human female. It begins at puberty and continues until menopause which occurs at about ages 45 to 55. Menopause is the physiological cessation of menstruation, therefore the end of childbearing.

Pregnancy is the state or condition of being pregnant from the time of conception to childbirth. The duration of pregnancy in women is approximately 280 days. Embryology is the study of the embryo, the early, developing stage of the living organism. Embryonic life begins at conception, with the fertilization of the ovum, and is sustained by the placenta where it grows within the amniotic sac within the mother's body.

From the beginning of the third month of pregnancy until birth, the developing child is called a fetus. During pregnancy the mother's metabolism changes owing to the demands made on her body systems. Her lungs must provide more oxygen and her heart must pump more blood. The kidneys must excrete nitrogenous wastes from the fetus and the mother's body.

During pregnancy, the mother needs proper nutrition to provide for the growth of the fetus as well as to maintain the health of all organs as the body is prepared for labor and birth.

Following the birth of the child, the mother should maintain her health, and that of her child by attention to nutritional needs, and by specific exercises to tone and strengthen her muscles.

**The Endocrine System**

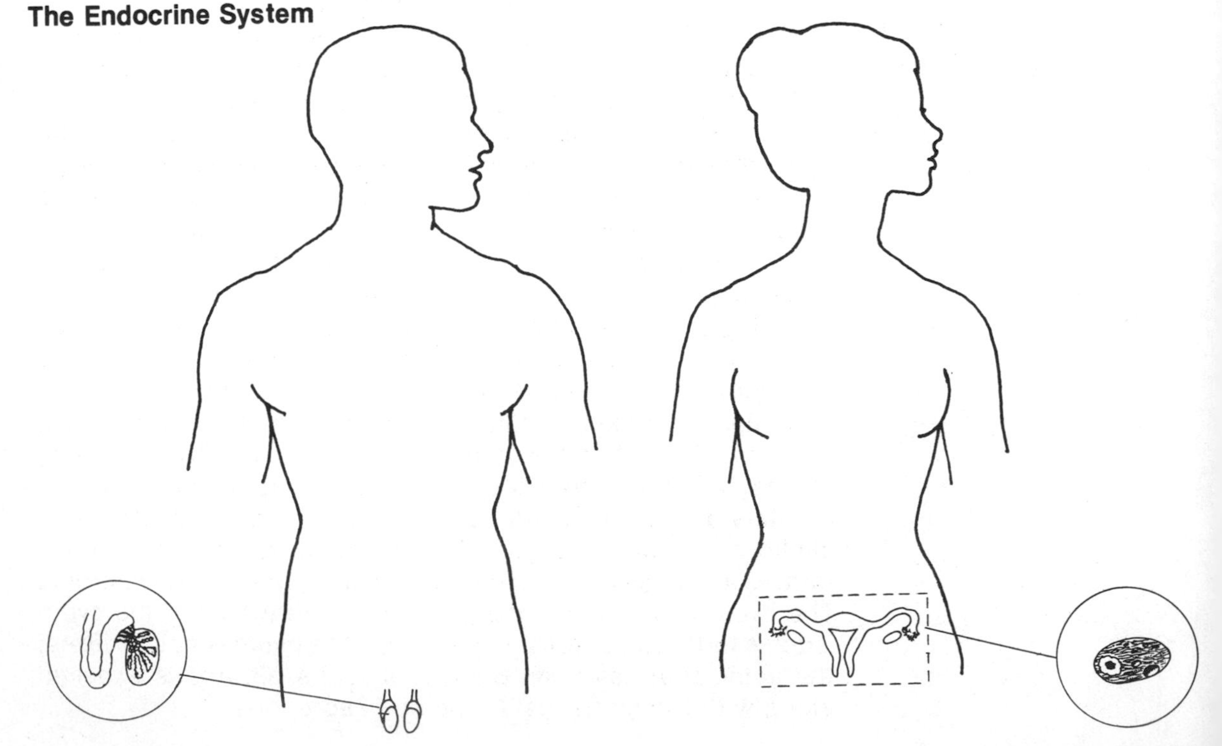

*Testes (in male)*

*Ovary (in female)*

**QUESTIONS FOR DISCUSSION AND REVIEW**

1. What is the reproductive system?
2. What is a gonad?
3. What is the difference between an embryo and a fetus?
4. What is the difference between asexual and sexual reproduction?
5. What is ovulation?
6. What is a zygote?
7. What is the approximate duration of pregnancy in women?
8. When does embryonic life begin?

**ANSWERS TO QUESTIONS FOR DISCUSSION AND REVIEW**

1. The reproductive system is the generative apparatus necessary for organisms to reproduce organisms of the same kind or species.
2. A gonad is a sex gland, the ovary in the female and the testes in the male.
3. From the beginning of conception until approximately the third month of pregnancy the developing child is called an embryo. After that time it is called a fetus.
4. Asexual reproduction as in some one-celled organisms means that no partner is needed to reproduce. In humans and animals reproduction is sexual and requires a male and female to reproduce.
5. Ovulation is the discharge of a mature egg cell from the follicle of the ovary.
6. A zygote is the fertilized ovum, the cell formed by the union of a spermatozoon (sperm) with the ovum (egg).
7. Pregnancy lasts approximately 280 days.
8. Embryonic life begins with conception.

# PART III PREPARATION FOR MASSAGE

# Chapter 6 Sanitary Practices

**LEARNING OBJECTIVES**

After you have mastered this chapter, you will be able to:

1. Explain the need for laws that enforce the strict practice of sanitation.
2. Sanitize and sterilize implements and other items used in massage procedures.
3. Explain the difference between pathogenic and non-pathogenic bacteria.
4. Explain the importance of cleanliness of person and of surroundings as protection against the spread of disease.
5. Explain how various disinfectants, antiseptics, and other products are used most effectively.
6. Explain how various types of sanitizing equipment such as wet and dry sanitizers and ultraviolet rays are used.

**INTRODUCTION**

In more recent years great progress has been made in the control and prevention of disease. In the medical profession sanitation and sterilization are required procedures that are taken for granted. Every state has laws that make the practice of sanitation and sterilization mandatory for the protection of public health. In the personal service professions, every precaution must be taken to protect the health of clients as well as the health of practitioners. The nature of the personal service business determines the procedures for the extent of sanitation and sterilization. For example, in the cosmetology profession, a comb or brush used on one client may not be used on another until it has been thoroughly cleansed and sterilized. The esthetician (skin care specialist) must apply products only with sterilized applicators. The massage practitioner may not use the same kinds of implements or have need for the same sanitation procedures, however, appropriate and recommended procedures must be followed diligently.

The massage practitioner need not be a biologist to have some understanding of bacteriology and to be aware of the importance of impeccable cleanliness at all times. Contagious diseases, skin infections, and other problems can be caused by the transfer of infectious material by unclean hands and nails and by unsanitary equipment and supplies. Therefore, the primary concern is that any item (linens, apparatus) that comes in contact with the client is clean and sanitary. The practitioner's hands must be sanitized by washing with soap and warm water and rinsed with alcohol before touching each client. The premises must also be clean at all times.

## PATHS OF DISEASE AND INFECTION

*Bacteria* are minute, unicellular microorganisms exhibiting both plant and animal characteristics. They are also called *germs* or *microbes* and are most numerous in dirt, refuse, unclean water, and diseased tissues. Bacteria exist on the skin, in the air, in body secretions, underneath the free edges of the nails, and elsewhere. There are hundreds of different kinds of bacteria that can only be seen under a microscope. Bacteria are classified as either *nonpathogenic* (harmless) or *pathogenic* (harmful). Nonpathogenic bacteria, the beneficial and harmless type is the most numerous and performs useful functions, such as aiding the digestive process and other bodily functions. The saprophytes are an example of nonpathogenic bacteria.
Pathogenic bacteria, though not as numerous, are of greater concern to us because they produce disease. Parasites belong to this group because they require living matter for their growth and reproduction. We are primarily concerned with understanding and identifying pathogenic bacteria in order to deal with them more effectively. The following chart shows the three general forms of bacteria: *cocci, bacilli,* and *spirilla.* To the right of the name and shape of the bacteria are listed the types of bacteria and the common diseases or conditions with which they are associated.

Pathogenic bacteria become a menace to health when they are able to invade the body. Immunity is the ability to resist infection by harmful bacteria once they have entered the body. Healthy people are able to resist infection better than those with low resistance. Healthy skin is one of the body's most important defenses against invasion of harmful bacteria. Fine hairs in the nostrils, mucous membranes, and tears in the eyes also help to defend against bacteria. Inflammation (redness and swelling) is a sign that white blood cells (corpuscles) are working to destroy harmful microorganisms in the bloodstream. The body also produces antibodies, which inhibit or destroy harmful bacteria. *Antibodies* are any of a class of proteins produced in the body in response to contact with antigen (toxin, enzymes, etc.) that serve to immunize the body against specific antigens.

A *virus* is defined as any of a class of submicroscopic pathogenic agents that are capable of transmitting disease. A virulent substance has the power to invade tissues and to generate harmful toxins.

The massage practitioner must refuse to perform a service for a client who has a contagious disease or infection and suggest that the client see a physician. The practitioner also has a duty to protect his or her own health. For example, the practitioner's hands may pick up bacteria from the client's skin. If the hands are not cleaned, bacteria can be spread.

The best protection against the spread of disease is to keep yourself and your surroundings clean. To maintain high standards of cleanliness requires constant supervision. Board of health regulations should be observed in maintaining clean massage facilities at all times.

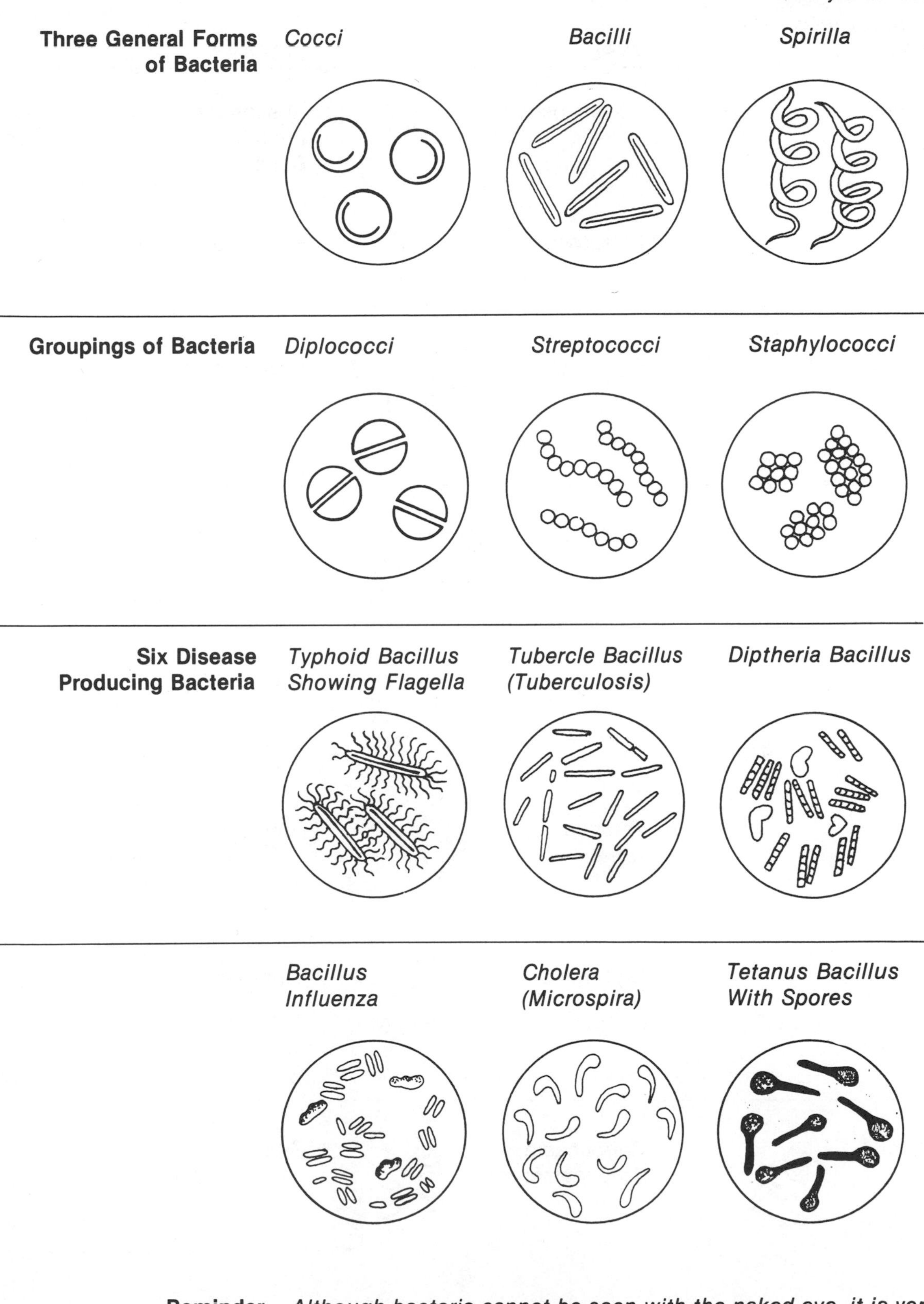


**Reminder** *Although bacteria cannot be seen with the naked eye, it is very important to practice cleanliness and sanitation at all times, to prevent the spread of contagious disease.*

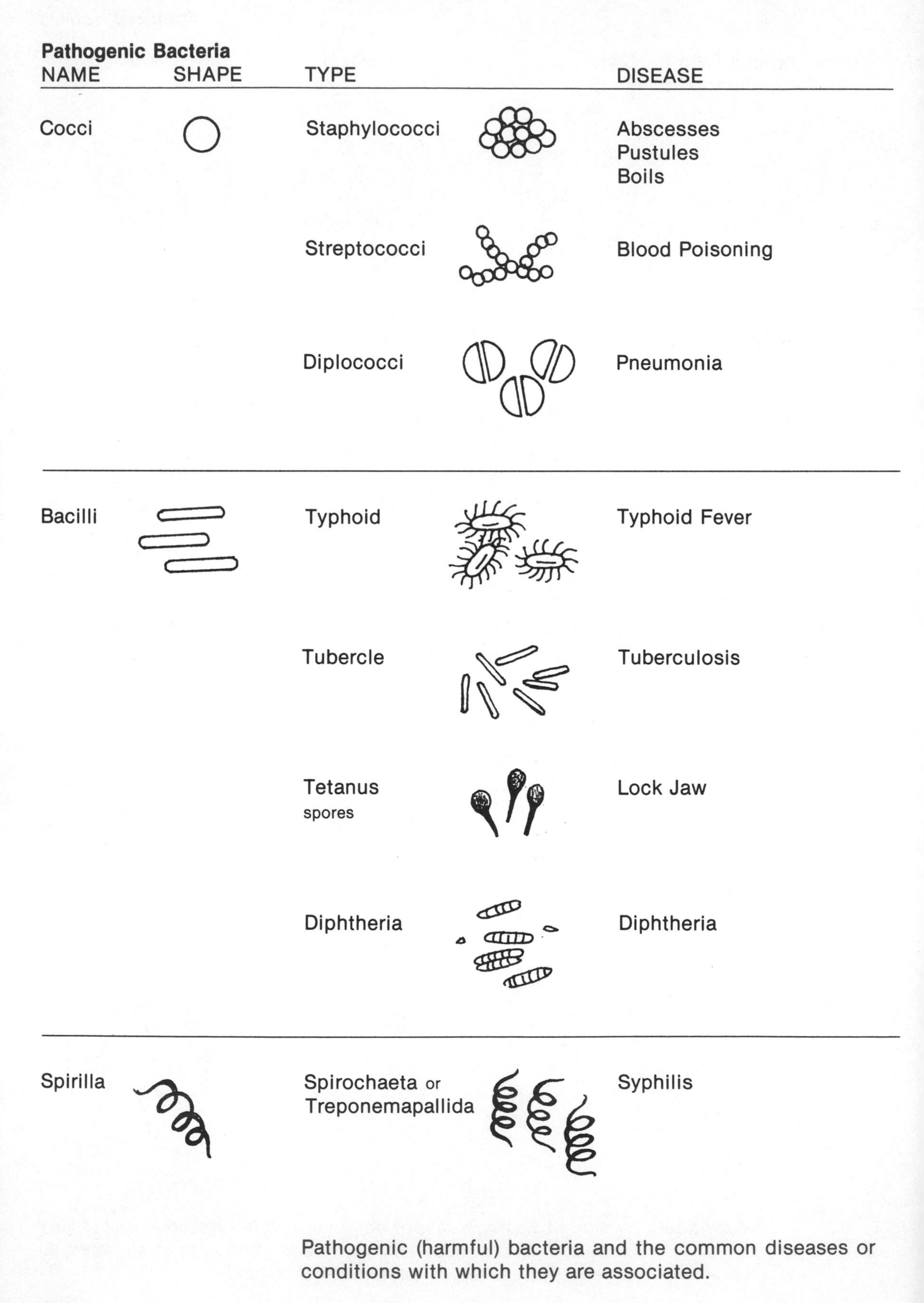

**Pathogenic Bacteria**

| NAME | SHAPE | TYPE | DISEASE |
|---|---|---|---|
| Cocci | | Staphylococci | Abscesses<br>Pustules<br>Boils |
| | | Streptococci | Blood Poisoning |
| | | Diplococci | Pneumonia |
| Bacilli | | Typhoid | Typhoid Fever |
| | | Tubercle | Tuberculosis |
| | | Tetanus<br>spores | Lock Jaw |
| | | Diphtheria | Diphtheria |
| Spirilla | | Spirochaeta or<br>Treponemapallida | Syphilis |

Pathogenic (harmful) bacteria and the common diseases or conditions with which they are associated.

## MAINTAINING SANITARY CONDITIONS

It is important to keep the salon or work area, dispensary, implements, and equipment in a sanitary condition. Supplies such as towels, blankets, and sheets should be clean and fresh for each client. Disposable products such as towels and sheets may be used and fresh ones supplied for each client.

Commercially designed cabinet sanitizers and ultraviolet-ray cabinets are convenient for keeping small implements, such as manicuring or pedicuring implements, sanitized until ready for use. Physical agents are:

*Moist heat.* This is the method of boiling objects in water at 212° degrees Fahrenheit (100°C) for about 20 minutes. A vessel known as an *autoclave* is sometimes used in the medical field for sterilization purposes.

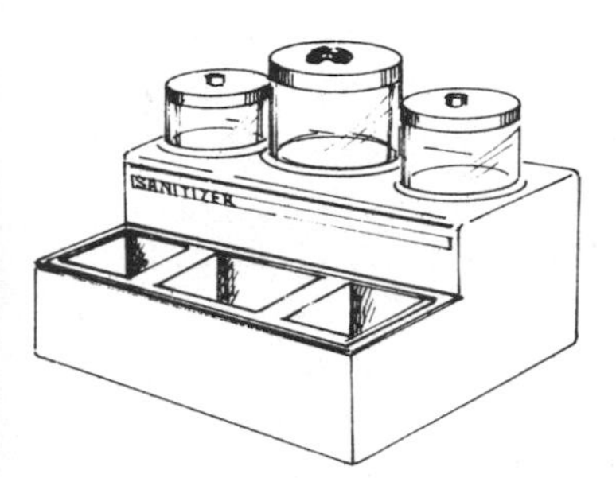


*Ultra Violet Ray Sanitizer*

*Dry heat:* This is a baking method that is also effective. Objects are placed in a dry cabinet sanitizer, and a small tray at the bottom of the cabinet is used to place a fumigant such as borax formalin.

*Ultraviolet-ray electrical sanitizers:* These are used to sanitize implements. Some implements can be washed with hot water and soap, immersed in alcohol, wiped dry, and then placed in a sterile container until needed.

Although the massage practitioner may not use a wide range of mechanical aids or electrical equipment, anything from body brushes to toenail clippers must be kept sanitized. There are disinfectants, antiseptics, and fumigants that kill or retard the growth of bacteria. Some are commercially prepared, economical to use, and quick acting. General antiseptics are alcohol, formalin, hydrogen peroxide, sodium hypochlorite, and boric acid. Disinfectants are stronger than antiseptics.

### Sanitizers

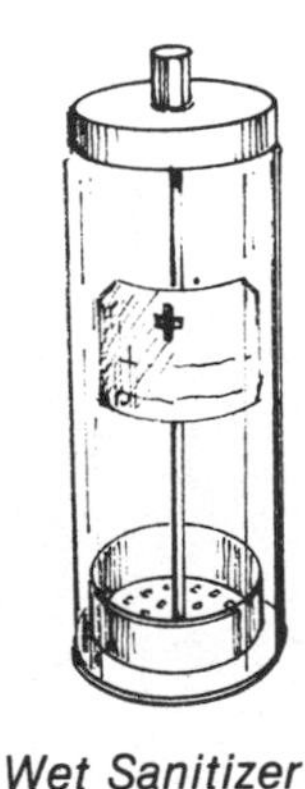

*Wet Sanitizer*

A *wet sanitizer* is any receptacle large enough to hold a disinfectant solution in which the objects to be sanitized can be completely immersed. A cover is provided to prevent contamination of the solution. Wet sanitizers can be obtained in various sizes and shapes.

Before immersing objects such as hand brushes in a wet sanitizer, be sure to:

Wash them thoroughly with hot water and soap.

Rinse them thoroughly with clear water.

This procedure prevents contamination of the solution. In addition, soap and hot water remove most of the bacteria.

After items are removed from the disinfectant solution, they should be rinsed in clean water, wiped dry with a clean towel, and stored in a dry or cabinet sanitizer until needed.

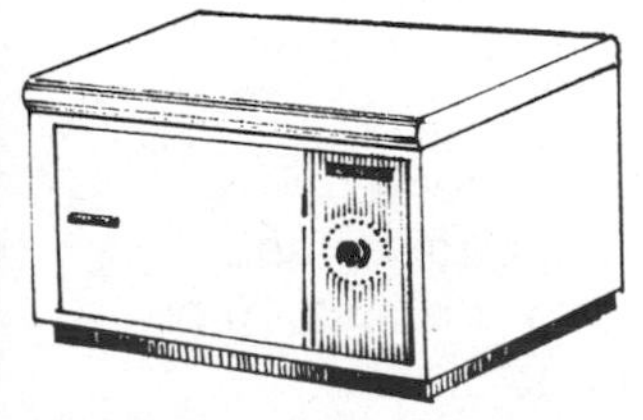

*Dry Cabinet Sanitizer*

A *dry* or *cabinet sanitizer* is an airtight cabinet containing an active fumigant. Sanitized implements are kept clean in the cabinet until needed.

Ultraviolet-ray electrical sanitizers are effective for keeping brushes and implements, such as manicuring and pedicuring tools, clean until ready for use. Implements must be sanitized before they are placed in the ultraviolet cabinet. Follow the manufacturer's directions for proper use.

**Disinfectants** Some disinfectants in general use are:

Quaternary ammonium compounds (quats).

Ethyl or grain alcohol.

Formalin.

*Quaternary ammonium compounds:* These are available in tablet or liquid form under different trade names. The advantages claimed for these disinfectants are short disinfection time, non-toxic, odorless and colorless, and stable. A 1:1000 solution is commonly used to sanitize implements. Immersion time ranges from 1-5 minutes, depending on the strength of the solution used. Implements such as manicuring and pedicuring tools, tweezers and spatulas can be immersed in this type of solution.

*Ethyl or grain alcohol:* This comes in liquid form. Electrodes and like implements can be sanitized in 70 percent solution.

*Formalin:* This is a safe and effective sanitizing agent which can be used as either an antiseptic or disinfectant. It is composed of 37 to 40 percent formaldehyde gas in water. A 25 percent solution is generally used for brushes. They are immersed for about 10 minutes. This preparation is 2 parts formalin, 5 parts water, and 1 part glycerine. The glycerine keeps metal from rusting. A 2 percent formalin solution can also be an effective sanitizing solution for the hands.

It is important to read directions on all containers when mixing any sanitizing agent.

**Approved Chemicals**

| NAME | FORM | STRENGTH | HOW TO USE |
|---|---|---|---|
| Sodium Hypochlorite (household bleach) | Liquid | 10% solution | Immerse implements in solution for 10 or more minutes. |
| Quaternary Ammonium Compounds | Liquid or tablet | 1:1000 solution | Immerse implements in solution for 20 or more minutes. |
| Formalin | Liquid | 25% solution | Immerse implements in solution for 10 or more minutes. |
| Formalin | Liquid | 10% solution | Immerse implements in solution for 20 or more minutes. |
| Alcohol | Liquid | 70% solution | Immerse implements or sanitize electrodes and sharp cutting edges 10 or more minutes. |

*Creosol or lysol:* (5—10 percent) can be used for the cleaning of floors, sinks, restrooms, etc. Commercially prepared solutions are available.

When in doubt about antiseptics and disinfectants approved for use in your salon or work area, consult your local health department or state board of health.

**SUMMARY OF PRECAUTIONS**

1. Keep yourself and your clothing clean.
2. Wash and sanitize your hands with soap, warm water, and mild alcohol before and after every client. A good hand brush should be used for scrubbing, particularly around the nails, then the hands should be rinsed with mild alcohol and wiped dry.
3. Keep all products, implements, and areas used during massage in a sanitary condition. This includes surfaces where items are placed.
4. Keep supplies (oils, lotions, creams, etc.) organized with caps sealed.
5. Never remove a product from its container with your fingers. Use a spatula. Be sure all products have correct labels to prevent using the wrong product.
6. Linens and towels should be laundered in hot water and soap. Chlorine bleach should be added for its germicidal benefits. Clean linens should be stored in closed cabinets. To prevent a "rancid" odor, sheets and towels should be laundered the day they are used. Generally, laundry products and fabric softeners will eliminate odor. However, once sheets and towels have become rancid, they should be discarded.

Some oils (peanut, olive, mineral, almond) tend to be hard to remove from fabric. Oil will usually wash out if sheets and towels are laundered immediately. When it is not possible to launder as often as needed practitioners should use disposable sheets.

7. Keep all areas of the work place and furnishings clean. This includes restrooms, dressing rooms, and work space.
8. The place of business should be well ventilated and kept at a comfortable temperature. Floors, walls, windows, and the like should all reflect your concern for cleanliness and pride in your place of business. Practitioners should know and practice all the rules of sanitation issued by their state board and department of health.

**QUESTIONS FOR DISCUSSION AND REVIEW**

1. Why do all states have laws pertaining to sanitation?
2. Why is it particularly important for a massage practitioner to practice rules of sanitation?
3. Why should the practitioner have some knowledge of bacteria?
4. What is the difference between pathogenic and non-pathogenic bacteria?
5. What is the main purpose of the body's production of antibodies?
6. Name three forms of pathogenic (harmful) bacteria.
7. What is the best prevention against the spread of harmful bacteria?
8. What should you do before using any disinfectant or antiseptic product?
9. Why are disinfectants used in the practice of massage?

10. What is the best method for keeping the hands and nails clean?
11. Which strengths of Creosol or Lysol are most suitable for cleaning floors, sinks, or restrooms?
12. What is sterilization?

**ANSWERS TO QUESTIONS FOR DISCUSSION AND REVIEW**

1. All states have laws pertaining to sanitation for the protection of the public. These laws protect both clients and practitioners.
2. The practitioner should practice the rules of sanitation because he or she is reponsible to safeguard the client's health as well as his or her own health.
3. The practitioner should have some knowledge of bacteria in order to fully understand the importance of preventing the spread of disease.
4. Pathogenic bacteria are harmful, while nonphathogenic bacteria are harmless and sometimes helpful.
5. The body produces antibodies to inhibit or destroy harmful bacteria.
6. Three forms of pathogenic (harmful) bacteria are cocci, bacilli, and spirilla.
7. The strict practice of sanitation is the best prevention against the spread of harmful bacteria.
8. Before using any disinfectant or antiseptic product, you should read the manufacturer's instructions and follow them.
9. Disinfectants are used in the practice of massage to keep all equipment, and the premises in a clean, sanitary condition.
10. The best method for keeping the hands and nails clean is to scrub them with a brush in warm, soapy water, rinse with mild alcohol then pat them dry.
11. Suitable strengths for Creosol and Lysol used to clean floors, sinks, and restrooms are 5 to 10 percent.
12. Sterilization is the procedure for making an object germ-free by destroying bacteria, both the harmful and harmless kinds.

# Chapter 7 The Consultation and Preparation for Massage

**LEARNING OBJECTIVES**

After you have mastered this chapter, you will be able to:

1. Prepare a checklist of supplies and equipment needed for therapeutic massage.
2. Describe various products and their uses.
3. Prepare a massage table.
4. Check and adjust lighting for the massage room.
5. Check all equipment for safety and readiness.
6. Adjust room temperature as required.
7. Conduct a consultation with a client.
8. Prepare the client's records.
9. Check the client's pulse rate and temperature.
10. Instruct the client in preparation procedures.
11. Drape a client properly and efficiently.
12. Instruct the client on positioning on the massage table.
13. Anticipate questions a client may ask.
14. Answer questions a client may ask before and following the massage.

**INTRODUCTION**

Because the practice of therapeutic massage is a part of the health field, it is important that a practitioner present himself or herself in a professional manner at all times. As a practitioner, your clothing must be appropriate for your work; neat, clean, and well fitting. You must be free of body and breath odors and have well-cared-for hands and nails. Your clients will expect you to project a professional image by your speech, by your appearance, and by your courtesy and good manners.

## YOUR PLACE OF BUSINESS

Clients coming into your place of business will be impressed by the environment and the people with whom they come in contact. Therefore the environment must be professional. In a massage establishment, space should be allotted for the exclusive practice of massage. While this is necessary for a client's privacy and comfort, it also gives a more professional image. Some practitioners go to their client's homes rather than maintain a studio and office space. However, it is better to have a business address from which to do business and to receive those clients who do not want to have the service at home.

### Studio Space

A massage room needs to be approximately 10 feet wide and 12 feet long. This allows enough space for all needed equipment as well as enough room to move around the massage table. It also allows space for a desk, chair, and supply table. A stool is also a handy item to have in the massage room, because there are times when the practitioner can sit down while working on the client's neck, face, feet, or hands. Sitting for a few minutes can give much needed rest when working long hours.

### Cleanliness in Your Workplace

Whether working in a small salon or studio with little space or a large, luxurious spa, the space and equipment must be kept clean and neat. The main concern is the protection of the client's health, and comfort.

### Equipment and Supplies

Equipment and supplies should be checked frequently to be sure they are in proper condition and that enough are on hand. For the safe operation of physical therapy apparatus, always follow the manufacturer's instructions and consider the needs and comfort of the client.

Each booth or room should have the appropriate furnishings and equipment for the treatments to be given. All equipment should be checked regularly for fitness and use and everything kept in a clean sanitized condition. Supplies such as oils, linens, and paper products should be selected and ready before the client enters the booth or room.

The following is a checklist of equipment and supplies generally needed. Add your own suggestions to this list:

**Massage room equipment**

Supply and linen cabinets
Chairs
Massage Tables
Stool
Bolsters and pillows
Bolster and pillow covers
Sheets
Blankets
Indirect lighting

**Changing room equipment**

Hangers (clothing)
Chair or bench
Small table

**Physical therapy equipment**

Anatomical wall chart
Standard weight chart
Standard height chart
Bathroom scales
Massage table
Heat lamp
Massage vibrator
Shower room
Shampoo slab
Bath cabinet
Foot basin
Bath tub
Wall plate
Electrical apparatus

**Exercise equipment**

- Stretching bars
- Weight lifts
- Stationary bicycle

**Supply Cabinet**

- Towels
- Sheets
- Pillows and cases
- Bolsters and covers
- Blankets or coverlets
- Disposable paper slippers
- Tape measure
- Room measure
- Mouth thermometer
- Facial cosmetics
- Talcum powder
- Massage creams, oils
- Moist hot packs
- Cold packs
- Cotton for facial cleansing
- Facial tissues
- Cotton-tipped swabs
- Sterilizing agents
- Table salt for salt glows
- Record cards
- Watch with second hand
- Robes or kimonos
- Alcohol or other sterilizing agents
- Anelegesic oil for sore or stiff muscles

## SELECTING PRODUCTS

There is such a wide range of products on the market that it may be difficult to choose the powders, oils, creams, or lotions you will want to stock. Quality is important. If you offer face massage, then you will need cleansers for different skin types, toners or freshening lotions (astringent), moisturizers, and products suitable for any special facial treatments you give. During the consultation or before applying to the face or body, it is best to determine if the client is allergic to any substance. When in doubt, give a patch test before proceeding with the application.

To give a patch test, first wash the area of the inner bend of the elbow with mild soap and warm water. Rinse the area, then use a cotton pledget to apply a small amount of the product to the skin. Allow 15 to 30 minutes to see if there is a reaction, such as signs of itching, inflammation and sensitivity, or a stinging sensation. If so, do not use the product. If there are no signs of inflammation or the above sensations, the product is considered mild enough to use.

Some people with allergies to fragrances and other cosmetic substances may need to have a patch test given 24 hours before a treatment. In such cases, the client will usually be under the care of a physician who can give guidance on which products to use and which to avoid.

### Oils and Powders

It is important to use fresh oil because rancid oil has a strong offensive odor. If oil gets on sheets and sets for a while, it will saturate the fibers and develop an offensive odor. If you buy oil in bulk, some should be transferred to smaller bottles. These bottles should be kept filled to the top because it is the air space in the bottle that causes the oil to become rancid. Mineral oils are not recommended for massage because they are a petroleum-based product and tend to dry the skin and clog the pores. A combination of such oils as coconut, sweet almond, apricot, olive, peanut, sesame, or sunflower oils are mild and easy to work with. A pleasant combination is coconut and almond oils. A good quality oil is the practitioner's most important product.

When oil does not have a pleasant smell but is not rancid, a few drops of oil of lemon, clove, cinnamon, or musk may be added. Usually a few drops of concentrate to a cup of oil will be enough to give a hint of scent. Oils and concentrated fragrances can be purchased from supply houses or are usually available at drug stores. Some practitioners like to mix their oils then place them in attractive, easy-to-handle bottles with dispenser tops. This prevents spillage.

While talcum powder does not provide the lubrication you get with oil, the same massage movements can be done effectively with powder, and some clients prefer powder. You must avoid inhaling talc when using it for massage.

There are excellent creams and lotions you may prefer to use. Always read the label to be sure you know the product's ingredients and that it is safe to use for massage. It is a good idea to have on hand a dictionary of cosmetic ingredients to look up familiar words. When possible, consult a pharmacist or dermatologist. The FDA (Federal Drug Administration) endeavors to control the distribution of products that contain harmful substances. However, what may be harmless to the majority of people, may cause an allergic reaction in someone with a sensitivity to a particular substance. Most nonprescription products are considered safe for the general public. Most practitioners keep a variety of lubricants on hand to better serve the needs and wishes of their clients. Alcohol is kept available for sanitation purposes. It is also used to remove excess oil from the client's skin following massage, before he or she dresses.

## THE MASSAGE ROOM

### Use of Music

While you may like music playing while you work, you must remember that some people find it distracting and prefer absolute quiet. You may wish to have a selection of soothing music available and ask the client what he or she prefers. Obviously, you should not attempt to match the rhythm of massage movements to the tempo of the music.

The client's comfort and confidence are of primary importance to the practitioner. It is good business to offer the client some kind of refreshment such as fruit or vegetable juice or herbal tea. Some salon owners provide coffee, tea or soft drinks for those who prefer them. A bowl of fresh fruit provides a hospitable touch.

### Temperature of the Massage Room

The temperature of the massage room should be comfortable. Generally, about 75° Fahrenheit is the temperature most clients like, and it keeps the practitioner from getting uncomfortably warm while working. The room should be warmed in advance because it is easy for the client to become chilled, especially after oil has been applied to the skin.

**Lighting**

It is difficult for either the practitioner or the client to be comfortable when the lighting in the room is harsh and glaring. Also colored lights such as red or blue can make the client feel uncomfortable. Reflective or soft natural light is preferred. Dimmer switches enable you to change the light easily. Avoid direct overhead lighting or any light that could shine directly into the client's eyes.

**The Massage Table**

A professionally designed massage table is essential because it allows the practitioner to move about or to change positions easily and when necessary, without breaking the rhythm of the massage movements. The table must be the right height in order to give the practitioner the leverage needed and to prevent fatigue of his or her back, neck, arms, and shoulders.

The height of the table is determined by the height of the practitioner so that he or she is not at a disadvantage when reaching and applying pressure. A good indicator for the proper height of a massage table is to stand in an erect, yet relaxed manner and measure the distance from the floor to the ulner (little finger side) side of your forearm. This is approximately the optimum height for the table. Another way to test the height of a table is to place the palm of your hand flat on the table. While doing this, you should be able to hold your arm straight at your side.

The width of the table should be 28 inches with an additional inch allowed for padding, or approximately 29 inches wide. Tables narrower than 27 inches do not give enough arm support for large clients. Tables wider than 30 inches become awkward when the practitioner is required to reach to the opposite side of the client.

A good length for a massage table is 76 inches long. Most tables are about 68 to 72 inches long, which may be too short for tall clients. The padding on the massage table should be firm so that pressure applied by the practitioner to the client, is absorbed by the client's body and not pushed into the table. About 1½ to 2 inches of high density foam is the best material to use. Padding should extend beyond the edge of the framework of the table by about half an inch all around to ensure the comfort of the client, who might place a hand or foot over the edge. Because it is durable and easy to keep clean, good quality vinyl is the best covering. Vinyl does not deteriorate when it comes in contact with oil and can be cleaned with a mild disinfectant after use.

When choosing a table, remember it is your main piece of equipment and, next to your hands, the most important regarding your comfort and that of your clients. One of your concerns should be that the table is stable and firm. If you have a situation where you will be working in an office or studio, a nonportable table is your best choice. If your situation is temporary, or if you prefer the freedom of taking your equipment with you, choose a good portable table. Regardless of your choice, check the construction carefully. The table should not shake, rock, or squeak.

Seldom will new equipment display these problems, but you must consider what will happen after it has been used for several hundred treatments.

Always buy equipment from a reputable company that stands behind its products. Be sure the items you purchase are guaranteed to hold up with reasonable use.

Tables comes in a variety of designs. Several studio and portable models have legs that can be adjusted up or down by removing and replacing wing nuts or thumb screws. These are advantageous if people of different heights use the same table, or if various techniques used require different table heights. Some studio tables have a height adjustment button and are operated by hydraulic force or electricity. Though costly, this type of table is very useful when dealing with the elderly or disabled, who might have difficulty getting on a table of normal height.

Often the bed of a massage treatment table will fold up or down in a variety of configurations. This is to accommodate specific therapy situations and may be of no use to the general massage practitioner. An exception is the head piece that adjusts up or down in order to alleviate cervical strain. Accommodations for the face may be in the form of a hole in the end of the table or a padded part attached to the end of the table. These additions allow the client to lie face down with the cervical spine straight, taking the strain off the neck and upper back.

## POSITIONING THE CLIENT ON THE MASSAGE TABLE

You may have clients coming to you for massage who will have different problems. Some client will be unable to lie face downward and others will not be able to lie flat on their backs without some kind of extra support. For this reason, extra supports should be a part of your professional equipment. For example, if a client is not able to get up on the massage table or lie down, you can use a chair and pillows to comfortably seat the person. You can then give a massage to the back quite easily.

A situation you might encounter is that of a pregnant woman who cannot lie on her back or face down without support. In such cases it is helpful to have on hand foam cushions in various shapes and sizes. These are made of fairly high-density foam and covered with vinyl for easy cleaning.

Firm bed pillows may also be used. Bolsters as wide as the table and 6 to 8 inches in diameter can be used under the client's knees when she is lying on her back. A smaller bolster may be placed under her ankles when she is lying face down. This positioning with bolsters or pillows provides more comfort for the client who has reduced flexibility in the ankles, knees, or lower back.

Another consideration for positioning the client face down is to have a half-circle-shaped support to place under the client's chest to take the pressure off the cervical spine while in the prone position. This support should hold the chest 3 to 4 inches off the table while allowing the head to rest forward comfortably.

Some people need support under the abdomen when they have severe back discomfort. Elevating the midsection and abdomen 6 to 8 inches in this manner helps you to work on the back more effectively. A person who is unable to lie back with the head resting on the table will need support at head and neck as well as the small of back and back of legs.

A variety of supporting pillows or bolsters as part of your equipment will enable you to position and support your client when necessary. All bolsters must have removable cloth slipcovers. Fresh ones are used for each client. Bolsters and pillows can also be placed under the bottom sheet next to the table to avoid contact with the client's skin.

## THE CONSULTATION

During the consultation, the practitioner is usually able to determine what the client wants and needs. If the client is under the care of a physician, this should be noted. The practitioner guides the client and explains premassage procedures, such as the reasons for taking the client's pulse and temperature before massage treatment. Attentiveness is particularly important when the client is coming to you for the first time and may tend to feel apprehensive.

## QUESTIONS THE CLIENT MAY ASK ABOUT BENEFITS OF MASSAGE

During the consultation, the client usually will want to know how the massage treatments will be beneficial. Being able to answer the client's questions adds to the practitioner's credibility as a professional and helps to put the client at ease.

The following is a review of the benefits of massage that may be of interest to clients:

*Circulatory system:* Massage improves the circulation of the blood throughout the body, thus improving the supply of oxygen and nutrients to all cells, tissues, and organs. It helps to remove metabolic wastes from the body and can be beneficial in decreasing blood pressure.

*Digestive system:* Massage aids in relaxing the abdominal and intestinal muscles and improves functioning of the digestive system. Massage stimulates the liver and kidneys and helps to alleviate faulty elimination.

*Lymph vascular system:* Massage helps to increase lymph circulation, aids in the elimination of metabolic wastes, and stimulates the immune system.

*Muscular system:* Massage stimulates and tones muscles. It helps to relieve soreness and stiffness in muscles and joints and strengthens connective tissues. It aids in relaxation, relieves fatigue, and provides relief of muscle spasms.

*Nervous system:* Massage increases the blood supply to the nerves and brain. It stimulates motor nerve points, alleviates stress and tension, and promotes a sense of well-being.

*Skin:* Massage increases the supply of blood to the skin, thereby nourishing tissues. It improves skin tone, helps to firm facial muscles, and helps to keep the sebaceous (oil) glands functioning normally.

**KEEPING RECORDS**

It is necessary to keep records of all services. Records should be accurate, and complete and should provide information concerning treatments given, products used, and the state of the client's health. All data should be recorded with each treatment, including any special information that may be needed as a reference.

A copy of the data card can be given to the client and one kept for your records. Keeping accurate records of the client's condition, tolerance, and reactions permits you to render more effective treatments and to accomplish better results.

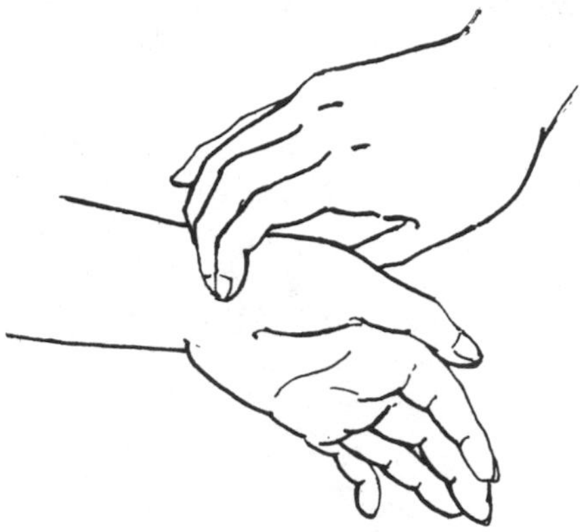

The pulse rate of an adult female is 80 beats per minute. The pulse rate of an adult male is 78 beats per minute. The pulse is taken while the client is lying down and after he or she has been resting for a short time.

*Position for palpating the radial pulse*

Your concern for the client's well-being helps to establish mutual confidence.

The practitioner never discusses or gives out personal information about clients, and all records should be kept in a secure place. A physician does not divulge information about a client's personal matters without the consent of the client and then only in cases where the exchange of such information is for the client's benefit. The practitioner often works closely with a client's physician when dealing with certain physical conditions, therefore the confidence of both client and physician must be respected.

When the practitioner feels that a client's physician should be consulted before beginning massage treatments, he or she should talk this over with the client.

**PREPARING THE CLIENT FOR THE MASSAGE**

It is important to keep the client informed about what is being done and why. This is especially important if it is the client's first visit to the place of business and/or first massage. The client's height and weight may be recorded if relevant to the treatment. This step is essential if the client is having massage as part of a weight loss program. The client's temperature and pulse rate are taken and recorded if necessary to the treatments being given.

**HOW TO TAKE THE CLIENT'S PULSE RATE**

1. Place three fingers (not the thumb) on the inside of the client's wrist and palpate the radial artery to feel the beat of the pulse.
2. Count the number of beats for a full minute on the second hand of your watch, or for 15 seconds x 4 (or 60 seconds).
3. Record the pulse rate.

## HOW TO TAKE THE CLIENT'S TEMPERATURE

The client may not understand why pulse rate and/or temperature is taken and recorded. It can be explained by stating that an abnormally high temperature or pulse rate can be indications of health conditions where massage treatments may not be advisable. A marked elevation in body temperature tends to increase the pulse rate.

Under normal circumstances when the client is well, it is not necessary to take the pulse rate and temperature. However, if during the consultation the client appears flushed, unusually warm, and does not feel well, then it is best to take temperature and pulse rate.

### Taking Temperature

Normal temperature is about 98.6 Fahrenheit. The most convenient way to take temperature is by way of the mouth.

1. Wash your hands in warm soapy water and rinse them well.
2. Lower the mercury in the thermometer below the 98° mark, hold the thermometer firmly between your thumb and forefinger and give your wrist a quick snap.
3. Rinse the thermometer under cold running water.
4. Insert the bulb end of the thermometer into the client's mouth beneath the tongue. Have the client keep his or her lips closed for about three minutes.
5. Remove the thermometer from the client's mouth and wipe it from top to bottom with a tissue.
6. Locate the column of mercury on the triangular edge of the thermometer, and note the point where it has stopped. This should give you an accurate reading of the client's temperature.
7. Record the temperature on your chart, and explain the results to the client.
8. Wipe the thermometer from top to bottom with a piece of cotton moistened with soap and water, then rinse it under cold water and immerse it in a sterilizing agent, such as 70% alcohol.

## CONSULTATION FORMS

When filling in consultation forms it is important to be tactful. If a client questions why you are asking certain questions, explain your reasons. For example, on the form you ask: "What do you do with the majority of your time? (hobbies, outside work)." The client's answers give the practitioner clues as to what area of the client's body may be carrying stress. Question: "Have you had any surgery?" The client's answer to this question gives the practitioner clues to health problems and contraindications that may be indicated. The question: "Have you received massages before?" This question allows the practitioner to determine what the client's expectation and preference may be. The question, "How did you find out about our massage services?" The client's answer to this question gives the practitioner information about the kind of advertising that is most effective.

NAME OF BUSINESS ____________________

Name ____________________ Date of Birth ____________________
month day year

Address ____________________ Telephone ____________________
Street No.

____________________ Business Phone ____________________
City State Zip

Occupation ____________________

What do you do with the majority of the rest of your time? (hobbies, outside work) ____________________

____________________

Your general condition of health ____________________

Have you had any serious illness ____________________ If so please describe it ____________________

Have you had any operations ____________________ If so, for what ____________________

Have you had any traumatic accidents or broken bones ____________________

Heart Condition ____________________ Blood Pressure ____________________

Are you on medication? ____________________ Is so, what ____________________

Do you use supplements? ____________________ If so, what ____________________

Do you wear contacts? ____________________ Are you currently being treated by a doctor, chiropractor or other practitioner? ____________________ If so, for what ____________________

Doctors or Chiropractors

Name ____________________ Name ____________________

Address ____________________ Address ____________________

____________________ ____________________

Telephone ____________________ Telephone ____________________

May I have permission to contact your doctor? ____________________

Why did you come for a massage? ____________________

____________________

Have you received any massages before? ____________________ When ____________________

Where ____________________ By Whom ____________________

What do you expect from this massage? ____________________

____________________

How did you find out about our massage services? ____________________

I understand the massage services are designed to be a health aid and are in no way to take the place of doctor's care when it is indicated. Information exchanged during any massage sessions is educational in nature and is intended to help you become more familiar and conscious of your own health status and is to be used at your own discretion.

____________________ ____________________
Date Your Signature

**BODY DIAGRAMS**

Body diagrams of the male and female figure are helpful when the client has some painful sore or stiff areas that may require special attention. Give the client a few minutes to indicate these areas on the diagram, then discuss the condition and explain how massage may be beneficial.

*On the diagrams below, mark as follows:*

*for any painful area*
*shade in any stiff or sore areas*
*areas of other concern and describe the condition which is occurring*

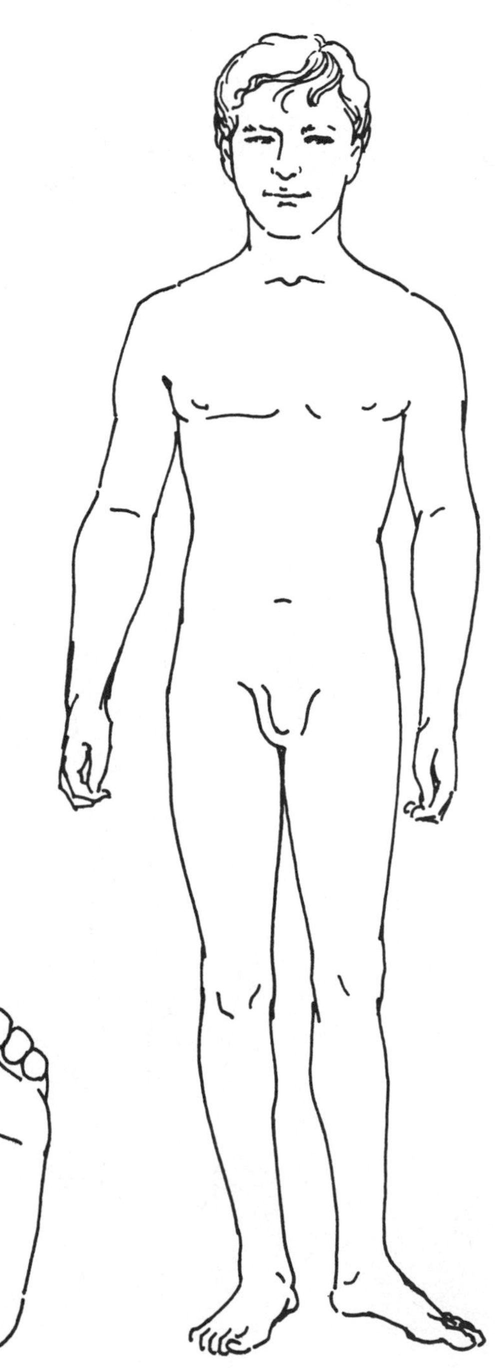

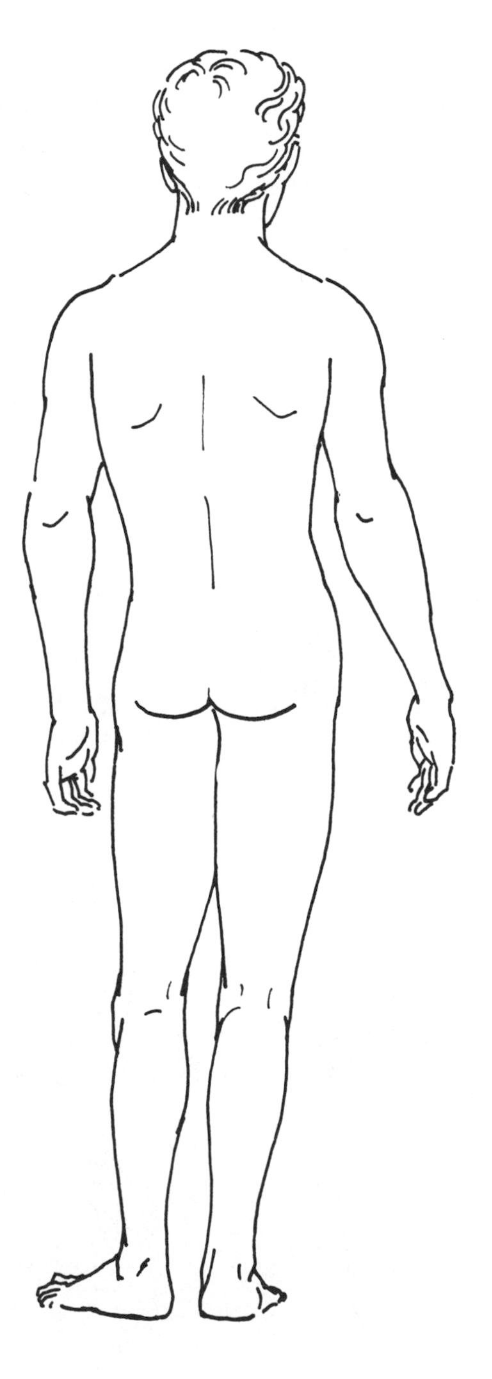

*On the diagrams below mark as follows:*

*for any painful area*
*shade in any stiff or sore areas*
*areas of other concern and describe the condition which is occurring*

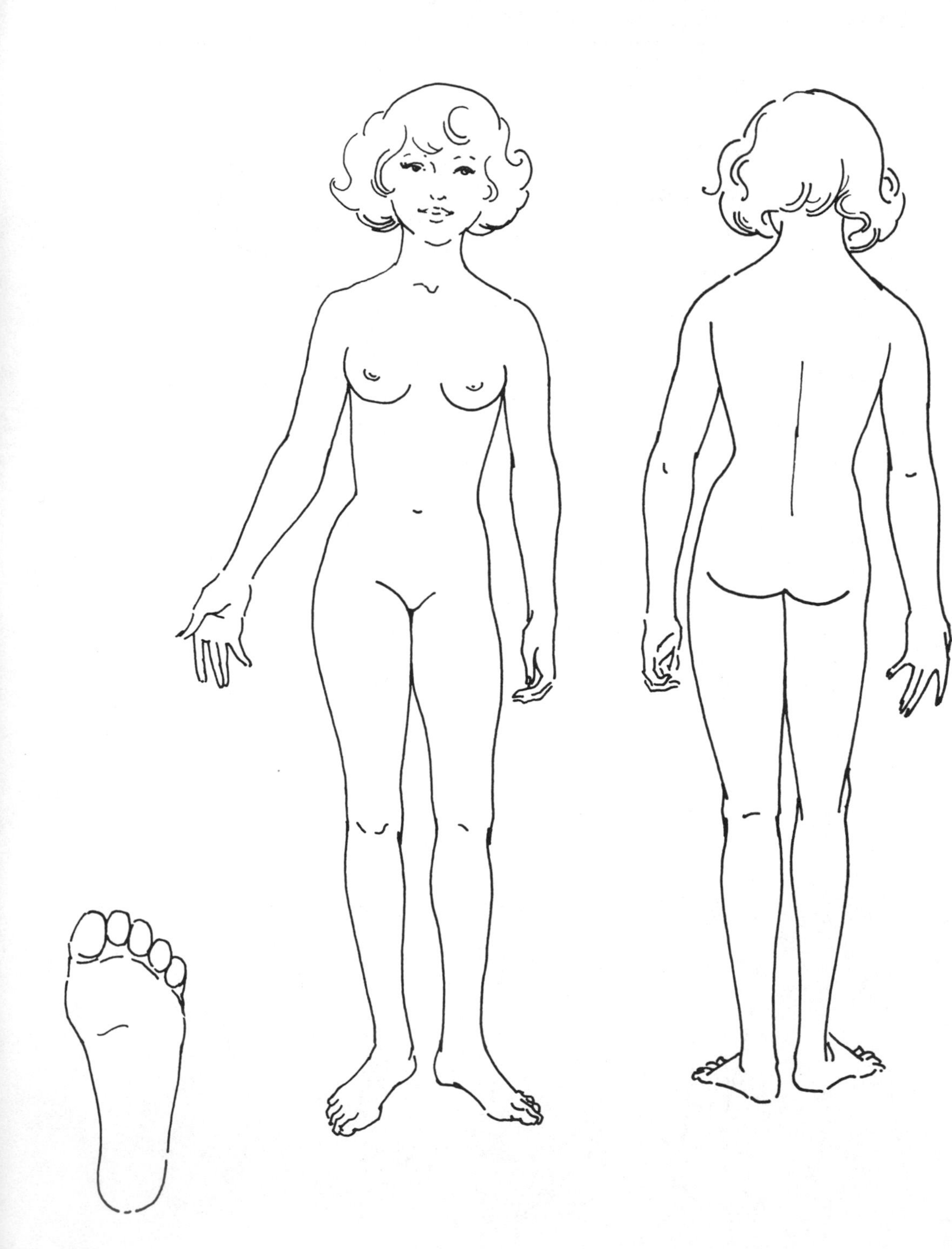

**Information Card**

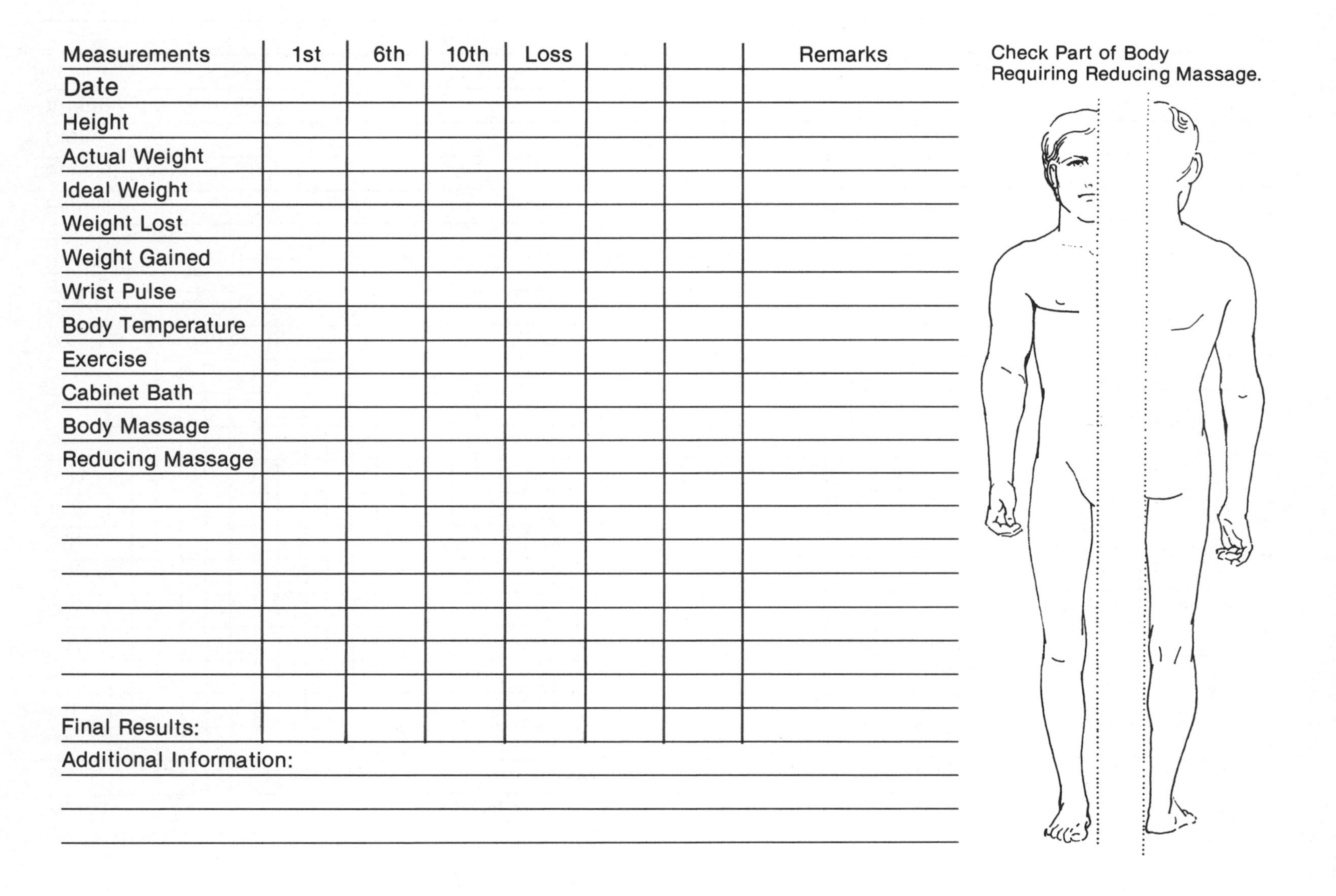

| Measurements | 1st | 6th | 10th | Loss | | | Remarks |
|---|---|---|---|---|---|---|---|
| Date | | | | | | | |
| Height | | | | | | | |
| Actual Weight | | | | | | | |
| Ideal Weight | | | | | | | |
| Weight Lost | | | | | | | |
| Weight Gained | | | | | | | |
| Wrist Pulse | | | | | | | |
| Body Temperature | | | | | | | |
| Exercise | | | | | | | |
| Cabinet Bath | | | | | | | |
| Body Massage | | | | | | | |
| Reducing Massage | | | | | | | |
| | | | | | | | |
| | | | | | | | |
| | | | | | | | |
| | | | | | | | |
| | | | | | | | |
| | | | | | | | |
| | | | | | | | |
| Final Results: | | | | | | | |

Additional Information:

Check Part of Body Requiring Reducing Massage.

Name Address Tel. Date

| Month | 1 | 2 | 3 | 4 | 5 | 6 | 7 | 8 | 9 | 10 | 11 | 12 | 13 | 14 | 15 | 16 | 17 | 18 | 19 | 20 | 21 | 22 | 23 | 24 | 25 | 26 | 27 | 28 | 29 | 30 | 31 | Total |
|---|---|---|---|---|---|---|---|---|---|---|---|---|---|---|---|---|---|---|---|---|---|---|---|---|---|---|---|---|---|---|---|---|
| Jan. | | | | | | | | | | | | | | | | | | | | | | | | | | | | | | | | |
| Feb. | | | | | | | | | | | | | | | | | | | | | | | | | | | | | | | | |
| Mar. | | | | | | | | | | | | | | | | | | | | | | | | | | | | | | | | |
| Apr. | | | | | | | | | | | | | | | | | | | | | | | | | | | | | | | | |
| May | | | | | | | | | | | | | | | | | | | | | | | | | | | | | | | | |
| June | | | | | | | | | | | | | | | | | | | | | | | | | | | | | | | | |
| July | | | | | | | | | | | | | | | | | | | | | | | | | | | | | | | | |
| Aug. | | | | | | | | | | | | | | | | | | | | | | | | | | | | | | | | |
| Sept. | | | | | | | | | | | | | | | | | | | | | | | | | | | | | | | | |
| Oct. | | | | | | | | | | | | | | | | | | | | | | | | | | | | | | | | |
| Nov. | | | | | | | | | | | | | | | | | | | | | | | | | | | | | | | | |
| Dec. | | | | | | | | | | | | | | | | | | | | | | | | | | | | | | | | |

Age

Occupation

No. of Visits

Source

| Payment | Date | Amount |
|---|---|---|
| | | |
| | | |
| | | |
| | | |
| | | |
| | | |
| | | |

Medical Examination: Date Doctor Address

Doctor's Advice Regarding:

Facial Massage

Body Massage:

Exercise:

Special Treatment (Baths)

Diet:

Additional Information

## DRAPING PROCEDURES

The process of using linens to keep a client covered while performing a massage is called DRAPING. This procedure allows for the client to be totally undressed and at the same time retain comfort, warmth and modesty. It gives the practitioner the freedom to massage all parts of the body unincumbered by the client's clothing.

Proper draping insures that the client stays warm. Perspiration, oil and being in a reclining position all increase the rate at which the body loses heat. The proper temperature for a massage room is 75°-80° F. If the area is cooler than this, extra precautions should be taken to make sure the client remains warm. It is much easier for a person to get chilled than for them to warm up. If a person is chilled, it is nearly impossible for them to relax.

Two items to keep on hand to deal with these cool situations are a twin sized electric mattress pad to put on the table under the sheet and a flannel blanket or sheet to put over the client after he or she is on the massage table and is properly draped.

By using proper draping and only uncovering the portion of the body that is being massaged and, by always concealing the client's personal parts, the practitioner maintains a professional and ethical practice while preventing embarassment to either the practitioner or the client.

There are several methods of draping. All methods consist of techniques of maintaining personal privacy while first, getting the client from the dressing area to the hydrotherapy area and/or the massage table. The next step is using adequate draping while client's receive their massage. And finally keeping the client well covered while he or she gets up from the massage table and returns to the dressing area.

For reasons of safety and liability, it is advisable that the practitioner assist the client onto the table at the beginning of a massage, into a sitting position and off the table at the end of the massage. Draping procedures should include techniques that allow these movements to be accomplished while keeping the client modestly covered.

## METHODS OF DRAPING

There are several methods of draping that are easy and effective. In this chapter we will discuss three methods. Practice each of these until you are proficient. You may choose one style that works best for you or you may combine portions of one method with another. While learning these various draping procedures refer to the step by step directions and the illustrations included in this chapter. The beginner should be careful to follow directions carefully and practice until he or she can drape a client smoothly and efficiently. It is also important to know how to instruct the client in how to change positions during the draping procedures.

**Method 1—Diaper Draping**

For this technique you will need a regular bath sized towel (two towels if the client is female) and a covering for the table. The table covering may be a small flat sheet, a cot sized fitted sheet or a disposable paper sheet. The towel may also serve as the wrap the client uses to get from the dressing area to the table.

Diaper draping is suitable when the environment is very warm (80° F or warmer) so there is no chance of the client becoming chilled. This technique also insures that the genital area is very well concealed.

**Method 2—Top Cover Method**

This method uses a table covering as in Method I along with a top covering that is large enough to cover the entire body. A large beach sized towel or one half of a sheet will serve this purpose well. The minimum size for the top cover is 72 inches long and 32 inches wide.

This cover sheet may also serve as the wrap the client uses to get from the dressing area to the table.

The use of this type of draping insures warmth and modesty while allowing easy access to each body part.

**Method 3—Full Sheet Draping**

This method employs the use of a full sized double flat sheet (minimum width 80 inches) to cover the table and wrap the client. When using this method it is necessary to supply an additional wrap for the client to get from the dressing area to the table. After the client is on the table, this wrap is used to secure the sheet and to cover the client when he or she turns over and when getting up after the massage.

The following is a list of items that may be used in the draping process.

**Sheets**

Full double flat sheets. (minimum width 80")

Cot sized fitted sheets

½ of full double sheets. Cut and hemmed to use as a table covering or a cover sheet.

Disposable sheets to use as table coverings when laundry is a problem.

Towels

Bath sized towels for diaper draping and for personal use after hydrotherapy.

Beach sized towels for body covers.

Terry cloth wraps to wear to and from the dressing area.

Miscellaneous

Pillow cases for covering pillows and bolsters.

Flannel sheets to use when extra warmth is needed.

Twin sized electric mattress pad for use on the table when warmth is a problem, such as when working in the home where it is too cool.

Remember that any materials coming in contact with the client's skin must be freshly laundered and sterile. Clean linens must be used for each client.

**Draping from the Dressing Area to the Massage Table**

This is the first step in the draping process and requires some form of wrap to be worn from the dressing area to either the hydrotherapy area or to the massage table. The method of draping during the massage as well as the size and sex of the client will determine the type of wrap that is used. For diaper draping, a bath sized towel may be sufficient. In the cover sheet method, the cover sheet may be used. Terry cloth wraps can be provided instead of a towel for the client to wear in any method of draping. These wraps can be purchased in a department store or uniform department. The woman's wrap fastens above the breasts while the man's wrap is a shorter version that wraps around and snaps at the waist. The length is usually just above the knees. These wraps are convenient because they secure and unfasten easily when the client is on the table, and they are easy to put back on after the massage. Wraps are available in small, large and extra large sizes for men and women.

When using a wrap or a towel, the client arranges it so the open side is situated at the side of the body. As the client sits on the edge of the table, the wrap is lifted out of the way to avoid sitting on the wrap. The wrap is then unfastened as the client is instructed to lie down. As the client lies down, the wrap is smoothly slipped from under the body. In this way the client is lying down on the table with the wrap covering the body, not underneath.

An alternative to this procedure is to have the client lie on the table then unfasten the wrap. Have the client lift the body slightly as you carefully slip the wrap from underneath.

Having gotten the client on the table, lying down and covered by the wrap, you are ready to proceeed with the draping of your choice and the massage.

When the massage has been completed and it is time for the client to get up and get dressed, a procedure must be followed that will maintain his or her privacy in a relaxed and efficient manner, while at the same time insuring the client's safety. The following illustrations will be helpful.

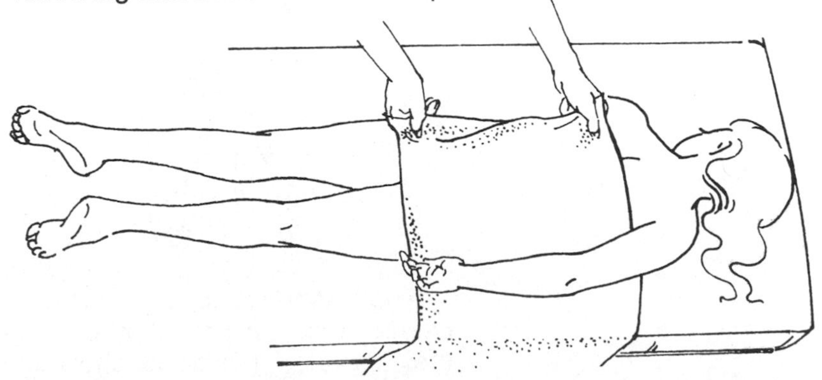

*The same wrap that the client wears from the dressing area to the massage table is used. The wrap is placed across the client's body and other draping removed. Instruct the client to lie on one side and arrange the wrap in such a way that it covers the back of the body with most of the wrap in front.*

**Draping**
*(Continued)*

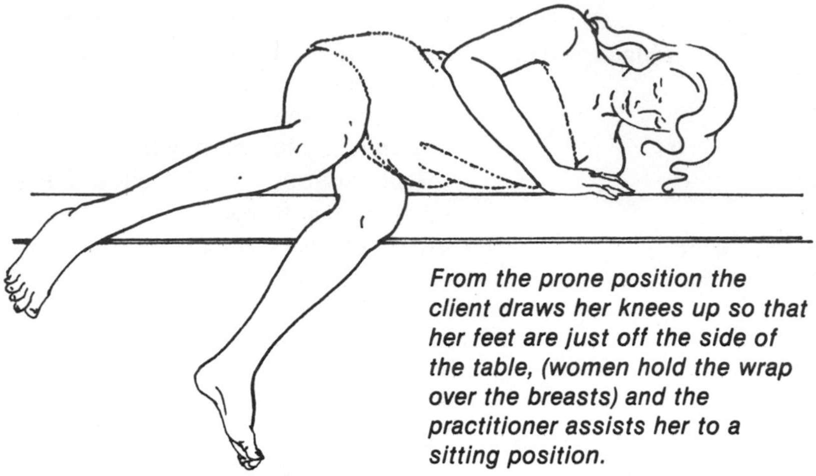

*From the prone position the client draws her knees up so that her feet are just off the side of the table, (women hold the wrap over the breasts) and the practitioner assists her to a sitting position.*

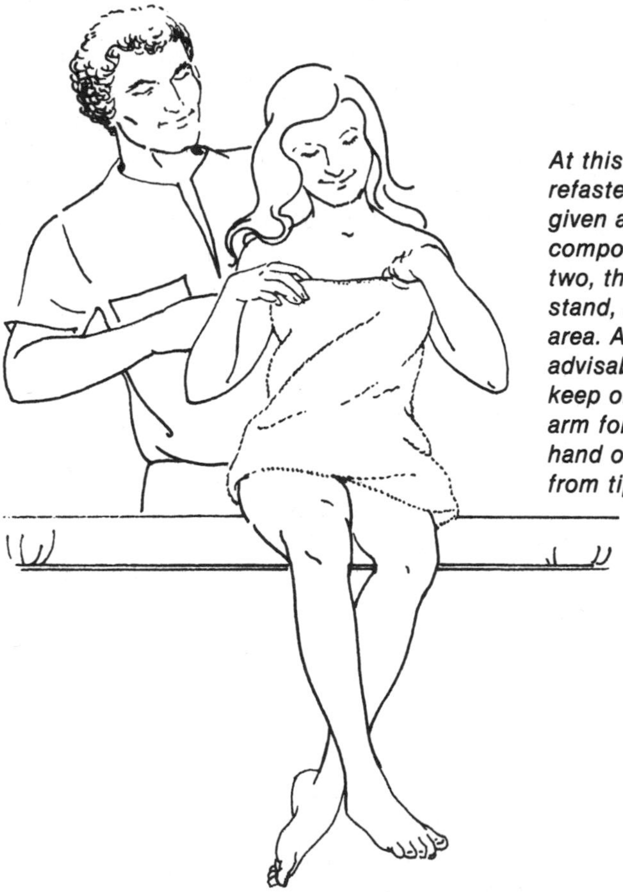

*At this point the wrap is refastened while the client is given a chance to regain composure. After a moment or two, the client is instructed to stand, and return to the dressing area. As the client stands, it is advisable for the practitioner to keep one hand on the client's arm for balance and the other hand on the table to prevent it from tipping.*

It is important to be courteous and attentive toward your clients from the time they enter your place of business until they leave. You should show concern for their safety and comfort at all times. Some clients will want and expect help when getting on or off the massage table, others will indicate that they prefer helping themselves. When in doubt, ask. For example you might say: "May I assist you?" or "Let me help you, Mrs. -----."

**Alternate Method**

An alternate and less desirable method is to leave the massage area while the client undresses, gets on the massage table and uses the wrap (or towel) as a cover. At the end of the massage the practitioner leaves the room and allows the client to get off the table without assistance. This method is considered less professional because it increases the chances that the client could be injured when getting on or off the table.

***Method 1 The Diaper Draping Method***

Follow the illustrations for this method until you are able to remember how to do the entire procedure in a smooth and efficient manner.

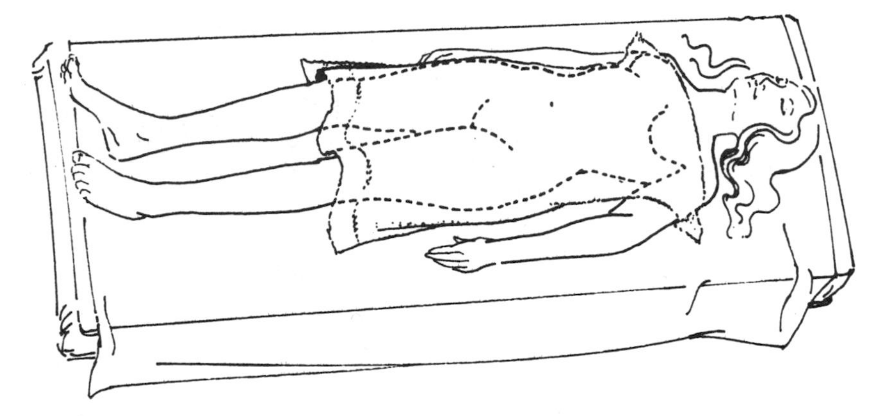

*A large terry towel is used for a covering. The towel must be long enough to cover the chest. It will come to just above the knees.*

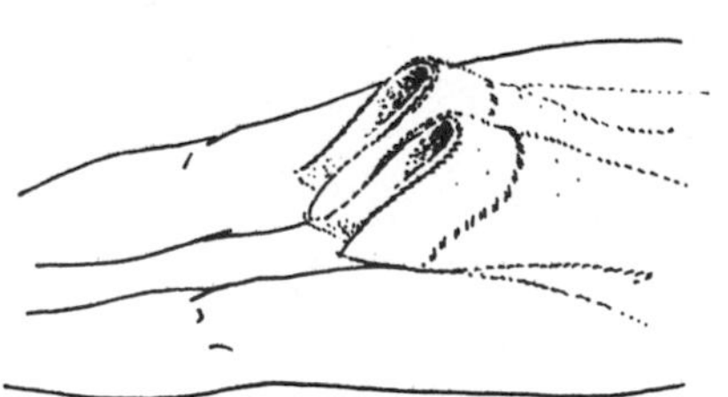

*Fold the lower end of the towel into four smooth folds.*

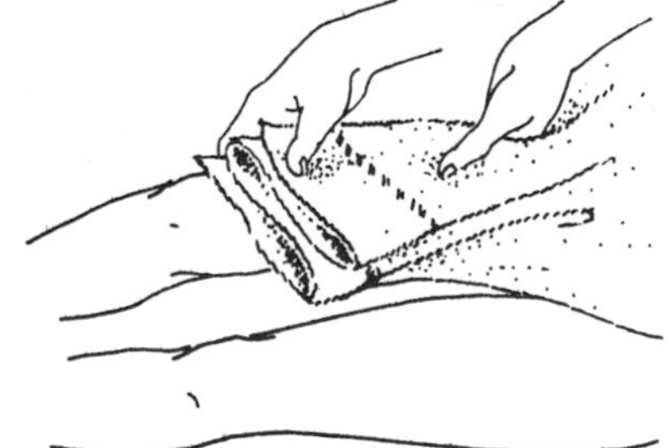

*The folds taper to fit the contours of the body.*

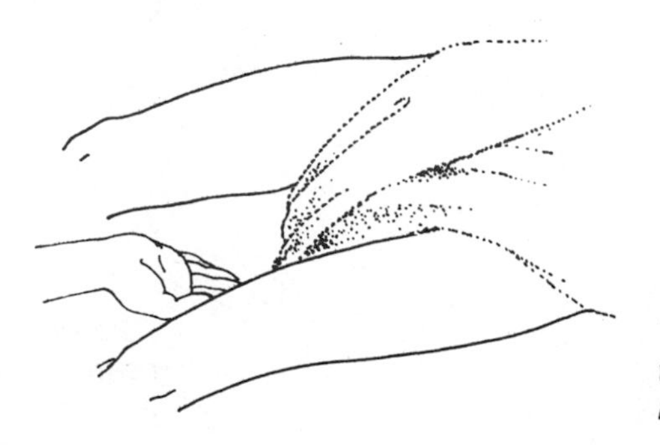

*The client's leg is raised enough to allow the end of the towel to be tucked under the sacrum.*

**Draping**
*(Continued)*

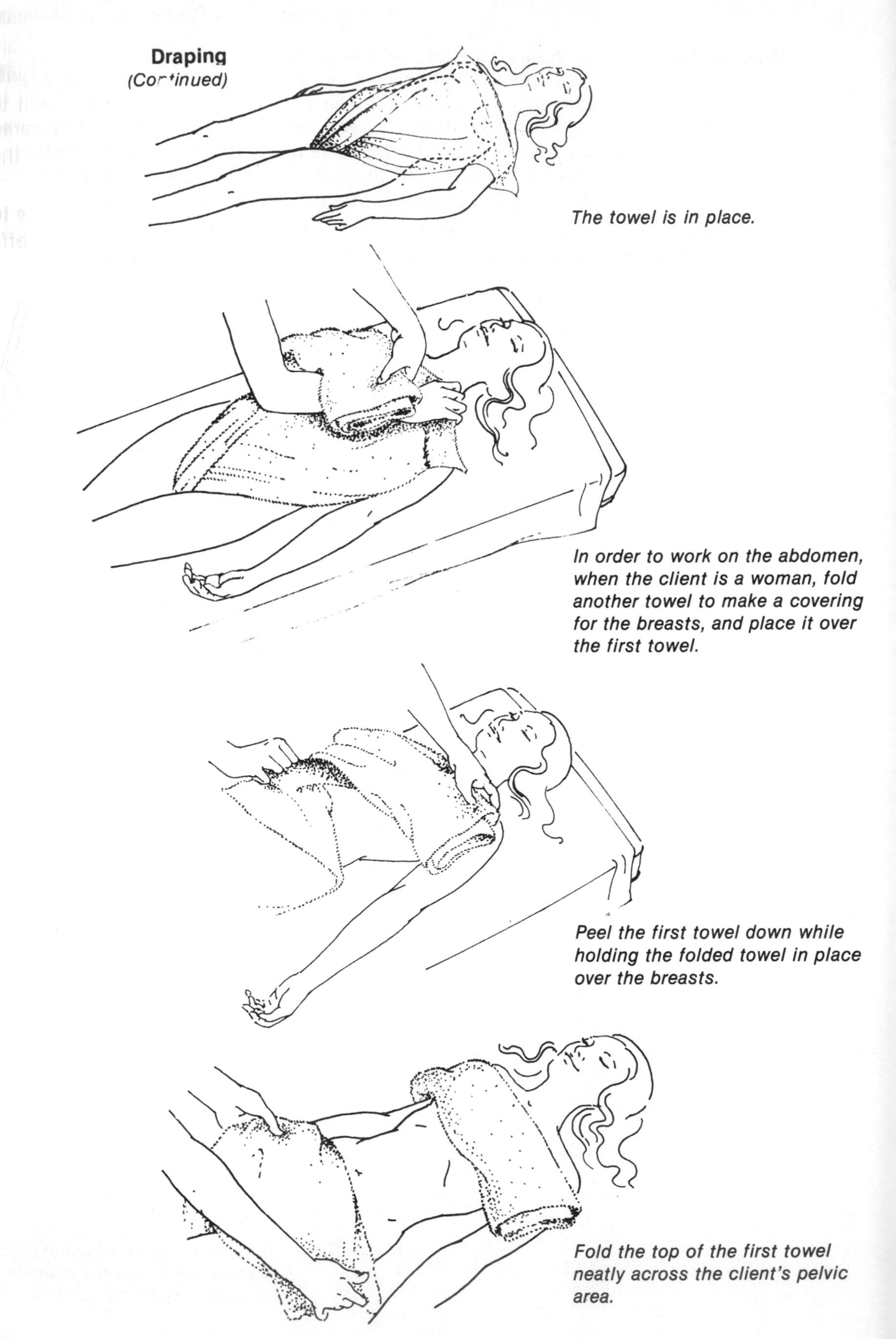

*The towel is in place.*

*In order to work on the abdomen, when the client is a woman, fold another towel to make a covering for the breasts, and place it over the first towel.*

*Peel the first towel down while holding the folded towel in place over the breasts.*

*Fold the top of the first towel neatly across the client's pelvic area.*

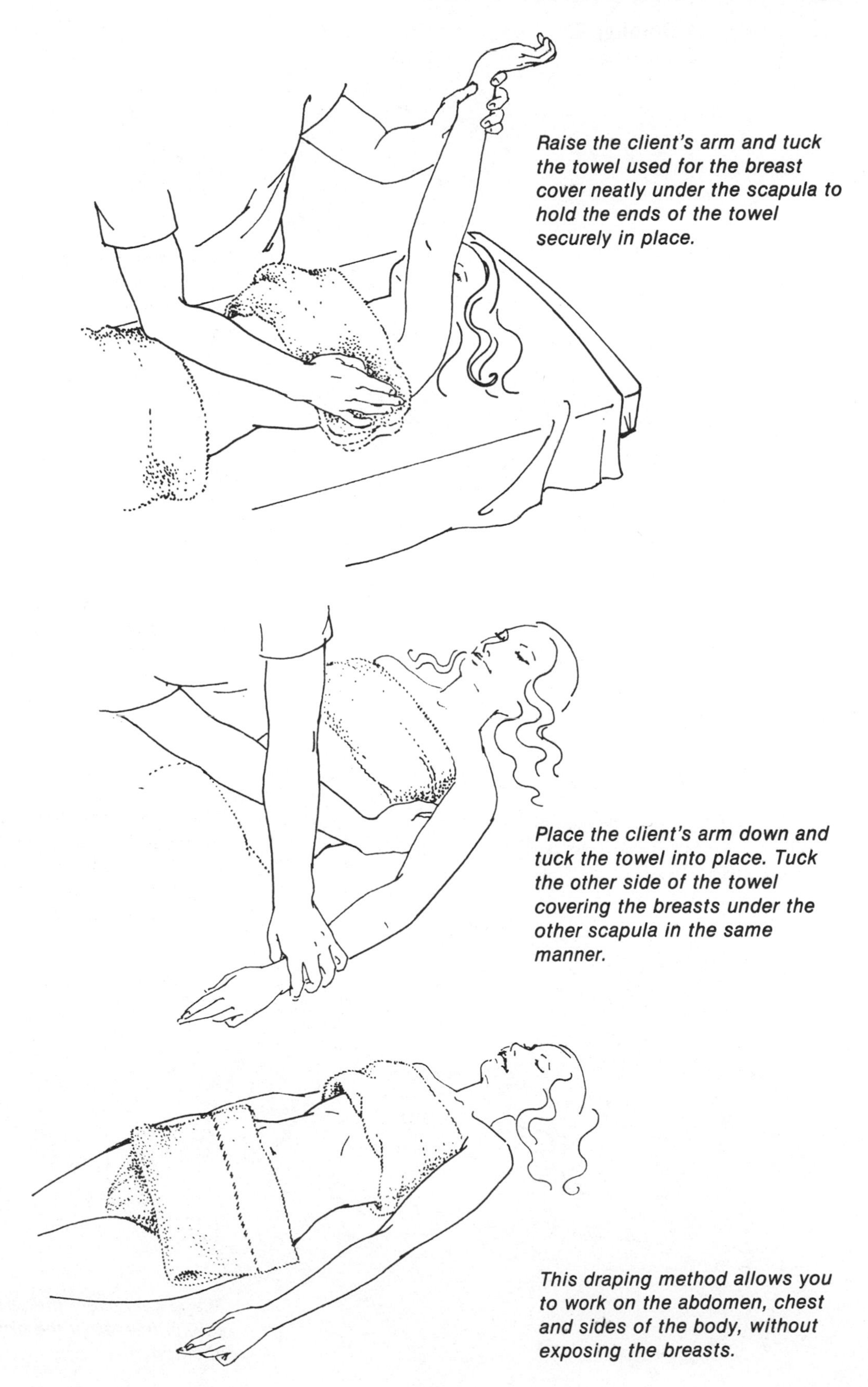

*Raise the client's arm and tuck the towel used for the breast cover neatly under the scapula to hold the ends of the towel securely in place.*

*Place the client's arm down and tuck the towel into place. Tuck the other side of the towel covering the breasts under the other scapula in the same manner.*

*This draping method allows you to work on the abdomen, chest and sides of the body, without exposing the breasts.*

## Draping
*(Continued)*

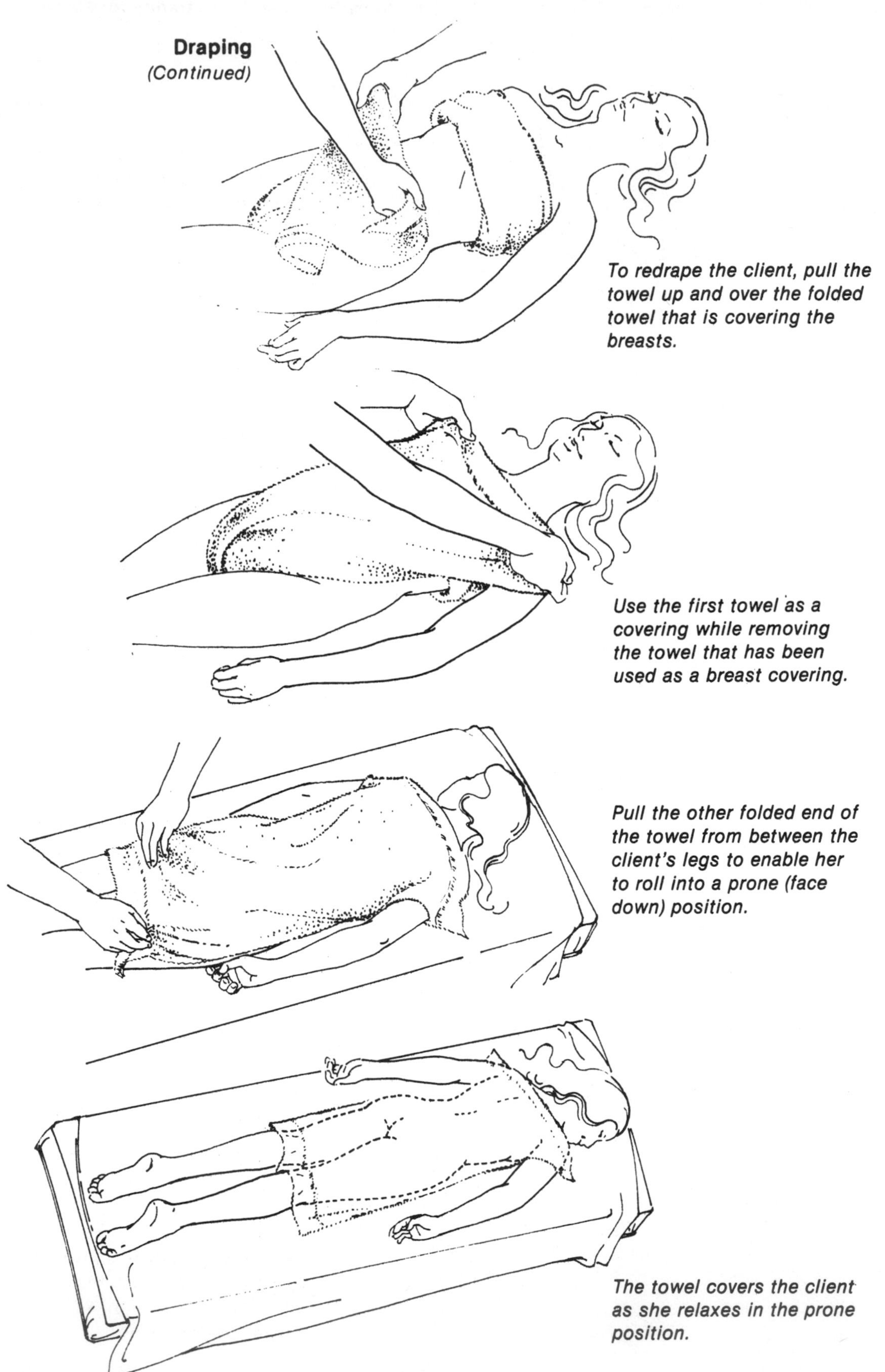

*To redrape the client, pull the towel up and over the folded towel that is covering the breasts.*

*Use the first towel as a covering while removing the towel that has been used as a breast covering.*

*Pull the other folded end of the towel from between the client's legs to enable her to roll into a prone (face down) position.*

*The towel covers the client as she relaxes in the prone position.*

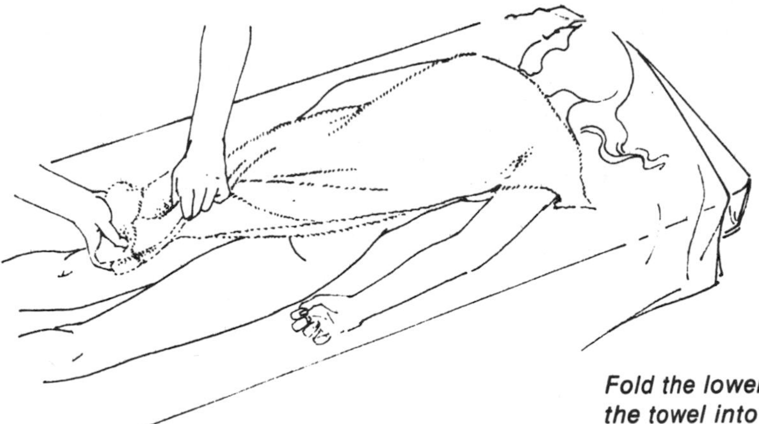

*Fold the lower portion of the towel into four folds again.*

*Lift the client's leg and tuck the towel under the leg near the groin area so that it is held securely in place.*

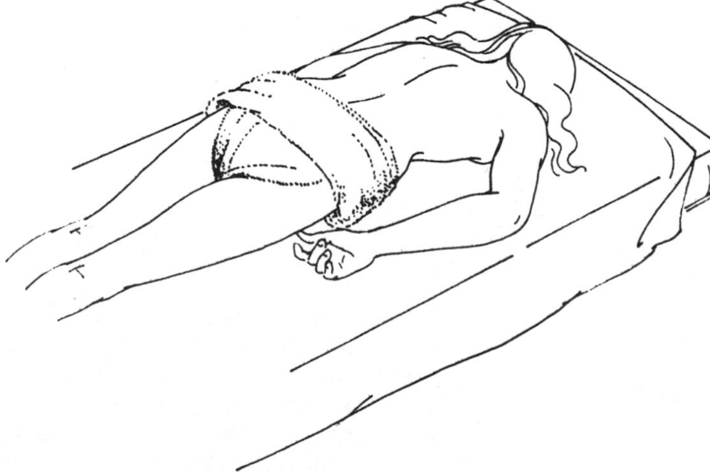

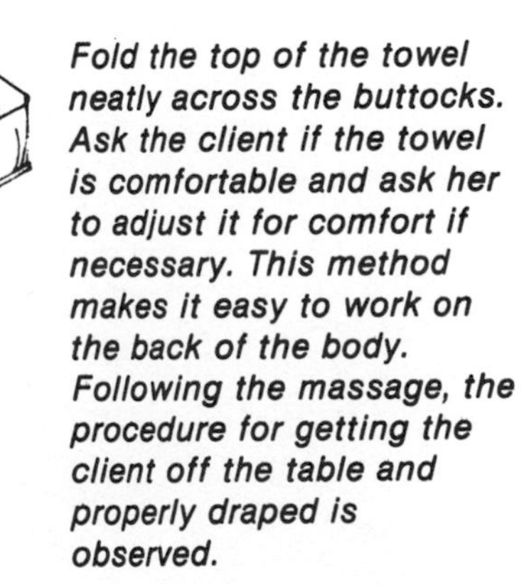

*Fold the top of the towel neatly across the buttocks. Ask the client if the towel is comfortable and ask her to adjust it for comfort if necessary. This method makes it easy to work on the back of the body. Following the massage, the procedure for getting the client off the table and properly draped is observed.*

**Method 2**
**The Top Cover Method**

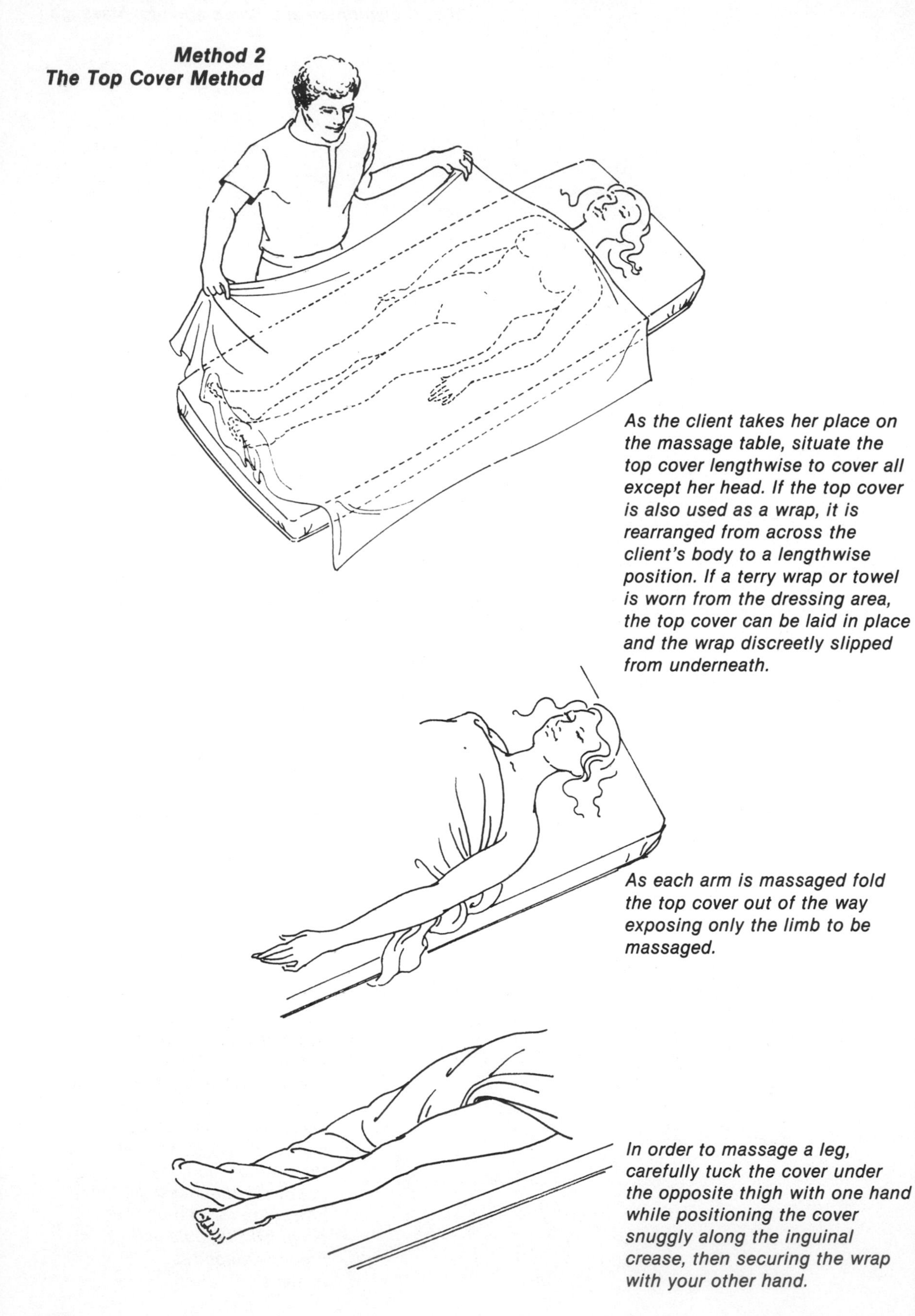

*As the client takes her place on the massage table, situate the top cover lengthwise to cover all except her head. If the top cover is also used as a wrap, it is rearranged from across the client's body to a lengthwise position. If a terry wrap or towel is worn from the dressing area, the top cover can be laid in place and the wrap discreetly slipped from underneath.*

*As each arm is massaged fold the top cover out of the way exposing only the limb to be massaged.*

*In order to massage a leg, carefully tuck the cover under the opposite thigh with one hand while positioning the cover snuggly along the inguinal crease, then securing the wrap with your other hand.*

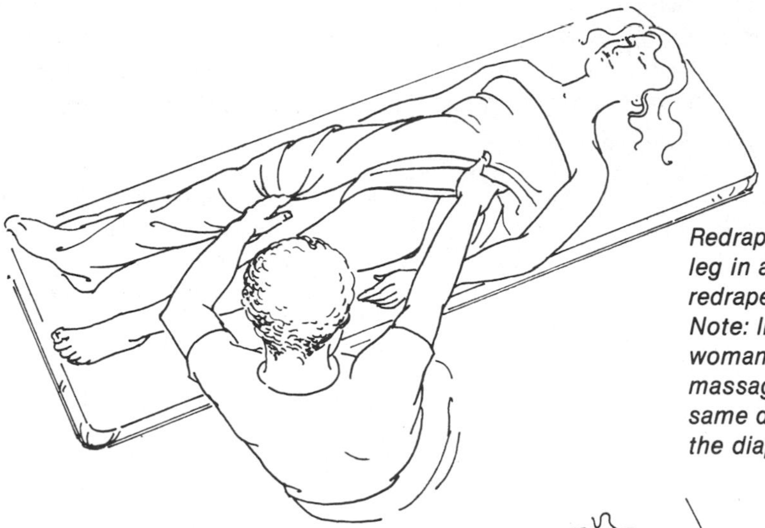

*Redrape the leg and do the other leg in a similar manner then redrape the leg.*
*Note: In order not to expose a woman's breasts when massaging the torso, use the same draping procedures as in the diaper draping method.*

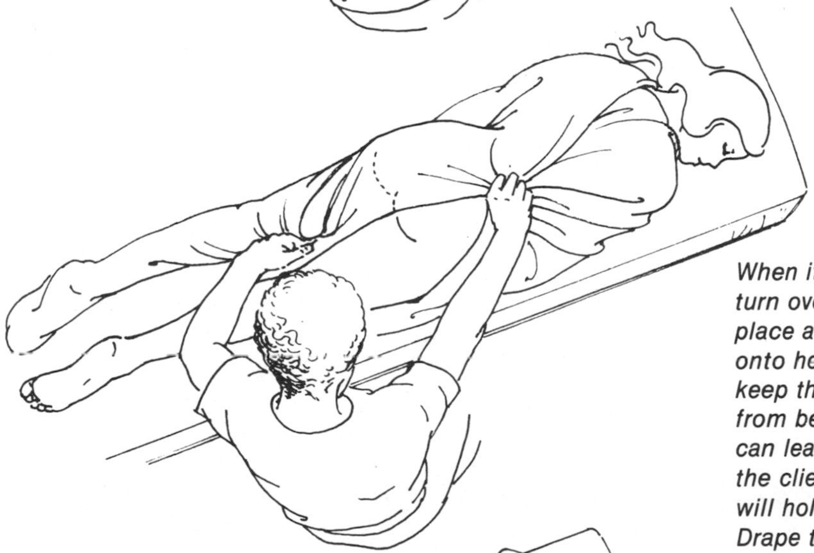

*When it is time for the client to turn over, hold the top cover in place and instruct her to turn onto her abdomen. In order to keep the massage table linens from becoming disarranged, you can lean against the table while the client turns toward you. This will hold the linens in place. Drape the back of the legs in a similar fashion as the front of the legs.*

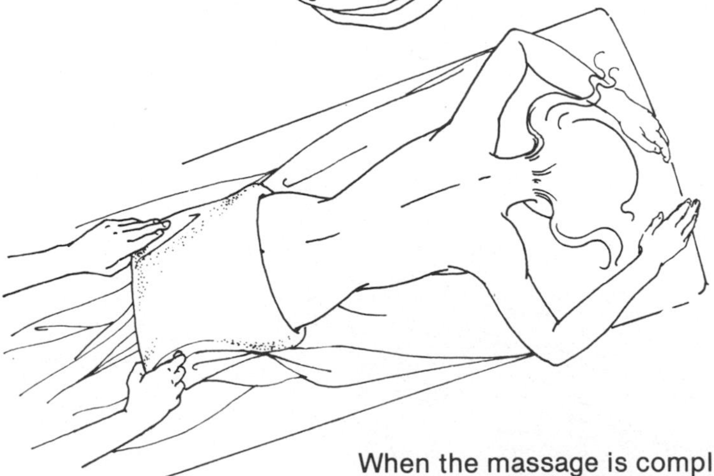

*To massage the back fold the cover down to expose the entire back.*

When the massage is complete and it is time for the client to return to the dressing area, use the top cover for a wrap by turning the cover sideways before having the client come to a sitting position. If you choose to use a separate wrap, put the wrap in place, and while holding it with one hand, peel the top cover from underneath the wrap.

**Method 3**
**Full Sheet Draping**

The following is a step-by-step description of the full sheet draping method. It incorporates the use of a double sized flat sheet and a separate wrap or towel. First, prepare the massage table by unfolding the double sized sheet and placing it on the massage table.

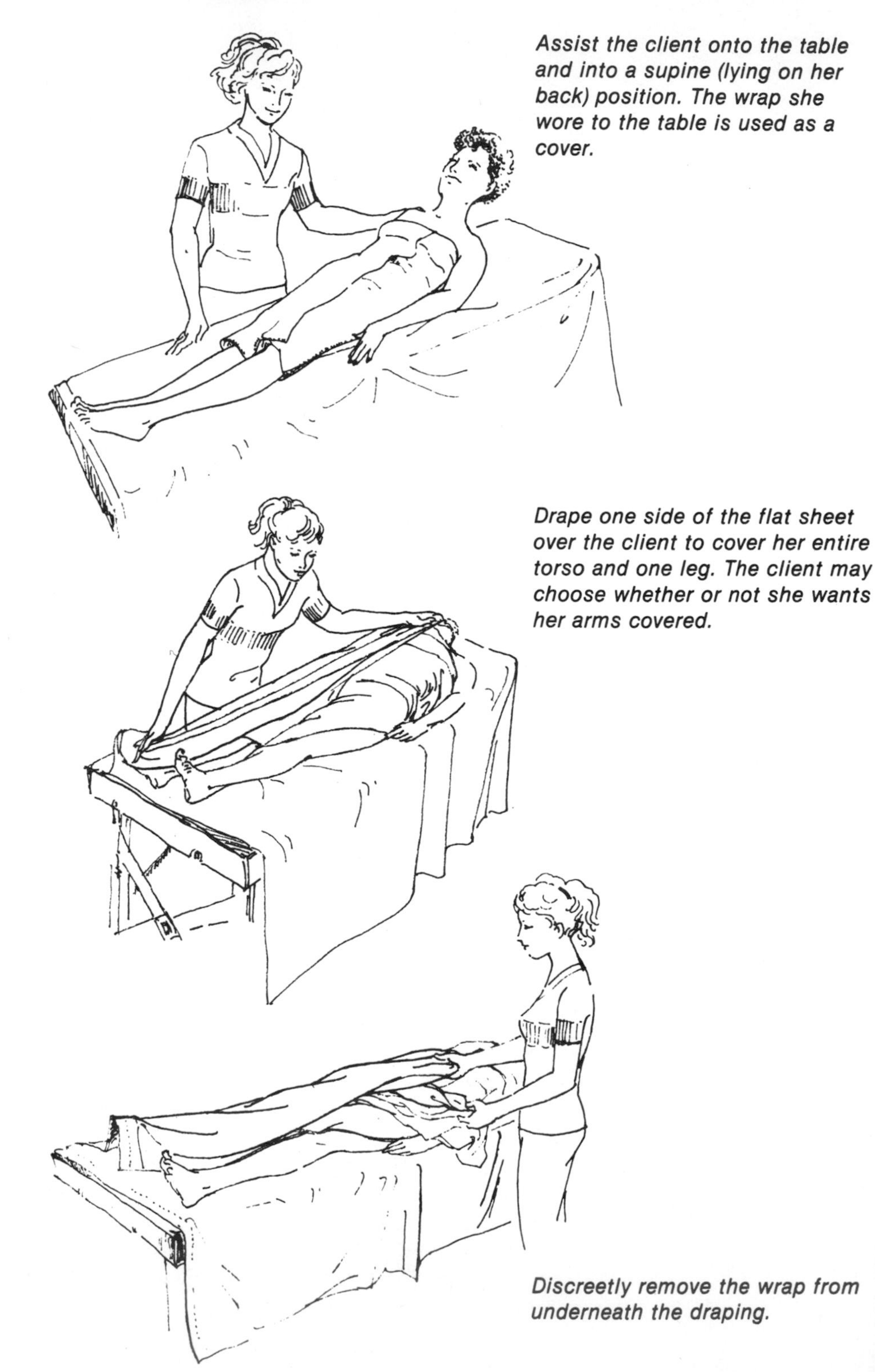

*Assist the client onto the table and into a supine (lying on her back) position. The wrap she wore to the table is used as a cover.*

*Drape one side of the flat sheet over the client to cover her entire torso and one leg. The client may choose whether or not she wants her arms covered.*

*Discreetly remove the wrap from underneath the draping.*

*Drape the other side of the flat sheet over the entire torso and the other leg.*

*The towel or wrap may be placed over the chest area to hold the drape in place. If it is not needed for this purpose, it may be placed aside for later use.*

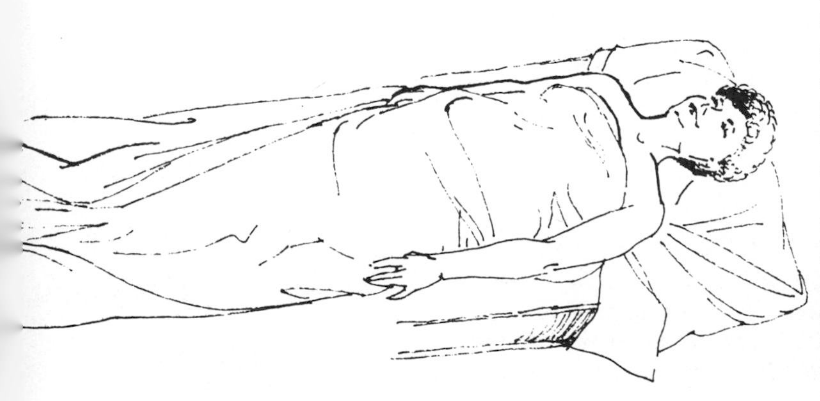

*If the client's arms are left outside the draping there is no problem. (a) If the client prefers having her arms uncovered, then proceed with undraping them by holding the top of the draping, lifting it slightly then reaching in with the other hand to grasp the client's wrist and lift her arm from beneath the drape. (b) After the arm has been massaged, the procedure is reversed, and the arm placed back underneath the draping at the client's side.*

**Draping**
*(Continued)*

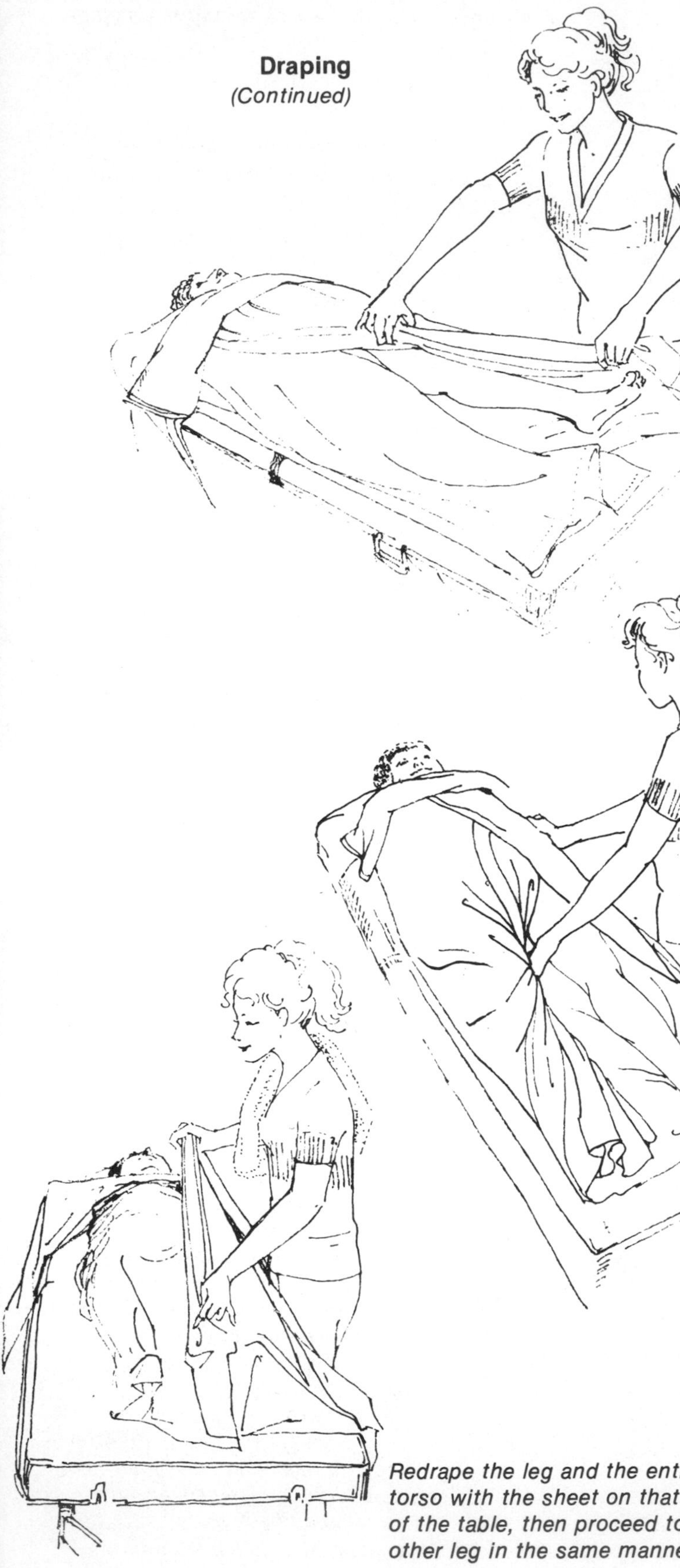

*Undraping the leg begins at the foot. Peel the sheet upward all the way to the illiac crest (hipbone). Remember that when initially draping the client, each leg was draped independently and was covered by only one layer of the draping sheet.*

*Carefully tuck the drape covering the opposite leg under that thigh with one hand, while arranging the rest of the draping with the other hand across the torso and the genital area. This method assures that the client will be well covered when massaging upward to the hipbone and when performing leg stretches.*

*Redrape the leg and the entire torso with the sheet on that side of the table, then proceed to the other leg in the same manner.*

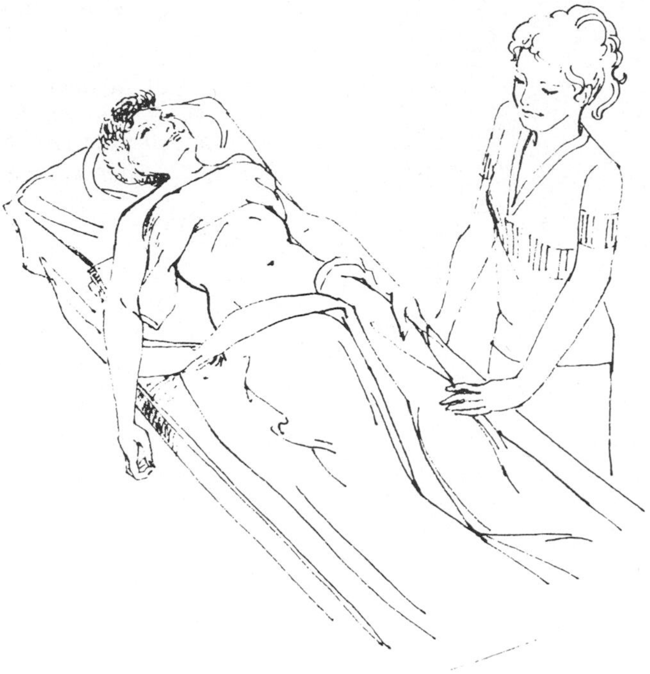

*Prepare to massage the upper part of the body by opening the draping to just above the pubic bone. When massaging a female client, fold the wrap (or towel) and use it as a breast covering. When massaging a male client, use the wrap to secure the draping at the level just above the pubic bone.*

*When it is time for the client to turn over, use the wrap to cover the personal parts of the body.*

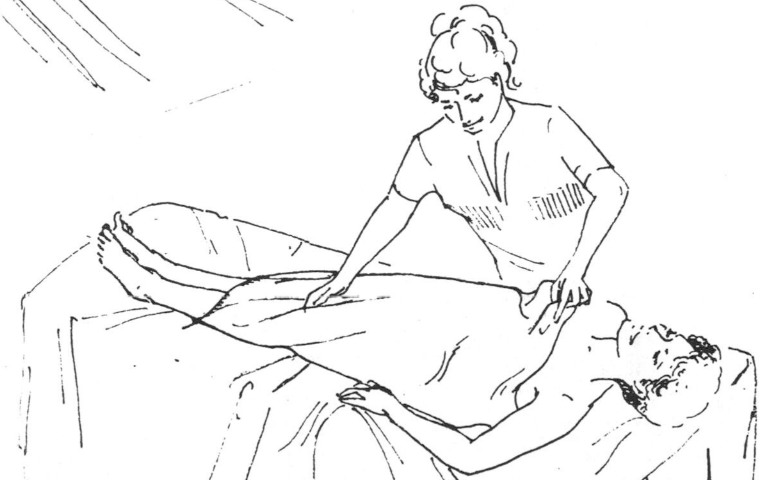

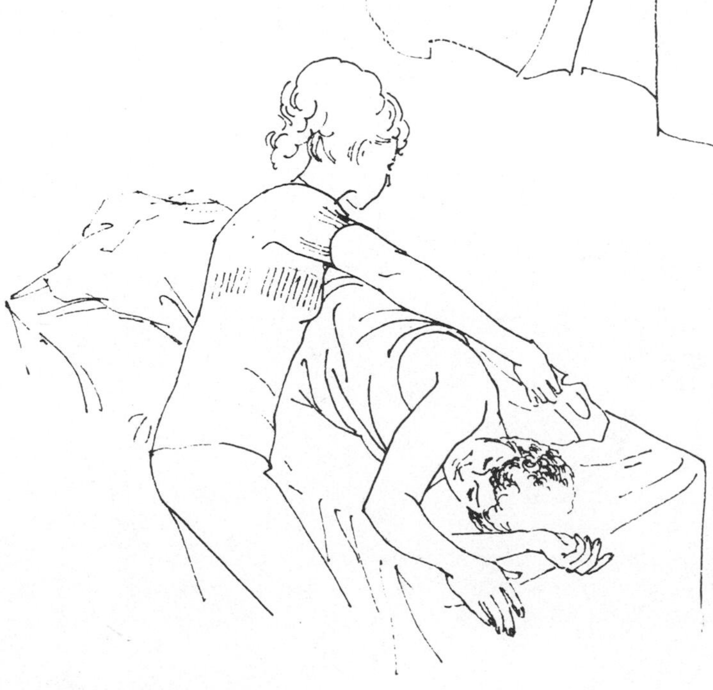

*(a) Remove all other drapings, while holding the wrap in place with your hands, and the flat sheet in place by leaning against the table.*

**Draping**
*(Continued)*

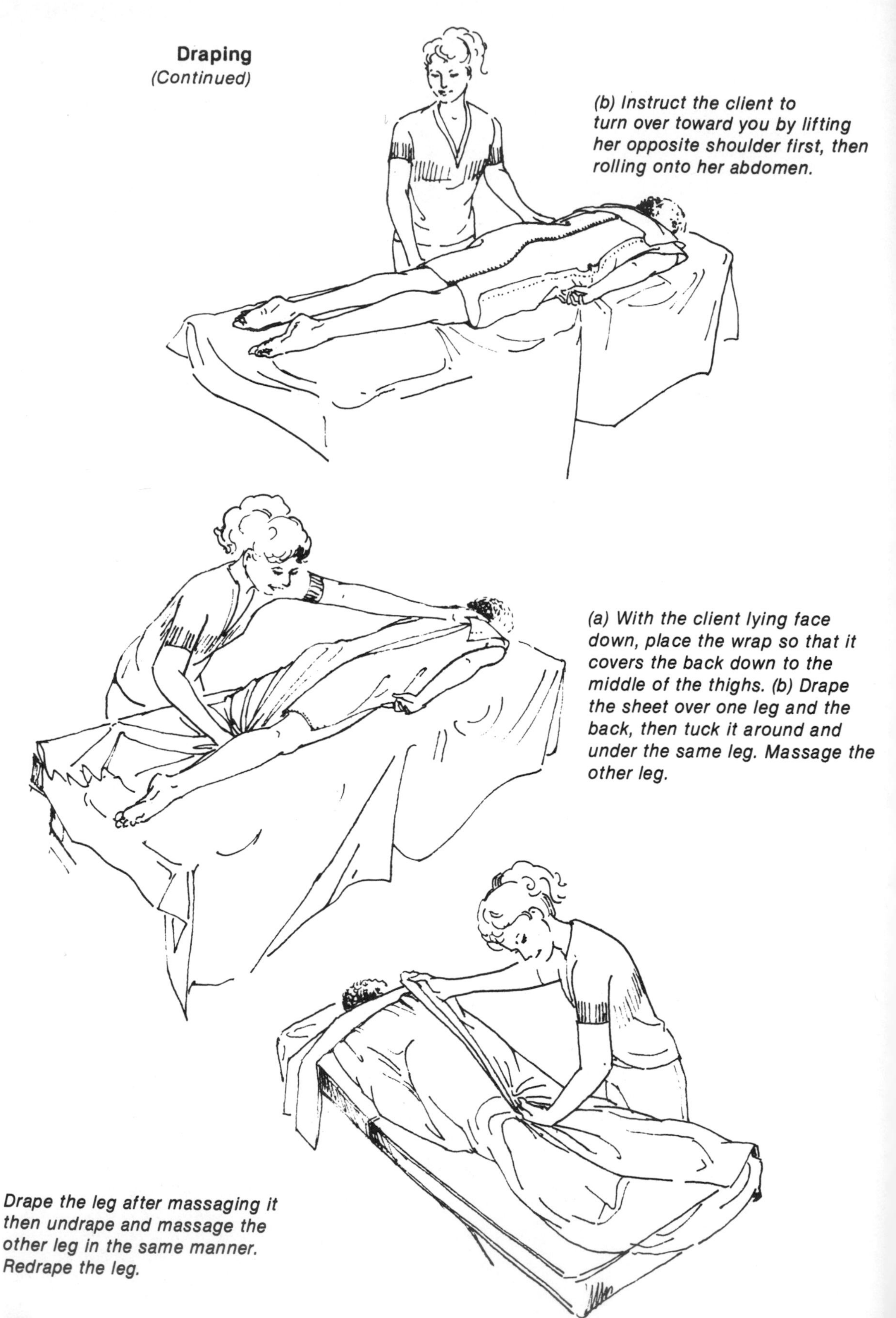

*(b) Instruct the client to turn over toward you by lifting her opposite shoulder first, then rolling onto her abdomen.*

*(a) With the client lying face down, place the wrap so that it covers the back down to the middle of the thighs. (b) Drape the sheet over one leg and the back, then tuck it around and under the same leg. Massage the other leg.*

*Drape the leg after massaging it then undrape and massage the other leg in the same manner. Redrape the leg.*

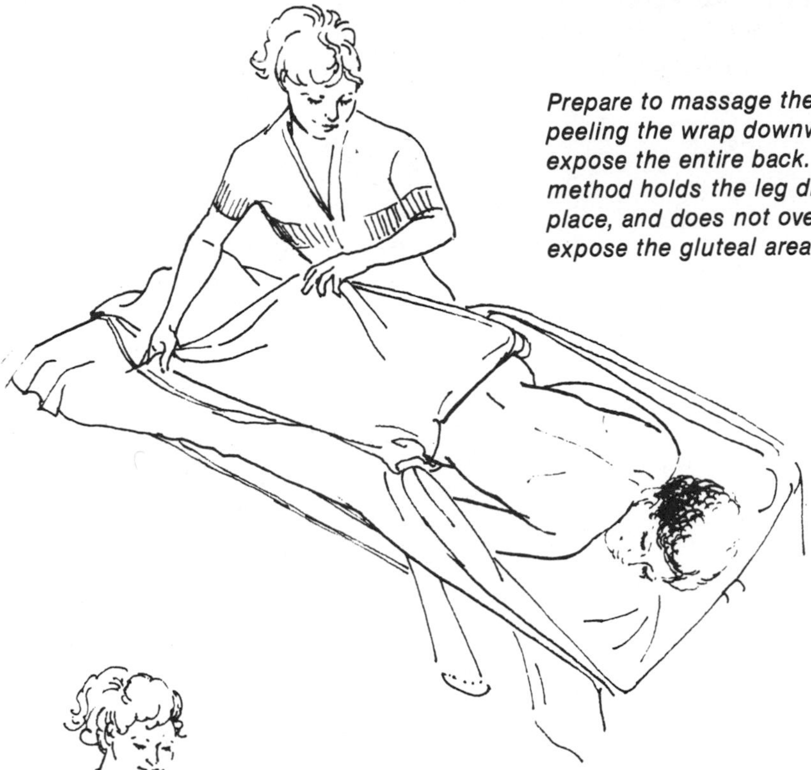

*Prepare to massage the back by peeling the wrap downward to expose the entire back. This method holds the leg draping in place, and does not overly expose the gluteal area.*

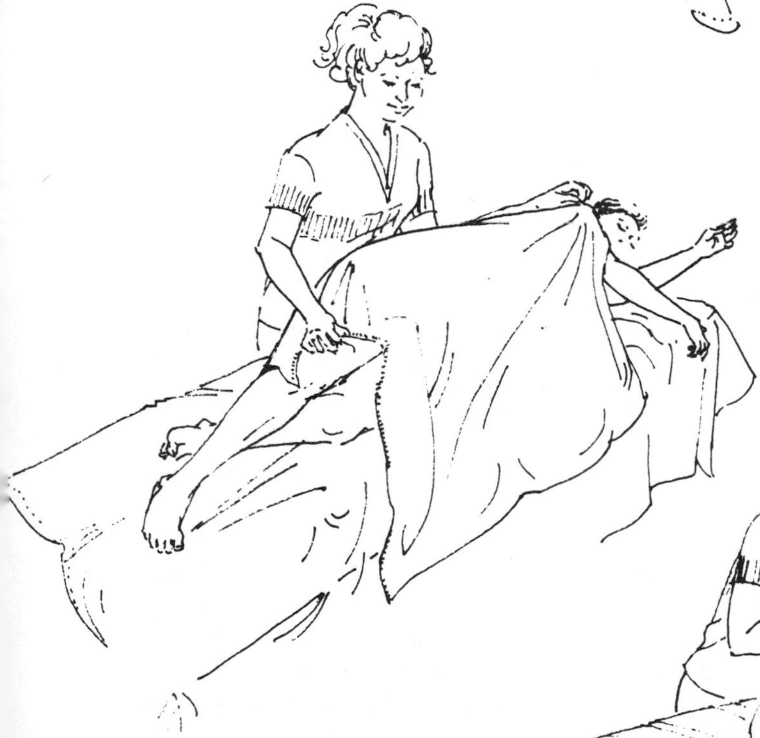

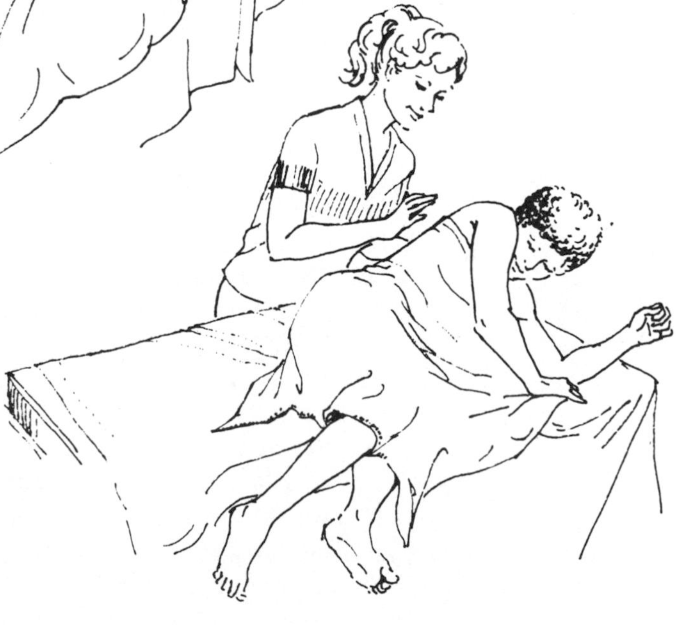

*After completing the massage, arrange the wrap in such a way that when the client turns on her side and sits up, she will be covered adequately. She will be able to arrange the wrap before getting off the massage table and wear it back to the dressing room.*

## QUESTIONS FOR DISCUSSION AND REVIEW

1. Why is it important to prepare a checklist of supplies and equipment before receiving clients.?
2. What kinds of products are usually used for body massage?
3. What is the approximate temperature for the massage room?
4. Why is it important to be able to adjust the height of the massage table?
5. What type of lighting is preferred in the massage room?
6. Why should the client be asked if he or she would like background music?
7. Why is it important to keep accurate records?
8. Why is the consultation important to the success of the massage treatment?
9. Why is it important to inform the client of premassage procedures?
10. Why should the massage practitioner anticipate questions the client may ask and be able to answer them?
11. Why is it important to be prepared to take the client's pulse rate and temperature before giving the massage treatment?
12. Why is it important to explain the draping techniques to the client?

## ANSWERS TO QUESTIONS FOR DISCUSSION AND REVIEW

1. Preparation is essential to good service, and it shows that you are professional.
2. Oils, creams, and powders are usually products used for body massage.
3. The massage room is usually most comfortable for clients when the temperature is around 75 to 80° F.
4. The height of the massage table should be adjusted to give the practitioner more leverage to do the massage efficiently. Correct height also prevents the practitioner from becoming fatigued too soon.
5. Soft, natural, indirect lighting is best in the massage room.
6. Some people find music distracting and prefer absolute quiet.
7. Accurate records are important to both the practitioner and client because special information may be needed for reference. Well-kept records also help the practitioner to determine and render the most effective treatments.
8. The consultation is important to obtain certain data regarding the client's health and to determine the most effective treatments.
9. The client may not understand why premassage procedures are necessary.
10. Being able to anticipate and answer questions the client may ask, gives the practitioner more credibility.
11. An abnormally high temperature or pulse rate may indicate conditions where massage is not advisable.
12. Explaining draping procedures and techniques to the client before, during and after the massage, adds to his or her confidence and prevents embarrassment on the part of the client or the practitioner.

# PART IV MASSAGE TECHNIQUES

# Chapter 8 The Effects, Benefits, and Contraindications of Massage

**LEARNING OBJECTIVES**

After you have mastered this chapter you will be able to:

1. Explain the physiological effects and benefits of massage.
2. Explain the psychological effects and benefits of massage.
3. Describe the effects of massage on the circulatory, muscular, and nervous systems of the body.
4. Describe the effects of massage on the skin.
5. Demonstrate how the practitioner establishes rapport with the client.
6. Explain the main contraindications for massage.

**INTRODUCTION**

There is much historical evidence to indicate that massage was one of the earliest remedial practices for relief of pain and for the restoration of healthy body functions. Massage is a natural and instinctive method by which minor aches and pains can be soothed away while bringing relief from nervous tension and fatigue.

The term "massage" is applied to different practices, but in this chapter the techniques of classic or Swedish massage will be covered. The effects of massage may differ from one client to another depending on the needs of the individual and the results to be achieved. You may do the same massage on two different people and get different results. In addition to physical effects, the client is also affected mentally and emotionally. There are many healthy people who believe that frequent massage helps them to remain physically, mentally, and emotionally fit. They enjoy the pleasant, refreshing, and invigorated feeling they get from a good massage.

Physiologically, a person's activity is divided into two modes: the action or active mode and the passive or resting mode. In the active mode a lot of demand is placed on the body's systems, and a great deal of energy is expended. Both mental and physical activity may be accelerated. This is when wear, tear, and aging of the body takes place. During the resting or passive mode or phase, the body can convert energy into rejuvenating and restoring body tissues. If a person feels sluggish and nonproductive, massage generally will induce relaxation and impart a renewed sense of well-being. Basically, this is due to the increase of nutrients (by way of the blood stream) to the system and the release and flushing out of cellular wastes.

## EFFECTS AND BENEFITS OF MASSAGE

Massage can have positive effects on the range of motion of limbs that have a limited range due to tissue injury, inflammation, or muscle strain. The client may have experienced discomfort or pain and have limited use of the limbs or may have stopped using the limb altogether. The limb will need to be taken through the range of motion passively and carefully and the range increased gradually.

Passive movement is the method by which joints are massaged with no resistance or assistance by muscular activity on the part of the client. Passive massage benefits circulation of the blood and lymph, nourishes the skin and relaxes the nerves. Active movement in massage refers to exercises in which the voluntary muscles are contracted by the client. Active exercise, such as participating in sports or a specific exercise regimen, helps to firm muscles, improve circulation, and aids the function of all internal organs.

There are indications that massage is beneficial in numerous conditions; however, in cases of injury or disease, the client's physician should be consulted before massage treatments are given. Massage has been credited with being of great benefit in helping patients recover from various illnesses or injuries. In some cases devices that use heat, light, cold, water, and electricity may be recommended by the client's physician. Many times a physician will recommend massage for both its physical and psychological benefits.

The nervous system can be stimulated, soothed, or toned depending on the type of massage movement applied.

1. Stimulating effect
   a. Friction (light rubbing, rolling, and wringing movement) stimulates nerves.
   b. Percussion (light tapping and slapping movements). Percussion increases nervous irritability. Strong percussion for a short period of time excites nerve centers directly.
   c. Vibration (shaking and trembling movements) stimulates peripheral nerves and all nerve centers with which a trunk is connected.
2. Sedative effect
   a. Gentle stroking, especially over reflex areas, produces the most effective results.
   b. Light friction and petrissage (kneading movements) produce marked sedative effects.

### Effects of Massage Upon the Muscular System

Massage encourages the nutrition and development of the muscular system by way of stimulation of its circulation, nerve supply, and cell activity. Regular and systematic massage causes the muscles to become firmer and more elastic while muscles too weak to be used voluntarily can be strengthened by massage treatments.

The supply of blood to the muscles is proportionate to their activity. It is estimated that blood passes three times more rapidly through muscles being massaged. Petrissage or kneading movements create a pumping action that forces the venous blood and lymph onward and brings a fresh supply of blood to the muscles. Strong vibrations cause rapid contractions of the muscles.

Massage prevents and relieves stiffness and soreness of muscles. Muscles fatigued by work will be more quickly restored by massage than by passive rest of the same duration. Massage aids in the removal of metabolic waste products and helps nourish tissues.

Facial massage helps to keep the facial muscles toned and aids in the prevention of premature lines and wrinkles.

**Physiological Effects of Massage**

Skillfully applied massage is one of the more effective means of influencing the structures and functions of the body. Depending on the type and manner of manipulation, a sense of mild relaxation, stimulation, or refreshment may ensue following massage. Under no circumstances should massage be applied so vigorously as to cause the client to feel exhausted, or result in bruised or sore tissues.

There are two effects of massage, mechanical and reflex, which may occur separately or together. The specific effects of any massage movement will vary with the degree of pressure applied to particular parts of the body.

Gentle stimulation of the sensory nerve endings in the skin, as in superficial stroking, results in reflex effects, either locally or in distant parts of the body. When direct pressure is applied to the muscles, blood, and lymph vessels, or to any internal structure, both reflex and mechanical effects are experienced by the body.

The immediate effects of massage are noticeable on the skin. Friction and stroking movements heighten blood circulation to the skin and increase activity of the sweat (sudoriferous) and oil (sebaceous) glands. Accompanying the increased flow of blood, there is a slight reddening and warming of the skin. Nutrition of the skin is improved. Massage treatments over a period of time impart a healthy radiance to the skin. The skin tends to become softer, more supple, and of finer texture.

The physiological effects of massage are not limited to the skin. The body as a whole benefits by the stimulation of muscular, glandular, and vascular activities. Most organs of the body are favorably influenced by scientific massage treatments.

**Effects of Massage upon the Nervous System**

The effects of massage upon the nervous system depend on the direct and reflex reaction of the nerves stimulated. Invigorating effects are experienced by the entire nervous system.

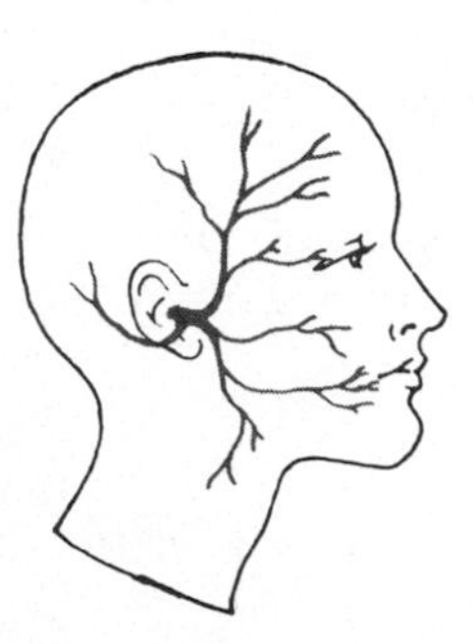

## Effects of Massage upon the Circulatory System

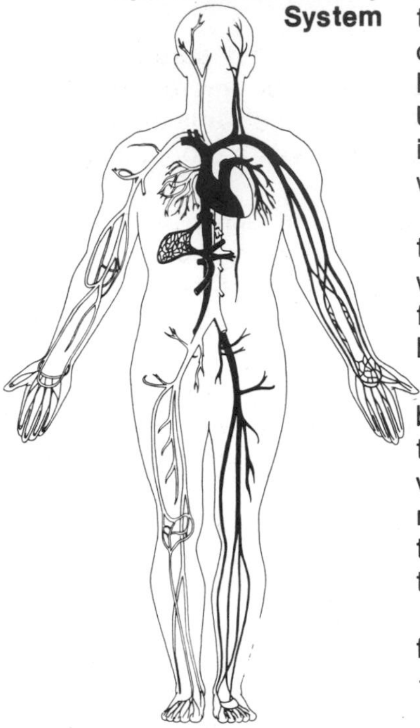

Scientific body massage procedures affect the quality and quantity of blood coursing through the circulatory system. With the increased flow of blood to the massaged area, better cellular nutrition and elimination are favored. The work of the heart is lessened due to the improvement in surface circulation. Under the influence of massage, the blood-making process is improved, resulting in an increase in the number of red and white blood cells.

An important principle to remember is to always massage toward the heart. Massage movements should be directed upward along the limbs and lower parts of the body and downward from the head, thereby facilitating the flow of blood back to the heart and other eliminatory organs.

Massage may influence the blood and lymph vessels either by direct mechanical action on the vessel walls or by reflex action through the vaso-motor nerves. Pressure against the vessels not only tones their muscular walls but also propels the movement of the blood. The vaso-motor nerves, by controlling the relaxing and constricting of the blood vessels, determine the amount of blood which will reach the area being massaged.

Massage movements affect blood and lymph channels in the following ways:

1. Light stroking produces an almost instantaneous though temporary dilation of the capillaries, while deep stroking brings about a more lasting dilation and flushing of the massaged area.
2. Light percussion causes a contraction of the blood vessels, which tend to relax as the movement is continued. Strong percussion should be used with care, since sudden dilation, if it continues, may lead to paralysis of the part massaged.
3. Friction hastens the flow of blood through the superficial veins, increases the permeability of the capillary beds, and produces an increased flow of interstitial fluid. This creates a healthier environment for the cells.
4. Petrissage or kneading stimulates the flow of blood through the deeper arteries and veins.
5. Friction and kneading aid the lymph circulation by draining the tissues of waste products.

Because massage requires a great deal of physical energy on the part of the practitioner, mechanical and electrical apparatus have been devised as aids to manual massage. The hand vibrator is an example. The same contraindications for manual massage also apply when any kind of helpful apparatus is used.

## Psychological Effects of Massage

The psychological effects of massage should not be underestimated. If the client feels healthier, invigorated, and more energetic, then the massage has been worth the effort. People with no health problems can have regular massages as much for psychological as for physical benefit.

Many people suffer from stress and find that massage promotes relaxation as it soothes away minor aches and pains. Some clients feel that regular massage keeps them looking more youthful and encourages them to pay more attention to proper nutrition, exercises, and good health practices.

Massage helps clients to become more aware of where they are holding tension, and where they have tight muscles or painful areas. The practitioner may discover these painful areas, and the client may not have been previously aware of them. By becoming in touch with, or aware of these areas of the body, the client can begin to focus on relaxing them on a daily basis. The client should be told that when muscles are tight there is constriction in the circulation to the affected area. Becoming aware of these trouble spots and treating them, is considered part of preventative maintenance.

## ESTABLISHING RAPPORT WITH CLIENTS

It is important to establish professional rapport with the client because the success of the massage treatment depends on mutual trust and respect. Clients like to feel that the practitioner regards people as individuals and has some insight into their feelings. A pleasant, confident, and professional manner on the part of the practitioner helps to put the client at ease so he or she can relax and enjoy the massage. This is particularly important when the client is having massage for the first time and does not know what to expect. The human touch itself can have a healing and therapeutic effect, and the practitioner's manner will help to dispel any sense of nervousness, shyness, or doubt on the part of the client.

It is also important that a practitioner establish good relations with physicians and build a reputation as one who cares about the welfare of his or her clients. Clients should be encouraged to report to their physicians when the massage treatments have been beneficial. Physicians want to know that you are working professionally and in the best interests of their patients, and generally they are happy to assist you with whatever information they can provide.

## CONDITIONS GENERALLY RELIEVED BY MASSAGE

Almost all healthy people occasionally have some physical condition that can be improved by massage. When relief is obtained, there is also a renewed sense of well-being. No matter how well a client may be, a good massage will leave that person feeling much better.

The following is a list of conditions most frequently relieved by regular massage treatment:

1. Tension is relieved in muscles. With the release of tension there is a lessening of stress, and the client feels better able to cope with emotional problems.
2. Mental and physical fatigue is relieved, leading to renewed energy and ambition.
3. Pain in the shoulders, neck, and back usually caused by strain is relieved.
4. Muscles and joints become more supple. Soreness and stiffness are relieved.
5. Muscles become firmer, and the figure is improved.
6. Circulation is improved, thus improving skin tone.

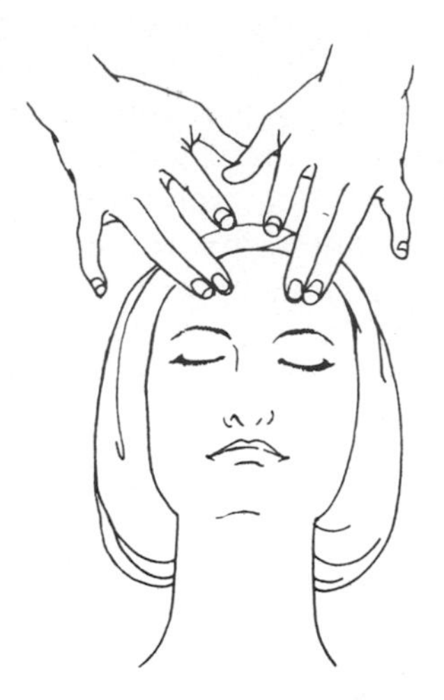

7. Digestion, assimilation, and elimination problems are often corrected.
8. Facial massage helps to prevent problem blemished skin, tones the skin, and softens fine lines.
9. Headache and eyestrain are often relieved.
10. Massage improves body metabolism.
11. Deep relaxation is induced and insomnia relieved.
12. Muscular spasms and internal cramps are relieved.
13. Obesity (overweight) and flabby muscles can be improved when combined with proper exercise and diet programs.
14. Pain in joints, sprains, and poor circulation are relieved.
15. Increased circulation of nourishing blood to the skin and other parts of the body encourages healing.
16. Mental strain is reduced resulting in better productivity.
17. Mildly-high blood pressure is temporarily reduced.
18. Renewed sense of confidence and control is experienced.

## CONTRAINDICATIONS FOR MASSAGE

While there are many benefits from therapeutic body massage, there are also contraindications of which the professional practitioner is aware.

*Contraindication* means the expected treatment or process is inadvisable. In massage it means that conditions may exist in which it would not be beneficial to apply massage to a part or all of the body. The practitioner must know not only when massage is advised but more importantly when it should be avoided, or when certain strokes or movements should not be used.

When you define massage as a form of touch that is applied in a therapeutic manner, then it is true that massage of some form is beneficial to nearly everyone. However, there are situations where particular manipulations may not only be uncomfortable for the client but could be dangerous.

The practitioner should make a special effort to understand fully the indications and contraindications in massage. Many conditions respond favorably to massage, while others can be aggravated or worsened by specific massage techniques. Such techniques would be contraindicated. This means that certain movements could do more harm than good.

During the first interview or consultation with a client, it is important to obtain information about the state of his or her health and determine any reasons why massage treatments might be inadvisable. When in doubt, caution is the best policy. The client can be asked (tactfully) to supply a physician's report and/or recommendations before beginning treatments, or the practitioner could ask the client's physician first, in case there are questionable circumstances.

The major contraindications include the following:

*Abnormal body temperature:* 98.6° F (Fahrenheit) 37° C (Celsius) is considered normal temperature, but it may vary depending on the time of day or other factors. Temperature can vary from 96.4° to 99.1° F (35.8° to 37.3° C). Some doctors and therapists say that massage is not recommended when temperature exceeds 99.4°. If the client feels abnormally warm or feverish, temperature should be taken to ascertain the advisability of massage treatment. Massage is contraindicated when the client has a fever, because generally fever indicates that the body is trying to isolate and eliminate an invading pathogen. The body is stepping up its own action in order to confine, narrow down, and eliminate the problem. Therefore massage would tend to work against the defense mechanisms of the body.

*Acute infectious disease:* Typhoid, diphtheria, influenza, severe colds, and the like would preclude massage. The client should seek his or her doctor's advice.

*Inflammation:* When there is inflammation in a particular area of the body, massage is not advisable because it could further irritate the area or intensify the inflammation. This is particularly true for spreading or penetrating types of manipulation. Inflamed joints do not indicate massage of the joint itself; however, there are some pressure point applications that are useful. "Therapeutic touch," which is simply placing your hands on or near the inflamed area, may be helpful.

Although working directly on an area may be contraindicated, working on a reflex or related area or working in an area proximal to the affected area can be useful because it tends to open up the natural healing properties of the body. A *reflex* is a point that is distant to the affected area yet, when stimulated, has an effect on that area.

There are numerous types of inflammations. A word with the suffix "tis," pertains to inflammation. For example, arthritis is an inflammation of the joints, neuritis is an inflammation of a nerve or nerves, dermatitis is inflammation of the skin, and so on. Caution must be used when a client has any kind of inflammation that could be worsened by massage. Also, you will not want to cause damage or to be held liable for a problem that results from a massage that you perform.

*Osteoporosis:* This is a condition that leads to deterioration of bone. In advanced stages bones become brittle, sometimes to the point that they are easily broken. This condition is prevalent in the elderly and in certain kinds of diseases. The symptoms of osteoporosis may include frailty and stooped shoulders. In women it can be due to reduced estrogen levels. It is best to obtain the advice of the client's physician before giving massage when osteoporosis is indicated.

*Varicose veins:* This is a condition where the veins break down because of back pressure in the circulatory system. The veins bulge and rupture, usually in the legs. Varicose veins are often the result of standing for long hours. Also, in women the pressure on the large veins in the pelvic area during pregnancy often contributes to this condition.

Blood is pumped through the veins by means of pressure originating in the heart and is helped along by contractions of muscle surrounding the veins. Veins are basically tubes consisting of a layer of endothelial lining and smooth muscle and are covered with connective tissue. When veins become abnormally dilated due to excessive back pressure, they rupture and are called varicose veins.

The client may not realize that development of varicose veins is often the result of gravity or obstructed venous flow, such as might happen in crossing the legs or other sitting postures that cut off circulation to the legs. This excessive back pressure causes veins to stretch to the extent that small valves within the veins, which normally allow blood to move only in one direction, collapse and lose the ability to stop the backward flow of blood. Blood then accumulates in enlarged portions of the vein. If the flow of blood becomes obstructed, clotting may occur. When this condition is accompanied by inflammation, it is painful and potentially dangerous. The client should see a physician because surgery is often helpful.

The practitioner will recognize varicose veins as bluish, protruding, thick, lumpy vessels usually found in the lower legs. Also, to be considered with caution are the small reddish groupings of broken blood vessels that often surround a small, protruding vein. Any deep massage on these areas may set a blood clot loose in the general circulation and cause a serious problem.

Inflammation of a vein accompanied by pain and swelling is called *Phlebitis.* If a blood clot forms, it can cause the dangerous condition known as *thrombophlebitis.* If a piece of this clot loosens and floats in the blood, it is called an embolus. If this embolus reaches the lungs, it can cause death by pulmonary embolism. If the embolus reaches the brain or the nourishing vessels of the heart, it can bring about stroke or cardiac arrest.

It is easy to see why massage would be contraindicated in cases of varicosities. However, massage proximal to the affected area might be very helpful, especially superficial (barely touching) techniques.

Phlebitis may be the result of surgery, or may be secondary to an infection or injury, or may have no apparent precurser.

*Aneurosa:* This condition is a localized dilation of a blood vessel or, more commonly, an artery. It can be caused by congenital defect, arteriosclerosis, hypertension, or trauma and is generally located in the aorta, thorax, and abdomen and sometimes in the cranium. Although this condition can appear, it is rarely encountered in the massage field, and if suspected, should be referred to medical attention.

*Edema:* Edema is another circulatory abnormality that generally appears as puffiness in the extremities but is sometimes more widespread. Edema is an excess accumulation of fluid in tissue spaces; it has numerous causes. In some instances massage is indicated and in others, it is not. If edema is the result of back pressure in the veins due to immobility, massage and mild exercise may prove helpful. If on the other hand, edema is the result of protein imbalance due to breakdown in the kidneys or liver, or is the result of increased permeability (allowing passage especially of fluids) of the capillaries due to inflammation, massage is contraindicated.

When edema is suspected, it can be easily detected by pressing a finger into the area. When the finger is removed and an indentation remains, edema is present. This indentation will take several seconds to return to the level of adjoining skin.

Edema can also result from an imbalance of factors that regulate the interchange of fluids between the capillaries and tissue spaces. Other causes can be related to heart or kidney disease, poison in the system (affecting histamine levels that cause increased capillary permeability), and obstruction of lymph channels. Obviously such conditions should be brought to the attention of a physician.

If edema is related to pregnancy and is caused by toxemia (poisons in the blood), then massage is contraindicated. The practitioner should not try to reduce edema by direct massage on the area until channels leading out of the area have been flushed open. This means that if edema is in the feet, it is advisable to open channels in the abdomen, groin, and thigh before massaging the feet. Another consideration is to work on reflexes to increase lymph activity.

*High blood pressure:* High blood pressure means pressure of the blood against the walls of the arteries. If the client has a history of high blood pressure, his or her physician should be consulted before treatment. The client may be taking medication to bring the condition under control. Unless it is severe, massage may be of assistance in relieving some of the hypertension that accompanies high blood pressure. Any massage that involves high blood pressure should be soothing and sedating. Low blood pressure is not a consideration in massage.

*Specific conditions or diseases:* It should be obvious to the practitioner that a client who is suffering from severe asthma (a chronic respiratory disorder), diabetes (deficient insulin secretion), or any type of heart or lung disease should be under the supervision of a physician. Massage would not be given without the physician's knowledge and advice. This is why it is important to take time during the first consultation (interview) to determine the client's state of health.

*Cancer:* Cancer is a disease that can become widespread through the lymphatic system. Because massage affects the lymphatics, any massage that tends to increase lymph flow is contraindicated for cancer patients. However, there are exceptions where limited massage may be included in the daily regimen. For example, many physicians believe that an essential for those who are severly ill is caring, understanding, and human touch. A person who has been diagnosed as having cancer knows what to expect and knows which part of the body is affected. The practitioner can limit the massage to simple reflex and touch therapy to provide comfort to the client. The practitioner must remember that malignancies and cancers are contraindicated to circulatory types of massage.

*Fatigue:* In cases of chronic fatigue the excretory system is already over burdened, and there is little to nourish those overworked and exhausted tissues. When a client is suffering from chronic fatigue, massage should be extremely light and superficial to induce rest and relaxation. Over a period of time, massage helps to restore the client's energy.

*Intoxication:* Intoxication is a contraindication because it can spread toxins and overstress the liver.

*Psychosis:* Psychosis is another condition where it is advisable to work directly under the supervision of the patient's doctor.

*Medication and drugs:* There are times when a client will be taking specific medication or drugs, and massage may or may not be recommended. Generally, the practitioner will not encounter drug-related problems unless he or she is planning to specialize in this kind of therapy. In this case, the practitioner should keep in mind that while most doctors do not specialize in massage, they recognize its benefits.

*Skin problems:* The following skin conditions are contraindications. Usually only the affected areas are of concern. For example, a minor laceration on the hand would not prevent massage of other healthy parts of the body. However, as has already been stated, when a condition is of a contagious nature, massage is not given. The following are various skin disorders:

| | | | |
|---|---|---|---|
| skin cancer | eczema | tumor | boils |
| sores | rashes | scratches | carbuncles |
| warts | skin tags | moles | acne |
| lumps | scaly spots | pimples | wounds |
| lacerations | burns and blisters | inflammation | scar tissue |
| adhesions | hypersensitive skin | stings and bites | |
| bruises | broken vessels | | |

*Hernia:* Hernia is a protrusion of an organ or part of an organ, such as the intestine protruding through an opening in the abdominal wall surrounding it. This is also referred to as a rupture, and massage is not recommended over or near the afflicted area.

*Frail elderly people:* Frail elderly people may have fragile bones and very sensitive skin. However, gentle massage may be beneficial.

*Scoliosis* (crooked spine): Massage must be recommended by the client's physician. Caution must be exercised.

## MASSAGE DURING PREGNANCY

During a normal, healthy pregnancy, massage may be found to be very beneficial in promoting relaxation, soothing nerves, and relieving strained back and leg muscles. Massage also tends to instill a feeling of well-being to both mother and unborn child. However, certain situations and conditions exist of which the practitioner must be aware.

Massage should always be soothing and relaxing. No heavy percussion or deep tissue massage should ever be done, likewise abdominal kneading or other deep abdominal massage should be avoided. Care should be taken late in term to position the mother in such a way as to assure the comfort of both mother and unborn child.

When the client is supine (face up), pillows are used under the knees and head.

When the client is on her side, pillows are placed under her head and upper knee or between her legs.

During the second and third trimesters, lying prone (face down) places pressure on the abdominal area. This position is not only very uncomfortable, it may be dangerous to the unborn child. A prone position is not advisable unless proper and adequate support is provided. If there is any question as to the state of health of either the mother or unborn child, the client's doctor must be consulted before massage is given.

## QUESTIONS FOR DISCUSSION AND REVIEW

1. What is "passive" movement massage?
2. What is "active" movement massage?
3. What are the immediate effects of massage on the skin?
4. Which massage movements produce a stimulating effect on the nervous system?
5. Which massage movements produce a sedative effect on the nervous system?
6. How does massage relieve sore and stiff muscles?
7. Why are all massage movements directed toward the heart?
8. Which massage movements increase the flow of blood and lymph?
9. What are the main psychological benefits of massage?
10. What are the main physiological benefits of massage?
11. Why is the practitioner's professional manner important to the client?
12. What is the meaning of contraindication as it relates to massage?
13. Why does the practitioner need to take the client's temperature?
14. What should the practitioner do when a client has a condition that appears to be a contraindication to massage?
15. How does massage benefit a woman during a normal, healthy pregnancy?

## ANSWERS TO QUESTIONS FOR DISCUSSION AND REVIEW

1. Passive massage movement is the method by which joints are massaged with no resistance or assistance by muscular activity of the client.
2. Active movement massage refers to exercises in which the voluntary muscles are contracted by the client.
3. The immediate effects of massage on the skin include increased circulation of the blood, which nourishes the skin, improves tone, and helps to normalize the functioning of the sebaceous (oil) glands.
4. Friction, vibration, and light percussive movements produce a stimulating effect on the nervous system.
5. Gentle stroking, light friction, and petrissage produce a sedative effect on the nervous system.
6. Massage relieves stiff, sore muscles by improving circulation of the blood to the body part. It also helps in the removal of waste products and supplies the cells with oxygen and nourishment.
7. Massage movements are directed toward the heart to facilitate the flow of blood back to the heart.
8. Light stroking, deep stroking, light percussion, friction, petrissage, and gentle kneading are all useful in increasing the flow of blood and lymph.
9. The client is benefitted psychologically by massage because he or she feels it is beneficial. Massage helps the client to feel healthier, invigorated, and more energetic.
10. The main physiological benefits of massage are stimulation of the muscular, vascular, and glandular activities of the body. Circulation is increased and soreness and stiffness of the muscles relieved.
11. A professional manner on the part of the practitioner helps to dispel any nervousness, shyness or doubt the client may have.
12. Contraindication means the expected treatment or process is inadvisable. In massage it refers to any condition in which massage is not advisable, as it would not be beneficial or might be dangerous.
13. The practitioner takes the client's temperature because massage is not recommended when the client's temperature is abnormally high. An abnormally high temperature may indicate the onset of illness or other health problems.
14. When the client has a condition that appears to be a contraindication to massage, the practitioner explains that it will be necessary to have a physician's recommendations and consent before massage treatments are given.
15. Massage benefits a woman during a normal healthy pregnancy by promoting relaxation, soothing nerves, relieving strained back and leg muscles and instilling a sense of well-being.

# Chapter 9 Classification and Mastery of Massage Movements

## LEARNING OBJECTIVES

After you have mastered this chapter you will be able to:

1. Demonstrate mastery of various hand exercises specifically for the benefit of massage practitioners.
2. Demonstrate correct standing posture and movements specifically for the benefit of massage practitioners.
3. Explain why it is necessary and desirable for the massage practitioner to develop coordination, balance, control, and stamina.
4. Explain why it is necessary and desirable for the massage practitioner to develop strong, flexible hands.
5. Describe the concepts of grounding and centering and how these practices benefit the massage practitioner.
6. Describe the four major categories of massage movements.
7. Explain Swedish (classic) massage techniques.
8. Demonstrate mastery of basic massage movements.
9. Demonstrate passive and active joint movements.
10. Explain and demonstrate rhythm, pressure, and duration as applied to therapeutic body massage.

## INTRODUCTION

In recent times the various movements used in body massage have been studied scientifically. Some movements are devised to induce relaxation while others are meant to invigorate and stimulate the body. The massage practitioner is primarily concerned with manual movements that have beneficial effects on the client's body and how to apply these movements correctly and effectively.

Massage is a strenuous practice and when done correctly, it requires a great deal of energy. By developing correct habits while learning, the practitioner can do much to lessen the effort and to prevent fatigue when doing several massages a day.

## BUILDING STRENGTH AND FLEXIBILITY OF THE HANDS

The practitioner's hands are the most important tools used in massage. Hand mobility is important to maintain a regular rhythm and to control the hands when doing slow or fast movements. Flexible hands aid in working on the contours of the client's body and in controlling both speed and pressure. In addition to well-trained hands, the practitioner must have a good sense of balance and body control in order to move easily while applying various massage movements. The following exercises will help to develop strength, control, balance, and flexibility of the hands.

## Hand Exercises

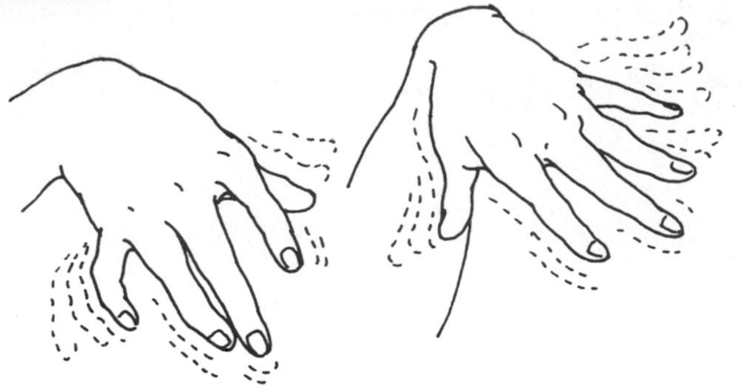

*Hold your hands at chest level and shake them vigorously for about 10 counts. This exercise warms and limbers the hands.*

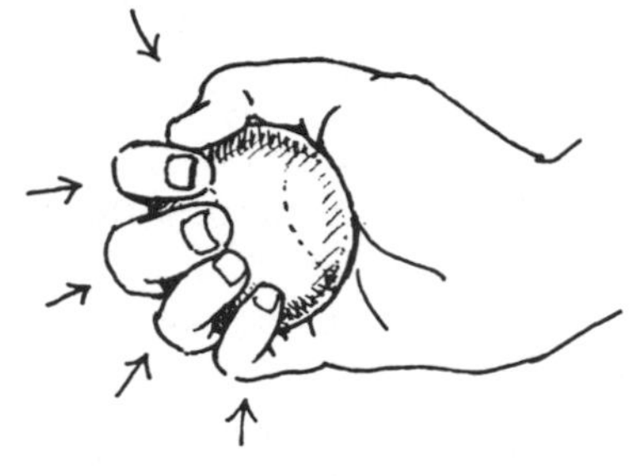

*Hold your hands at chest level. Use a small ball or clinch your hands into tight fists. Squeeze the ball or fists as hard as you can while counting to 10. Repeat this exercise several times. This exercise will strengthen your hands and wrists.*

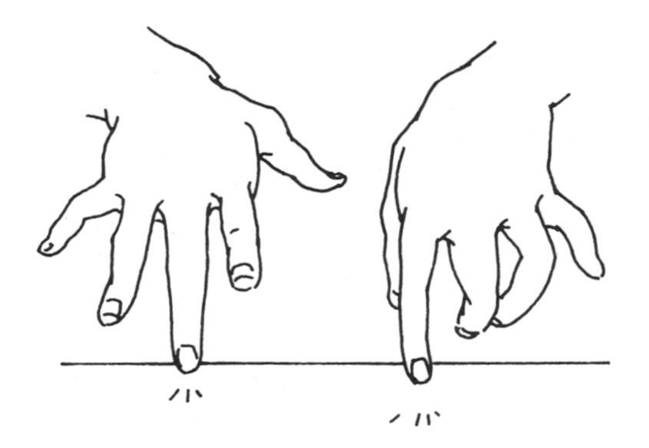

*Place both hands palms down on a flat surface such as a table top. Begin with the thumbs and count each finger to the little finger and back to thumbs. This exercise is similar to playing a piano or typing. It is excellent for improving coordination and hand control.*

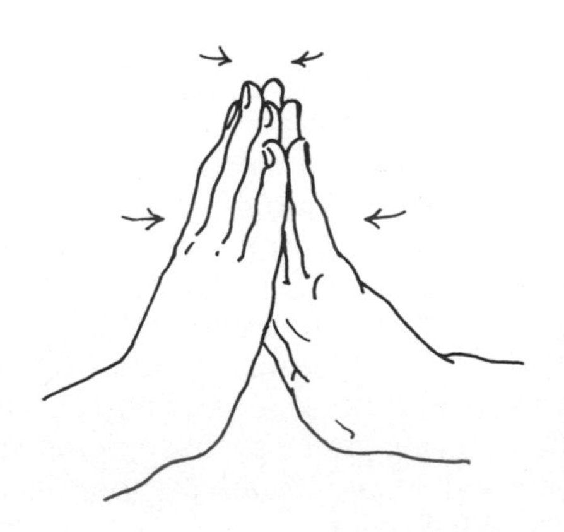

*Place your palms together at chest level. Press one hand against the other back and forth. This will make your wrists supple and strong. Repeat the presses about 10 times.*

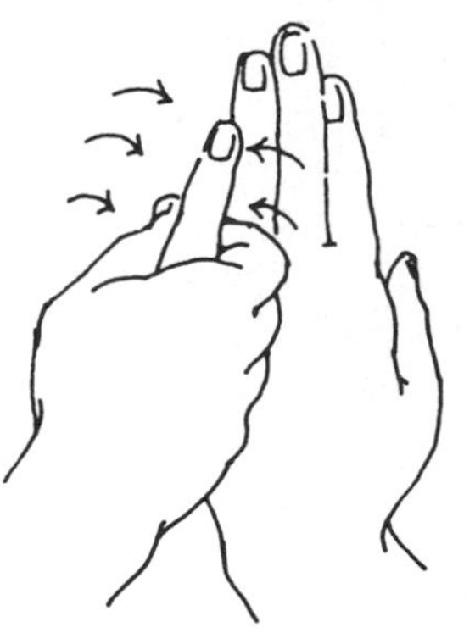

*Beginning with the thumb of the left hand, massage all the fingers of that hand by rubbing each finger from the knuckles of the hand to the tip of the finger. Repeat on the right hand. This exercise stimulates circulation and helps to keep the hands supple.*

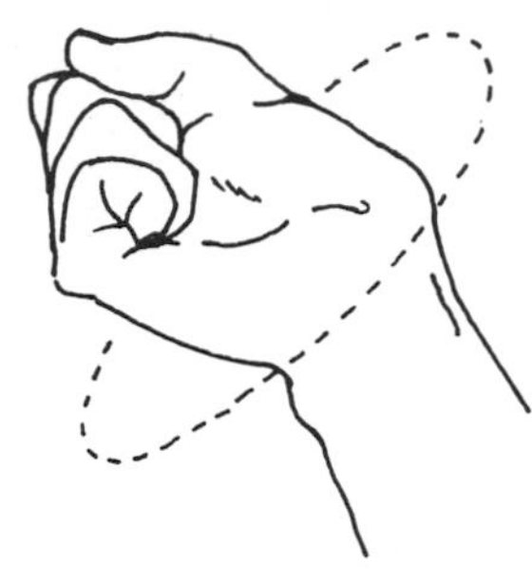

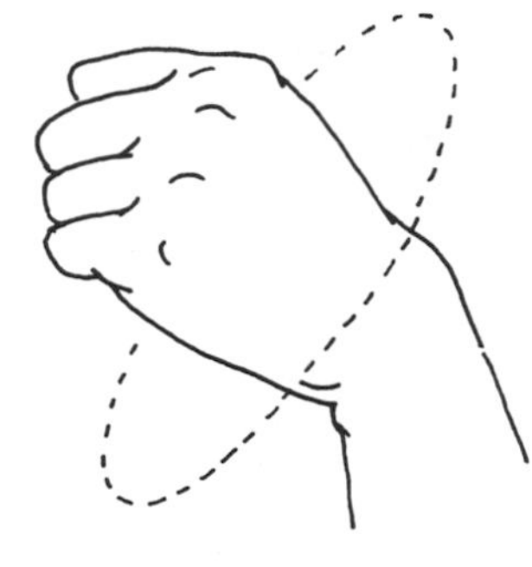

*Hold your hands in fists at chest level. Rotate both hands in circles forward 10 times, then reverse 10 times. This exercise strengthens and limbers the wrists.*

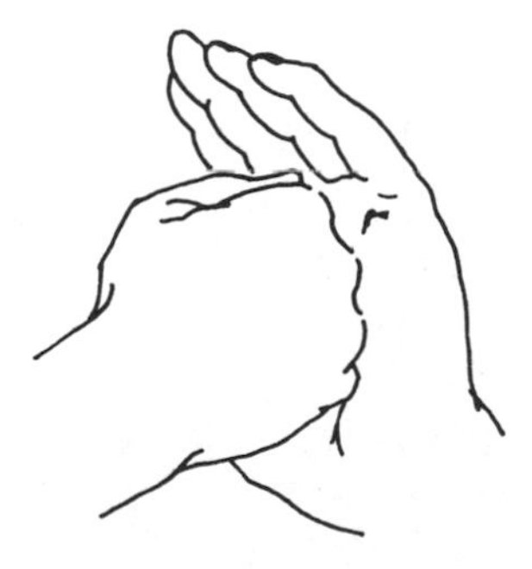

*Press the fist of one hand into the palm of the other with each hand resisting the other. Do this 10 times on each hand. This exercise will strengthen the entire arm and the hand.*

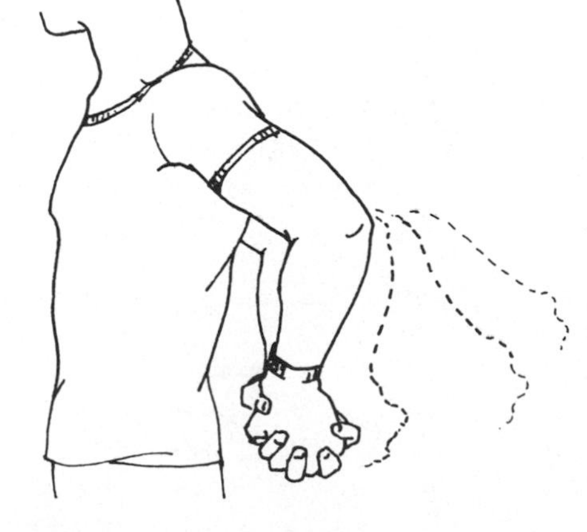

*Clasp your hands just below your waistline at the back of your body. Pull your arms upward while holding the tension for 10 counts. Pull your arms downward for 10 counts. This exercise strengthens the muscles of your arms, shoulders and hands.*

Do these exercises everyday, or every other day, to keep your muscles strong and flexible.

## POSTURE AND STANCES

Correct posture and stances (standing positions) are important to the practitioner because they aid balance and allow the delivery of firmer, more powerful, more direct massage strokes. Correct posture is essential to conserve strength and prevent backache due to stress on the practitioner's arms and shoulders during the massage procedure. Good posture helps to sustain energy when it is necessary to work long hours because it enables the practitioner to move around the table more freely and easily while maintaining the flow of movement and energy.

The most common stances are called the "horse" and the "archer."

### Horse Stance

For the horse stance both feet are placed in line with the edge of the massage table. For example, this is the most comfortable stance when doing petrissage on the legs or back.

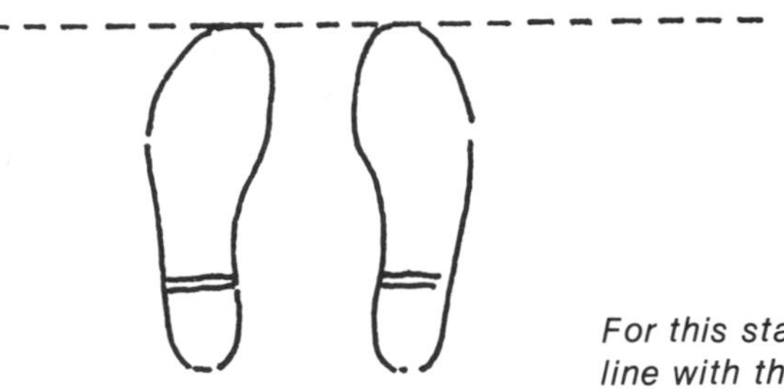

*For this stance the feet are in line with the edge of the table.*

### Archer Stance

The archer stance is the most commonly used, especially when the practitioner's shoulders are at an angle (other than parallel) with the edge of the table. For the archer stance an imaginary line is drawn through the center of one foot, at the arch and passes through the other foot at mid-heel and, the third toe.

In either stance knees should be kept flexed slightly because stiff, rigid knees contribute to fatigue. Keeping the spine fairly erect and bending from the waist allow for easier movement around the massage table. Correct stances make it easier to shift weight from foot to foot so movement is smooth, as in dancing. Correct stances also give the practitioner more body power when leaning into the movements and enables easier use of hands and arms when giving a massage.

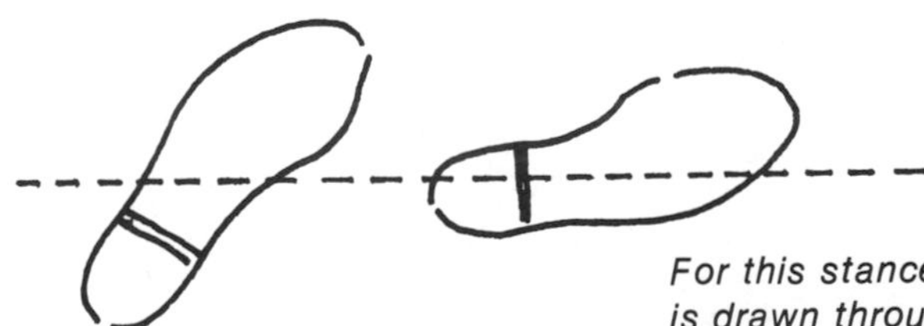

*For this stance an imaginary line is drawn through the center of one foot at the arch and passes through the center of the other foot at mid-heel and third toe.*

## EXERCISES FOR STRENGTH, BALANCE AND BODY CONTROL

There are two techniques called "centering" and "grounding" that are important to the practitioner because they provide a base from which to work.

*Centering:* Centering is based on the concept that you have a geographical center in your body; the pelvic area, located about two inches below the navel. The Chinese refer to this as the "dan tein." Centering gives you a certain confident sense of balance and self assurance. Many of the ancient writings about martial arts mention this concept. Being centered means you feel self-assured and emotionally stable. Being uncentered means you feel insecure and unstable. Feeling centered (in control) is of value because it is important to be able to handle problems that arise without becoming frustrated or emotionally involved. Centering is accomplished by concentrating on the geographical center (dan tein) and on being self-assured.

*Grounding:* Grounding is based on the concept that you have a connection with the client and that you function as something of a grounding apparatus, helping the client to release unwanted tension and feelings of stress. Grounding is achieved by mentally visualizing yourself as having the ability to draw from a greater power or energy. Try thinking of yourself as a tree rooted to the ground. Controlled breathing is also helpful. The concepts of grounding and centering will become more clear as you master the following exercises.

### Exercise 1 Grinding Corn

This exercise is based on the idea a practitioner must be able to reach the full length of the part of the client's body that is being worked on and to be able to shift the weight easily from one foot to the other while maintaining good posture. The exercise is called 'grinding corn" because the movement is similar to using an old-fashioned hand corn grinder. You may also think of it as a movement similar to polishing a car. Use your imagination.

***Procedure***

Place your feet apart (about the width of your shoulders), and tilt your pelvis forward and upward. Bend your knees, and sink down until you are in a demi-knee bend. Do not go all the way down to a squatting position. Keep your back straight, and don't allow your head to jut forward. If you have had dance training you will recognize this stance as the plie (bending knees) that dancers practice to improve their posture, balance, and coordination. While maintaining this posture, hold your hands in front of your body (palms down) about the level of your waistline. Now begin to move both hands toward the right forming a wide oval. This will look as if you are ready for a karate move.

After you get the feel of the standing position and hand movements, begin to move the right hand clockwise and the left hand counterclockwise. Shift your weight from foot to foot. Keep making the ovals (keeping your back straight) until you are comfortable with the movement. Lower your hands about six inches by bending your knees into a deeper knee bend. Continue practicing. As you continue the exercise, become aware of the centering concept previously described and allow your movements to be initiated from the pelvic area (about two inches below the navel), with the rest of your body following through. Remember this is your geographical area or center which allows your entire body to move with balance and strength.

As you master these techniques and continue to practice them, your arms, hands and shoulders will become less fatigued because of the support supplied by the rest of your body.

**Exercise 2**
**The Wheel**

The wheel is sometimes referred to as the "Buddhist Wheel" because of the forward and backward motion of the body.

***Procedure***

First, take a deep breath exhaling slowly. Repeat this several times. This exercise helps you to relax. Take a comfortable stride with feet apart. Turn the left foot out at a 45-degree angle. Shift most of your weight to the left foot while bending the left knee slightly. With the left heel remaining on the floor, step forward with the right foot, keeping the weight resting on the ball of the right foot. Remember to keep your hips and shoulders facing forward and your knees bent. The right foot should be forward about 15 to 20 inches. Shift your weight first to the right foot then back to the left, in a rocking motion. Once you have the feel of the stance, take a deep breath and exhale slowly while placing your hands about six inches apart with palms facing. Begin making circles with your hands while imagining that you have a large wheel suspended in front of you. The top of the wheel is about shoulder level and the bottom is at the level of your pubic bone. Continue the movement while taking several deep breaths, and then without breaking your rhythm, turn your right foot to a 45 degree angle and take one step forward. Repeat the exercise several times.

To complete the exercise, bring your feet together so that your weight is distributed evenly. Turn your palms facing downward and allow your hands to float down to your sides. Stay in this position for a few seconds to experience the feeling. As you master this movement, you will find that it is best accomplished by concentrating on originating the movement from the pelvic area (center or dan tein) and moving straight forward and backward while allowing the rest of your body to follow.

**Exercise 3**
**The Tree**

This exercise emphasizes the importance of posture and concentration and is combined with centering, grounding, and correct breathing.

***Procedure***

Stand with your feet together with your shoulders relaxed down and back. Pull your buttocks downward slightly. This will cause your pelvis to tilt upward. Take a deep breath and exhale slowly. Begin the exercise by turning the left foot out (bending the left knee), and shifting all your weight to the left foot. Keep your upper body erect. Move the right foot straight forward so that when the right leg is extended, the ball of the right foot rests lightly on the floor. Bring both arms up to about shoulder level to form a circle. This should look as if you are trying to reach around a large tree. Your fingers will be pointing toward each other, about two inches apart. Keep your head up, chin level, and gaze ahead. As you hold this pose, the leg bearing your weight may feel weak and begin to tremble. However, by maintaining the pose for about three minutes at a time and practicing your breathing exercises, you will soon experience a sense of renewed strength and power.

Change the pose to the left foot position (left foot forward) with your weight on the right foot, continue to breathe deeply, exhaling slowly. Alternate the right and left feet, continuing to practice until you feel completely in control. To finish the exercise, bring your feet to a side by side position with your weight distributed evenly and your back straight. Allow your arms to float down to your sides. Take a moment to experience what is happening to your body.

Although you may find these exercises tiring and sometimes boring, remember there is no easy way to accomplish erect posture, body strength, coordination, and proper breathing without some effort. Keep foremost in your mind that your goal is to be able to perform efficiently as a master of massage techniques. As you begin to do professional massage, you will see how these exercises increase your feeling of self-esteem.

## INSTRUCTING THE CLIENT IN BREATHING FOR RELAXATION

When the client is on the table, relaxed and comfortable, encourage him or her to breath fully and deeply. Many people have never done this and may need some basic coaching. Help the client by using some of the following suggestions:

Tell the client to breath through the nose deeply so that the abdominal area expands first followed by the chest. Hold for a few counts, then allow the breath to flow outward. Maintain the exhalation for a short time, and repeat the exercise a few times. Observe the client's breathing, and synchronize your own breathing. Have the client continue breathing freely for a few minutes to encourage relaxation and stress reduction.

## CONTACT WITH THE CLIENT AND QUALITY OF TOUCH

In administering a massage there is much more to take into account than the application of strokes to various parts of the client's body. The practitioner must be aware of contact with the client and quality of touch, the constitution or composition for the massage itself, the posture of the client and how the whole body is used in the application of the various movements, and the role the breath plays for both the practitioner and the client.

The way that "touch" is administered to the client determines the success of the massage and is often the reason a client will continue to return and ask for a particular practitioner.

From the time a client enters a massage establishment, the confidence and ability of the practitioner are communicated. The confidence shown through the initial contact "touch" instills a certain trust in the recipient that encourages relaxation.

It is important for the practitioner to maintain contact with the client throughout the course of a full massage. If the client is in a state of wakeful conversation with eyes open and is following the moves of the practitioner, then there is verbal and visual contact. However, if the client is in a state of relaxation with eyes closed, the sense of touch is the only communication. If the contact is broke, there is an immediate reaction on the part of the client and relaxation may change to anxiety.

## CLASSIFICATION OF MASSAGE MOVEMENTS

There are any number of massage manipulations and possible combinations of strokes so that a massage can be tailored to the needs of each client. Regardless of whether a massage routine is standard or specialized for the client, there is much more to applying strokes than the movement of the hands. The body and mind of the practitioner are also involved.

The following movements to be mastered are often referred to as the "classic" movements, and have stemmed from Swedish massage techniques. The massage practitioner must understand into which category specific movements fall. Most massage treatments combine one or more of these movements, as divided into the six major categories:

1. Touch.
   a. Superficial.
   b. Deep.
2. Effleurage or stroking movements.
   a. Superficial.
      - Feathering.
      - Applying oil.
   b. Deep.
      - Over large surfaces.
      - Over heavier muscles.
3. Petrissage or compression movements.
   a. Kneading.
   b. Fulling.
4. Friction (these are considered to be compression movements).
   a. Wringing.
   b. Rolling.
   c. Chucking.
   d. Compression.
   e. Circular friction.
   f. Transverse or cross fiber friction.
5. Percussion Movements.
   a. Tapping (tapotement).
   b. Slapping.
   c. Cupping.
   d. Hacking.
   e. Beating.
6. Vibration.
   a. Manual.
   b. Mechanical.
7. Joint movements.
   a. Passive.
   b. Active.
      - Active assistive
      - Passive resistive

Each manipulation is applied in a specific way for a particular purpose. The practice of massage becomes scientific only when the practitioner recognizes the purposes and effects of each movement and adapts the treatment in accordance with the client's condition and the desired results.

Control over the results of a massage treatment is possible only when the practitioner regulates the intensity of the pressure, direction of movement, and duration of each type of manipulation.

## UNDERSTANDING MASSAGE MOVEMENTS

The practitioner must understand the movement to be applied to a particular part of the body, for example:

Light movements are applied over thin tissues or over boney parts.

Heavy movements are indicated for thick tissues or fleshy parts.

Gentle movements are applied with a slow rhythm and are soothing and relaxing.

Vigorous movements are applied in a quick rhythm and are stimulating.

An important rule in massage is that most manipulations are directed towards the heart (centripetal). When a massag treatment movement is directed away from the heart, it is said to be centrifugal. The duration of a massage treatment should be regulated. Usually a therapeutic body massage takes about one hour, but some practitioners take less time. A prolonged massage can be fatiguing to some clients. When a student is learning massage, a full body massage can take an hour and a half to two hours. This is not unusual because it takes practice for movements to become smooth and efficient. After a while, an hour will be plenty of time to accomplish the desired results.

There are times when the practitioner will require more time, so the duration of massages vary. Knowledge and experience are necessary prerequisites to judge the client's special needs.

### Description of Strokes and Other Movements

*Touching:* The placing of the practitioner's hand, finger, or body part (such as forearm) on the client without movement in any direction. Touch is skillfully and purposely applied in order to achieve physiological (soothing) effects.

*Stroking:* The practice of gliding the hand over some portion of the client's body with varying amounts of pressure or contact according to desired results.

*Friction:* Massage strokes designed to manipulate soft tissue in such a way that one layer of tissue is moved over or against another.

*Percussion:* The rapid and alternate movement of the practitioner's hands in a striking motion against the surface of the client's body, using varying amounts of force and hand positions.

*Joint movement:* The manipulation of the joints or articulations of the client.

### Application of Massage Strokes

*Touching:* Light or superficial touch is purposeful contact in which the natural and evenly distributed weight of the practitioner's hand is exerted on a given area. The size of that area may be regulated as necessary by using one or more fingers, the entire hand, or both hands to achieve the desired results.

*Application:* Touch is the first technique in developing a therapeutic relationship. Touch may be in the form of a hand shake or a "pat on the shoulder." In the course of a massage, touch constitutes the first and last contact of the practitioner with the client. Some therapeutic techniques employ touch almost exclusively (jin shin do, accupressure, polarity, therapeutic touch, rieki). Touch can be remarkably effective in the reduction of pain, lowering of blood pressure, control of nervous irritability, or reassurance for a nervous, tense client. If a person has signs of contraindications for a basic massage, or is in a fragile condition, a complete treatment using touch exclusively is acceptable. The main objective of touch is to soothe and to provide a comforting connection that can be used when all else fails.

**Deep Touch Using Pressure**

Deep touch is performed with one finger, thumb, several fingers, or the entire hand. The heel of the hand, knuckles, or elbow can be used according to desired results. The application of deep pressure is used when calming or stimulating effects are desired. It may be used with other techniques such as cross-fiber friction, compression, or vibration. Deep pressure is useful in soothing muscle spasms and relieving pain at reflex areas, stress points in tendons, and trigger points in muscle. In addition to extensive use in trigger-point therapy, deep pressure is a technique often applied in reflexology, sport massage, accupressure, and shiatzu.

**Definitions of Movements**

Stroking may be done using a varying amount of pressure and length of strokes. Strokes glide over the client's entire body or body part (arm or leg). Generally the movement is toward the heart, with the return stroke being much lighter and away from the center of the body.

*Ethereal body or aura stroking:* This type of stroking is done with long smooth strokes where the practitioner's hands glide the length of the client's entire body or body part coming very close to but not actually touching the body surface. Generally the movement is in one direction only, with the return stroke being slightly farther from the body.

The application of this very soothing stroke is done only when the surrounding circumstances are very quiet, relaxed, and the patient receptive. It is often used as the final stroke of a massage.

*Feather stroking:* Feather stroking movements are done with the very tips of the fingers lightly touching the client. The practitioner may use very light pressure of the fingernails.

The application of feather stroking, sometimes called "nerve stroking," is usually done from the center outwards and is used as a final stroke to individual areas of the body. Two or three such strokes will have a slightly stimulating effect on the nerves, while many repetitions will have a more sedating response.

*Superficial stroking or effleurage:* Effleurage is a succession of firm and light strokes applied by passing the flat surface of the hand over a somewhat extended portion of the body. It is usually the first stroke used in massage. There are two varieties of effleurage: superficial and deep. Superficial stroking employs the lightest possible touch. In deep stroking the pressure becomes firmer as the hand glides over the surface of the body.

Superficial stroking is generally applied prior to any other movement. Slow, gentle, and rhythmic movements produce soothing effects. Rhythmic strokes should be applied in the direction of the venous and lymphatic flow.

Although superficial stroking appears to be simple, its technique is mastered only by long practice. The practitioner's hand should be relaxed in order to mold the part being massaged. The direction of movement should always be the same. Upon completion of the stroke, the practitioner's hand is elevated and directed to the starting point.

Superficial stroking is a valuable application for overcoming a general tired feeling or restlessness. This movement is particularly soothing to nervous or irritated people. Nervous headaches and insomnia (sleeplessness) are often relieved by gentle stroking of the forehead.

Deep stroking is especially valuable when applied to the muscles, but it is effective only when the part under treatment is in a state of relaxation. Then, the slightest pressure of the surface will be transmitted to the deeper structures. The movements are always directed from the end of a limb toward the center of the body. As pressure is applied to the veins and lymphatic vessels, their elastic walls tend to spread and permit a better flow of fluids to the heart. Deep stroking also aids disquamation (shedding) of dead surface skin cells.

The technique of effleurage, or stroking movements, is accomplished either with the fingers or palm of the hand.

1. Over large surfaces, such as the limbs, back, chest, and abdomen, the stroking movement is performed with the palm of one or both hands.
2. Over small areas, such as the eyes or hands, the stroking movement is performed with the fingertips.

**Step by Step Effleurage or Stroking Movements**

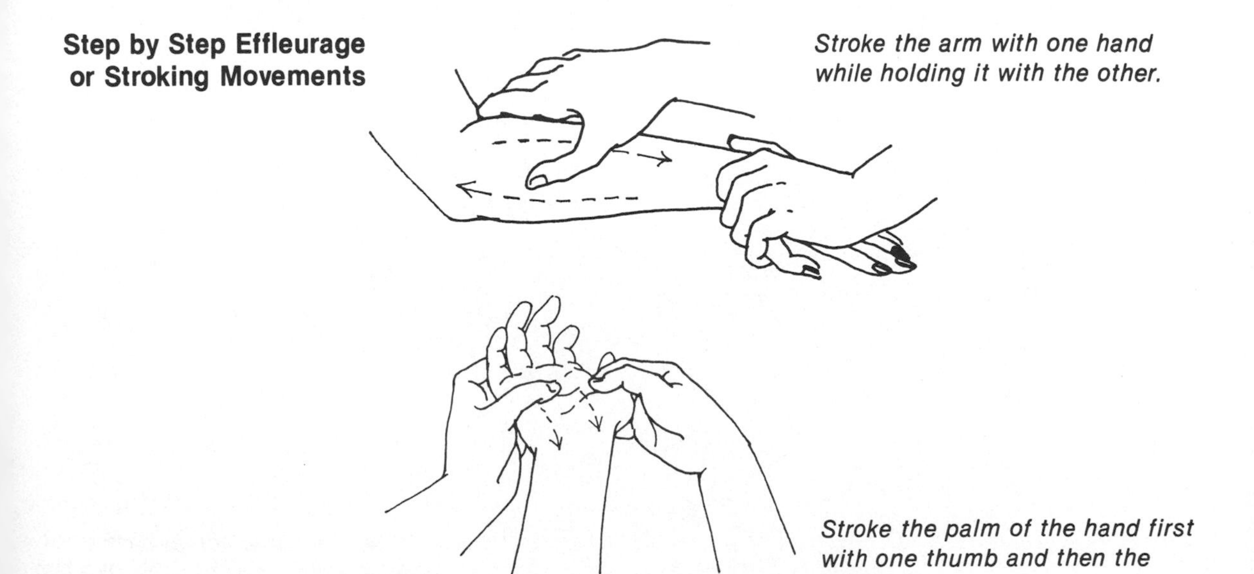

*Stroke the arm with one hand while holding it with the other.*

*Stroke the palm of the hand first with one thumb and then the other.*

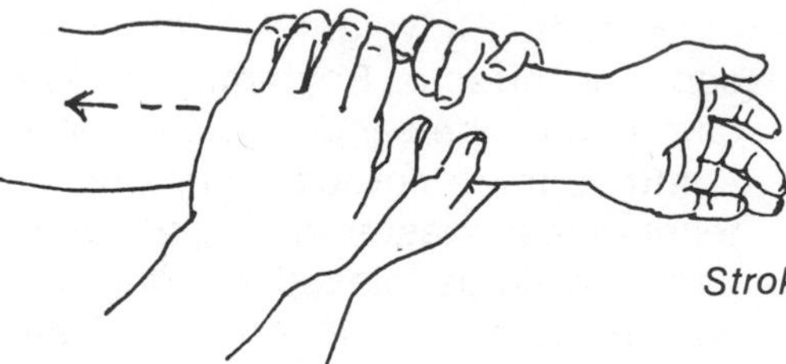

*Stroke the arm with both hands.*

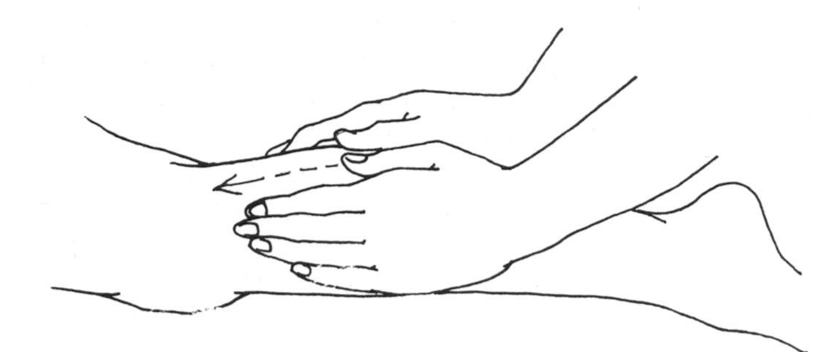

*Stroke the leg with both hands.*

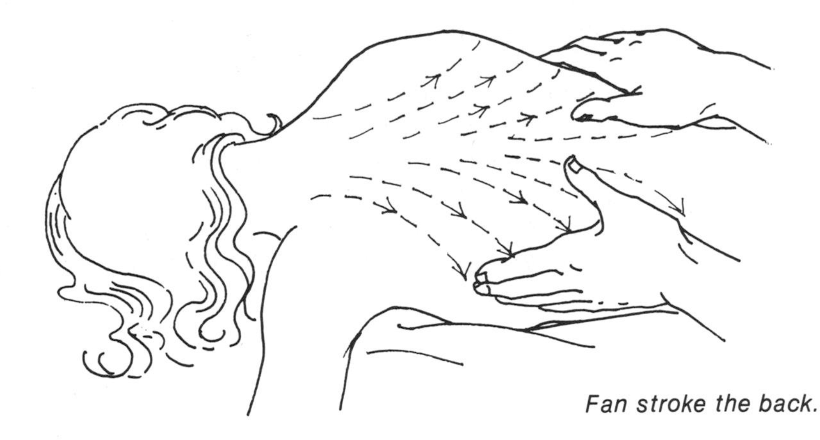

*Fan stroke the back.*

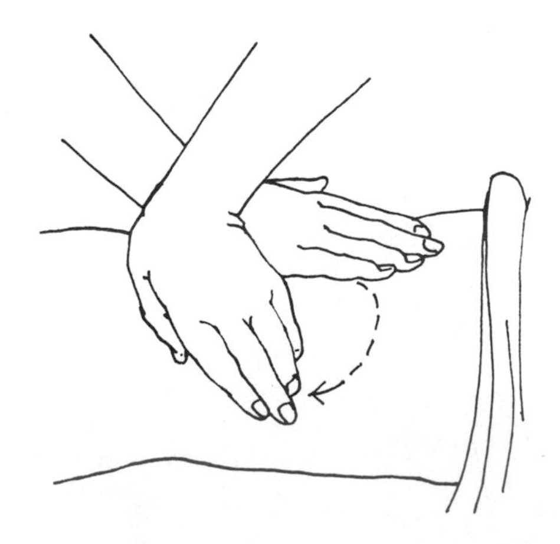

*Stroke the abdomen in a deep circular movement.*

## COMPRESSION MOVEMENTS

Other forms of friction sometimes classified by themselves are compression movements. As the name implies, these are pressing movements directed into muscle tissue by either palmar or digital compression. Palmar compression is done with the whole hand (palm side) or the heel of the hand over the large area of the body. Digital compression is done with a finger, a number of fingers or the thumb and involves digging deeply into muscle tissue to relieve and break down the buildup of tension.

Compression movements require a squeezing and rubbing action over the skin and its underlying structures. Within this classification are grouped the following movements: petrissage, friction, and vibration. Compression movements should be progressive, applied lightly at first then with gradually increased pressure. More pressure can be tolerated over thick and fleshy areas than over thin tissues or bony surfaces. The degree of pressure should never be so forceful as to cause the muscles to become tight. This application of gentle pressure to relaxed muscles yields better results than the use of tremendous force over tense muscles.

Compression movements have an invigorating effect upon the body. Petrissage or kneading serves a useful purpose in revitalizing dry and scaly skin by stimulating the flow of blood and lymph. These movements are particularly helpful in preventing muscle stiffness following prolonged exertion or exercise.

### Petrissage, or Kneading Movements

Petrissage, being a vigorous movement, is generally used for the massage of the back, abdomen, and extremities. In this movement, the skin and muscular tissues are raised from their ordinary position and then squeezed, rolled, or pinched with a firm pressure, usually in a circular direction. Heavy pressure is applied towards the heart (centripetal) to aid venous and lymphatic flow.

Over thick structures, such as in fulling of the arms, the flesh is grasped between the fingers and palm of the hands. Over smaller structures, such as the hands or fingers, the flesh is held between the thumb and fingers.

### *Step by Step Petrissage or Kneading Movements*

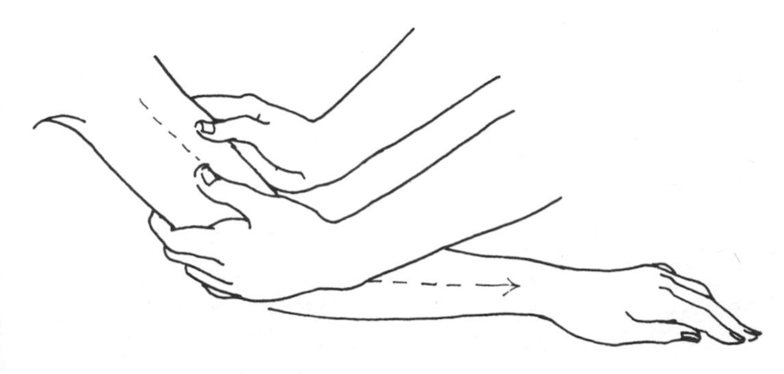

*Knead the muscles of the arm.*

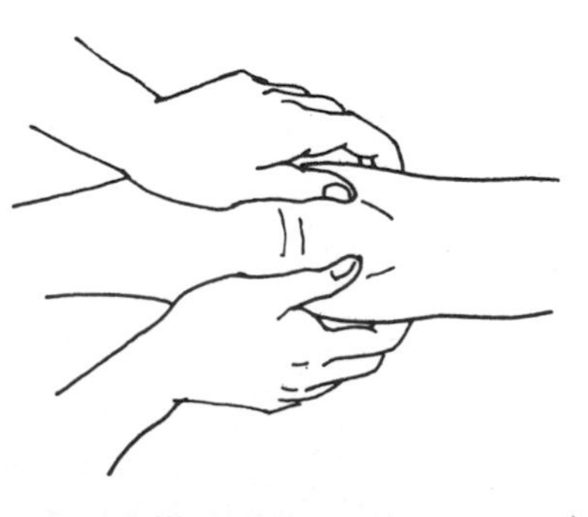

*For fulling movement, grasp the flesh between the fingers and palms of the hand.*

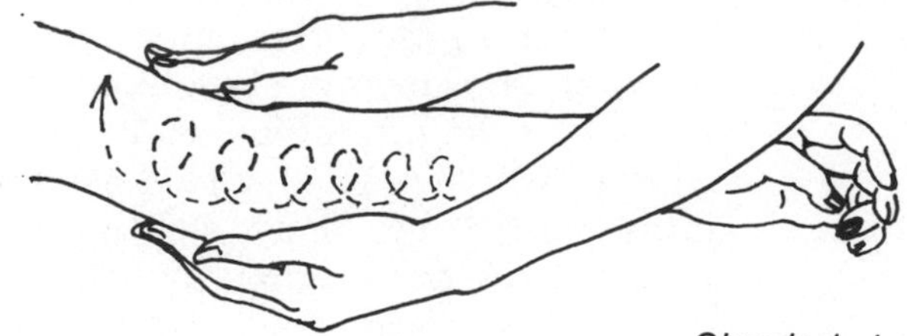

*Circularly knead the muscles of the arm.*

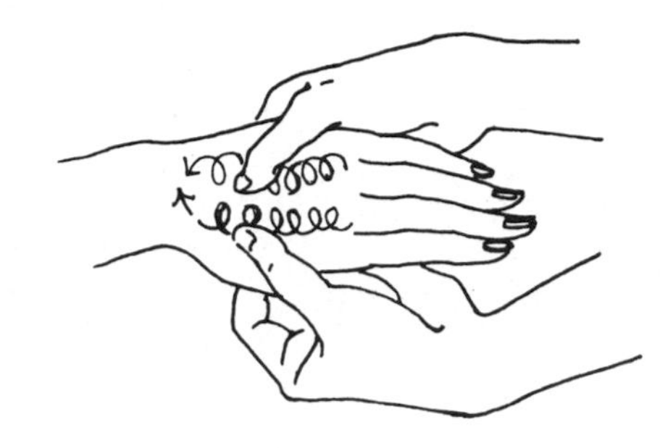

*Circularly knead the muscles of the hand.*

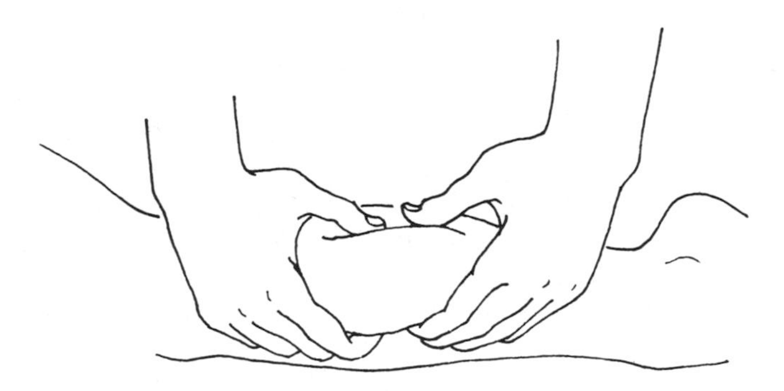

*Knead the calf muscles.*

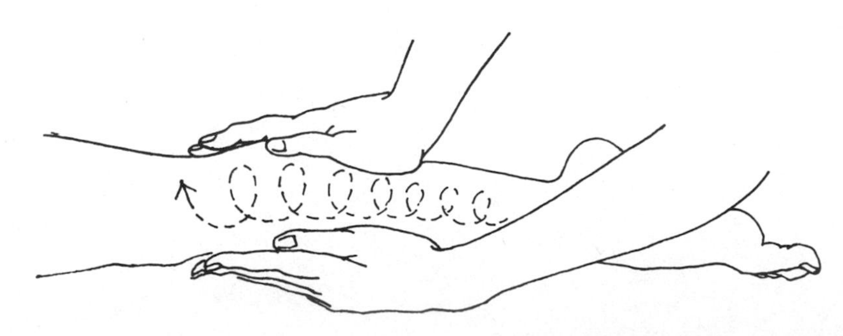

*Circularly knead the muscles of the leg and thigh.*

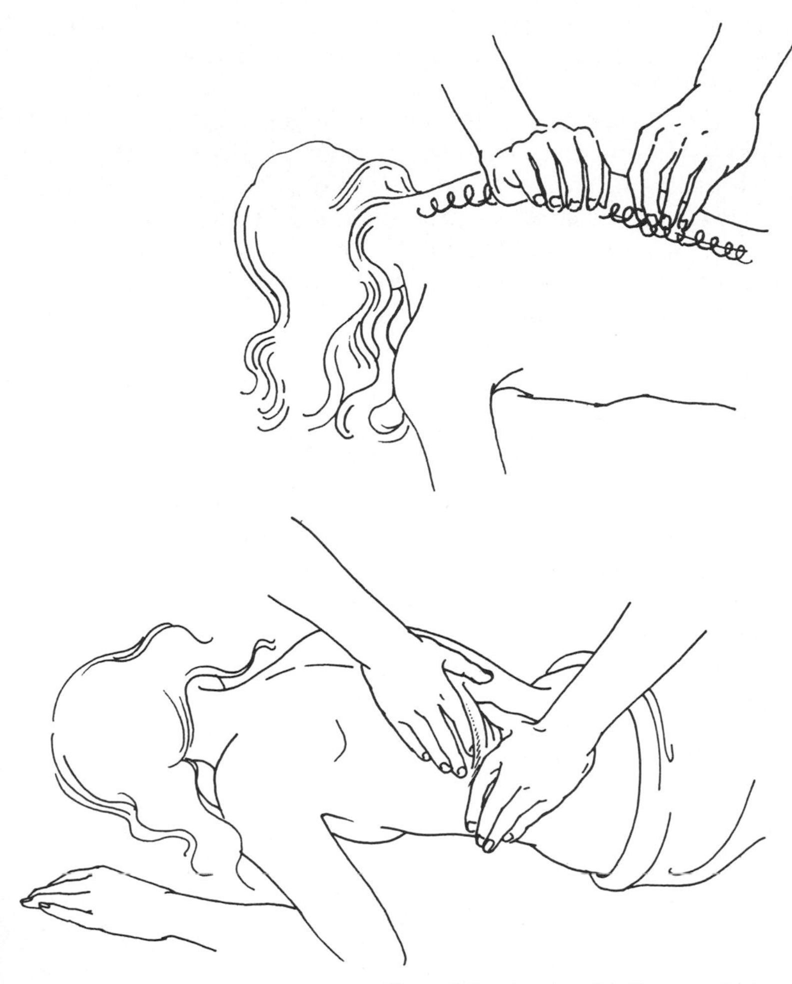

*Knead around the spine.*

*Knead the back with fingers and thumb, using a back and forth motion.*

*Knead the muscles of the abdomen.*

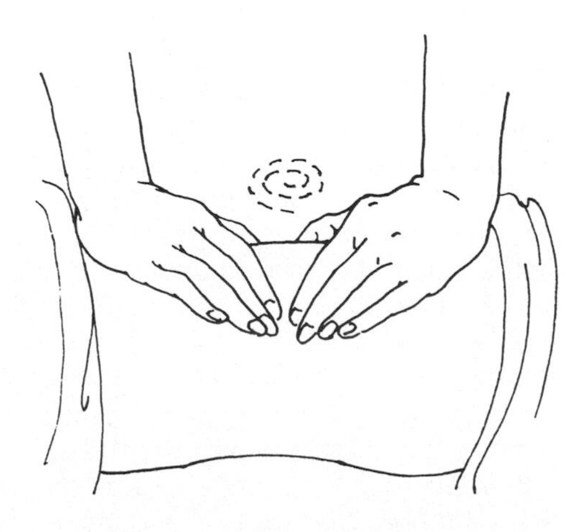

*Knead the muscles of the intestines.*

*Knead the abdomen with broad sweeping movements of both hands.*

## Friction Strokes and Movements

Friction differs essentially from kneading in that the hand is allowed to slip along the surface of the skin, instead of squeezing the part being massaged. Friction movements involve taking the more superficial layers of the flesh and moving them against the deeper tissues, whereas kneading is done by grasping the tissues and applying lifting and pulling movements to pull away from the skeletal structures, then squeezes in such a way as to milk out the body fluids. This is done in such a way that it also increases heat. As heat increases, the metabolic rate increases as well as the rate at which exchanges take place between the cells and the interstitial fluids (fluids situated within or between the tissues of an organ or body part). The added heat and energy also affect the connecting tissue surrounding the muscles, making them more pliable so they function more efficiently.

Friction also helps to separate the tissues and to break down tissue bundles. It softens the amorphous (massed) ground substance of the fluid between the different layers of fascia and increases the flow of blood to the area. With friction strokes the area usually becomes red. This indicates that more blood is being rushed to the surface of the skin. Friction also aids in absorption of the fluid around the joints.

Friction has a marked influence on the circulation and glandular activity of the skin. There are a number of different friction strokes that involve moving a more superficial layer of tissue against the adipose layer (connective tissue containing fat cells) just beneath the skin.

Rolling is a back and forth movement with the hands, in which the flesh is shaken and rolled in a quick direction across the axis, or the imaginary centerline of the body part.

Chucking, rolling, and wringing are variations of friction and are employed principally to massage the arms and legs. The chucking movement is accomplished by grasping the flesh firmly in one hand and moving the hand up and down along the bone, while the other hand keeps the limb in a steady position. It is a series of quick movements along the axis of the limb.

Wringing is a back and forth movement in which both hands of the practitioner are placed a short distance apart on both sides of the limb. It resembles the wringing out of a wash cloth. While the hands are worked downward, the flesh is twisted against the bones in opposite directions.

Friction is a massage movement requiring pressure on the skin while it is being moved over its underlying structures. Over muscular parts or fleshy layers, friction is applied with the palms of the hands. Over small surfaces, friction is applied with the fleshy parts of the finger tips.

Friction movements may be circular or directional. In circular friction the fingers or the palm of the hand contact the skin and move it in a circular pattern over the deeper tissues. Directional friction may be either cross fiber or longitudinal friction. Cross fiber friction, as the name implies, works perpendicularly across the muscle, tendon or ligament fibers. In longitudinal friction, the practitioner's hand moves in the same direction as the tissue fibers.

**Step by Step Friction Strokes**

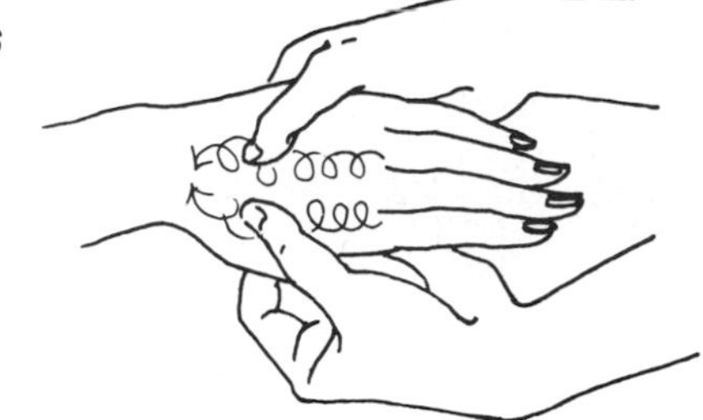

Apply circular friction to muscles of the hand.

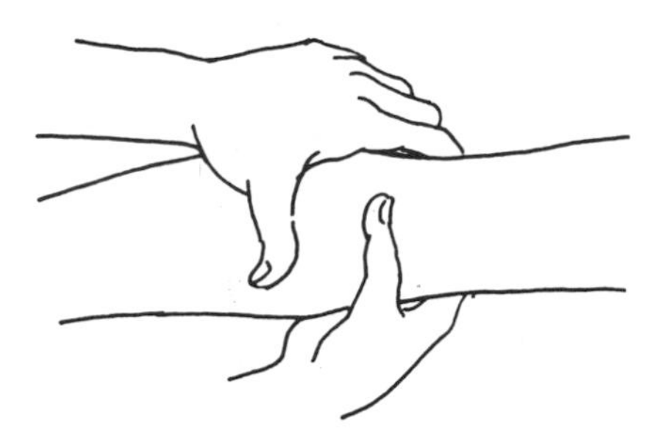

Apply circular friction to muscles of the arm.

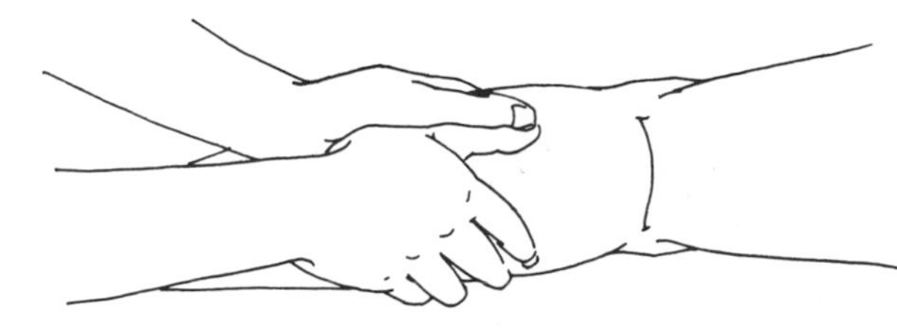

Apply circular friction to muscles of leg and thigh.

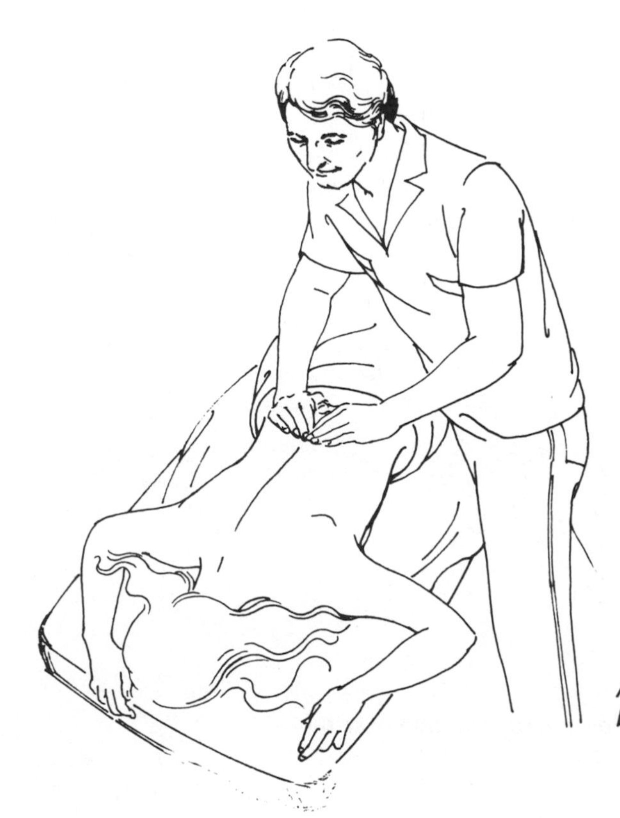

Apply circular friction over lower back and hips.

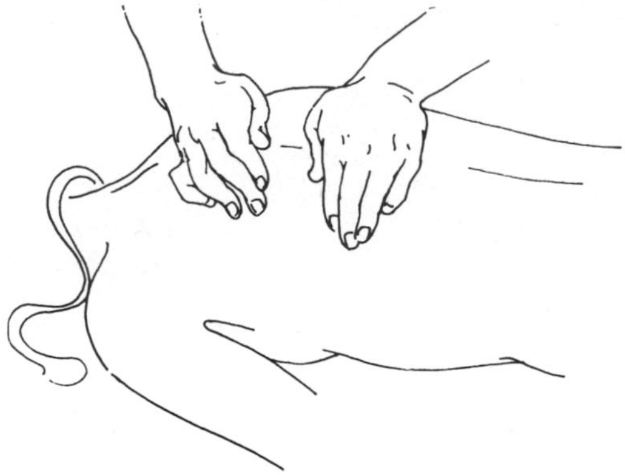

*Apply circular friction around the spine.*

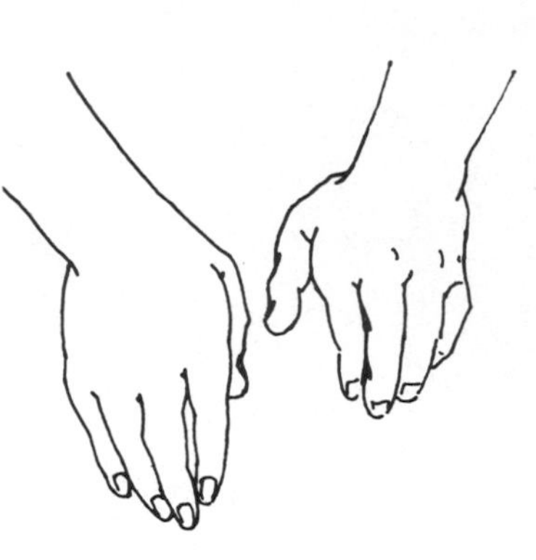

*Apply friction to the muscles of the abdomen.*

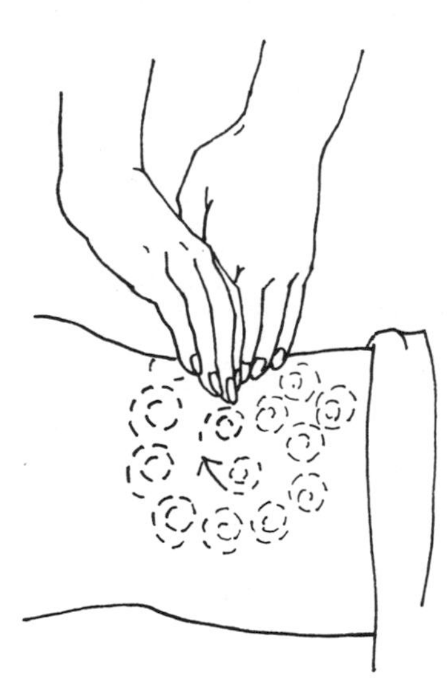

*Apply circular friction over the area of the intestines.*

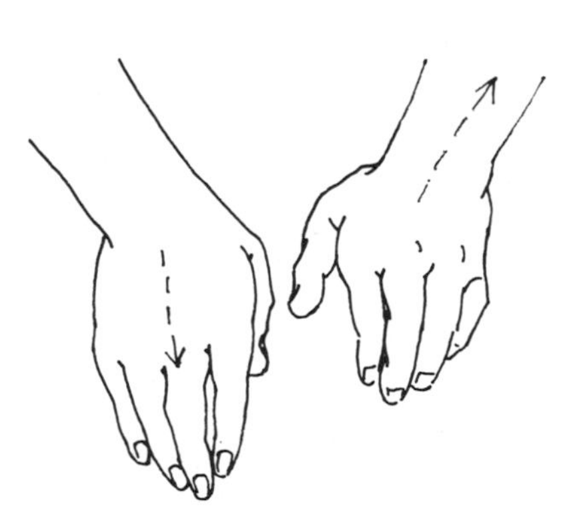

*Apply friction to the abdomen with broad sweeping movements of both hands.*

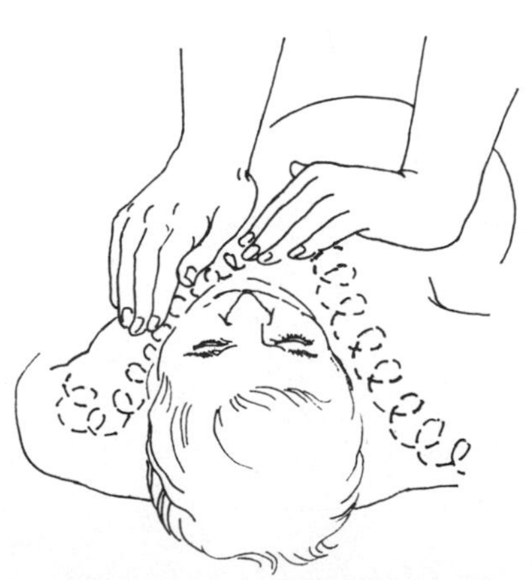

*Apply circular friction over the chest.*

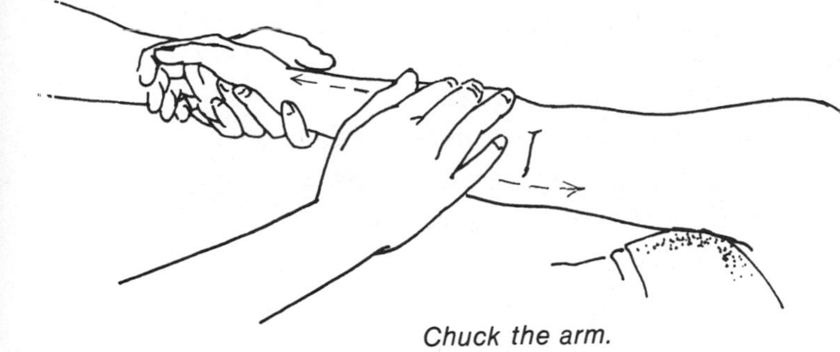

*Chuck the arm.*

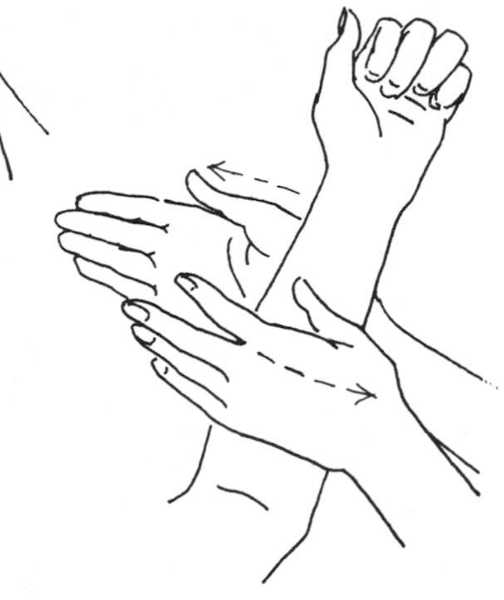

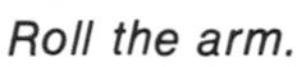

*Roll the arm.*

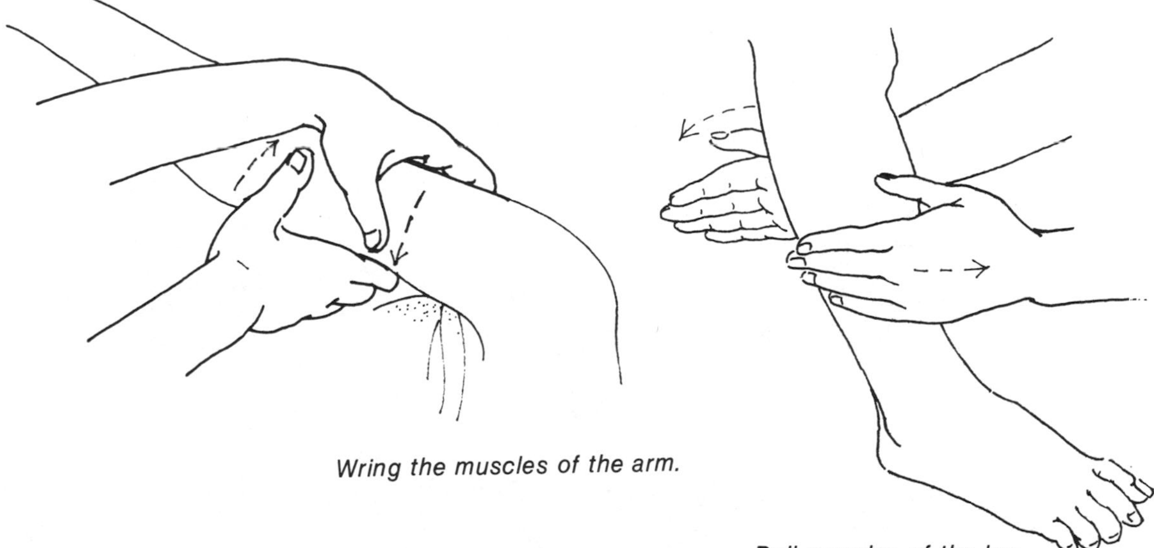

*Wring the muscles of the arm.*

*Roll muscles of the leg.*

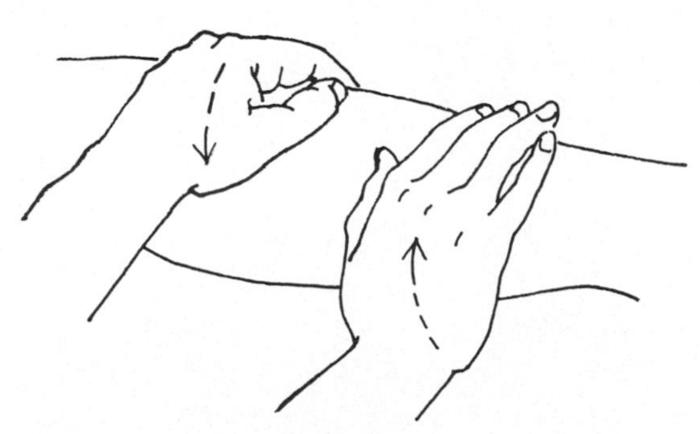

*Wring muscles of the thigh.*

## PERCUSSION MOVEMENTS

Percussion movements are executed with both hands simultaneously or alternately. The movements may be done in the following ways:

1. Tapping with tips of the fingers.
2. Slapping with flattened part of the hand.
3. Cupping with the cupped part of the hand.
4. Hacking with outer border of the hand.
5. Beating with the clenched hand.

Percussion movements include quick, striking manipulations such as tapping, beating, and slapping, which are highly stimulating to the body. The beating and slapping movements should be used with discretion, so the client is not over-stimulated by the treatment.

Tapping movements are employed on the face, chest, and back. Hacking and cupping movements are used when massaging the back, shoulders, arms, and legs. Beating and slapping, being vigorous forms of percussion, are usually limited to the stimulation of heavy muscles and adipose (fatty) tissue found over the back and buttocks.

The general effects of percussion movements are to tone the muscles and impart a healthy glow to the part being massaged. With each striking movement, the muscles first contract, then relax as the fingers are removed from the body. In this way, sagging muscles are strengthened and toned and fatty deposits reduced. Percussion movements should never be applied over muscles that are abnormally contracted, or over any sensitive area.

### Step by Step Percussion Movements

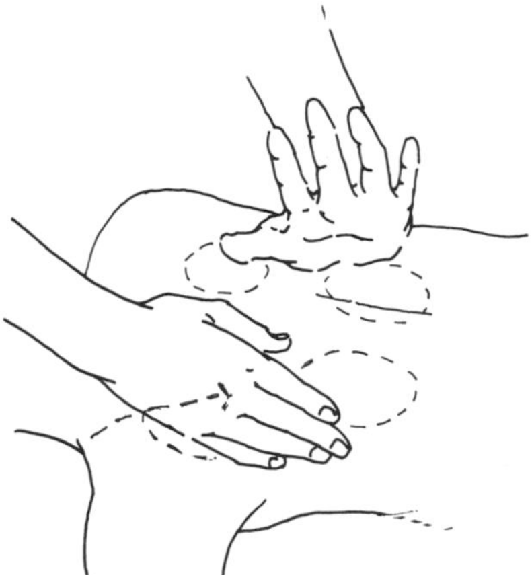

*Slapping movements on the back.*

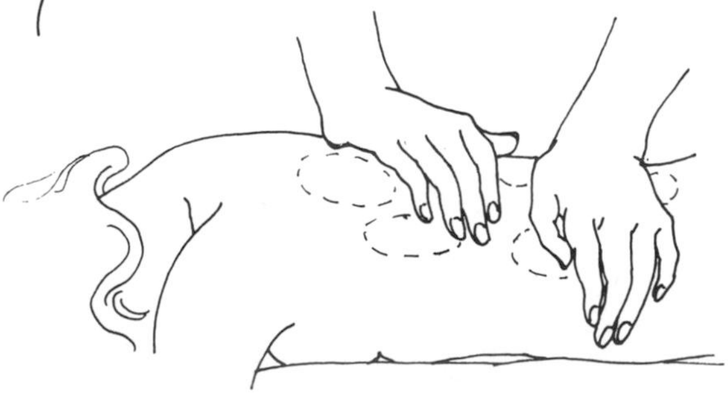

*Cupping movements on the back.*

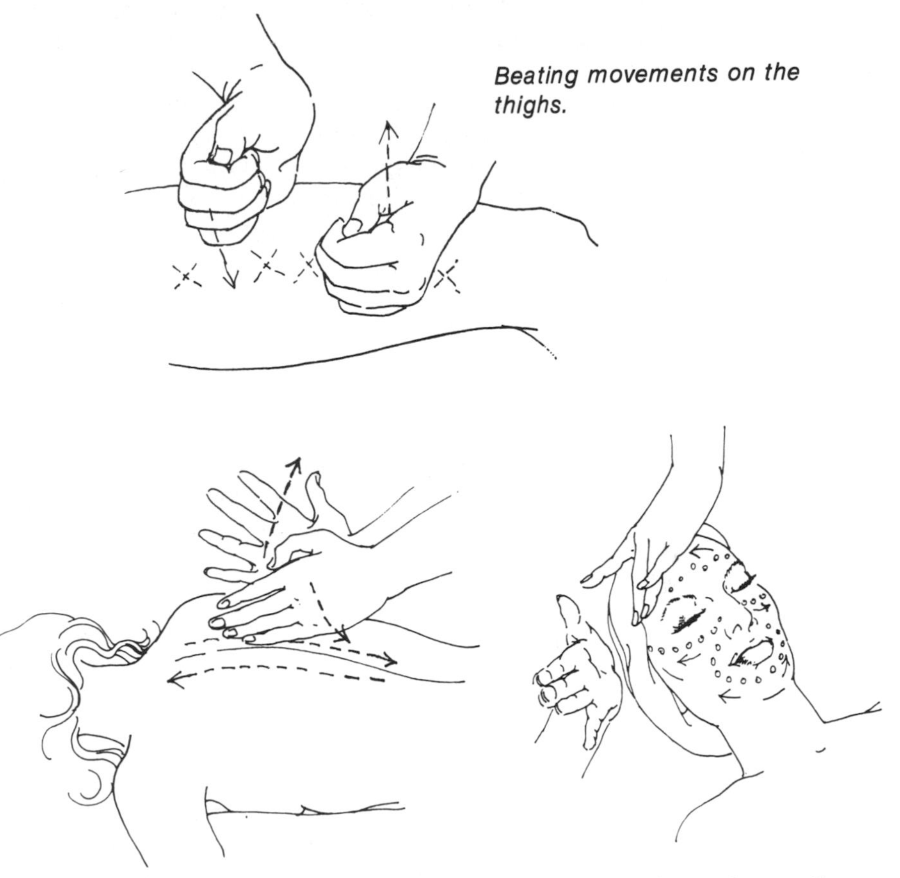

*Beating movements on the thighs.*

*Hacking movements on the back.*

*Tapping with fingertips on the face.*

**VIBRATION**

Vibration is a continuous shaking or trembling movement transmitted from the practitioner's hand and arm or from an electrical appliance to a fixed point, or along a selected area of the body. Nerve trunks and centers are sometimes chosen as sites for the application of vibratory movements.

The rate of vibration should be under the control of the massage practitioner. Manual vibrations usually range from 5 to 10 times per second, while mechanical vibrations can be adjusted to give from 10 to 100 vibrations per second.

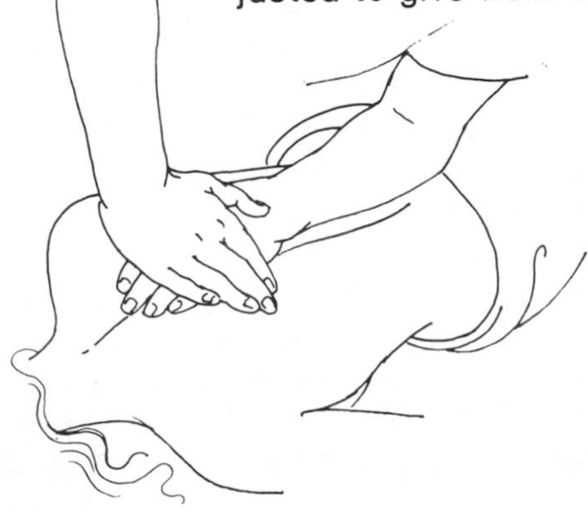

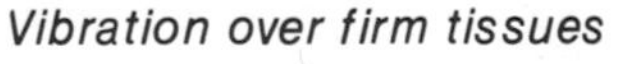

*Vibration over firm tissues*

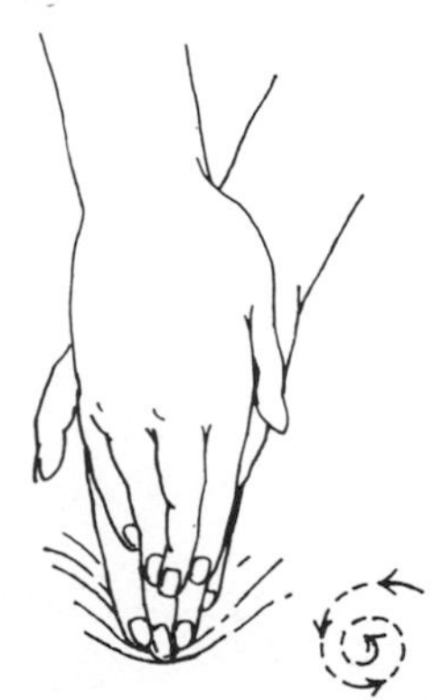

*Vibration over soft tissues*

The effects of vibratory movements depend not only on the rates of vibration but also on the intensity of pressure and duration of the treatment. This form of massage is soothing and brings about relaxation and release of tension when applied lightly. It is stimulating when applied with pressure. A numbing effect is experienced when vibrations are applied for a prolonged period of time.

Shaking is another movement classified as friction. It is a relaxing movement that helps find where the client may have tension in a part of the body. Shaking allows the client to release tension.

**JOINT MOVEMENTS**

There is a great variety of joint movements that can be used to manipulate any joint in the body including joints of the toes, knees, hips, arms and legs, the vertebrae, or even the less movable joints of the pelvis and cranium.

The basic classifications of joint movements are passive and active. The active joint movements involve the client actively participating in the exercise by offering resistance to the manipulation. For example, the practitioner straightens the client's arm while asking the client to tighten his or her biceps to hold against or resist the movement. Passive joint movements are done while the client remains quietly relaxed and allows the practitioner to stretch and move the part of the body to be exercised.

After the joint movements are completed, a few strokes of effleurage are applied to drain away waste materials that have been drawn out of the tissues. The procedure is followed by a light stroking movement from the proximal aspect (nearest to the center of the body) to the distal aspect (farthest away from center) of the part of the body being massaged. This is often the final movement of a massage routine for that part of the body. The body part is then redraped and the practitioner moves on to the next part of the body to be massaged.

Joint movements are used to manipulate the upper and lower extremities of the body. These movements are classified as follows:

*Passive joint movements:* the practitioner moves the joint, while the client's muscles are relaxed.

*Active joint movements:* The client performs the joint movement with or without the assistance of the practitioner. Active joint movements may be sub-divided into two categories: active resistant and passive resistant.

Active assistance joint movements are done on clients to restore lost mobility when they are having difficulty moving a limb. The client is instructed to perform a motion at the same time the practitioner assists through the movement. Active resistant joint movements help to strengthen muscles. The client is instructed to make a motion while the limb is held to resist movement. Joint movements may be applied with or without resistance, using either a forward, backward or circular motion.

## Step by Step Joint Movements of the Extremities

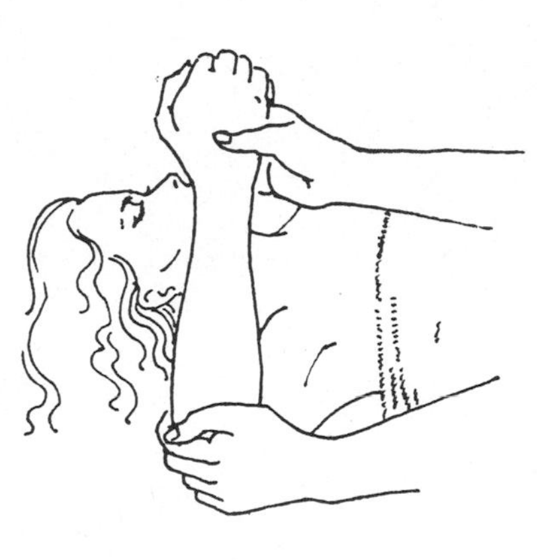

*Passive movement. Rotating the shoulder joint in a forward direction.*

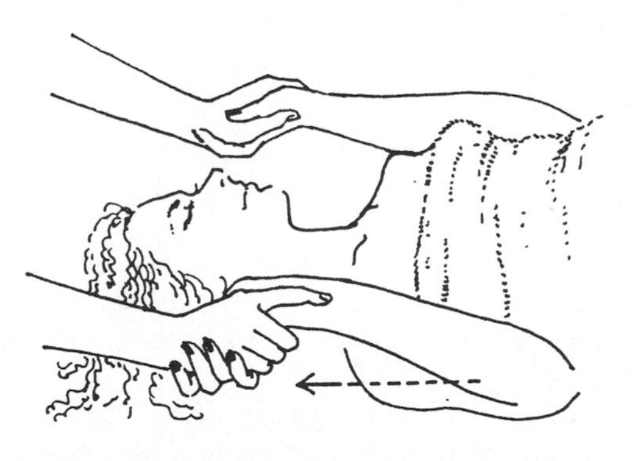

*Passive movement. Rotating the shoulder joint in a backward direction.*

*Active movement. Folding the client's arms to chest then stretching them above the head.*

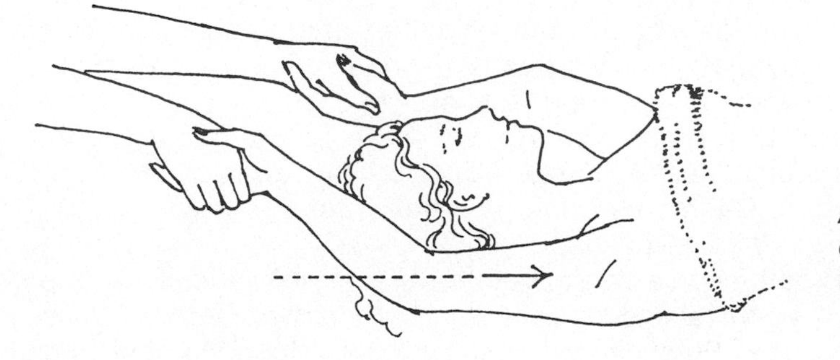

*Active movement. Placing the client's outstretched arms back to a folded position on the chest.*

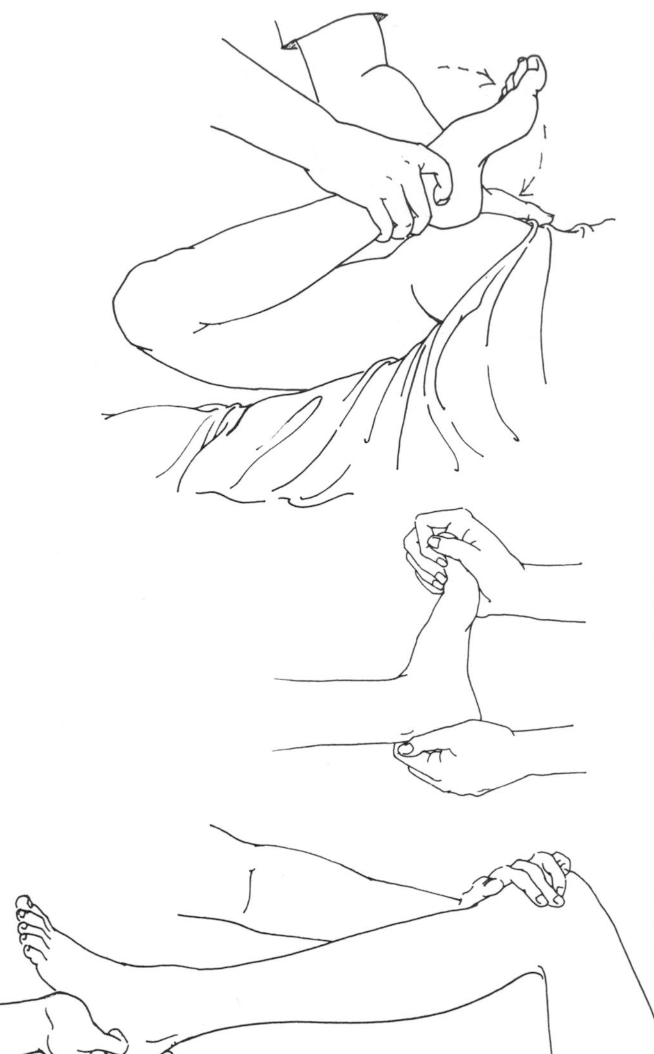

*Active movement. Bending the client's knee pressing the heel against the thigh, and then the knee to the chest.*

*Passive movement. Rotating the ankle joint in a forward and backward direction.*

*Passive movement. Rotating the knee joint in a forward and backward direction*

**RHYTHM AND PRESSURE IN MASSAGE**

People have individual vibrations and their own sense of rhythm. Practitioners need to develop this innate sense to help tune in to other people and work more effectively with them as individuals.

Research is now being done on the effect of different frequencies of vibrations and their effects on the human body. Included in this type of research is the effects of flourescent lights on learning and other abilities, and the healing effects of light and sound. The practitioner needs to remember that some people are high strung (tense), while others are very low key (relaxed). It is important to work with people according to their particular needs instead of working against their natural rhythm. Clients will return to the practitioner who is not only well trained, but aware.

Breathing is a part of your natural rhythm and is important to your stamina and to your ability to move easily while giving massage. Practice deep breathing by inhaling and exhaling slowly for short periods of time. Singing, swimming, yoga, running, and the like are all good exercises that strengthen the lungs and aid controlled breathing.

The practitioner must develop awareness of the right amount of pressure to be used for various techniques and throughout a treatment. It is important to begin to massage an area of the body cautiously, gently, and lightly then apply more pressure as you become aware of underlying structures and the condition of tissues. This also helps you to note tension and stress build-up and determine how to proceed according to the client's body condition and sensitivity. The rule is to increase the pressure as you work on an area, then decrease it as tension in the area begins to dissipate.

People have different thresholds of pain, so it is important not to work to a point that produces pain because if that threshold is crossed, the client may tense up and your work will be ineffective. Some body work may produce discomfort that is constructive; however, you should never hurt the client. Pain can damage the body.

The state of relaxation brought on by massage makes the client mentally receptive, as in hypnosis. When fully relaxed, the client can be guided by the practitioner through some mental or physical exercise to enhance or relieve a particular condition. For example, the practitioner may place his or her hands on the client and make suggestions such as "You will feel rested and relaxed," or "You will sleep better tonight because you will be free of tension. You will feel more relaxed than you have for some time." This type of positive suggestion should be made just before the client is fully awake.

Once you have mastered the basic skills for massaging each part of the body, you will soon be able to gauge rhythm, pressure, and duration of a massage. Remember that the first step in any massage procedure is preparation. This means preparing yourself by wearing comfortable clothes that allow you to move about easily, and by preparing your facility so that everything is in readiness before the client arrives. You need to also prepare yourself mentally and physically by doing deep breathing, exercising as necessary, and by thinking positively.

## QUESTIONS FOR DISCUSSION AND REVIEW

1. Name four basic movements used in massage.
2. What control should the practitioner have over the massage treatment?
3. Over which part of the body are light movements applied?
4. Over which parts of the body are heavy movements applied?
5. How should gentle movements be applied to produce a soothing effect?
6. How should vigorous movements be applied to produce a stimulating effect?
7. In which direction is massage generally applied?
8. What is effleurage?
9. Which kind of effleurage requires the lightest possible touch?

10. Which kind of effleurage requires firm pressure?
11. What are the benefits of superficial stroking?
12. What are the benefits of deep stroking?
13. In what manner are compression movements applied to the body?
14. Name three kinds of compression movements.
15. How should the practitioner regulate the pressure of compression movements?
16. How is the kneading movement applied in massage?
17. For what part of the body is the fulling movement recommended?
18. What are the benefits of compression movements?
19. What is the proper way to apply friction movements to the body?
20. Which forms of friction can be used to massage the arms and legs?
21. What is the proper way to apply vibratory movements to the body?
22. What is a safe rate of vibration?
23. How can the practitioner control the effects produced by vibratory movements?
24. Why is excessive vibration harmful?
25. What is the proper way to apply percussion movements to the body?
26. Name the various forms of percussion movements.
27. What are the benefits of percussion movements?
28. To which parts of the body should percussion movements never be applied?
29. To which parts of the body can light tapping movements be applied?
30. To which parts of the body can hacking and slapping movements be applied?
31. To which parts of the body can joint movements be applied?
32. Name two types of joint movements.
33. In which manner can joint movements be applied?

**ANSWERS TO QUESTIONS FOR DISCUSSION AND REVIEW**

1. The four basic movements are effleurage or stroking, compression, percussion, and joint.
2. The practitioner should regulate the intensity of pressure, direction of movement and duration of each type of manipulation to meet the client's needs.
3. Thin tissues and bony parts.
4. Thick tissues and muscular parts.
5. A slow rhythm produces a soothing effect.
6. A quick rhythm produces a stimulating effect.
7. Massage is generally applied in a centripetal direction, or towards the heart.

8. Effleurage is a stroking movement applied with the flat surface of the hand or fingertips over the body.
9. Superficial stroking.
10. Deep stroking.
11. Superficial stroking produces soothing effects and overcomes tiredness or restlessness.
12. Deep stroking develops muscles and stimlulates the venous and lymphatic flow.
13. Squeezing and rubbing action are applied over the skin and its underlying structures.
14. Three types of compression movements are petrissage, friction, and vibration.
15. Pressure is regulated by first applying light pressure, followed by gradually increasing pressure. More pressure is used over fleshy areas, less pressure over thin tissues and bony parts.
16. By grasping muscular tissue with one or both hands, then squeezing, rolling, or pinching with a firm pressure.
17. The arms.
18. Compression movement invigorates the body, stimulates the flow of blood and lymph, and prevents muscular stiffness following exercise.
19. The fingers or hands slip closely over the skin, and pressure is applied over the underlying structures in small circles or other directions.
20. Chucking, rolling, and wringing.
21. Vibration is applied with a continuous shaking or trembling movement by means of the practitioner's hands or an electrical vibrator.
22. Vibration is safe at a rate of 5-10 times per second by hand, 10-100 times per second by vibrator.
23. By controlling the rate of vibration, intensity of pressure, and duration of treatment.
24. Excessive vibration produces a numbing effect.
25. By quick striking movements performed with both hands simultaneously or alternately.
26. Percussion movements are slapping, beating, hacking, cupping, and tapping.
27. Percussion movements tone the muscles, strengthen sagging muscles, and reduce fatty deposits.
28. Muscles that are abnormally contracted or over any sensitive area of the body.
29. Face, chest, and back.
30. Back, shoulders, arms, and legs.
31. Arms and legs.
32. Passive and active joint movements.
33. Joint movements can be applied with or without resistance, using either forward, backward, or circular motion.

# PART V MASSAGE PROCEDURES

# Chapter 10 Procedures for a Complete Body Massage

**LEARNING OBJECTIVES**

After you have mastered this chapter, you will be able to:

1. Determine the duration of massage movements for different parts of the body.
2. Understand and be able to explain the benefits of each movement.
3. Name massage movements and demonstrate how they are done.
4. Demonstrate a basic body massage (massage 1).
5. Demonstrate massage variations (massage 2).
6. Demonstrate advanced massage techniques (massage 3).
7. Use correct anatomical terms when describing the part of the body being massaged.
8. Demonstrate correct procedures for draping the client.
9. Demonstrate correct posture and stances for the massage practitioner.
10. Demonstrate professional courtesies toward clients before, during, and after massage.
11. Understand when and where certain massage movements should and should not be intensified.
12. Answer the client's questions concerning any aftereffects of massage.

**INTRODUCTION**

Before beginning a professional body massage, it is important to "tune in" to the client.

The massage begins when the client is positioned on the massage table and you, the practitioner, come in contact with his or her body. Once you undrape and apply oil to the part of the body to be massaged, you must remember to keep in contact with the client's body throughout the procedure. You try not to break the circuit of touch once it has been established between you and your client. Your goal is to maintain a constant flow without surges or breaks as long as contact is maintained. You do this because once contact is lost, it can be somewhat startling to the client when you reestablish contact. Generally the person receiving the massage will have his or her eyes closed and will be in a relaxed, dreamlike state as the massage progresses. As long as you maintain contact, the client will not be distracted from the relaxed state or psychic connection, so it is important not to break contact until the massage is finished and the final strokes lightly feathered off.

Should a situation arise where it is necessary to leave the client, this should be explained. Some clients are very much aware of the movements of the practitioner, so it is best to limit conversation. Another reason for continual contact with the client is that it allows him or her to become in touch mentally with that part of the body being massaged. For example, if a hand is being massaged, and the practitioner moves to an arm, as soon as contact is made, the client becomes aware of the arm and is anticipating the massage. This is why abrupt movements should be avoided at all times.

If you are massaging the client's arm and he or she is in a state of deep relaxation, and if the arm is dropped suddenly; contact is broken. This interrupts the pleasant state you have worked so hard to establish, and the client may not be able to relax again. There should be no element of surprise as the massage moves from one part of the body to another. To sum up, if you are to maintain trust on the part of the client, contact must be maintained throughout the massage procedure. The client usually comes to you for the purpose of relaxation and for the general sense of well being that he or she receives from a good massage.

### CONTACT WHILE APPLYING OIL

When you are ready to apply the massage oil to the client's skin, lay the back of your hand lightly against the part of the body to be massaged. Put enough oil in the palm of your hand to apply a thin film over the body part on which you are to work. Do not apply oil directly from the container to the body surface because it will feel cold to the client and will cause discomfort. Rub your hands together to warm the oil to body temperature. This also makes it easier to spread the oil over the client's skin. Your hands should glide easily over the skin without dragging or pushing the underlying muscles.

To apply oil efficiently, use long superficial strokes (effleurage) that cover the entire area to be massaged. As the oil is smoothed, strokes can become firmer. Effleurage is used to apply the oil and at the same time encourage the flow of body fluids toward the center of the body. Strokes should be continuous, pushing in the direction of the heart then gliding back to the starting point. A good general rule is to lead with the little finger (ulnar) side of your hand, with the hand relaxed, yet firm, so that even when passing over an obstacle such as the knee or shoulder, the hand is in complete contact with the client's skin.

### THE MASSAGE SEQUENCE

Sequence refers to the pattern or design of a massage. Developing a good sequence is especially important because it coordinates and organizes the massage so there is smooth progression from one stroke to the next, and from one body part to the next. It provides a framework for a thought out, logical progression and at the same time allows for flexability and creativity.

The sequence of the overall massage is designed in a logical progression that leaves the client with a feeling of completedness. Although a sequence may vary according to the situation, a pattern should be used that insures that every part of the body is massaged properly and thoroughly.

Massage movements for adjacent areas as well as bi-lateral body parts should follow in sequence. For example, when beginning with the hand the massage should progress to the arm and then to the shoulder. Then massage the other hand, arm and shoulder, followed by massage of both shoulders, the neck and the head. Finally, massage the chest, abdomen, one leg and foot, followed by massage of the other leg and foot. This completes the massage for the front of the body.

There are many possibilities for "putting it all together" therefore it is important to follow a plan that insures completeness and balance.

Developing a sequence also insures a thorough massage that is balanced between one body part and another. Following is an example of an effective sequence to be used on each body area.

1. Make contact with, and undrape the body part to be massaged.
2. Apply massage oil with light effleurage.
3. Apply effleurage to accustom the body to your touch. Effleurage also flushes out the lymph and venous blood.
4. Apply petrissage, kneading the tissues to warm them. This also enables you to become aware of any areas of tension or congestion in the muscles.
5. Apply effleurage to again flush the area.
6. Apply friction by using any of the recommended friction techniques.
7. Apply effleurage to the area again because this flushes the area again while linking and integrating the segmented parts back into the whole.
8. Do joint movements to restore mobility by reinforcing the possibility of movement. At the same time joint movements stretch the muscles and connective tissues, and lubricate the joints.
9. Apply effleurage to flush out the loosened debris and to give a feeling of length to the body part.
10. Apply feather strokes. This stimulates the peripheral nervous system, smoothes the energy field and says "goodbye" to that part of the body.
11. Redrape the part of the body that has been massaged, undrape the next part and continue until the client has been given a thorough massage.

## PROFESSIONAL RULES TO REMEMBER

Knowledge of the restrictions and limitations of massage are as important as the knowledge of its proper use. A well trained practitioner knows when a massage treatment is indicated, how it can be modified for the greatest benefit to the client, and under what circumstances it should not be applied.

Before beginning the massage routines in this chapter, review the basic rules for safe and effective massage procedures.

1. Wash your hands thoroughly with soap and hot water and rinse and dry them before and after each treatment.
2. Avoid chilling the client by contact with cold hands or by having the temperature of the room too low for comfort.
3. Allow the client to have a short rest period before and after the massage.
4. Never apply massage so vigorously that it causes fatigue in the client.
5. Keep your nails short and smooth to avoid scratching the client's skin.
6. Avoid heavy, rapid or jarring movements that might convey fear of injury to the client.
7. Never use any form of heavy stroking against the venous blood supply.
8. Never massage the body immediately after the client has eaten a meal.
9. When the client is obese it may be necessary to apply massage with more strength but not to the point of discomfort for the client.
10. Everything used in massage treatments should be clean and sanitary.

## PROCEDURE FOR A GENERAL BODY MASSAGE

### Massage 1

The Massage 1 routine is flexible in that some steps can be omitted and others included. The student should follow the instructor's directions.

The main objective is to give a beneficial massage that is suited to the client's desires and needs.

1. Preliminary steps:
   a. Obtain all necessary supplies and arrange as needed.
   b. See that the client has all items needed to prepare for the massage.
   c. Direct client to the dressing room and explain preparation procedures.
   d. Record necessary information about the client's health, weight, etc.
   e. Obtain and record the client's pulse and body temperature.
   f. Wash and sterilize your hands.
   g. Provide a cap, headband, or drape the client's head to protect hair.
   h. Assist the client onto the massage table or into the facial chair.

2. Facial massage (optional):
   a. Apply cleansing cream or lotion with spreading, stroking, and rotary movements. If removing makeup, use a second cleansing application. Follow with astringent.
   b. Remove cleanser with tissues or warm, moist towels.
   c. Apply massage oil or cream.
   d. Do facial massage procedures.
   e. Remove excess oil or cream followed by skin freshening lotion or astringent.
3. Exercise (optional):
   a. Demonstrate the recommended exercises with or without mechanical apparatus.
   b. Begin with simple exercises and increase them progressively in difficulty and duration.
   c. Supervise the client in the performance of exercises.
4. Hydrotherapy (optional):
   a. Select bath most suitable for the client.
   b. Adjust the bath equipment and accessories.
   c. Take temperature of the bath.
   d. Assist the client as necessary to enter the bath.
   e. Control temperature of the bath and duration.
   f. Attend the client as necessary during the bath. Give water to drink, and take pulse if necessary.
   g. Assist the client as needed following the bath.
   h. Allow the client to rest for a short period following the bath.
5. Preparation for body massage:
   a. Assist the client onto the massage table and into a supine (face-up) position.
   b. Wash and sterilize your hands.
   c. Apply massage oil, cream, or other lubricant over part to be massaged first.
   d. Drape the client's body with sheet or towel with the exception of the part to be massaged.
6. Order of treatment (overview):
   The following procedure is suggested for a basic massage. However, it may be varied to suit the convenience of the practitioner and the needs of the client.
   a. Begin with the arms, right then left.
   b. Proceed to front of the legs, right then left.
   c. Continue movements over chest, neck, and abdomen.
   d. The client will turn over to assume a prone (face down) position. Begin with the back of the legs, right then left. Finish the massage with the back of the body.

Following the massage the client should be allowed to rest for a short period then be assisted from the table.

## Step by Step Procedures for Massage 1

The following step-by-step procedure helps you to learn basic massage techniques quickly. Massage oil is applied and all preliminary steps observed.

### *General Arm Massage*

1. Raise the client's arm.
2. Stroke the arm three times.
3. Bend the elbow and rest it on the table.
4. Press the metacarpal bones back and forth.
5. Knead each finger, hand, and arm three times.
6. Rotate each finger.
7. Stroke the arm once.
8. Roll the arm three times.
9. Apply cupping and hacking movements of the arm.
10. Stroke the arm lightly three times.

### *Arm Movements for Body Massage*

Depending on the client's requirements, the following movements may be included or omitted.

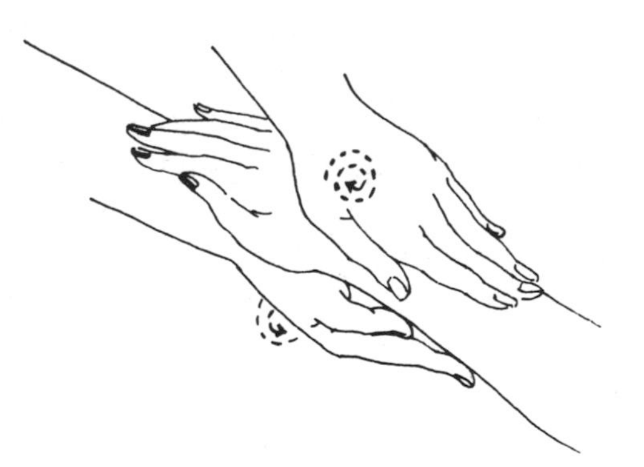

*Circular rubbing movements of the hands.*

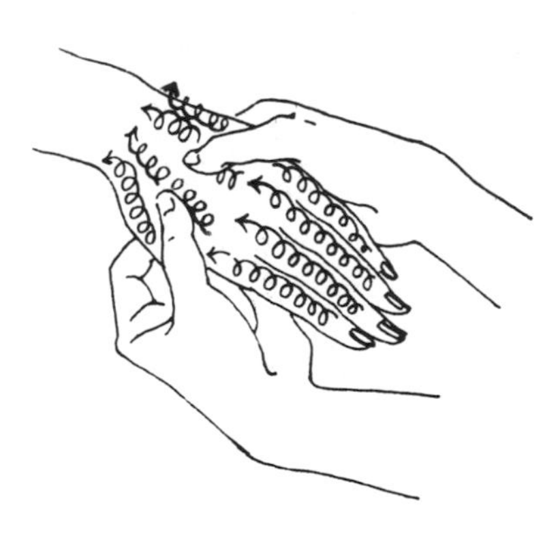

*Circular kneading of the fingers and hand.*

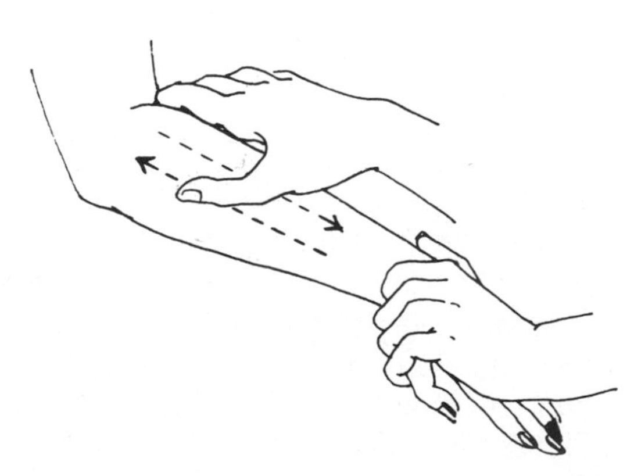

*Chucking the arm.*

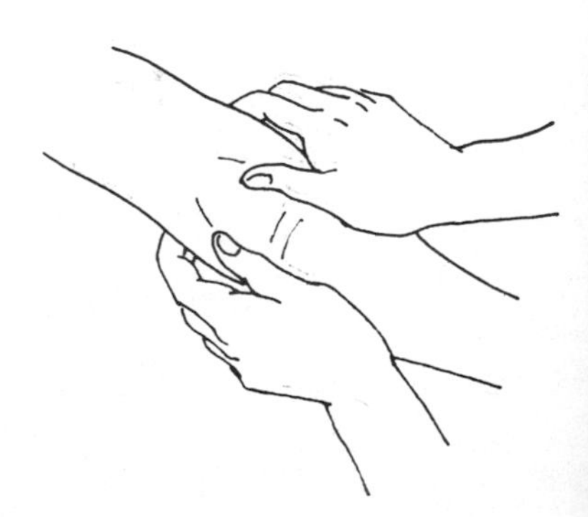

*Fulling the arm.*

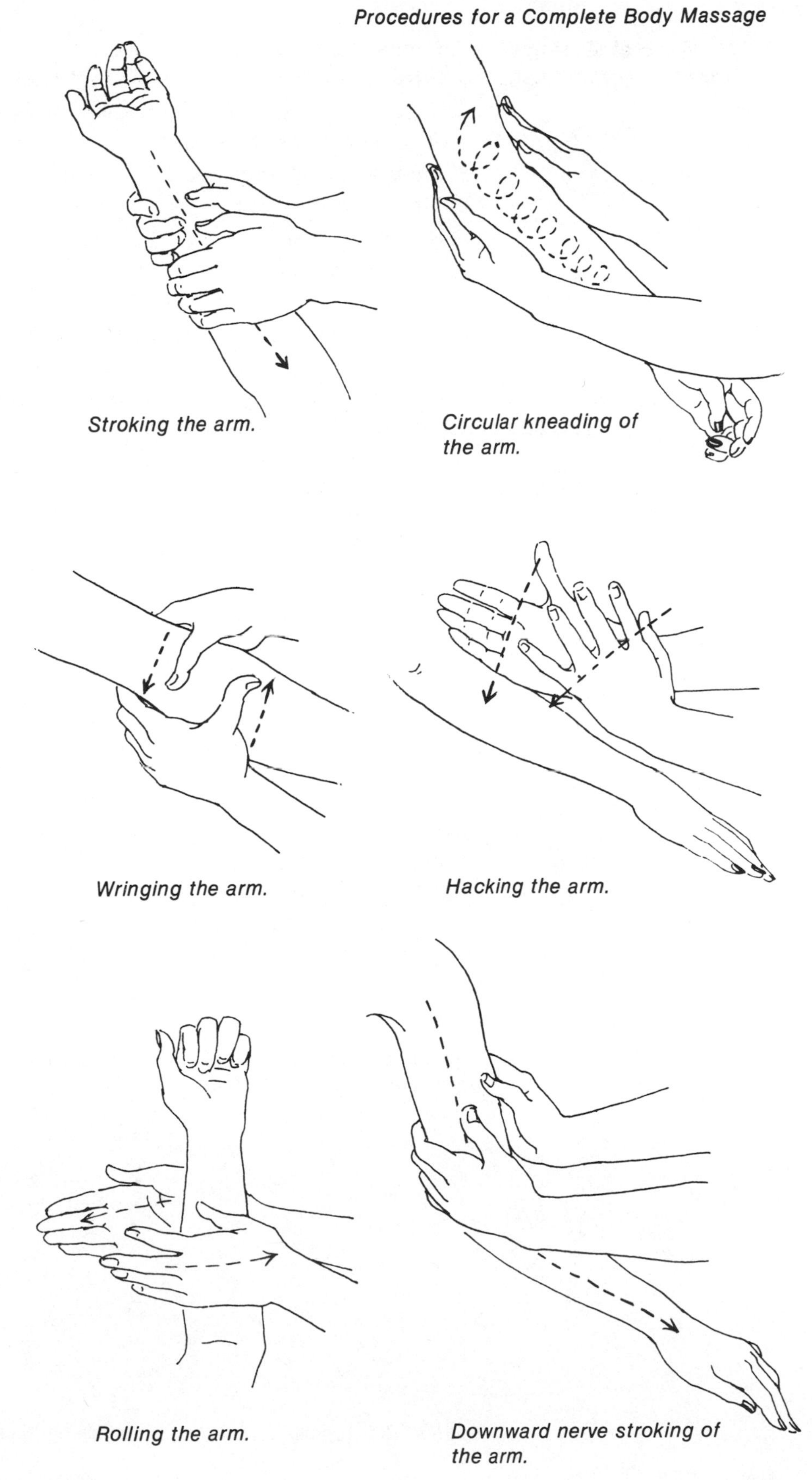

Stroking the arm.

Circular kneading of the arm.

Wringing the arm.

Hacking the arm.

Rolling the arm.

Downward nerve stroking of the arm.

**General Massage for the Foot and Leg**

1. Stroke the leg three times.
2. Press metatarsal bones of the foot back and forth.
3. Knead each toe, around foot, ankle, and over leg three times.
4. Rotate each toe three times.
5. Vibrate the leg and foot.
6. Stroke the leg once.
7. Raise the knee.
8. Roll the leg three times.
9. Stroke the leg three times.
10. Apply hacking and cupping movements to the leg.
11. Stroke the leg lightly three times.

***Massage for the Foot and Leg***

Depending on the client's requirements, the following movements may be included or ommitted.

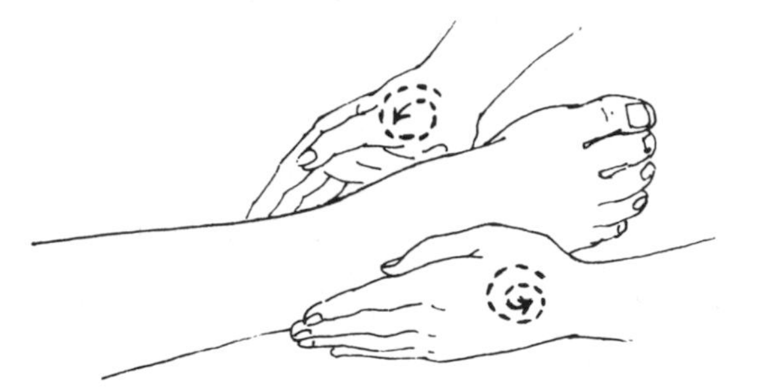

*Warming the foot and ankles with circular rubbing movements.*

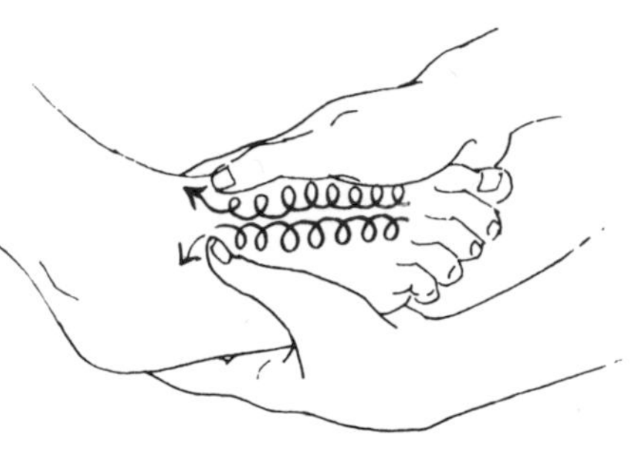

*Circular kneading of the foot.*

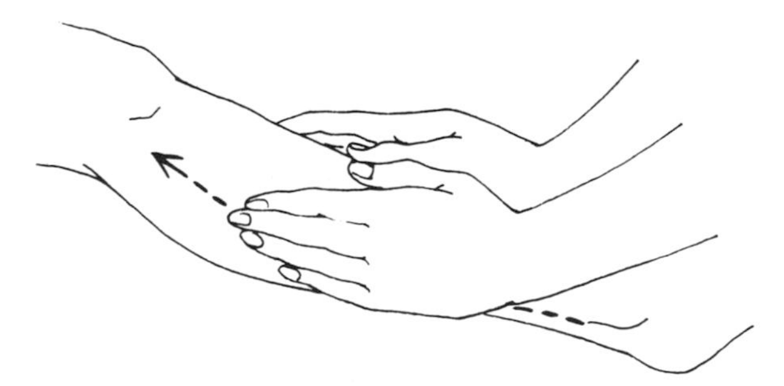

*Stroking the leg upward with both hands.*

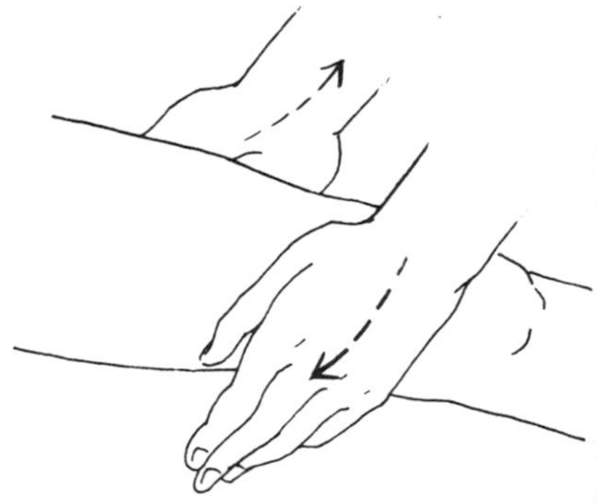

*Rolling the muscles of the thigh.*

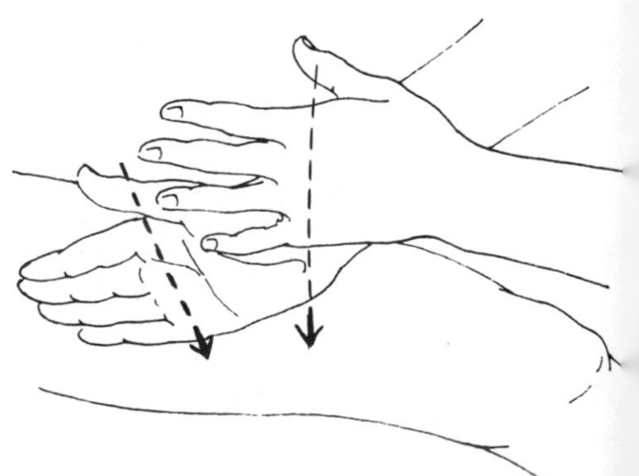

*Beating the muscles of the thigh.*

*Hacking the muscles of the thigh.*

*Circular kneading of the leg and thigh.*

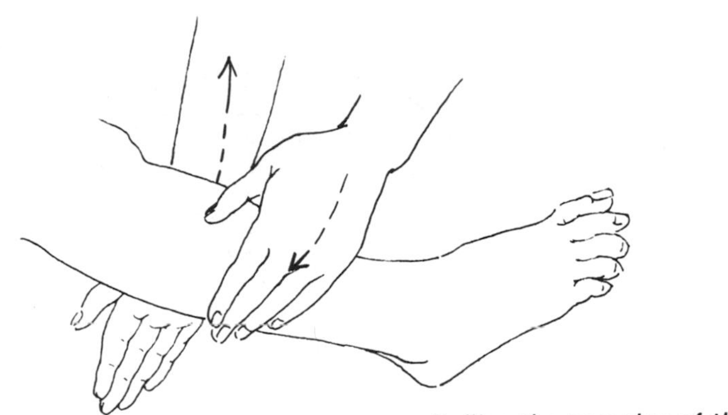

*Rolling the muscles of the leg.*

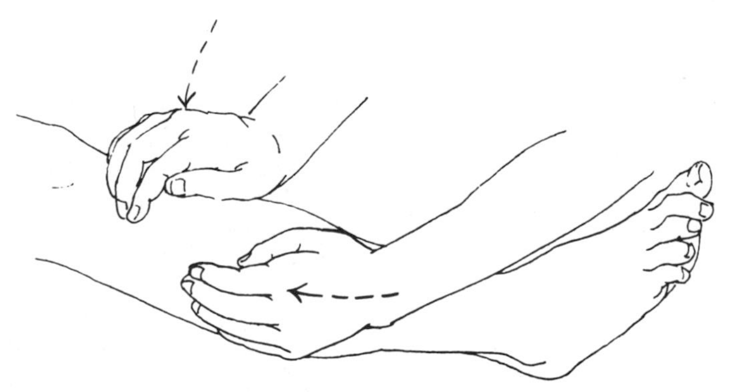

*Cupping the leg and thigh.*

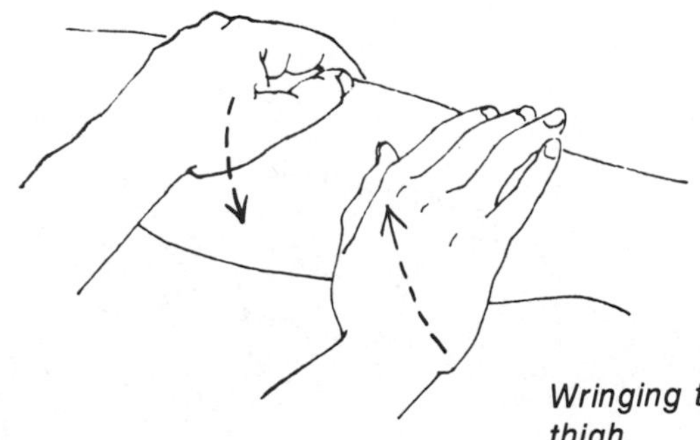

*Wringing the muscles of the thigh.*

**General Massage for the Chest and Neck**

1. Stroke the back of the neck once.
2. Knead back and sides of the neck.
3. Rub the chest area three times, going from side to side, coming up under each arm and down between the breasts.
4. Stroke the chest three times.
5. Apply hacking and cupping movement around the collar bone.
6. Stroke the chest lightly three times.

***Chest and Neck Movements***

Depending on the client's requirements, the practitioner may include or omit any of the following movements.

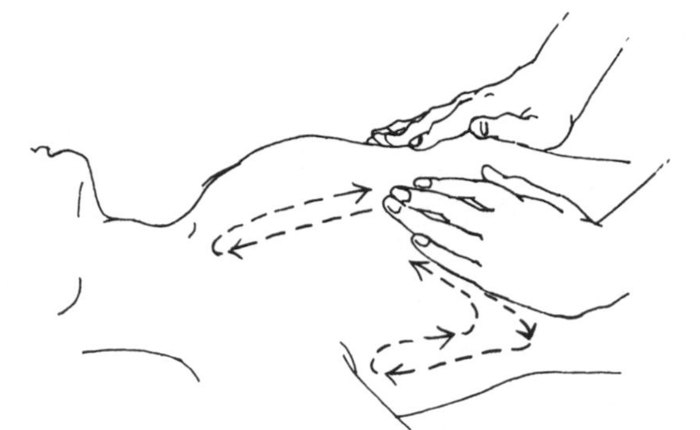

*Stroking the chest with both hands, from center of chest across lower ribs (a); up under the arms (b); down under the arms (c); towards center of chest (d); up center of chest (e); and then down the center of the chest (f).*

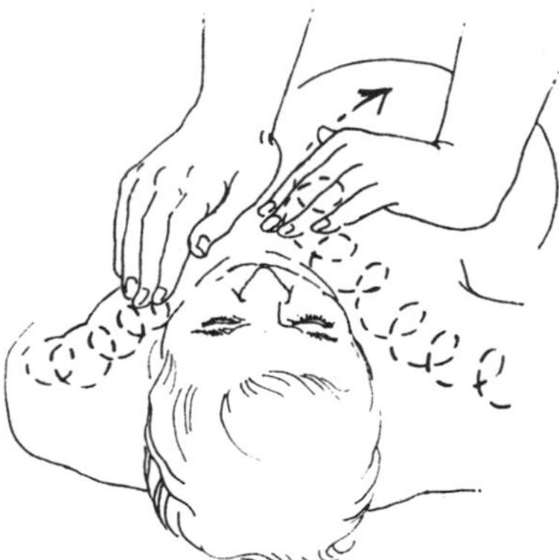

*Circular friction over the chest.*

*Stroking the upper shoulders and neck with both hands, from upper arms towards the center of the chest (a); back to the upper arms (b); up the side of the neck (c); and then down under the shoulders (d).*

*Kneading the back of neck.*

**General Massage Movements for the Abdomen**

1. Stroke the abdominal area three times.
2. Knead the abdominal muscles back and forth three times.
3. Vibrate the abdominal area with a circular motion over colon, intestines, stomach, and liver.
4. Stroke abdomen lightly three times.

***Abdominal Movements for Body Massage***

Depending on the client's requirements, the practitioner may include or omit any of the following movements.

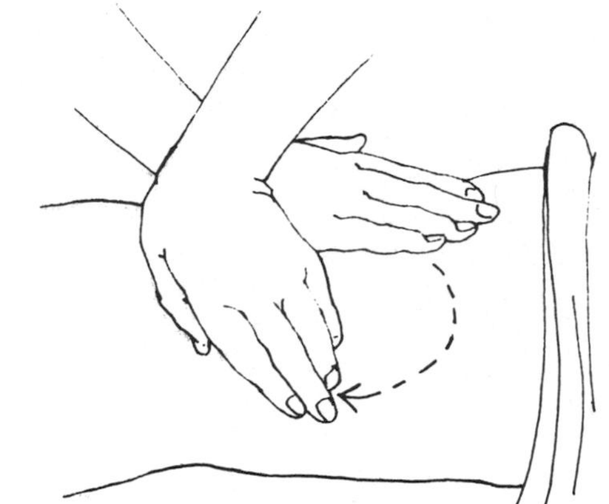

*Stroking the abdomen with deep circular movement.*

*Kneading the abdomen downward.*

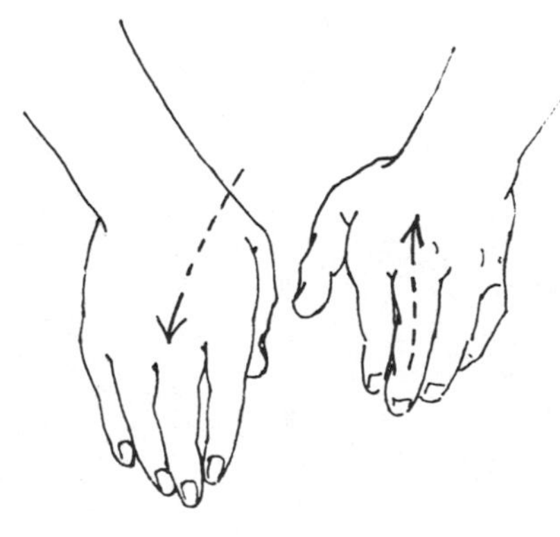

*Kneading the muscles over the abdomen.*

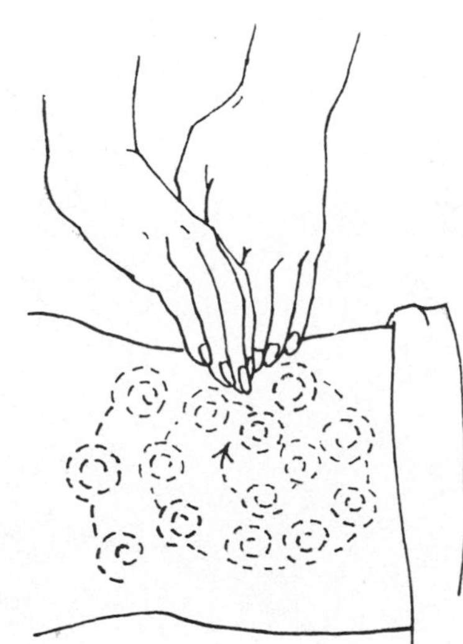

*Vibrating over the abdominal organs.*

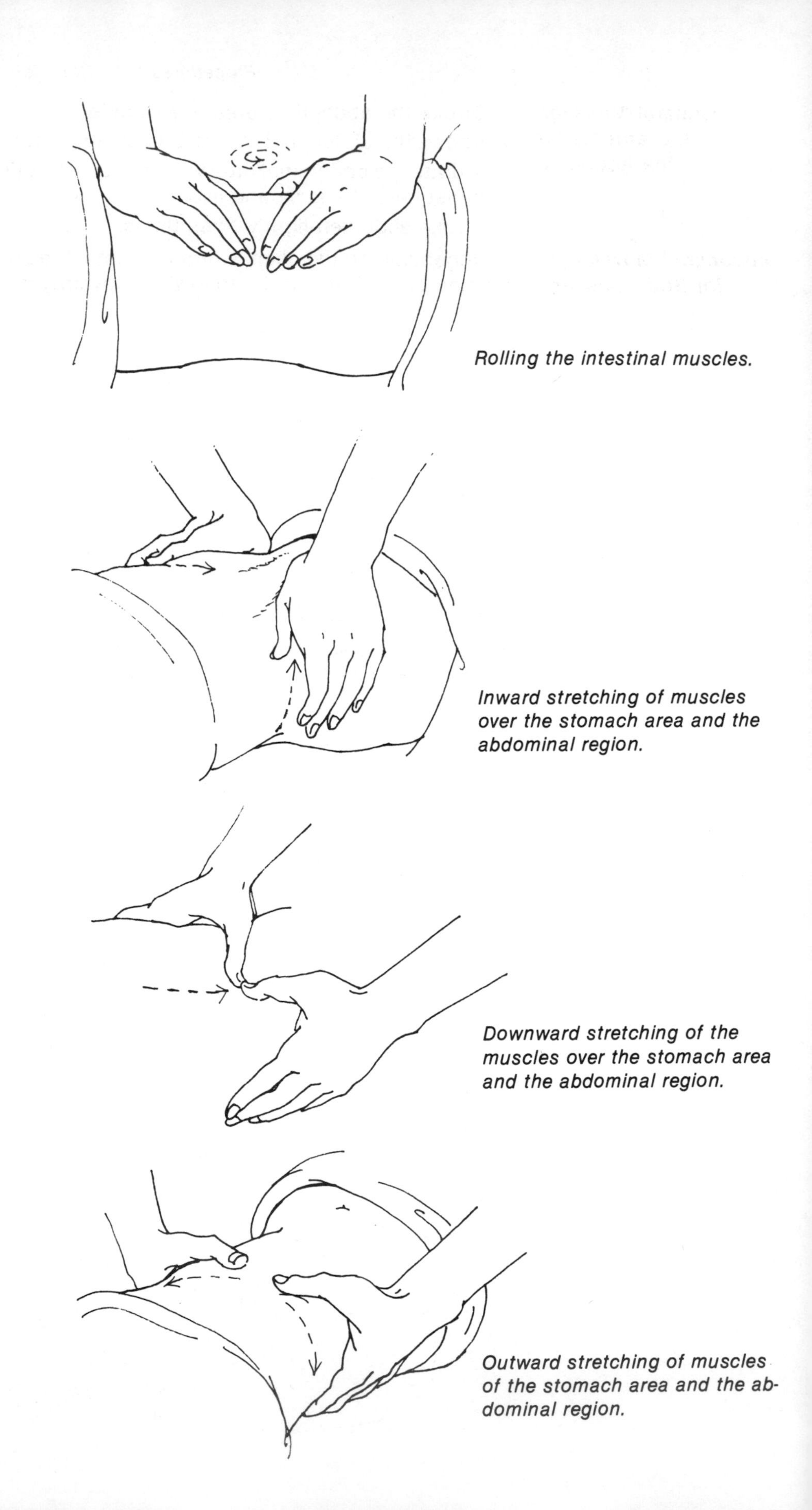

*Rolling the intestinal muscles.*

*Inward stretching of muscles over the stomach area and the abdominal region.*

*Downward stretching of the muscles over the stomach area and the abdominal region.*

*Outward stretching of muscles of the stomach area and the abdominal region.*

**CHANGE OF POSITION**

The client turns over to a prone, face downward position. Apply massage oil or cream to the back of the legs and body.

**General Massage for the Back of the Legs**

1. Move legs apart and stroke each leg three times.
2. Knead each foot from toe to heel.
3. Rub each leg from the heels to the hips.
4. Knead and vibrate the hips and buttocks.
5. Stroke each leg three times.
6. Apply hacking and cupping movements to each leg, from ankles to hips and back again.
7. Stroke each leg lightly three times.

***Back of Leg Movements for Body Massage***

Depending on the client's requirements, the following movements may be included or omitted.

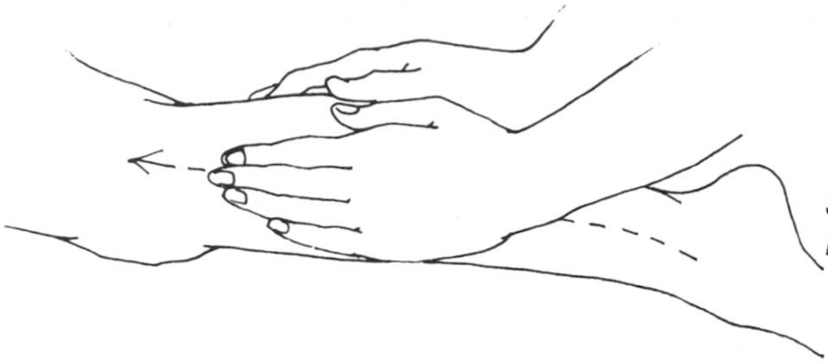

*Stroking the leg upward with both hands.*

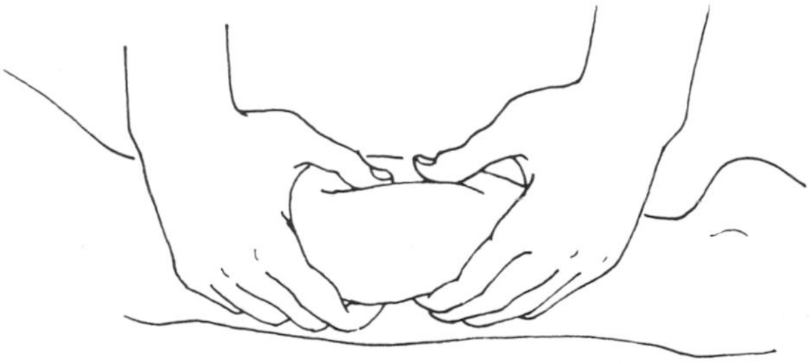

*Kneading calf muscles.*

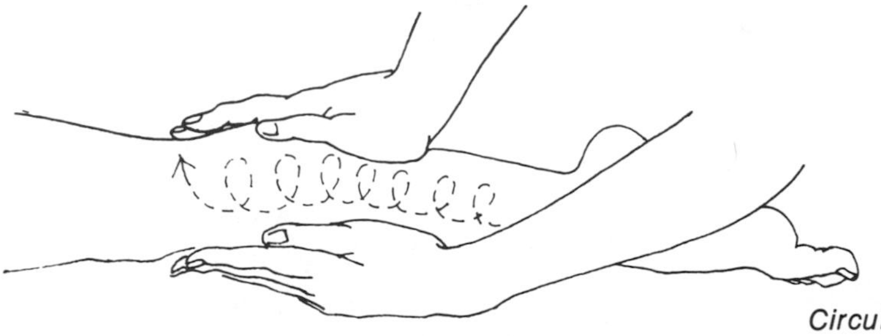

*Circular kneading muscles of leg and thigh.*

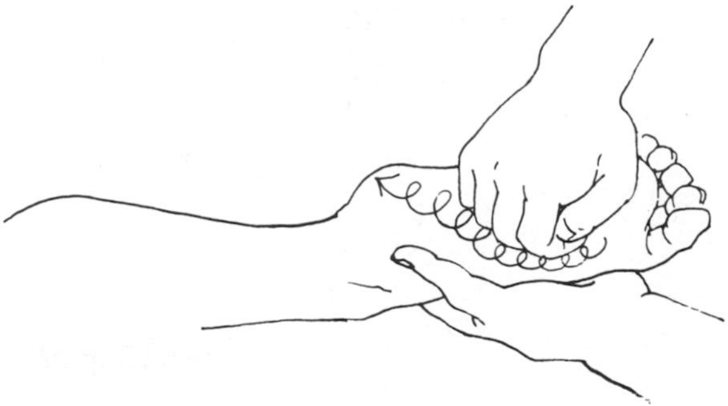

*Kneading the sole of the foot.*

**General Massage for the Back of the Body**

1. Stroke the back five times up and down the spine on each side of the body.
2. Place the hands flat on each side of the spine, and stretch them outwards toward the shoulders. Stroke five times.
3. Continue Step 2 to cover the entire back.
4. Vibrate each vertebra three times.
5. Knead the entire back and each side of the spine.
6. Stroke the back three times.
7. Apply light hacking movements over the spine, gluteal muscles, and between the shoulders.
8. Stroke the back lightly five times.

***Back Movements for Body Massage***

Depending on the client's requirements, the following movements may be included or omitted.

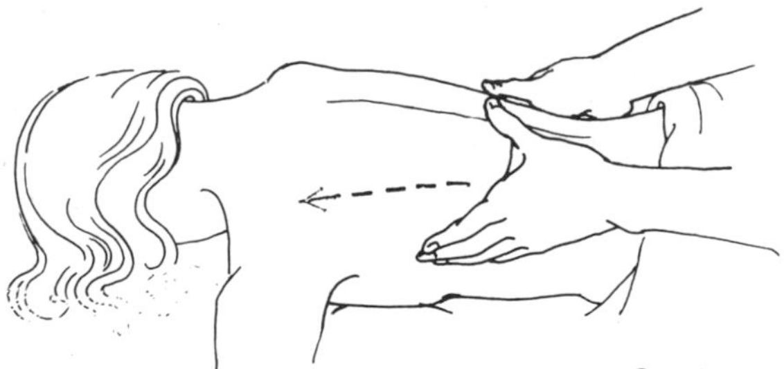

*Stroking the entire back.*

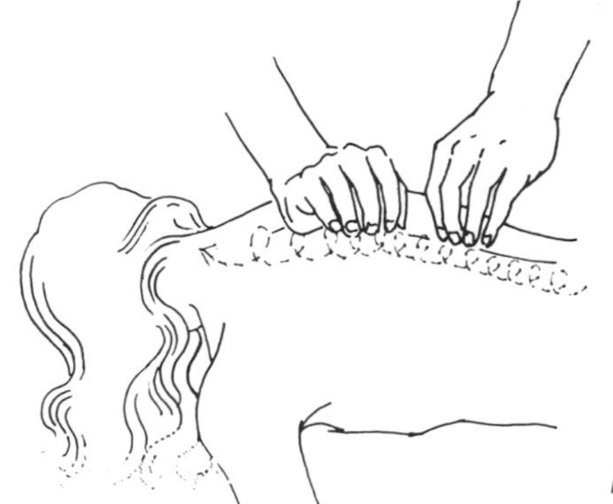

*Kneading around the spine.*

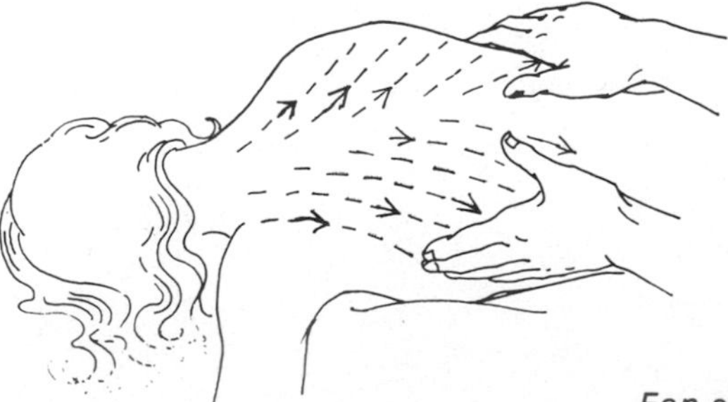

*Fan stroking of the back.*

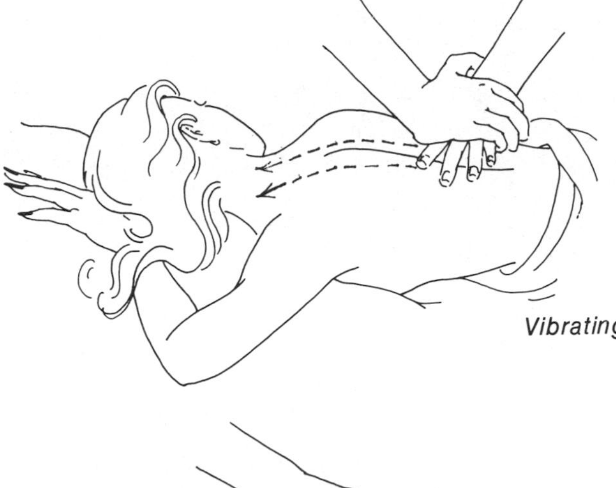

*Vibrating over each vertebra.*

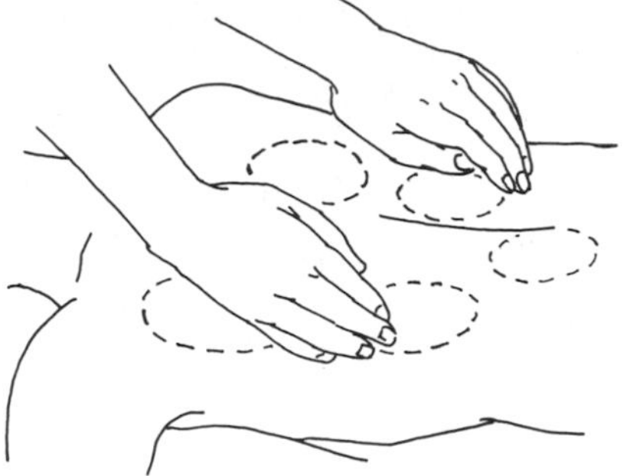

*Cupping along the back.*

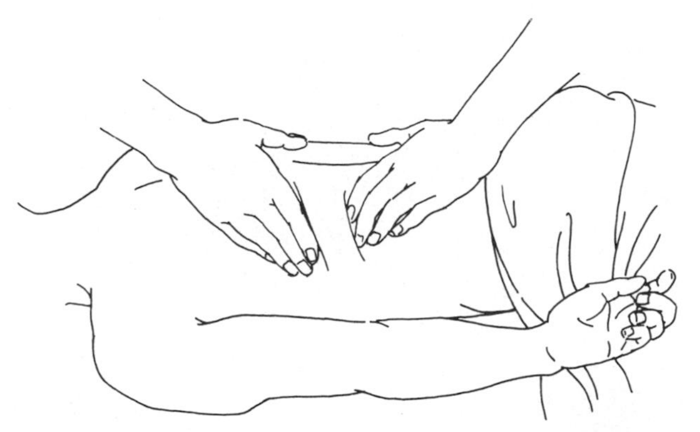

*Kneading of the fleshy tissue of upper back.*

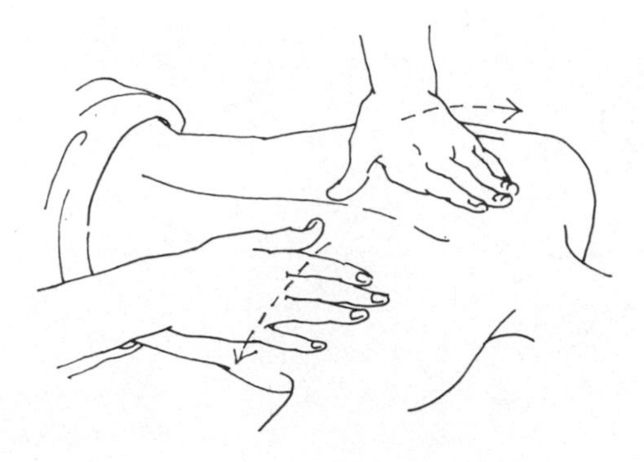

*Outward stretching of the muscles of the back.*

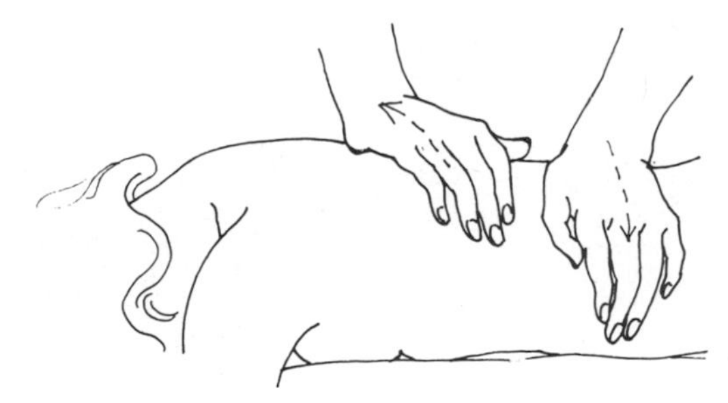

*Stretching the muscles of the lower back in a backward and forward movement.*

*Slapping the back.*

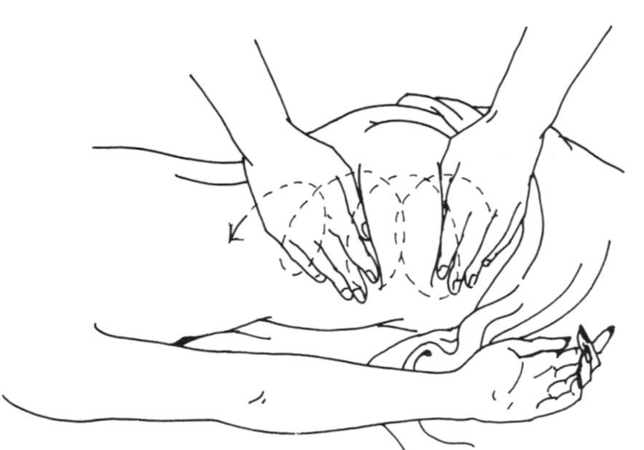

*Applying circular friction over the lower back and hips.*

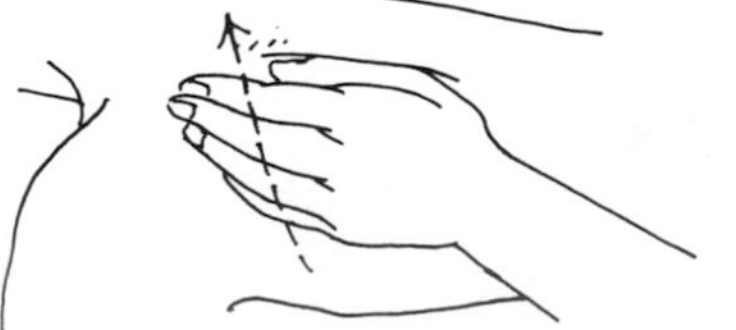

*Inward stretching of the muscles of the back.*

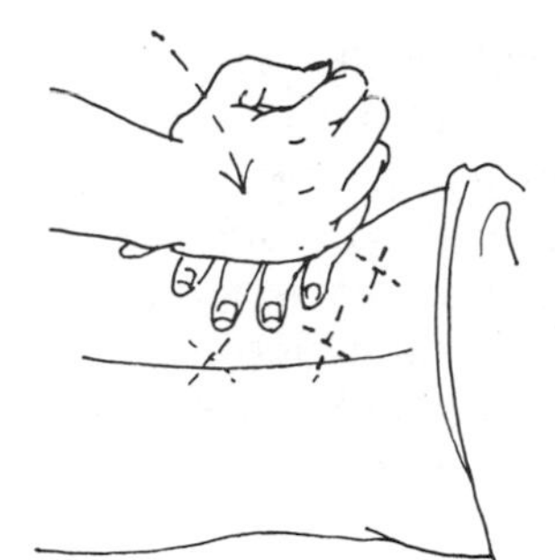

*Beating the lower back.*

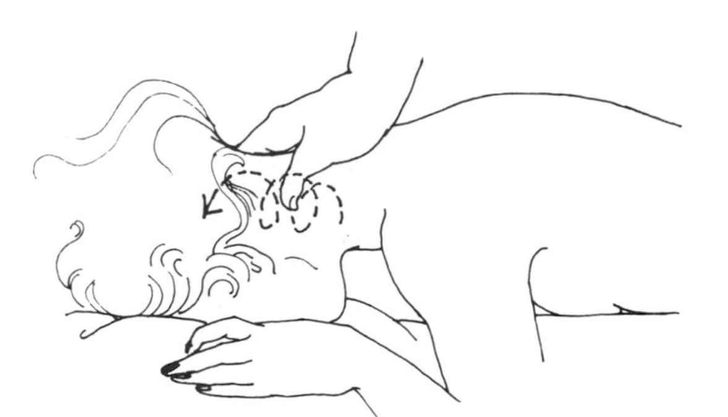

*Circular kneading of the back of the neck.*

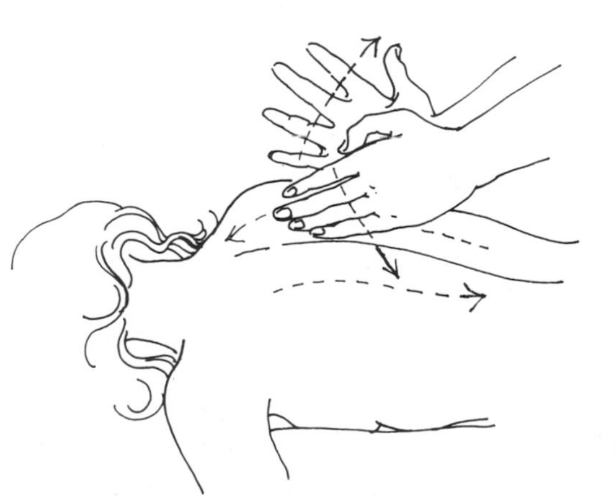

*Hacking over the spine.*

**COMPLETING THE TREATMENT**

1. Use tissue to remove massage cream or other lubricant from the client's body.
2. Apply alcohol or astringent lotion over the client's back. Ask the client to turn over and continue applying lotion over front of the body.
3. Cover the client's eyes, and permit him or her to relax in a reclining position.

**FINAL CONSIDERATIONS**

1. Complete the client's record card.
2. Suggest supplementary services and answer any questions the client may have.
3. Place supplies in their proper place, discard used items.
4. See that all equipment and items, including massage table and bath, are properly prepared before the next client arrives.

## PROCEDURE FOR PROFESSIONAL BODY MASSAGE

### Massage 2

Massage, like any other skill, requires practice and patience to learn all the basics before attempting to build speed, and before trying new techniques. By the time you have mastered Massage 1, you should be familiar with most of the terms for the various movements used in basic body massage. Massage 2 incorporates additional techniques to help you increase efficiency, remember sequence of movements, and to readily identify movements and anatomy by proper names. While doing massage, pay attention to your hand positions, and how you stand and move.

Massage 2 enables you to review what you have learned, but allows for even more creativity in varying massage routines. Before beginning the massage concentrate on projecting the manner, attitude and appearance of the professional massage practitioner. Read directions carefully for each step. This routine is not illustrated. Once you have learned how to give a complete massage correctly and efficiently, you will not need to refer to your notes, illustrations, or written guides. Your aim is to be able to give the complete massage in a knowledgeable and professional manner.

### Preliminary Steps

1. Prepare all facilities and products.
2. If this is the client's first visit, be ready to greet her or him on time and introduce yourself. In many places of business the practitioner is addressed by his or her first name. For example, when introducing yourself to a new client you might say, "Good morning Mrs. Mason, I'm Carolyn. I'll be working with you today." You do not address the client by his or her first name unless it is customary to do so, or if the client has asked that you use his or her first name.
3. Put first time clients at ease by showing the facilities and explaining the services.
4. The first step with any client is the consultation or interview (see Chapter 7). Have the client fill out the information sheet first, and review it with the client to obtain more direct information. Discuss the client's needs and expectations and the kind of massage he or she prefers. This is the time to be observant of the client's physical condition and determine what benefits should be derived from the massage.
5. When appropriate, take the client's temperature and blood pressure. Explain why these procedures are done.
6. Explain to the client how he or she is to prepare for the massage. Show the client to the shower or hydrotherapy area, depending upon which services that client has decided upon. Provide proper draping for the client from the dressing area to the massage table.
7. Assist the client (as necessary) to the massage table, and explain the position, either supine or prone, he or she should assume. Drape the client appropriately and provide extra support (towels or bolster) under knees or head if necessary.

There are many possibilities for varying massage techniques for different clients. The following massage procedure will help you to become more proficient and creative.

**Step-by-Step Procedures for Massage 2**

1. Begin with the client lying supine on the massage table. Make initial contact (tune in) by first placing your hands on the frontal eminence of the client's forehead or the back of the neck, at the base of the head. If you prefer, you may begin by placing your hands on the client's shoulders. Hold the touch for a few seconds without moving.
2. Massage the neck
   a. Apply oil with a bi-lateral effleurage stroke beginning at the sternal notch and continuing over the shoulders, up the trapezius and the back of the neck to the occipital ridge.
   b. Turn the client's head to one side supporting it with your hand. Continue effleurage strokes, leading with your little finger and beginning just inferior (below) the mastoid process (boney bump below and behind the ear). Continue down the lateral aspect of the neck, over the shoulder and back up the trapezius to the occipital ridge. Repeat 3 to 5 times.
   c. Thoroughly petrissage that side of the neck paying attention to any tight areas.
   d. Repeat effleurage on neck and shoulders.
   e. Apply circular friction to any congested or tight areas.
   f. Repeat effleurage.
   g. Turn the client's head to the opposite side and repeat the movements as you did in steps b through f.
   h. Return the client's head to the central position and apply bi-lateral petrissage and friction to the neck and shoulders.
   i. Do the following joint movements: Move the head back with the chin up then lower the chin down to the chest. Move the head with the ear, first to the right shoulder, then to the left. Rotate the head to its full range of motion (lateral rotation). The spine remains in a straight line.
3. Massage the face.
   a. Touch the frontal eminence and hold for 30 seconds.
   b. Ask the client to inhale slowly, exhale, and continue breathing deeply.
   c. Apply digital effleurage with your thumb from the centerline of the face to the hairline. At the hairline, work gradually down to the eyebrow and across the eyes (the supraorbital and suborbital ridges).
   d. Apply circular friction from the temples to the jaw. Massage along the hairline and in front of the ear, carefully massaging the temporal and mandibular joints.

   e. Apply directional friction downward along the mandible, and circular friction under the mandible.
   f. Apply light palmar friction on the cheeks.
   g. Apply light effleurage from the centerline of the face to the hairline.
4. Massage the scalp.
   a. Without using oil, apply gentle friction movements over the entire scalp.
   b. Apply digital vibration using all five digits bilaterally. This is done in such a way as to move the scalp over the cranium and not the hair over the scalp.
   c. Smooth the hair into its natural contour.
   d. Repeat the effleurage strokes on the neck for a few seconds, feathering off the strokes to finish this part of the massage.
5. Massage the arms.
   a. Undrape one arm to make contact and apply oil on the client's arm from wrist to shoulder using light effleurage.
   b. Locate the handle at the wrist, and put the client's arm in slight traction by holding it with the wrist handle. Apply effleurage, leading with your little finger. Apply more pressure from wrist to neck, then lightly stroke as you return to the wrist. Repeat three to five times.
   c. Change your hand so that you are holding the client's arm (the same one you are working on) with the opposite hand at the wrist handle. Do effleurage again three to five times.
   d. Hold the thumb side handle (the client's wrist) with the arm that is closest to the client. Begin effleurage leading with your little finger up from the wrist, up the arm, over the shoulder, and up to the back of the neck. Rotate your hand as it travels over the client's shoulder; at the same time apply slight traction to the handle. Proceed up the back of the neck then down under the shoulder (trapezius area), then glide back to the starting point at the wrist. Repeat three to five times.
   e. Change the handle to your other hand, the ulnal side, of the wrist. Lead with your little finger, apply effleurage up the medial aspect of the arm over the shoulder, around and down into the axillary portion of the arm, then return to the wrist. Repeat three to five times.
   f. Using both hands, grasp the arm at shoulder level and apply petrissage directing individual movements toward the shoulder while moving down the arm to the client's hand.
   g. Wring and roll (using both hands) from the shoulder, moving down the arm and giving special attention to the muscles of the forearm. Repeat effleurage to the arm.

6. Massage the hand.
   a. Apply petrissage to the palm of the client's hand.
   b. Apply friction to the palm.
   c. Apply petrissage to the back of the hand.
   d. Apply friction to the back of the hand.
   e. Do petrissage on each digit, including a joint movement.
   f. Apply joint movement. Support the client's hand and rotate all fingers clockwise and counterclockwise. Extend and flex the fingers, wrist, and elbow.
   g. Rotate the shoulder joint clockwise and counterclockwise. Extend the arm straight above the client's head to stretch the entire arm. Apply traction at the wrist while moving the arm from a position above the client's head and back down to the side.
   h. Shake and vibrate the arm and hand.
   i. Apply a final effleurage of the arm and hand, and rotate the shoulder.
   j. Apply lateral effleurage, then feather downward with superficial strokes from the neck, down the arm, to the fingertips.
   k. Redrape the client as necessary, and repeat the arm and hand massage for the other side.
7. Massage the feet.
   a. Move to the feet maintaining contact by using a light brushing stroke. Pause momentarily to allow the client to sense where you are before you begin massaging the feet. Undrape one foot and leg up to the hip.
   b. Use just enough oil to allow your hands to work smoothly.
   c. Apply effleurage to each aspect of the foot so as to strip out the venous fluid. Stroke from the toes up to and past the ankle on the top and side of the foot.
   d. Apply petrissage and friction to the bottom of the feet and from the ball of the foot to the heel. Use a closed fist or heel of the hand to do the pressing movements.
   e. Apply kneading movements from the toes up to the ankles.
   f. Apply small circular friction movements between each of the tendons on the top and sides of the foot.
   g. Apply digital friction to each toe and between toes.
   h. Beginning with the toes, incorporate joint movements, first individually, then together. Apply plantar and dorsal flexion of the toes, then to the entire foot. Rotate the foot and ankle then separate the toes (phalanges) and wring and roll the foot.
   i. Repeat this entire procedure on the other foot and leg.

   Note: The practitioner may choose to work on adjacent parts of the body in sequence (from one part to the adjacent part) rather than interrupting the flow of movement.

8. Massage the front of the legs.
   a. Apply oil with light and continuous effleurage.
   b. Apply effleurage with both hands, leading with the little fingers beginning at the ankle. Apply effleurage to the lateral side of the leg by leading with one hand on the lateral side of the leg, followed by the other hand on the medial aspect of the leg. Your hands should span the entire front of the leg. Hand pressure may be increased with each effleurage stroke and feathered back to the starting point. The hand courses up the leg, over the hip, and turns as it returns to the starting point (the ankle). The medial hand progresses to the groin and turns as it returns lightly along the medial aspect of the leg to the beginning point at the ankle. Repeat these movements three to five times.
   c. Apply petrissage, beginning at the ankle and proceeding up the leg along the fleshy parts along the side of the tibia to the knee. Apply digital petrissage to the tendon areas around the patella. The thigh may require several passes up and down with this stroke because it is a large area.
   d. Repeat effleurage.

   *Optional position with the knee joint:* The following is an optional position for leg massage. In this position, the entire calf and thigh can be massaged easily. Position the client's foot flat on the table with the knee bent and the foot 16 to 18 inches from the buttocks. Wrap the foot with the drape and brace the leg either with your knee or by sitting on the table near the client's toes to keep the leg from sliding.

   e. With the leg in the bent-knee position, apply effleurage from ankle to knee.
   f. Apply petrissage from ankle to knee.
   g. Repeat effleurage from ankle to knee.
   h. While keeping the knee bent, apply a variety of friction techniques from ankle to knee. Pay special attention to areas that seem to be more congested or tight. Apply rolling, wringing, or cross-fiber friction in areas of tension.
   i. Apply effleurage to the leg from ankle to knee.
   j. Keeping the leg in the bent-knee position, apply effleurage from knee to hip, groin, and gluteal crease.
   k. Apply petrissage to the entire thigh. Make several passes to cover the entire circumference of the leg.
   l. Apply friction followed by effleurage to the entire leg.
   m. Apply joint movements. Grasp the ankle with one hand, and place the other hand just below the knee. Move the knee toward the chest while flexing it to the maximum. Pay attention to the degree of flexibility, and move the limbs firmly, but not forcefully, to their maximum range of movements. It is beneficial to have the client breathe deeply then exhale as you apply downward pressure on the knee.

n. Move your hand around to grasp the ankle at the level of the Achilles tendon, then elevate the foot toward the ceiling to extend the leg and flex the hip. Flex the hip to its maximum range of movement by moving the foot toward the client's head.

o. Flex the client's knee by bringing it toward the chest, then rotate the bent leg laterally, retaining slight pressure on the knee to maintain full range of motion as the leg rotates outward. Return the leg to the table by continuing the hip rotation and slowly straightening the leg. Your hand should support the back of the leg to prevent hyperextension as the leg is returned to the table. Repeat this procedure two times.

p. Repeat the above procedure by moving to the foot of the table and grasping the heel (handle) with the lateral hand (the one toward the outside of the leg you were working on). Rotate the foot and leg in the hip socket. This movement will be back and forth, and the foot movement will resemble a windshield wiper.

q. Place your other hand over the client's instep and apply slight traction. Shake the leg up and down. Keep the heel on the table to avoid hyperextension of the knee.

r. Apply effleurage to the entire leg three to five times.

s. Apply feather (nerve) strokes from hip to toes, three to five times.

t. Redrape the leg and proceed to the other foot. Repeat the entire procedure on the other leg.

9. Massage the Abdomen and Chest.

This part of the massage requires some special considerations. The need for draping usually varies when working with male and female clients. Women, for reasons of modesty may prefer having their breasts draped at all times. It is best to ask the female client what she prefers. Professional standards recommend that draping procedures (as directed in Chapter 7) be followed.

The following massage description refers to techniques used on the fully exposed torso with added comments when using breast draping.

In preparation for massage of the abdominal region, use a bolster or pillow to elevate the client's knees and support them so that the abdominal muscles will remain relaxed. Draping should be open enough to allow massaging down to the top of the pubic bone, but secure enough to avoid exposure of the genital area.

a. To begin, stand to the client's right to apply oil to the abdomen, chest and sides of the body.

b. Do effleurage strokes on the abdomen and chest, over the shoulders around and down the axillary areas, then down the sides to the crest of the illium. Massage back to the center with a turn of your wrist and repeat the movements.

When using breast draping, this stroke glides up as far as the drape will allow then laterally over the ribs and down to the illiac crest. Massage should not be done directly over the sensitive area of the nipples on men or women.

c. Do circular effleurage on the abdomen in a clockwise direction following the path of the colon. On this stroke, one hand remains in constant contact doing circular massage. The other describes a semi-circle beginning at the lower right of the client's abdomen, moving up the right side to the rib cage, across the abdomen just below the rib cage, then down the right side to an area just medial of the hip bone. Abdominal massage should always encourage the natural flow of the large intestines. Repeat the abdominal massage movements several times.

d. To more thoroughly massage the large intestine, apply circular friction to its entire length. Begin in the area of the lower left part of the abdomen. The circles should be on an oblique (deviation to the vertical or horizontal line) plane of the surface of the abdomen so that pressure is increased and decreased repeatedly over an area about two inches square, and at the rate of about 100 circles per minute. This movement encourages the contents of the colon toward the rectum. Proceed slowly back along the course of the colon all the way to the cecum, the first portion of the colon.

e. Knead the entire abdomen, massaging not only the abdominal muscles, but also stimulating the action of the abdominal organs.

f. Grasp as much of the abdominal tissue as possible and gently lift and shake it.

g. Do alternate hand strokes or shingles. Stand to one side of the client and reach over to the opposite side. Alternately pull your hands over the client's body toward you. As one hand nears completion of the stroke, the other begins a stroke. This movement begins just below the crest of the illium (hipbone) and may continue all the way over the shoulder and up the neck. When working with breast draping, it is necessary to adjust the drape to continue this movement up to the axillary area and back down to the hip. When massaging the area of the ribs, flex your fingers slightly and rake gently between the ribs with your fingertips.

h. Move to the head of the table for the following stroke. This is referred to as the "caring stroke" and is a complete stroke for the torso. This stroke can only be done when not using breast draping. Begin by placing your fingers (pointing toward each other) with palms flat on the client's skin at the uppermost aspect of the chest. Stroke downward with the little fingers leading, over the chest and abdomen to the pubic bone. Rotate your hands over the client's hip bone, around the gluteus medius, around the sides and back up to the axillary area. Rotate your hands as you continue upward, around the shoulders, up the trapezius muscles to the back of the neck, ending at the occiput. Rotate your hands as you move them back down to the starting point. Repeat the movement several times. This completes the massage of the front of the body.

At this point ask the client to turn over to a prone position. Be sure to follow proper draping procedures. Make the client comfortable by supplying a pillow or bolster to support the head, neck, back, chest, feet, or ankles as necessary.

10. Massage back of legs.
    a. Undrape one leg. This massage is similar to the procedures for the front of the legs.
    b. Make contact with the client's skin and apply the oil with light effleurage strokes.
    c. Apply effleurage, leading with your little finger of the lateral hand (medial hand following). Increase the pressure on the upward stroke with each pass. Repeat three to five times.
    d. Apply petrissage to the calf and thigh upward to the crest of the ilium.
    e. Repeat effleurage three to five times.
    f. When there are particularly tight or tense areas, go over them with more specific friction movements such as compression, wringing, rolling, and deep friction. Using the heel of the hand can be quite effective over the gluteal muscles and the hamstrings.
    g. Repeat effleurage.
    h. Apply joint movements. Grasp the client's ankle and move the foot toward the buttocks with gentle pressure to flex the knee and to stretch the muscles on the front of the thigh. Continue by making increasingly larger circles with the ankle to rotate the hip joint. Return the foot to the table.
    i. Apply percussion (optional) over the leg.
    j. Repeat effleurage as a finishing stroke, gently changing to feather (nerve) strokes.
    k. Redrape the leg and repeat the entire procedure on the client's other leg.
11. Massage for the back.

    No massage is complete without a good back massage. It is important to give a good back massage because the client usually expects and looks forward to this part of the massage. There are hundreds of manipulations that may be done on the back. They range from extremely superficial stroking to deep tissue work using elbows and even knees when necessary for articulations of the spine and ribs. The following is a basic soothing routine that is guaranteed to leave the recipient in a calm, relaxed state.

a. Follow proper draping procedures.
b. Stand to the side of the client. Apply oil with effleurage strokes.
c. Beginning at the top of the gluteal cleft, apply long effleurage strokes. Your little fingers will lead with the rest of your fingers pointing toward the spine. Apply long gliding strokes up the spine to the nape of the neck.
d. Move your hands out and over the shoulders and down the sides to the hips. Rotate your hands and return to the starting point. Repeat the movement five to eight times. Use equal pressure on pulling and pushing strokes.
e. Apply petrissage. Begin with the gluteal region on the opposite side of the client from where you are standing. Knead the side of the body from below the hips up into the axillary area. Move hands to a position nearer to the spine (midway between the spine and extreme side of the body), then knead back down to the gluteal area. Work along the spine to include the trapezius muscles, the upper shoulders, and the neck.
f. Begin at the neck with alternate-hand strokes (shingles) from the side of the body to the spinal process. Move down to the top of the thigh then back up to the top of the shoulder. Change sides and repeat the effleurage strokes.
g. Flex the client's elbow (closest to you), and place the client's hand on the table about six inches from the armpit. Some practitioners prefer to place the client's hand in the small of his back to abduct and elevate the scapula. In this position a number of kneading and friction movements can easily be performed on all sides of the scapula. Special attention should be given the teres, trapezius, the rhomboids, and the infraspinatus muscles.
h. Apply joint movement. With the client's hand still in position at the side, grasp the top of the shoulder with one hand. Place your fingers neatly into a notch near the coracoid process, and use this hold as a handle. Place the other hand just inferior to the scapula so the inferior angle of the scapula fits neatly into the "V" formed between your thumb and index finger. Lift and rotate the scapula away from the rib cage. Although this may seem unnecessary, it is very effective in relieving a number of stress-related shoulder problems. Rotate the shoulder several times in both directions.
i. Abduct the elbow so the upper arm is at a square angle from the body and the forearm is relaxed at an angle from the upper arm. Support the arm with both of your hands just proximal to the elbow, and gently swing the hand up and down, allowing the shoulder to rotate in a relaxed manner. Replace the hand and arm to the side of the body. Repeat all the movements on the other side of the back.

j. Repeat petrissage on the entire back area.
k. Repeat effleurage on the entire back area.
l. Apply wringing friction to the back, moving back and forth across the back and working all the way up the neck and back down.
m. Apply circular friction on each side of the spine on the erector spine muscles.
n. Do "hand walking" bilaterally along the spine. Begin at the base of the spine just above the sacrum. Use the full palm side of your hand to apply deep effleurage from the spine to the side of the body. This is almost a compression stroke that slides. Use considerable weight on the strokes as you walk your hands up the client's back. Less weight is used in the area of the kidneys and the eleventh and twelfth ribs. Proceed with the walking movements up the back all the way to the area of the first thoracic vertebrae, then back down to the sacrum.
o. Do sacrospinalis vibration. Place the first two fingers of one hand to either side of the base of the client's spine, about two inches apart. Bend your fingers slightly, so they dig in on the medial edge of the sacrospinalis muscle and along each side of the spinus process. Place your other hand on the top of the hand resting on the client's back, and press down firmly while vibrating slowly (about 120 vibrations per minute) from side to side along the client's body. Slowly glide both hands up to the spine, vibrating (jiggling) each spinal process back and forth about three to ten times. Pay attention to any area along the spine that seems especially tense. These areas should be given extra attention. Work all the way up the spine to the seventh vertebrae in this manner.
p. Move to the head of the table. Use either the thumbs or heel of your hand to stroke up the shoulder (as you did with two fingers), then back down to the sacrum. Repeat the entire process three or more times. If muscle tension persists, go over the areas with more compression and circular and cross-fiber friction.
q. At this time a number of percussion movements are optional. Hacking may be done lightly over the entire back including the gluteals, and the back of the legs. Beating movements may be applied over the thicker portions of the body. To end a stimulating massage, light slapping may be applied over the entire body.
r. A caring stroke completes the back massage. Remember that a caring stroke is an all inclusive effleurage that is applied by standing at the head of the massage table. Place your hands on the upper back so that your fingers nearly touch in the area of the first and second thoracic vertebrae. Apply gliding strokes down the entire length of the spine. Your hands glide over the gluteals and return

up the lateral portion of the torso to the axillary area, slide smoothly over the deltoids up the trapezius to the occiput, and return to the starting point. Repeat the movements several times.

12. To complete the massage of the entire body, lightly place one hand on the sacrum and the other at the top of the spine and hold the position for several seconds. Allow the client to relax quietly without being disturbed for about 10 minutes. Assist the client to a sitting position. Be sure draping is properly placed and assist her from the massage table as necessary. Show the client to the dressing area. After the client is dressed, take time to answer any questions or make recommendations.

**PROCEDURE FOR Massage 3**

Each time you give a massage you may find yourself becoming more innovative and more confident of your techniques. However, it is important to think before acting. The following illustrated massage routine provides an opportunity to review what you have learned from beginning massage movements to more advanced routines. The illustrations are designed to help you to remember to think of the part of the body you are working on in correct anatomical terms. For example, when massaging the arm, are you working on the lateral aspect of the arm, or the medial aspect of the arm? The point is to know (not guess), exactly what you are doing and why.

**Step by Step Procedure for Massage 3**

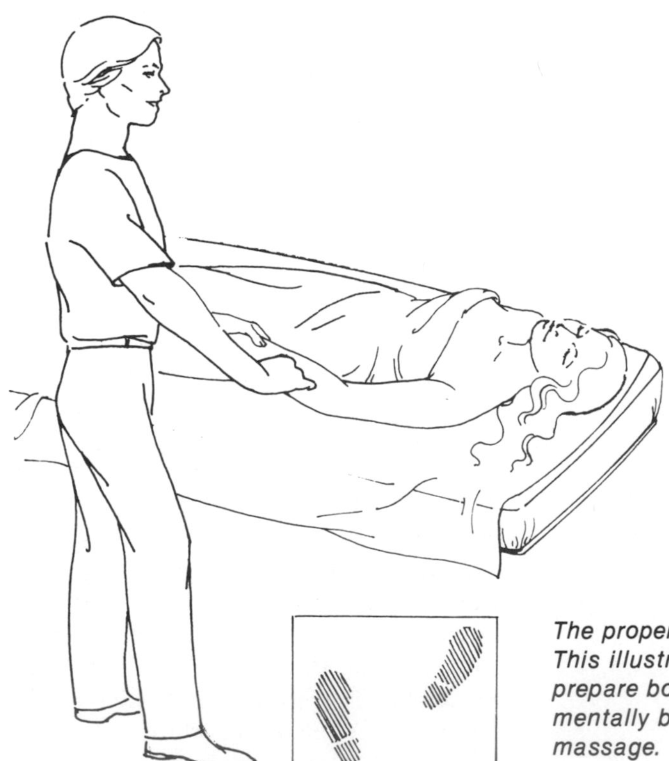

*The proper stance is important. This illustration reminds you to prepare both physically and mentally before beginning the massage.*

*Note the correct hand position and handle (the hand) to apply effleurage to the lateral aspect of the arm.*

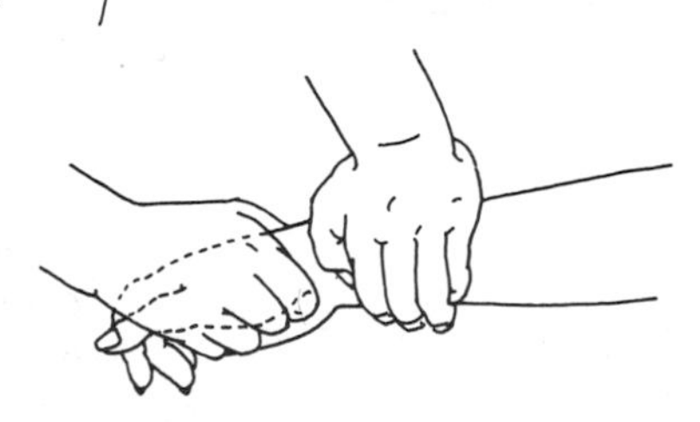

*Note the hand position and handle to apply effleurage to the medial aspect of the arm. Apply effleurage to the medial aspect of the arm.*

*Apply effleurage to the lateral aspect of the arm with your little finger leading. The stroke is continuous, up over the arm, over the shoulder, and back to the starting point. Use more pressure on the stroke up to the shoulder and a lighter more superficial pressure on the return stroke. The client's arm is held in slight traction throughout the stroke. An alternative is to place the arm on the table for this stroke.*

*Correct hand position for effleurage of the medial aspect of the arm.*

*Begin effleurage movements, leading with the little finger.*

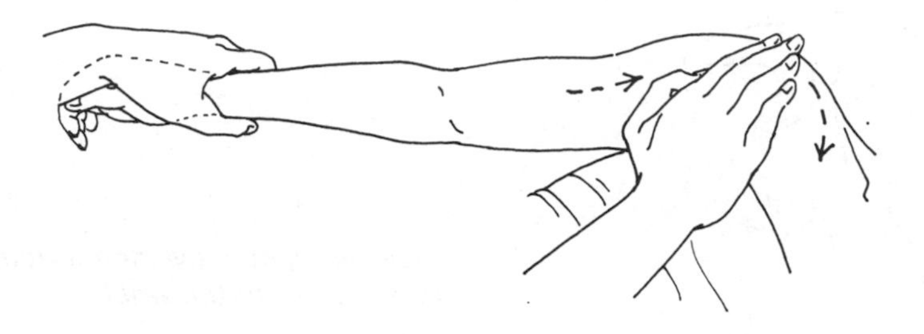

*Effleurage movements are continued up and over the shoulder then back down the arm.*

*Effleurage movements are continued up and over the shoulder (axillary area) for a slight joint movement and stretch.*

*Apply petrissage from the shoulder and continue down the arm.*

*Continue petrissage down the arm to the wrist.*

*Petrissage is followed by more effleurage, moving up the arm.*

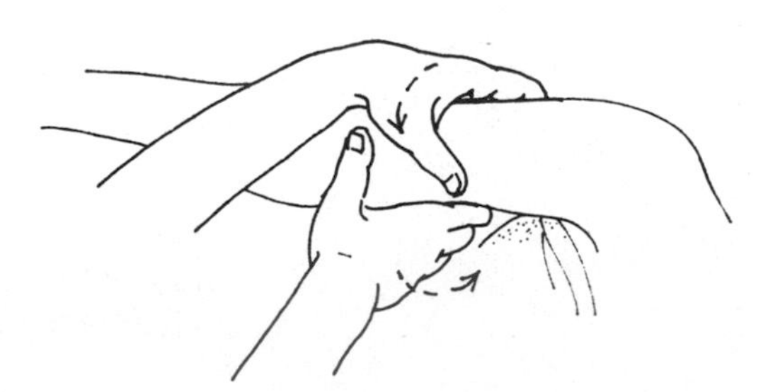

*Apply wringing movements from the shoulder to the wrist.*

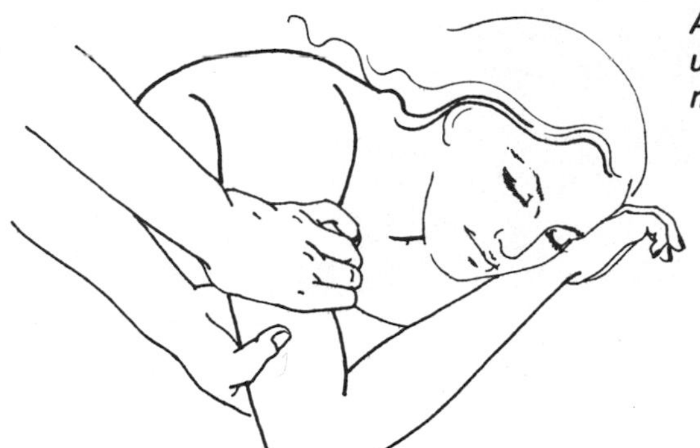

*An alternate position may be used for the wringing movements.*

*Do rolling movements from the shoulder to the wrist.*

*Use the client's hand as a handle for shaking the hand during petrissage and applying friction to the hand.*

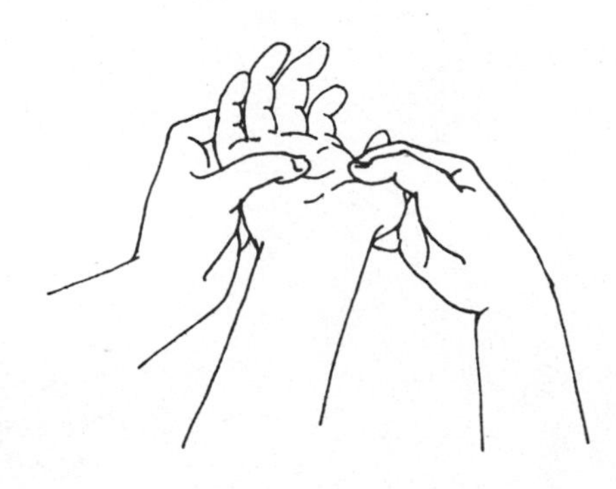

*Apply friction and petrissage to each of the fingers, spreading the metacarpals.*

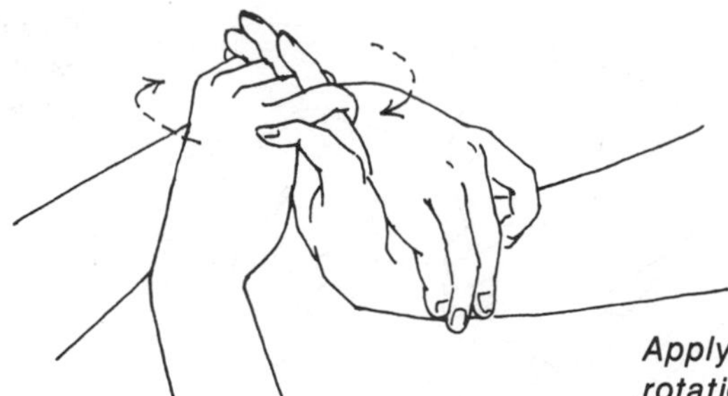

*Apply joint movements and rotation. Note the interlacing of the fingers.*

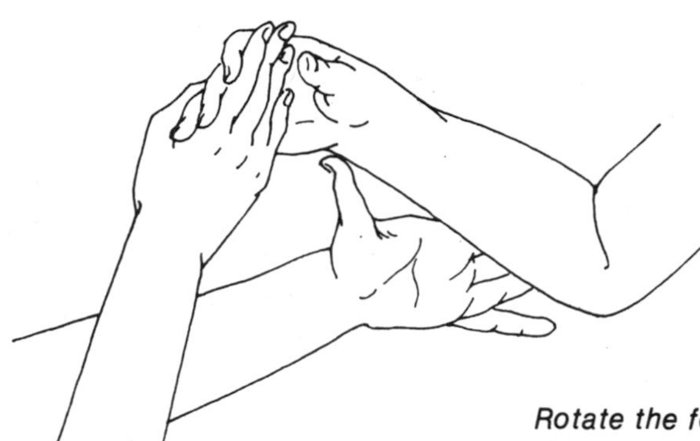

*Rotate the forearm. Note how the fingers are used to steady the client's elbow.*

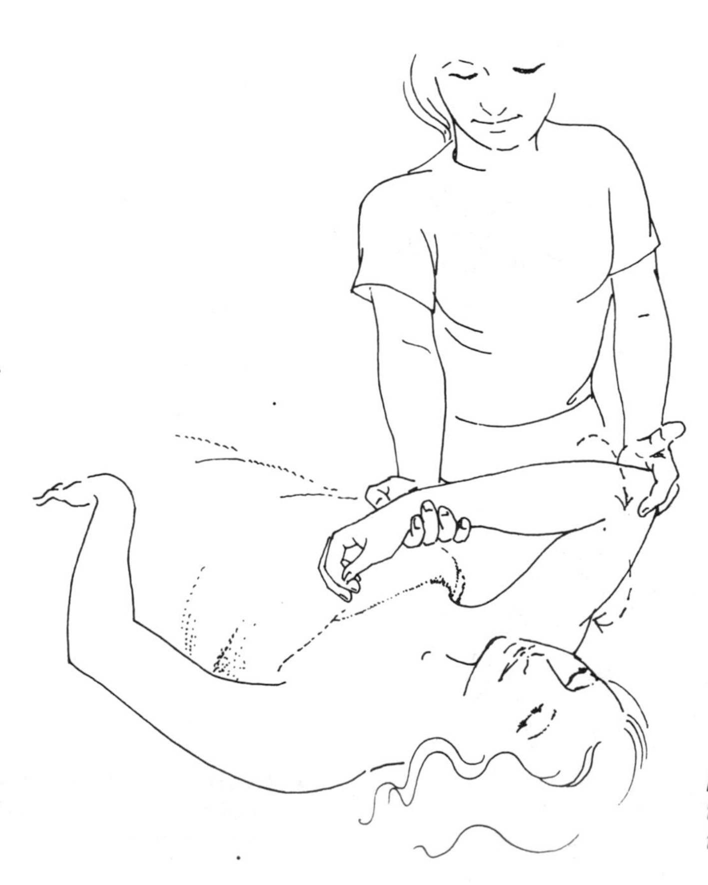

*Rotate the shoulder. Note how the fingers are used to steady the elbow.*

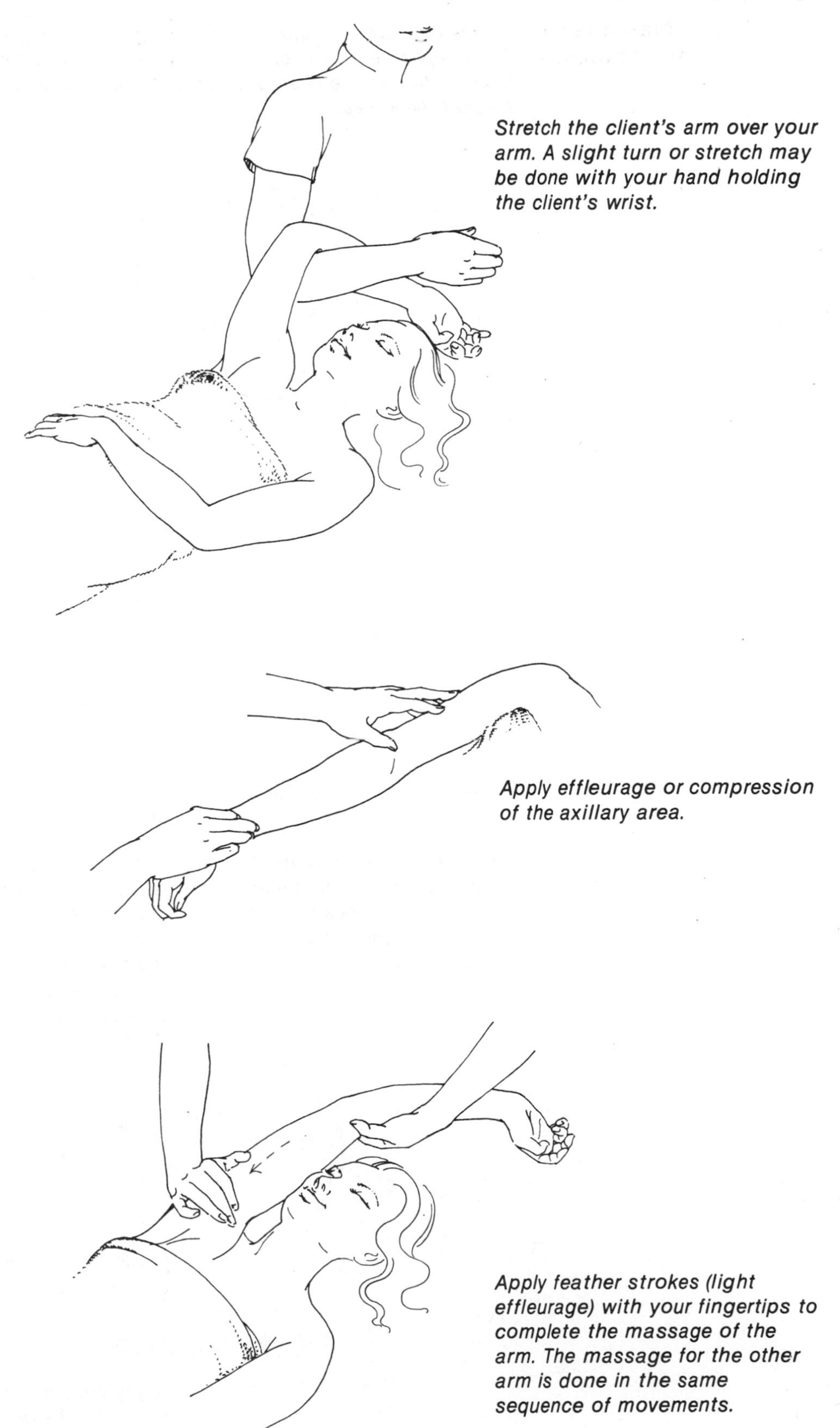

*Stretch the client's arm over your arm. A slight turn or stretch may be done with your hand holding the client's wrist.*

*Apply effleurage or compression of the axillary area.*

*Apply feather strokes (light effleurage) with your fingertips to complete the massage of the arm. The massage for the other arm is done in the same sequence of movements.*

## Massage for the Abdomen

*This is the correct position and draping for massage of the abdomen. Oil is applied before beginning the massage. A folded towel is used to cover the female client's breasts. A bolster may be used to support the knees.*

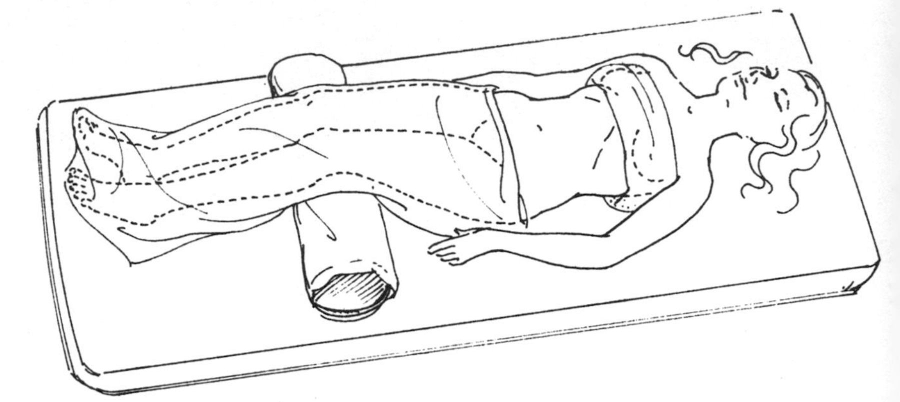

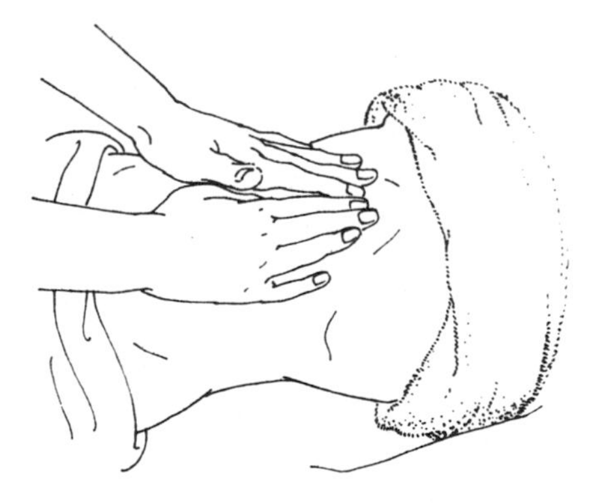

*Apply effleurage movements (leading with the little finger). The movement goes up, out, around, and down, then back to the center of the abdomen.*

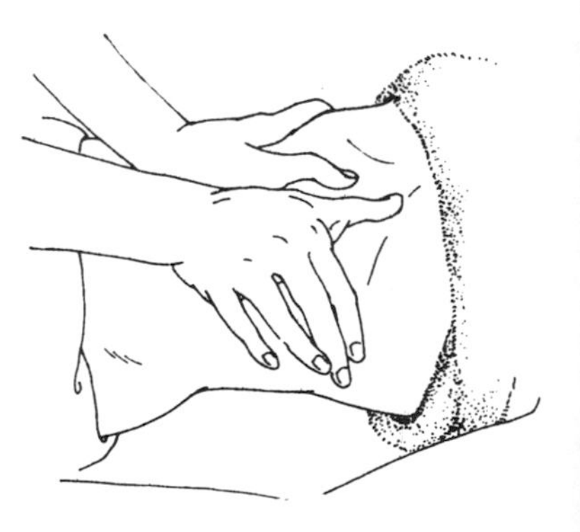

*The effleurage movements are repeated. When draping is not used to cover the chest (male clients), this stroke may include the entire trunk, continuing to the sternal notch, around to axillary area, and back down to the hips.*

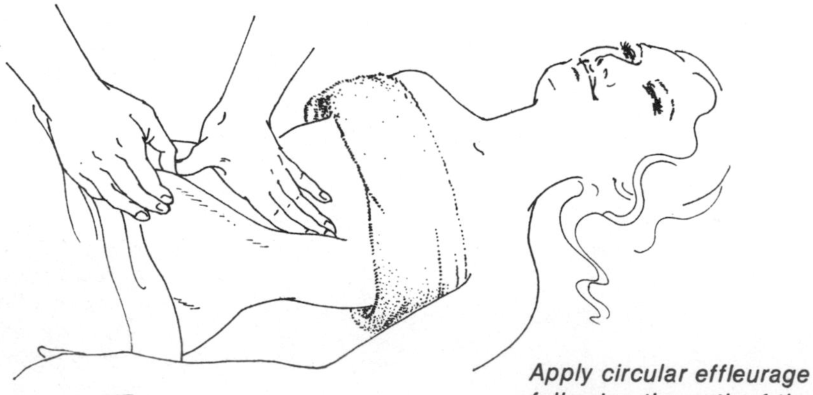

*Apply circular effleurage following the path of the colon.*

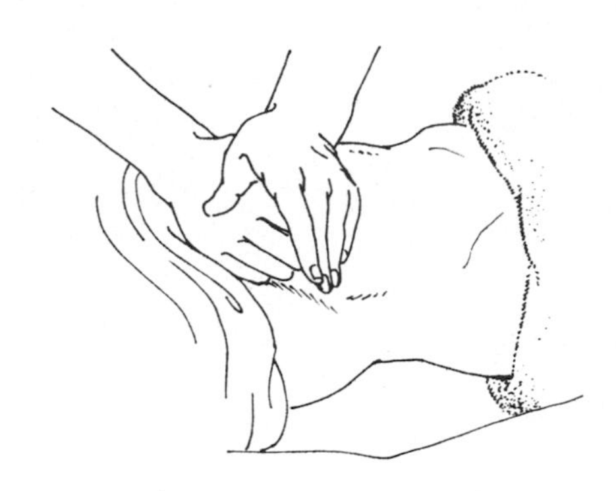

*Apply friction in small circles following the colon in reverse.*

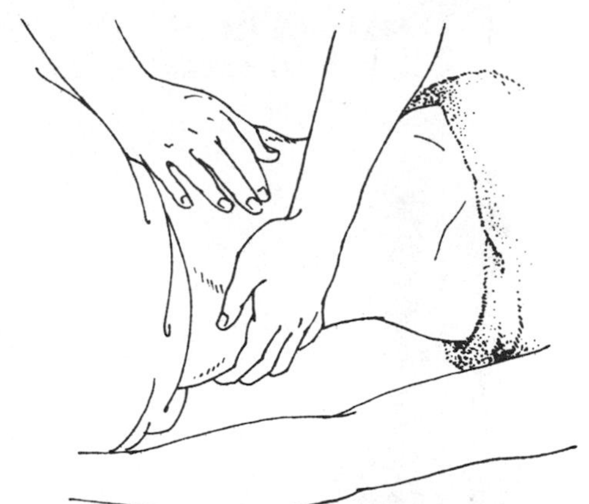

*Alternate hand stroking movements (shingles) are applied from trochanter to axilla. Note: Shingles is the name often used to describe alternate hand effleurage in which one hand repeats the stroke as the previous hand is about to complete the stroke.*

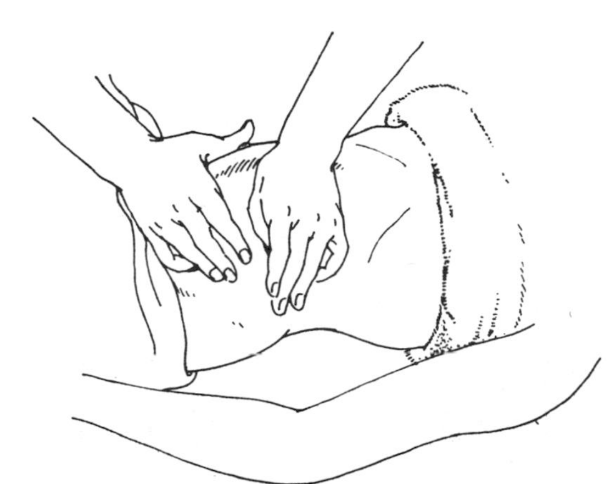

*Apply petrissage to the abdomen.*

*Apply a shaking movement. Grasp the skin of the abdomen and shake it gently. This movement stimulates the action of the large and small intestines.*

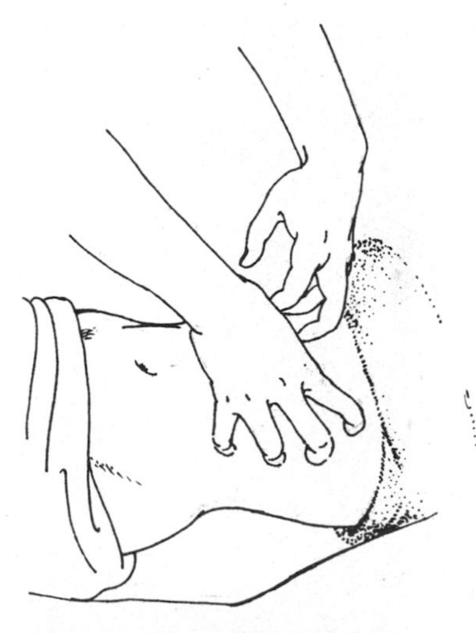

*Apply a raking movement several times with the tips of the fingers across the ribs and abdomen.*

**Massage for the Anterior Leg**

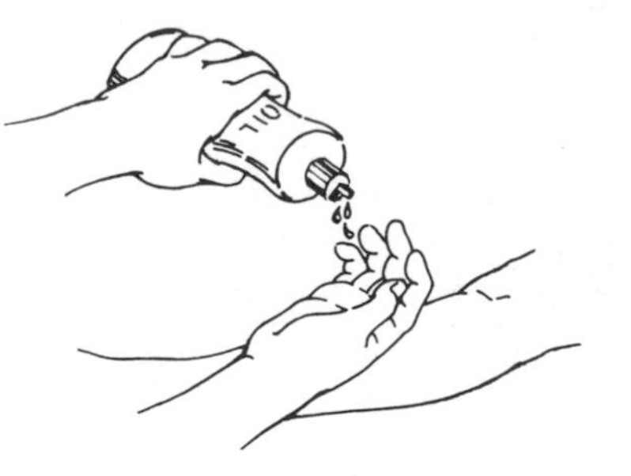


*Before beginning massage movements, undrape the leg and apply oil. With the back of your hands, maintain contact with the client's skin as you prepare to apply the massage oil.*

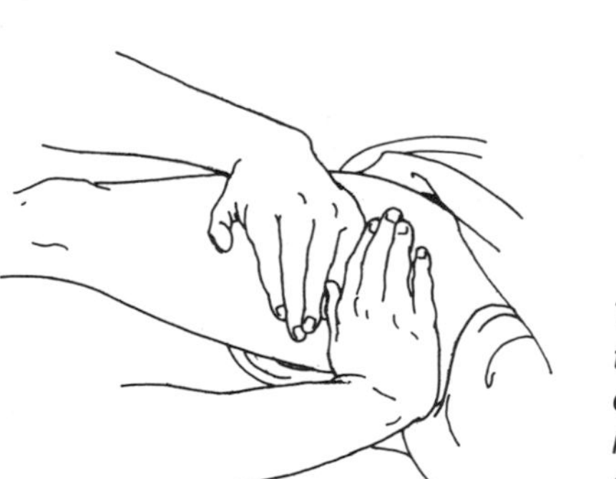

*Apply effleurage (leading with the little finger).*

*The leading hand should be on the lateral side of the leg in order to travel up and over the ilium and return back to the starting point.*

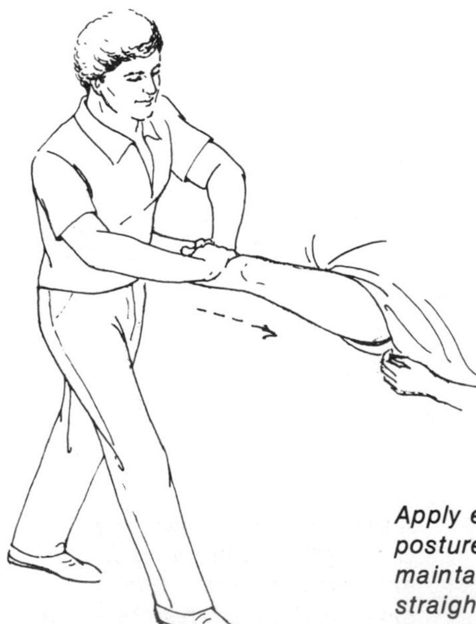

*Apply effleurage to the leg. Good posture and stance should be maintained and the back kept straight, with knees slightly flexed.*

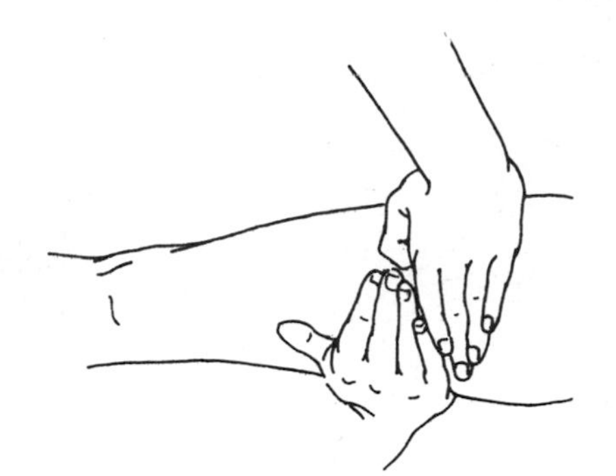

*Effleurage is continued. Note the position of the hands for effective effleurage.*

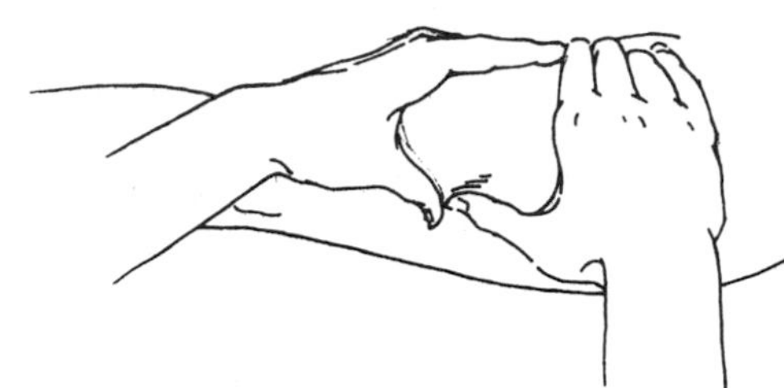

*Apply petrissage to the anterior leg.*

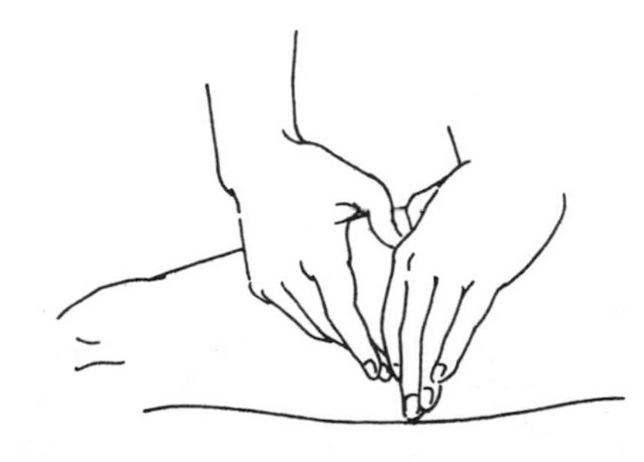

*Continue petrissage and wringing movements.*

*Continue wringing movements from thigh to ankle.*

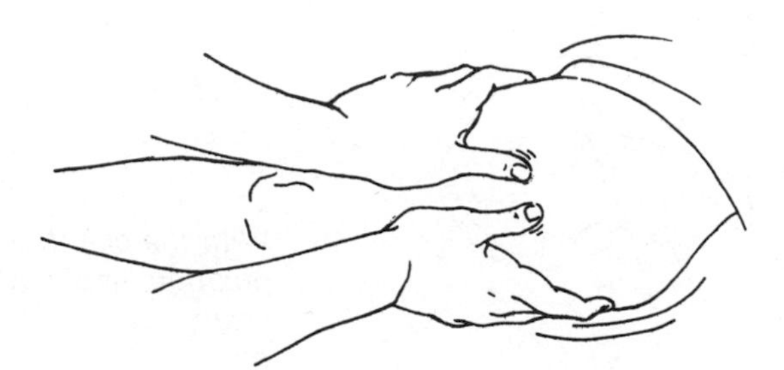

*Apply fulling (compression) movements.*

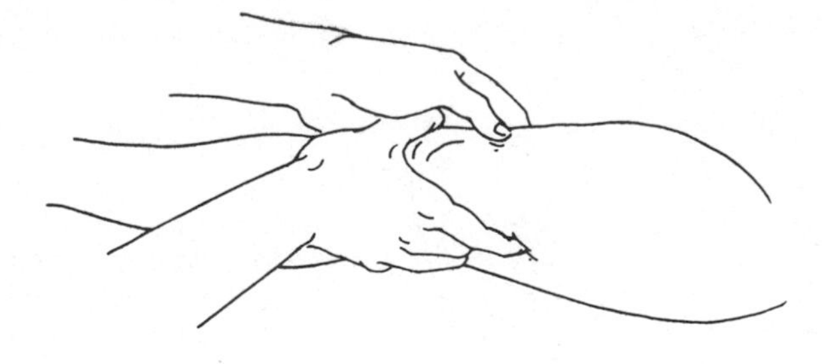

*Manipulate the kneecap by tracing circles with your thumb in opposite directions.*

*Apply friction along the tibia.*

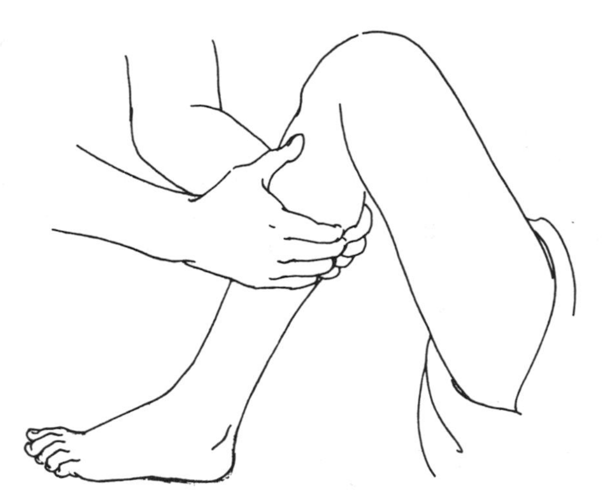

*Have the client assume the bent-knee position for petrissage, then apply wringing, rolling, and effleurage movements to the calf.*

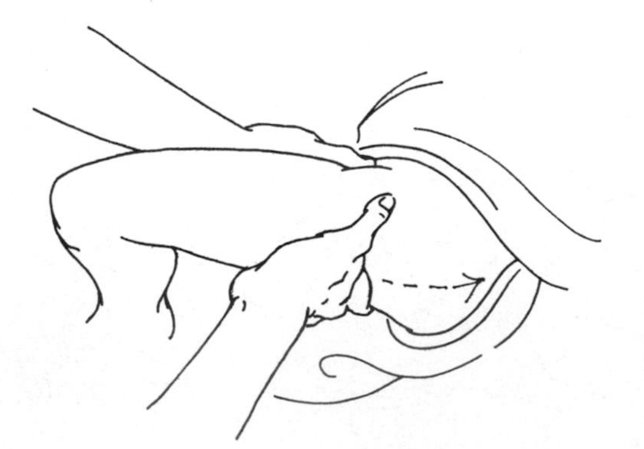

*With the client in the bent-knee position, apply effleurage to the thigh.*

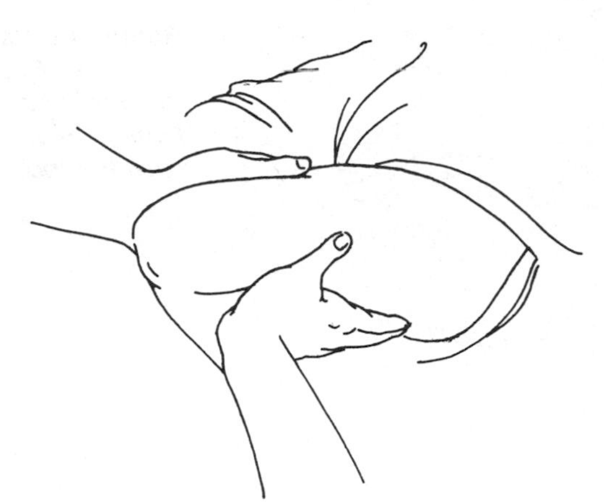

*Apply chucking to the thigh. With the client in the bent-knee position, manipulate soft tissue of the posterior aspect of the thigh and apply effleurage, petrissage, or rolling movements to the leg.*

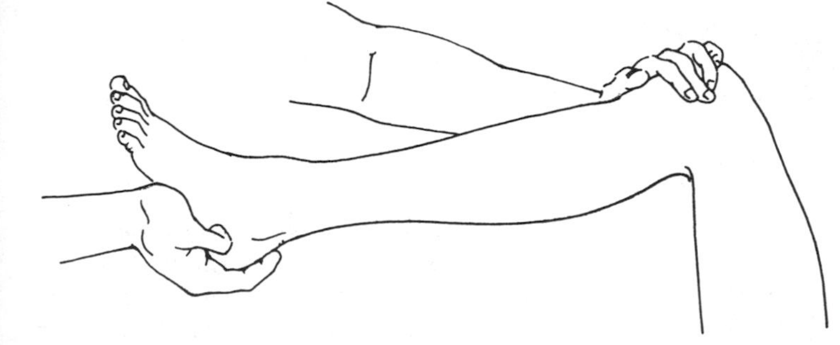

*Apply joint movements. The client's knee may be moved all the way to the chest, or this position may be used for joint rotations of the hip and knee in the range of motion. Note the position of the hands at the heel and knee.*

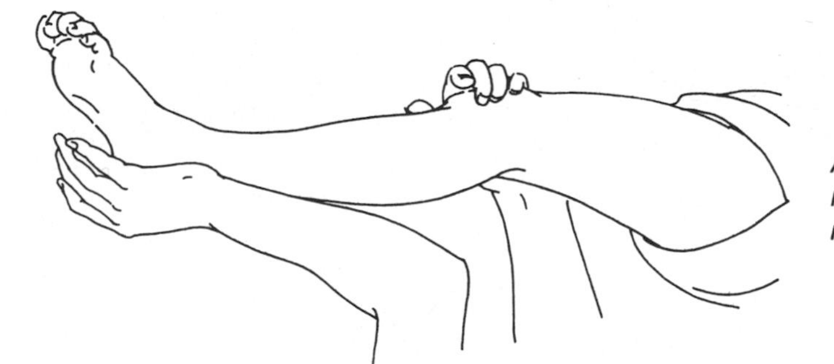

*Apply hamstring stretching movements in an up and down manipulation.*

*Continue the stretching movements. Note how the hand is placed to support under the knee to avoid hyperextension of the leg.*

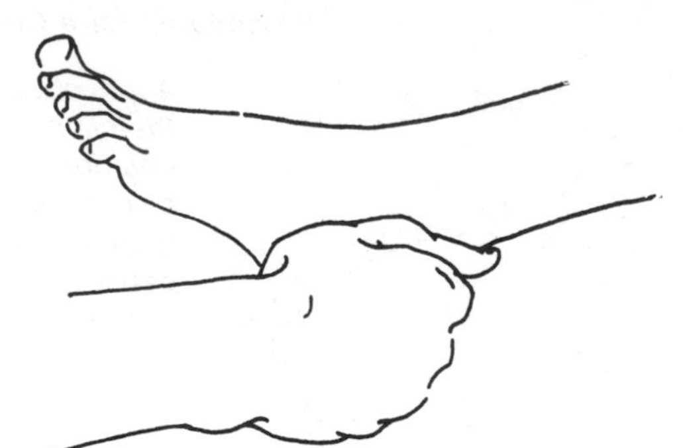

*Rotate the hip using the heel as a handle. While cupping the heel in your hand, do a back and forth (windshield wiper) movement with the foot.*

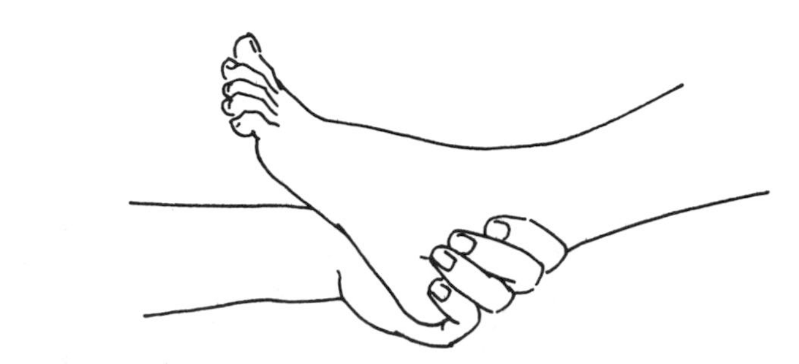

*Apply pulling and shaking movements. In cupping the heel, note the position of the hand as seen on the other side of the foot.*

*Apply stretching and shaking movements. This completes the sequence of movements for the anterior leg. Redrape the leg and proceed to massage the other leg.*

## Massage of the Posterior Leg

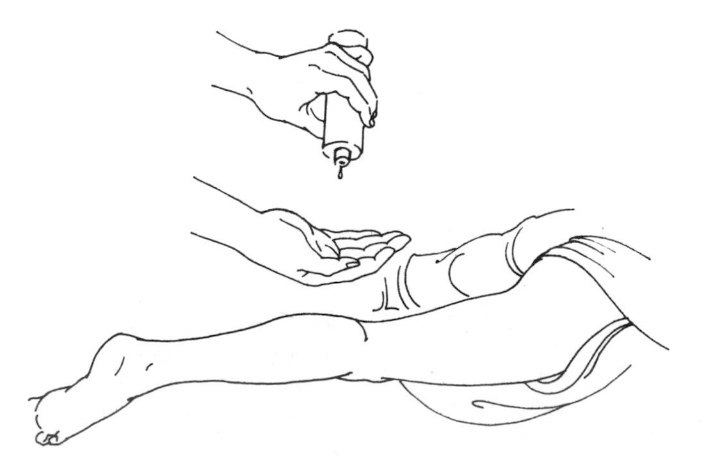

*Before beginning massage movements, prepare the posterior leg by undraping and applying oil. Keep the back of your hand against the client's skin while pouring the oil into your hand.*

*Apply effleurage movements, leading with the little finger. Stroke towards the heart. Note: The leading hand is on the lateral aspect of the leg in order to travel up and over the gluteal muscles and the iliac crest and back down the lateral side of the leg. At the same time, the medial hand travels up to the gluteal crease and back down the medial side of the leg. Both hands return to the starting point to repeat the stroke three or more times.*

*Apply petrissage on the entire leg.*

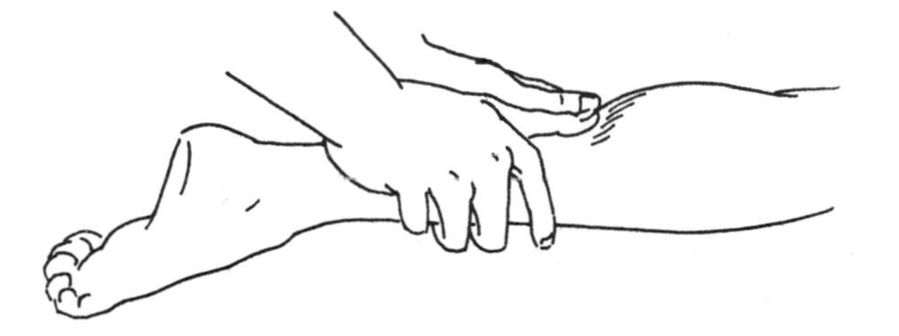

*Apply fulling or compression strokes to the entire leg.*

*Apply wringing movements to the leg.*

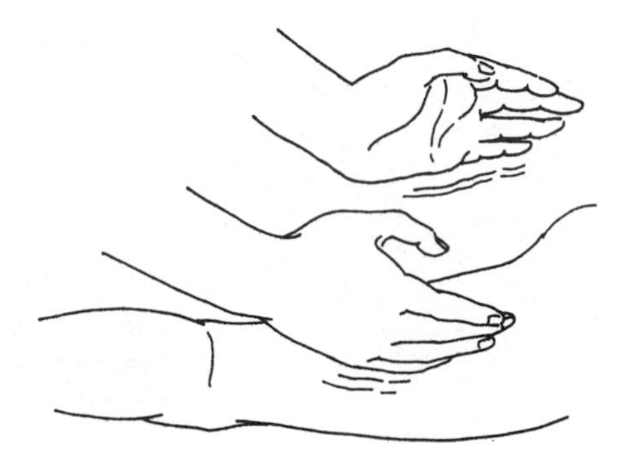

*Apply percussion movements to the posterior leg. Hacking can be done on the leg but should not be applied to the back of the knee.*

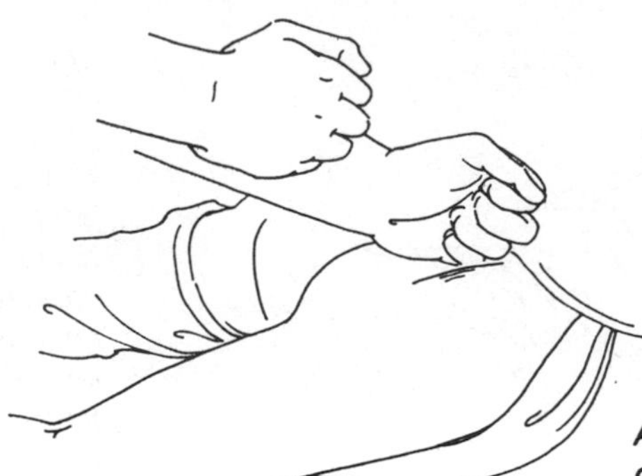

*Apply percussion (beating) to the gluteal area.*

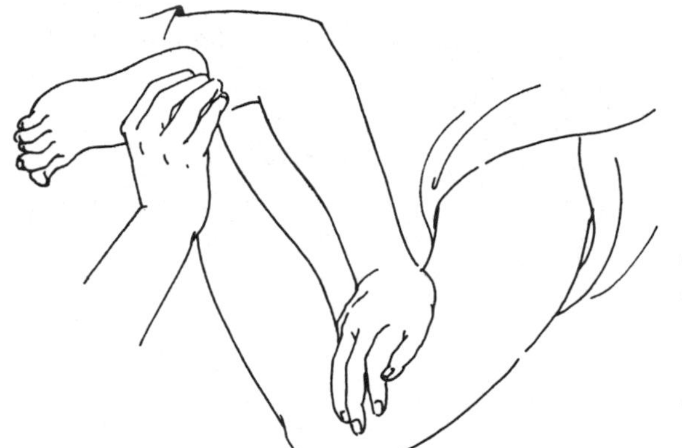

*Joint movements and flexing the leg give more extensive massage to the foot and posterior leg. Caution should be exercised to prevent over-flexing the knee.*

*Apply joint movements.*

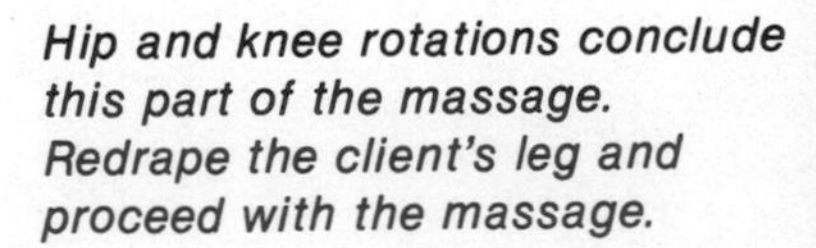

*Hip and knee rotations conclude this part of the massage. Redrape the client's leg and proceed with the massage.*

## Massage for the Back

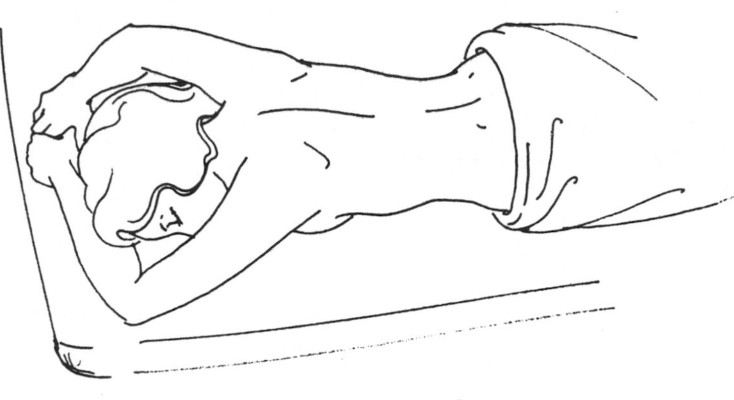

*Prepare for the massage by adjusting the draping and applying oil to the back. Apply effleurage beginning at the gluteal cleft. The fingers of one hand should be touching the other at the midline of the back.*

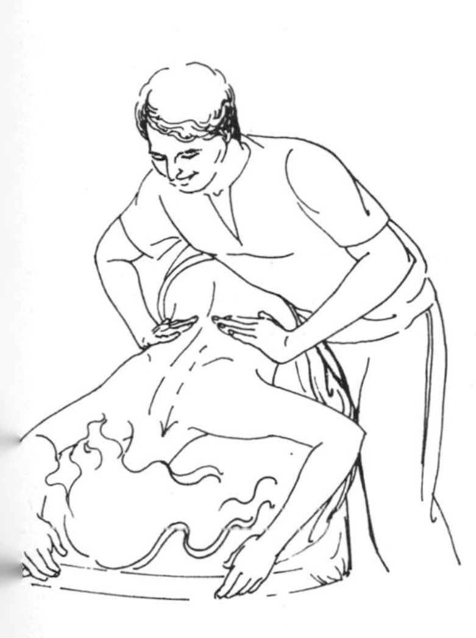

*Proceed with effleurage up the back, with little fingers leading.*

*Continue with effleurage strokes up the back and over the shoulders.*

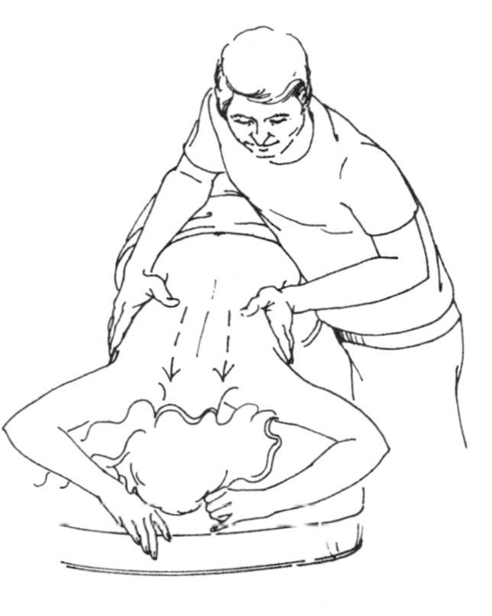

*Continue with effleurage strokes back down the sides, returning to the starting point. Pressure is consistent throughout the entire stroke.*

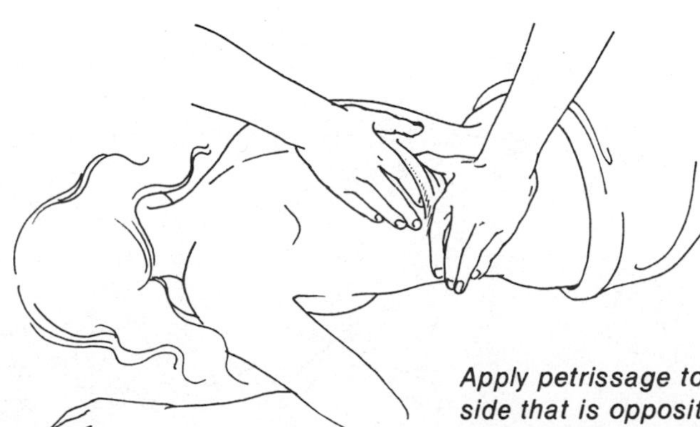

*Apply petrissage to the entire side that is opposite you. This takes several passes.*

Petrissage includes the trapezius muscles.

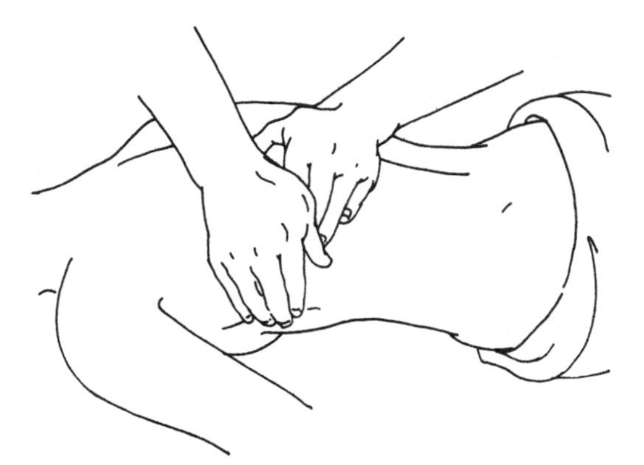

*Apply alternate hand stroking movements (shingles) up and down the entire side.*

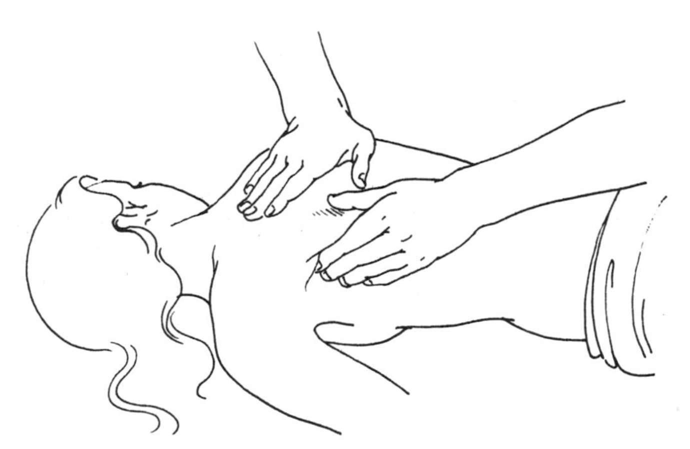

*Friction movements are applied around the scapula on the side opposite you.*

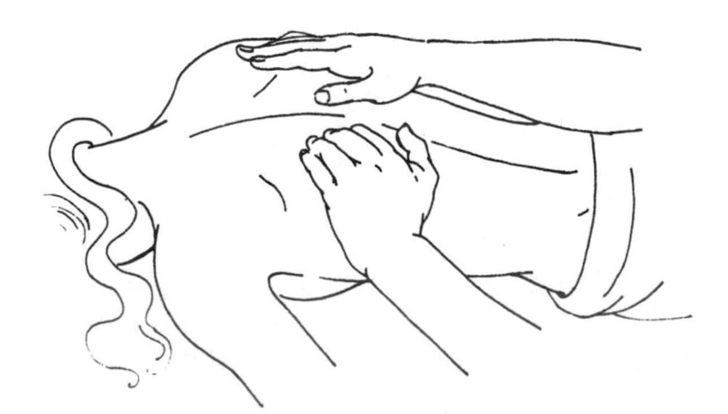

*Move around to the other side of the table to continue friction (compression) on the same scapula.*

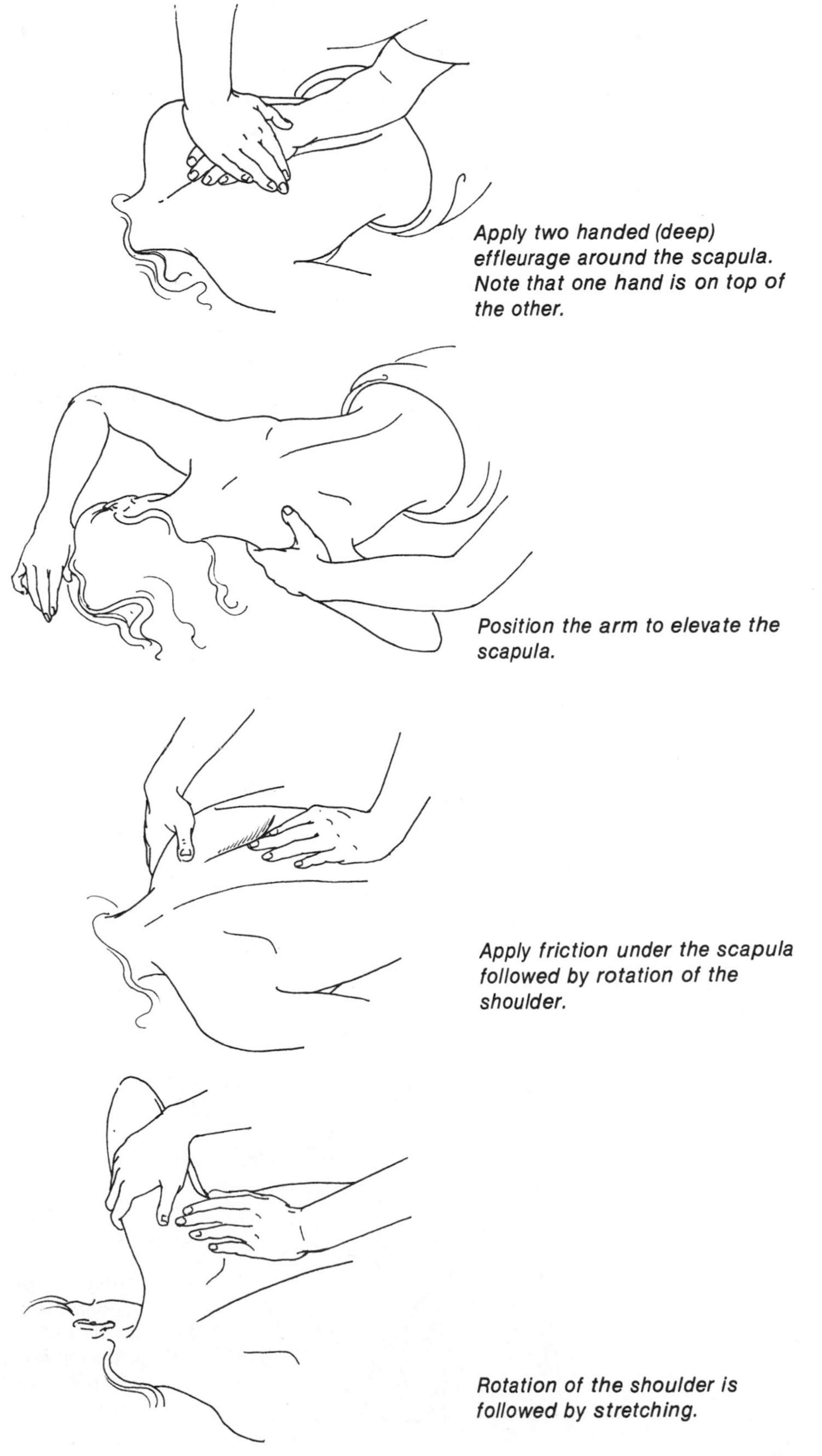

*Apply two handed (deep) effleurage around the scapula. Note that one hand is on top of the other.*

*Position the arm to elevate the scapula.*

*Apply friction under the scapula followed by rotation of the shoulder.*

*Rotation of the shoulder is followed by stretching.*

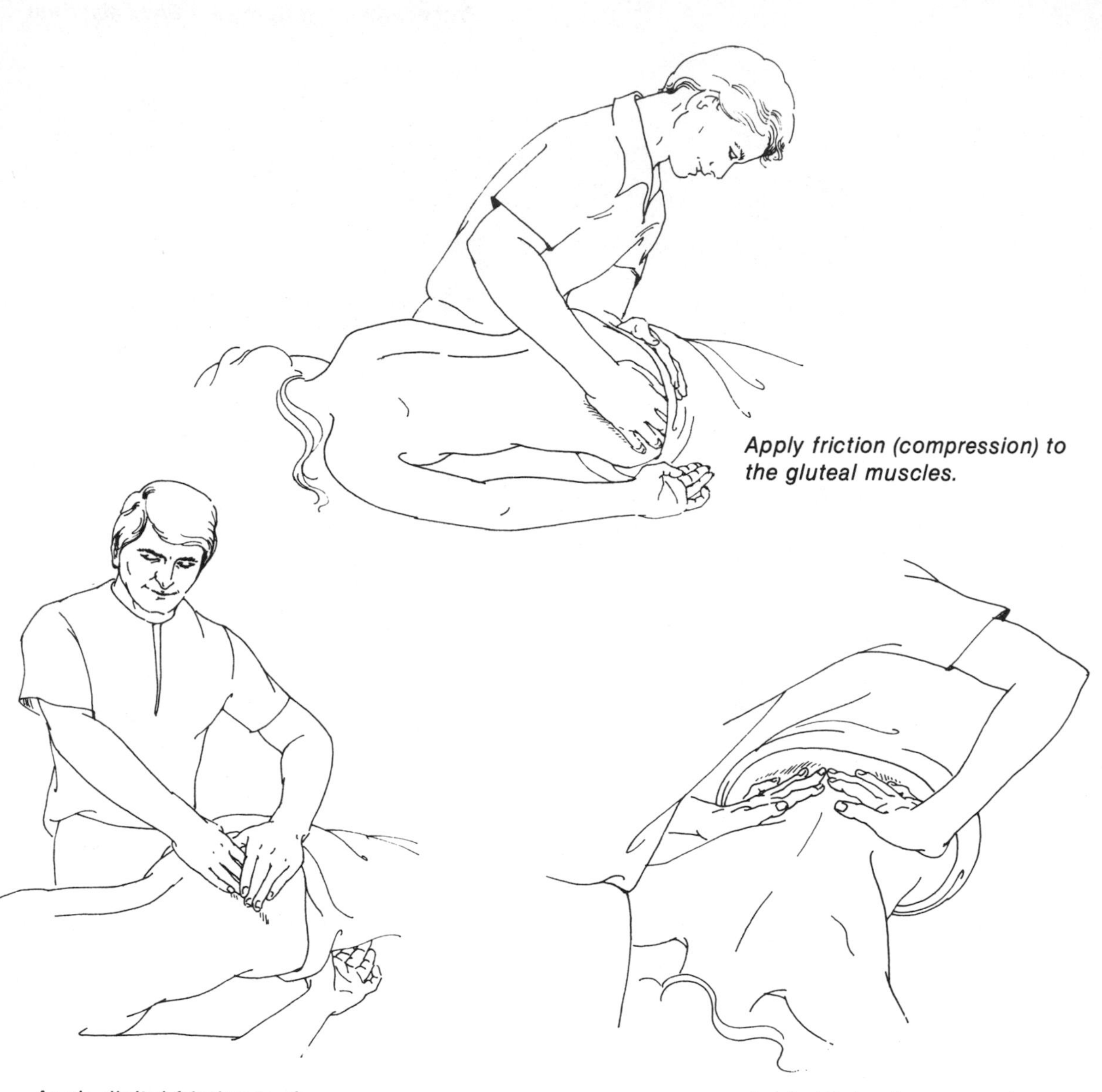

*Apply friction (compression) to the gluteal muscles.*

*Apply digital friction to the gluteal muscles.*

*Apply bilateral compression to the gluteal muscles.*

*Apply effleurage movements (caring strokes) from a position at the head of the client. The little finger leads the stroke, beginning at the nape of the neck.*

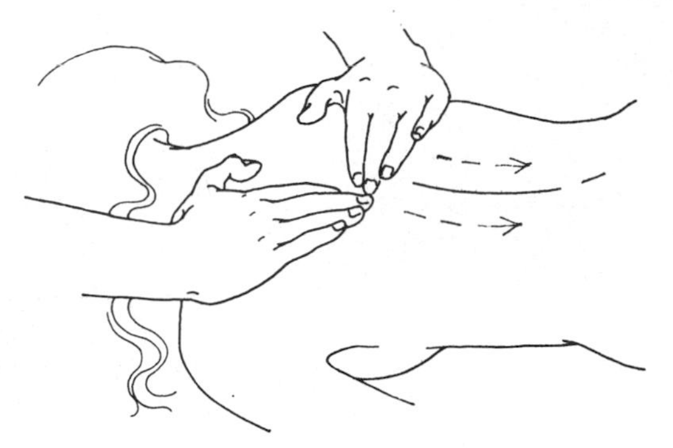

*Continue effleurage movements down the back, over and around the gluteal muscles, back up the sides, then over and around the shoulders to the nape of the neck.*

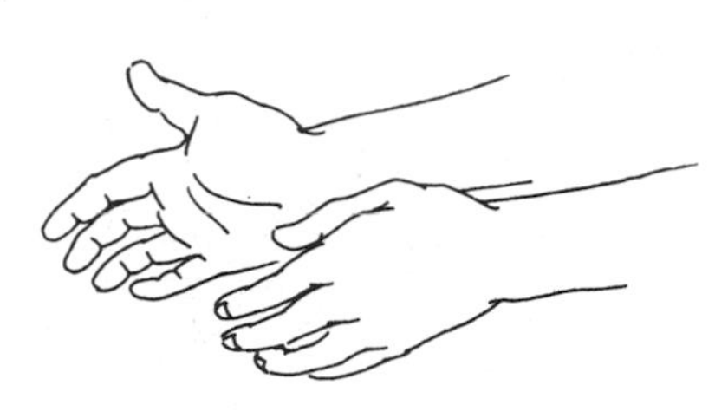

*Apply percussion movements to the gluteus muscles.*

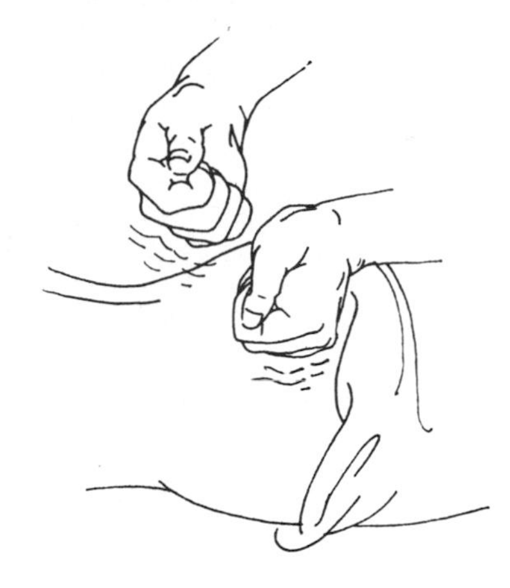

*Apply percussion with beating movements to the gluteal muscles.*

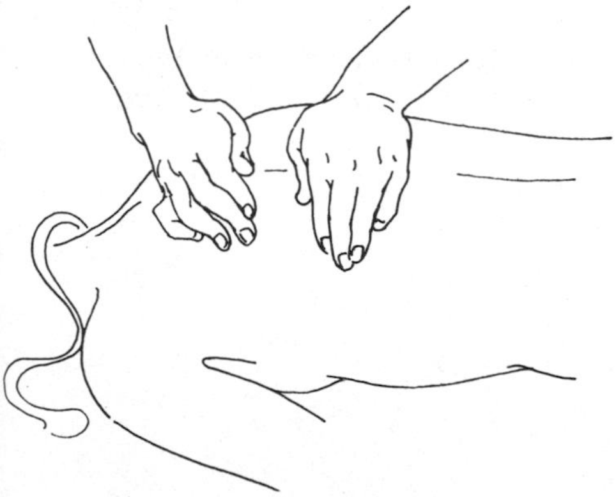

*Apply percussion with cupping movements over the lungs.*

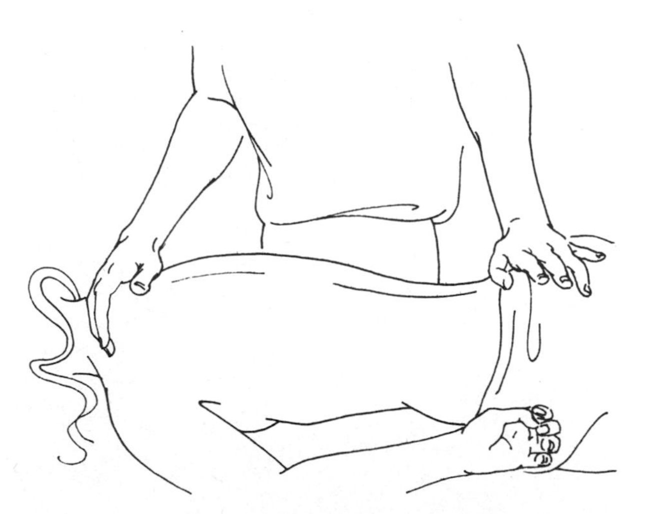

*A light touch at the base of the spine, at the base of the neck, or top of the head is a nice way to say "hello" or "goodbye" to the client's body.*

This completes the massage of the back. Redrape and proceed with the massage.

## Massage of the Feet

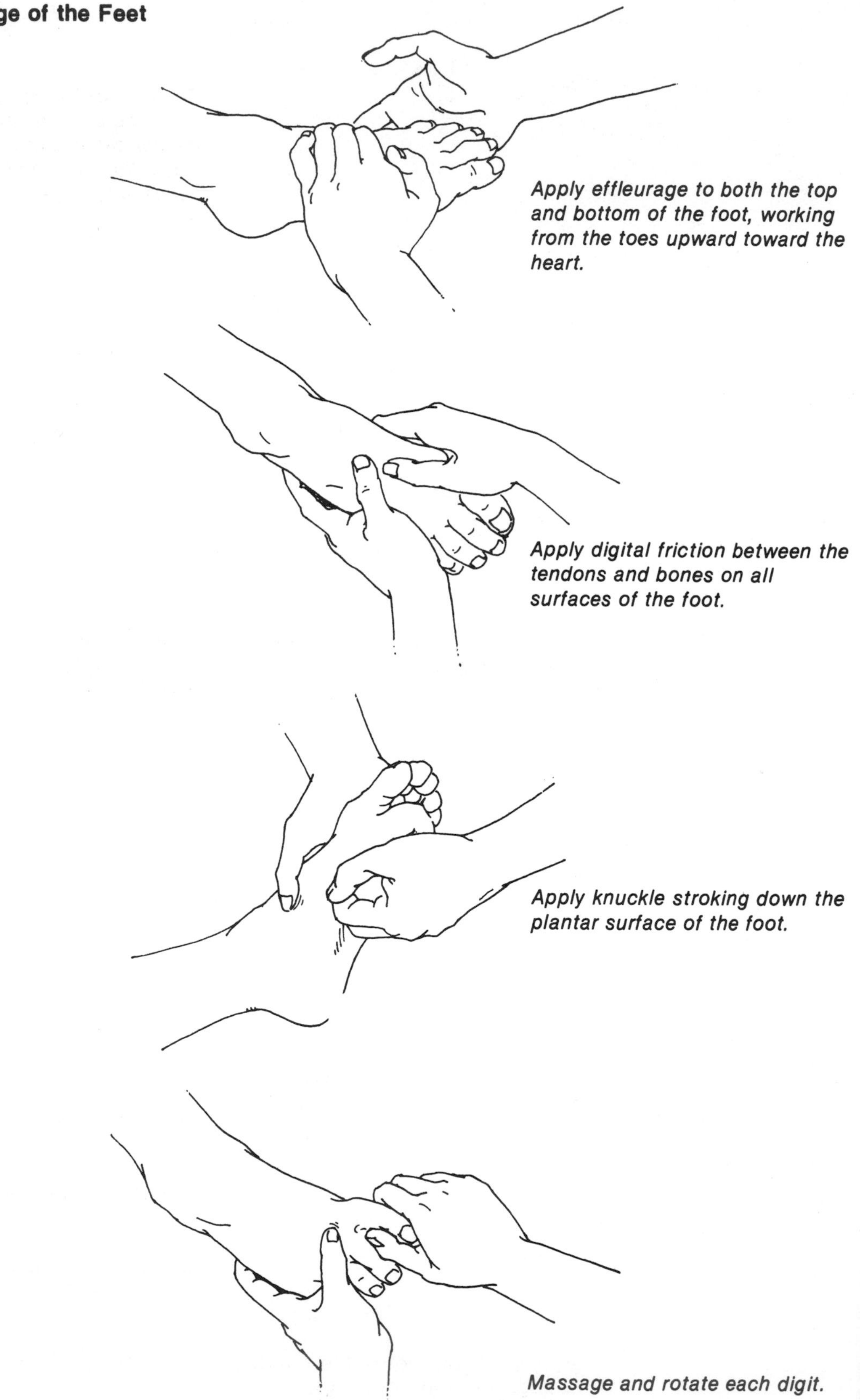

*Apply effleurage to both the top and bottom of the foot, working from the toes upward toward the heart.*

*Apply digital friction between the tendons and bones on all surfaces of the foot.*

*Apply knuckle stroking down the plantar surface of the foot.*

*Massage and rotate each digit.*

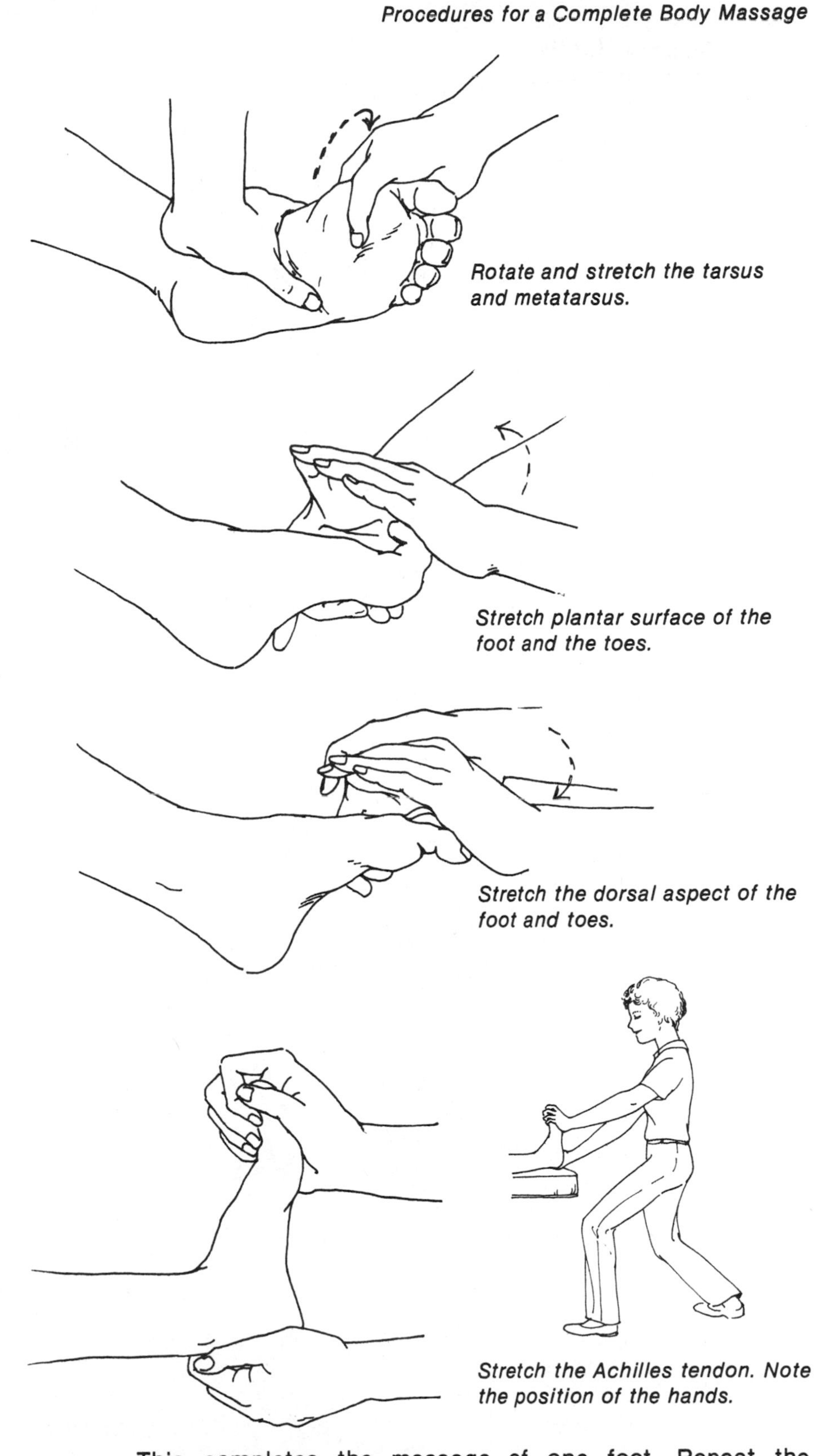

*Rotate and stretch the tarsus and metatarsus.*

*Stretch plantar surface of the foot and the toes.*

*Stretch the dorsal aspect of the foot and toes.*

*Stretch the Achilles tendon. Note the position of the hands.*

This completes the massage of one foot. Repeat the massage on the other foot.

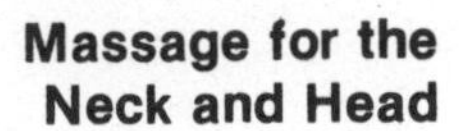

## Massage for the Neck and Head

*Apply bilateral effleurage (beginning at the sternal notch). Use the hands simultaneously, leading with the little fingers.*

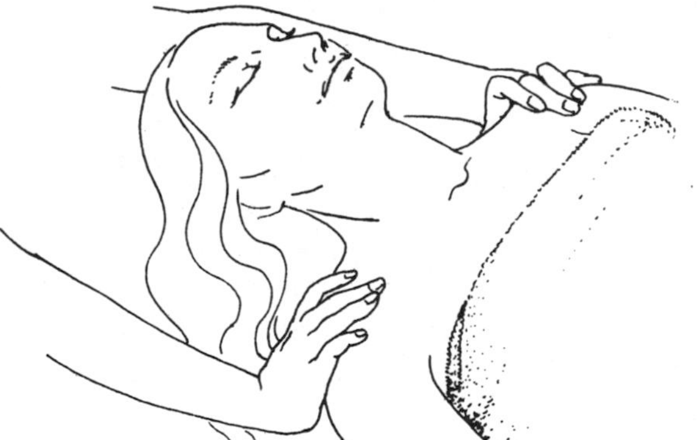

*Continue effleurage from the sternal notch, over the shoulders, and along the trapezius.*

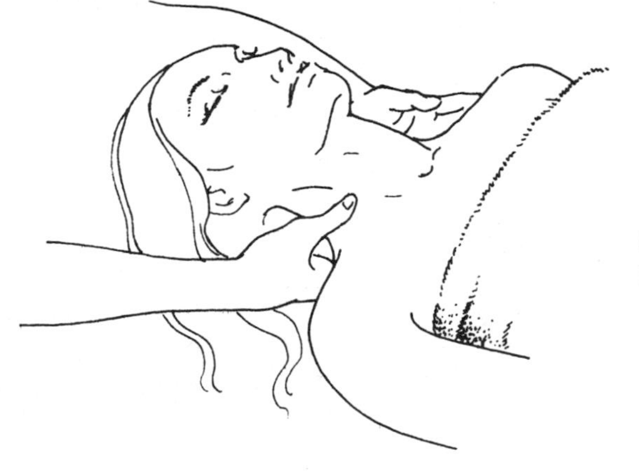

*Continue the movement up to the occipital ridge.*

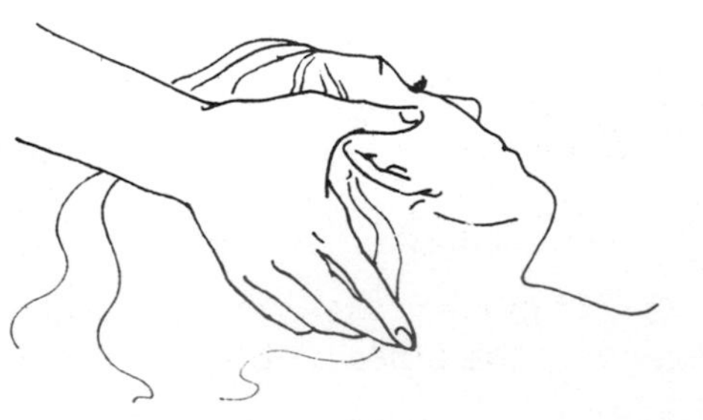

*Note placement of the hands in the "handle" position supporting the head.*

*Apply effleurage, leading with the little finger, just below the mastoid and continue down the neck.*

*Continue the movement across the shoulder and around the deltoid.*

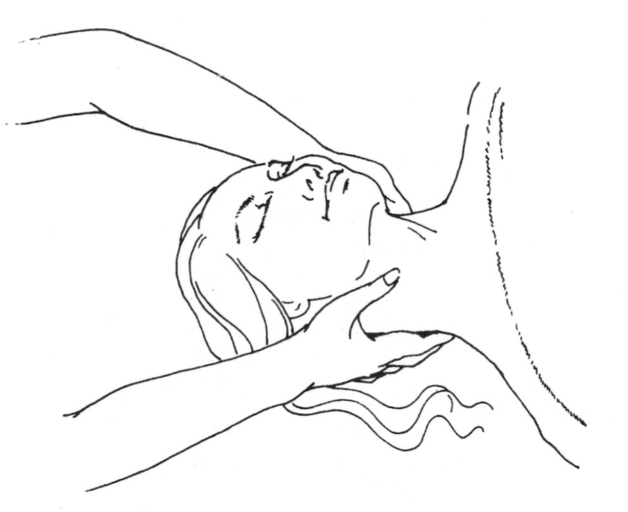

*Apply petrissage to the neck and shoulders.*

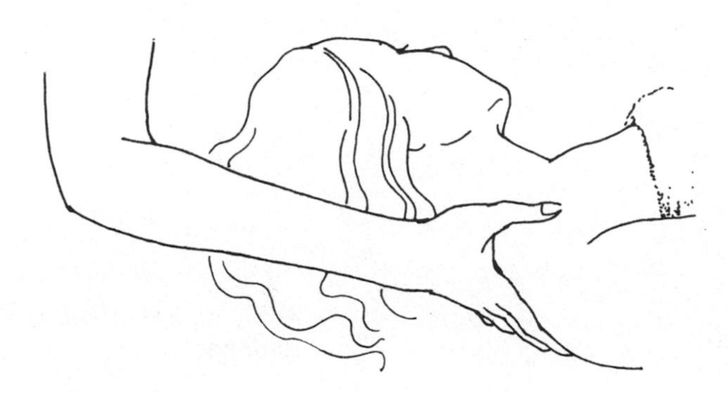

*Apply friction to the neck and shoulders.*

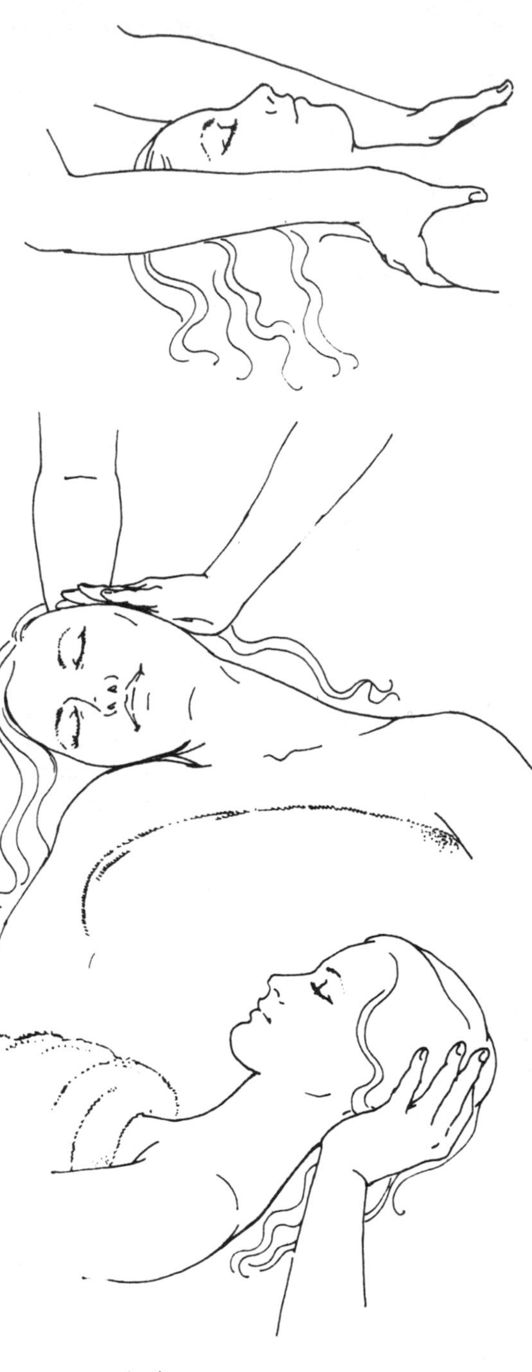

*Apply bilateral compression to the shoulders.*

*Apply passive joint movements by moving the head from side to side.*

*Apply passive joint movements by rolling the head forward. Note placement of the hands on the client's head.*

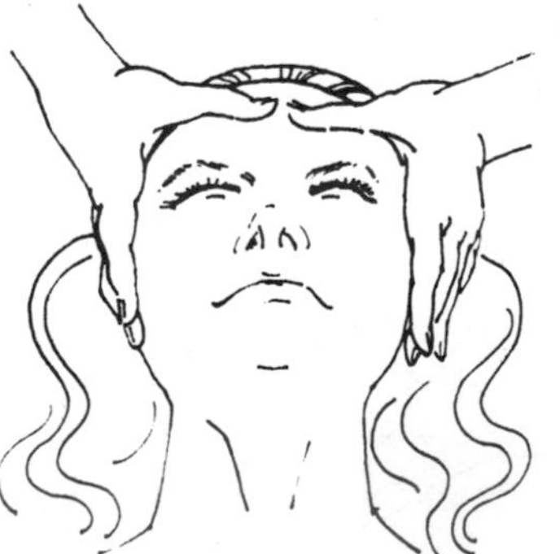

*Apply digital effleurage to the forehead.*

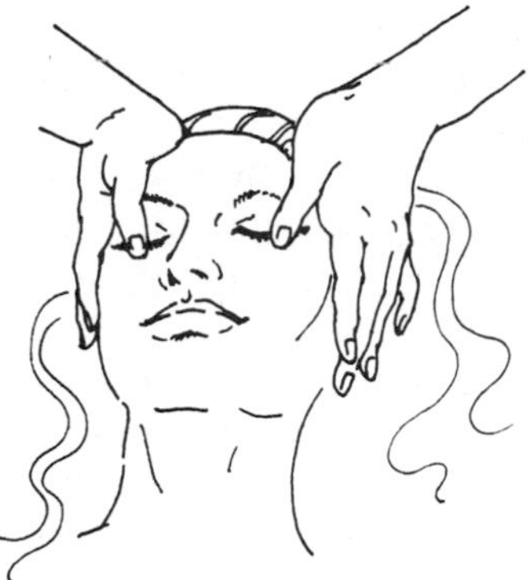

*Apply effleurage to the forehead and orbits.*

*Apply effleurage to the cheeks (zygomatics).*

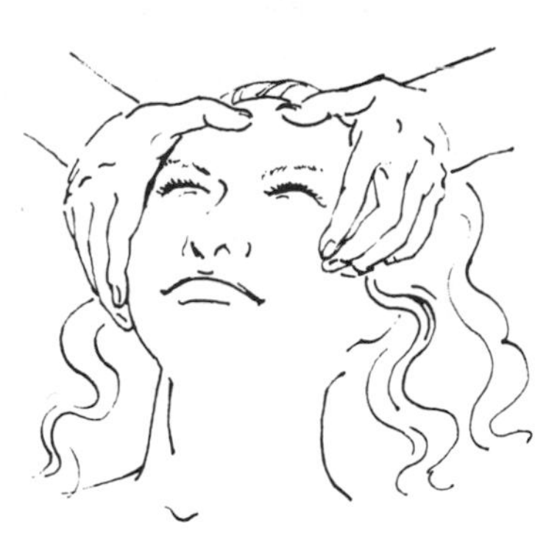

*Apply friction around the cheeks.*

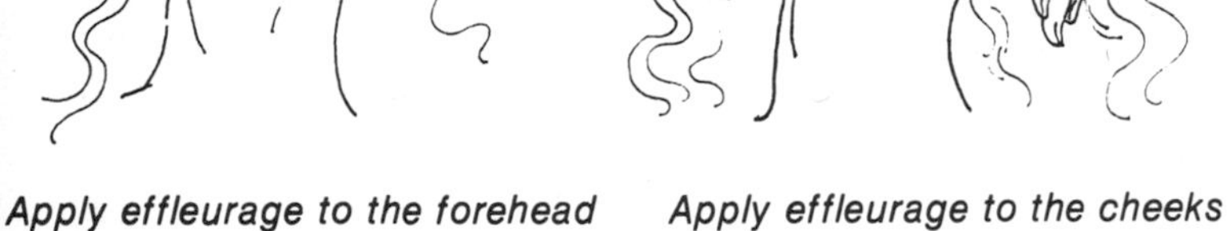

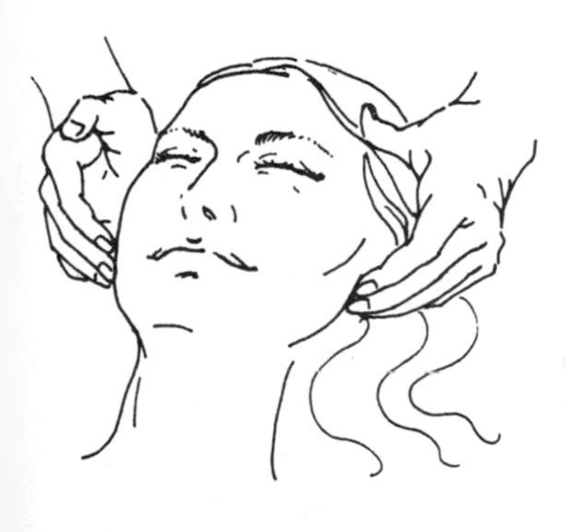

*Apply friction around the mouth (mandible) and jawline.*

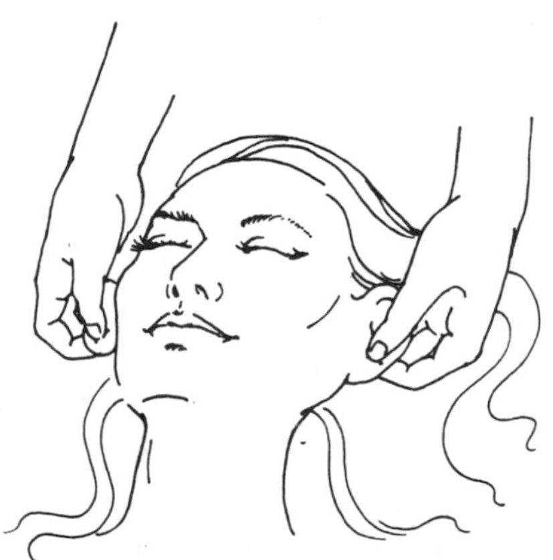

*Massage the ears with light friction movements applied with forefingers and thumbs.*

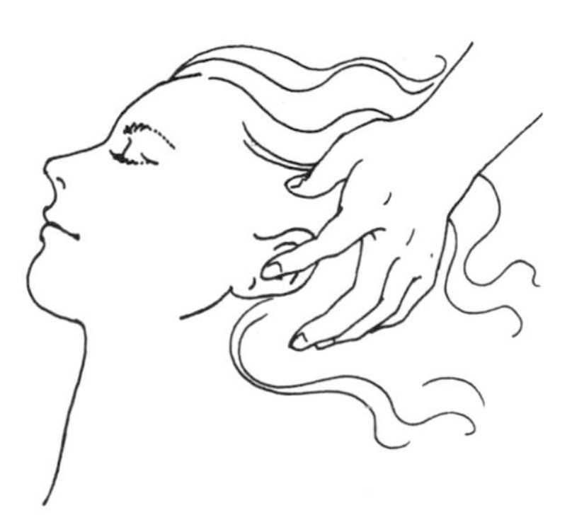

*Massage in and around the ears with light friction movement.*

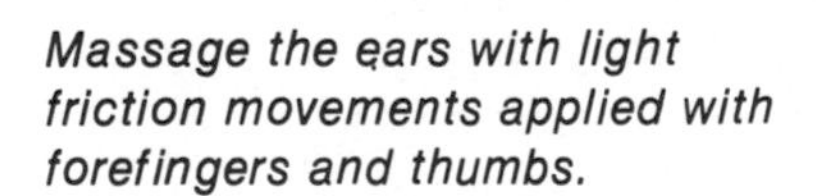

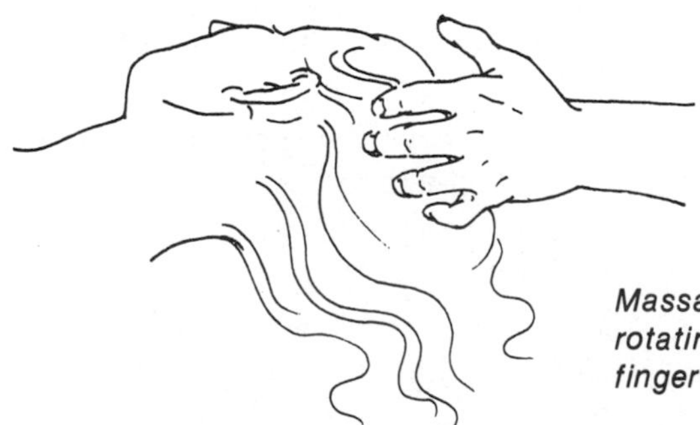

*Massage the scalp by making rotating movements with the fingertips.*

Following the scalp massage, smooth the client's hair in its natural contours. This completes the massage for the head and neck.

## COMPLETION OF THE MASSAGE

Following the massage, the client should be allowed to rest a short while before going out to face the world again. This rest period is beneficial especially if you have done body work to the extent that some changes have taken place in the client's physical structure. A few moments of relaxation will help to integrate these changes into the client's psychological and neurological senses.

It is important to instruct the client in what to do and what to expect following the massage, especially clients who come to you for the first time. For example, when you ask the client to drink plenty of water to keep the system flushed out, explain that a massage, when done properly, can cause a lot of turmoil within the body tissues and that on the cellular level an increased rate of exchange of body fluids takes place. That increase means that some metabolic wastes have been expired from the cells and have been put into the general systemic circulation. This waste material has to be dealt with because it puts an extra burden on the excretory system. If this waste is not flushed out it will be reabsorbed into the tissues. An increase in the intake of water and other healthful fluids will assist in the process of elimination by supplying more fluids for the kidneys, the colon, the lungs, and for perspiration.

You will need to give some guidelines as to the amount of water the client should drink. It is difficult to suggest a certain amount but usually four quarts a day is about right. If the treatment was given in the afternoon, the client should drink about two quarts of water that day and four quarts the following day.

### Aftereffects of Massage

Some clients experience certain aftereffects following massage and should be told that this is no cause for alarm. Usually the effects are felt following the first or second massage. Some people complain of a slight headache, upset stomach and nausea, or the feeling they get with the onset of a cold. Such reactions are due to an increase in metabolic waste material in the circulatory system. The particular symptom the client experiences depends on the organs that are being overtaxed. The intensity of the massage movements should be limited until the client has built up more tolerance. The client will seldom have a symptom that lasts for any length of time, however. He or she should be told to call you if there is a problem.

## QUESTIONS FOR DISCUSSION AND REVIEW

1. How often should the practitioner wash his or her hands with soap and water?
2. How can the practitioner prevent the chilling of the client's body?
3. How can the practitioner avoid scratching the client's body?
4. How can the practitioner prevent the client from becoming fatigued?
5. In which treatment does the practitioner require considerable strength?
6. Which massage movements should be avoided because they convey fear of injury to the client?

7. Is it better to massage the body before or after a meal?
8. What is the average duration of a local massage?
9. In which conditions should massage never be applied?
10. What preliminaries require attention before body massage?
11. Which position does the client usually assume first for body massage?
12. What is the usual order of massage movements?
13. What are the final considerations after completing body massage?
14. Why should the client be advised to drink plenty of water?

**ANSWERS TO QUESTIONS FOR DISCUSSION AND REVIEW**

1. The practitioner should wash his or her hands before and after each treatment.
2. Chilling of the client's body can be prevented by keeping the room warm and by making sure your hands are warm before contacting the client's skin.
3. Scratching the client can be avoided by filing the nails short and smooth.
4. By not applying massage too vigorously. Allow the client to rest for a short period before and after the massage.
5. In the treatment of obesity.
6. Heavy pressure, rapid movement or jarring contact cause fear and should be avoided.
7. Before the client has eaten a meal.
8. The average duration of a massage is about an hour.
9. Massage should never be applied when there is injury or abrasion of the skin, fever, inflammation of joints or veins, or when other contraindications are present.
10. Before a body massage, check facilities for readiness, obtain and arrange supplies and check self for readiness. Obtain necessary information regarding client's needs and wishes, advise the client regarding preparation procedures and assist as necessary, record the client's pulse and body temperature when necessary, and obtain client's weight and measurements (if program requires).
11. Generally, the massage begins with the client in supine (face up) position.
12. The usual order of massage begins with arms or back; proceeds to front of legs and continues over chest, neck, and abdomen. Stroking, kneading, rotary rolling, hacking, and cupping movements are generally applied in massage of the arms.
13. The final considerations of massage involve completing the client's record card, suggesting supplementary services, placing supplies in their proper places, discarding refuse, and arranging the massage table and bath for the next client.
14. The client should drink plenty of water to keep the system flushed out.

# Chapter 11 Face and Scalp Massage

**LEARNING OBJECTIVES**

After you have mastered this chapter, you will be able to:

1. Select and prepare the appropriate products and items needed to give a basic face or scalp massage.
2. Explain the benefits of face or scalp massage.
3. Explain contraindications for face and scalp massage.
4. Demonstrate correct procedures for cleansing the face.
5. Demonstrate correct procedures for giving a face massage.
6. Demonstrate correct procedures for giving a basic scalp massage.

**INTRODUCTION**

Face massage benefits the skin by stimulating blood to the tissues thereby nourishing the skin. Massage helps to tone the skin and keep underlying muscles firm. It also helps to keep sebaceous (oil) glands and the sudoriferous (sweat) glands functioning normally. The cleansing procedure removes surface as well as deeply embedded soil and helps to prevent problem blemishes such as blackheads, whiteheads, and pimples.

Practitioners may give a basic face and scalp massage as part of the complete massage service. Some clients may request one or both of these services while others may not. Whether or not to include face or scalp massage can be determined during the consultation.

The face and scalp massages included in this chapter are basic cleansing and relaxing procedures.

**FACE MASSAGE**

A face massage may consist of basic cleansing of the skin and gentle, relaxing massage movements, or it might include more extensive procedures using machines and various products. A complete face massage may be given as part of the therapeutic body massage, or it may be limited to a few rotary movements at the temples, around the forehead, and at the base of the skull. Generally, the massage practitioner gives only the basic, cleansing facial.

An esthetician specializes in face massage and skin care. An esthetician may work with a dermatologist in the treatment of skin problems or in a salon where nonmedical, preventive skin care treatments are given. The esthetician does a variety of manual massage movements and may also use various machines and apparatus such as vaporizers, brushing and suction machines as well as an assortment of products to achieve the desired results. Many estheticians are also qualified to give therapeutic body massage.

Whether the practitioner gives a partial or complete face massage, it is important to understand correct procedures. As with body massage, once the basic movements are mastered, the massage can be varied.

**The Consultation**

During the consultation it can be determined whether or not the client would like a face massage. Some women prefer not having their makeup disturbed. The client may have a skin condition such as an allergy which would be a contraindication for face massage. If the client has a healthy skin and wishes a face massage, the following items to be used for the facial should be prepared in advance:

mild cleansing cream or lotion

mild astringent or skin freshening lotion

a small towel or cape for the client's shoulders

cotton pads and pledgets to apply and remove cosmetics

cotton tipped swabs and facial tissues to remove makeup from eye area and the lips

a towel or headband to protect the client's hair

Cotton pads should be prepared and moistened in cool water then placed in a sterile container until needed.

***Cleansing Procedures***

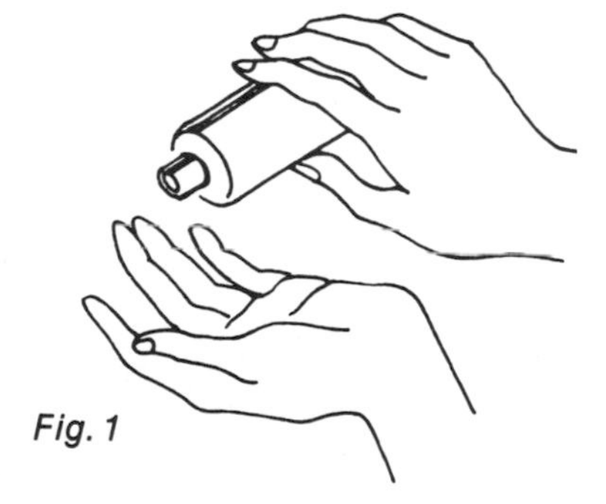

Fig. 1

*1. The practitioner's hands must be sanitized before touching the client's face. Wash the hands with mild soap and warm water and rinse them thoroughly. Wipe the hands with alcohol and dry them carefully. Nails should be a reasonable length and smooth so they will not scratch the client's face during the facial procedure.*

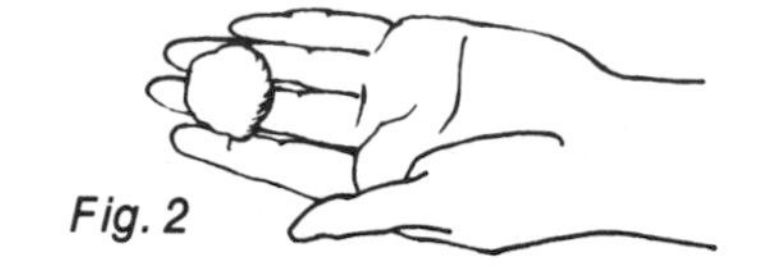

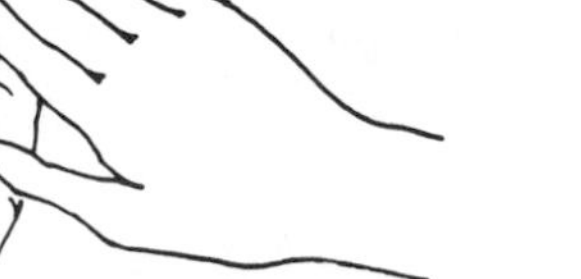

Fig. 2

*2. Apply about one level teaspoon or less of the cleansing product to the fingers of either the right or left hand.*

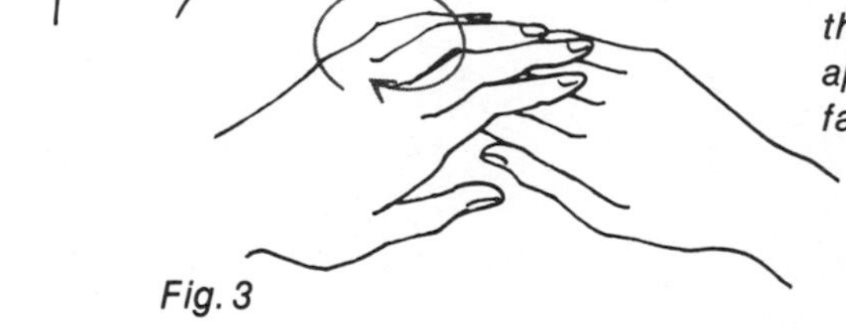

Fig. 3

*3. With the other hand, distribute the product over both sides of the fingers. You are now ready to apply the product to the client's face.*

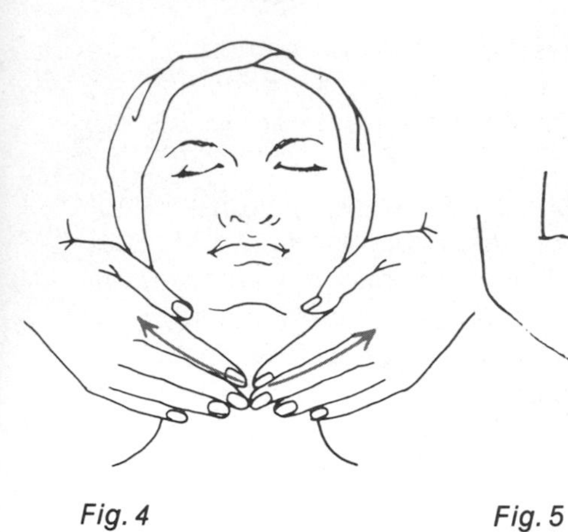

Fig. 4

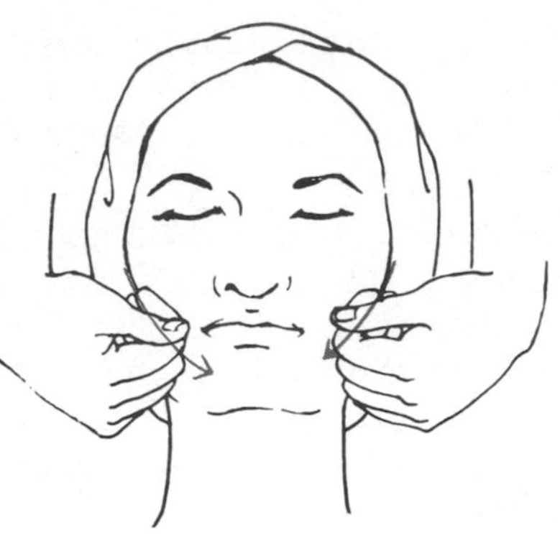

Fig. 5

*4. Place both hands palm down on the client's neck. Slide the hands back toward the client's ears until the finger pads rest at a point directly below the earlobes.*

*5. Reverse the hands so the back of the fingers are resting on the skin. Slide the fingers along the jawline to the chin.*

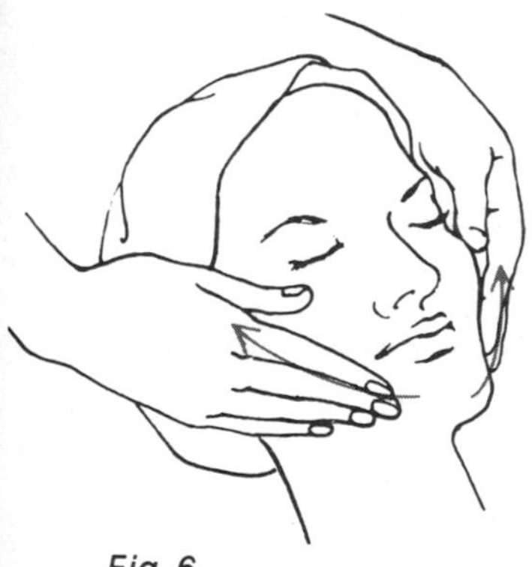

Fig. 6

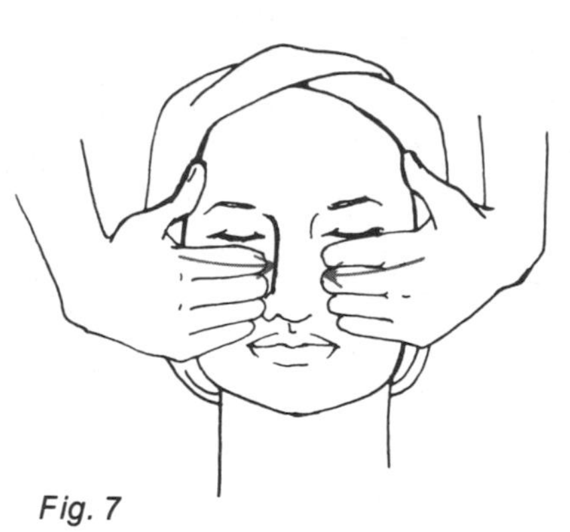

Fig. 7

*6. Reverse the hands again, and slide the fingers back over the cheeks until the finger pads come to rest directly in front of the client's ears.*

*7. Reverse the fingers again, and slide them forward over the cheekbones to the nose.*

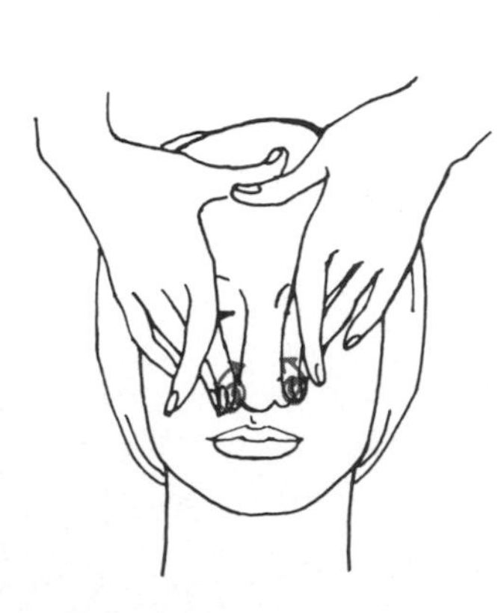

Fig. 8

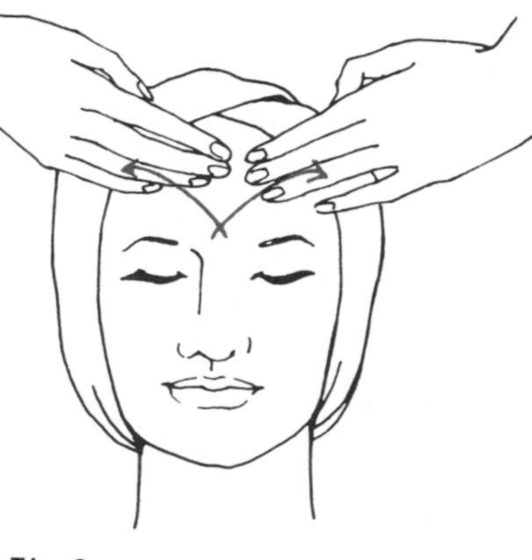

Fig. 9

*8. With the pads of the middle fingers, make small circular motions on the flairs of the nostrils.*

*9. Slide the fingers up to the forehead and outward toward the temples, pause with a slight pressure on the temples.*

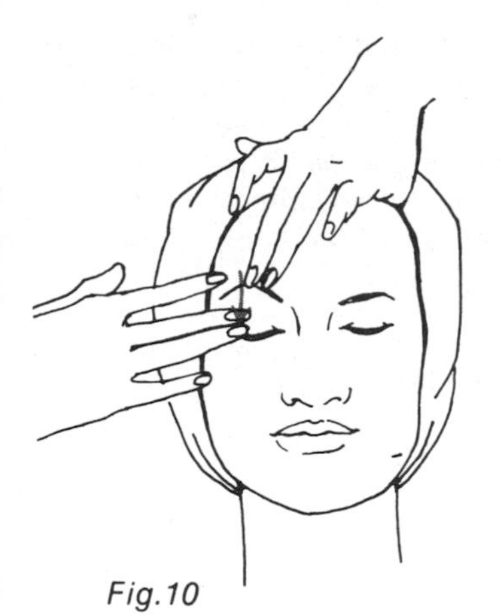

*Fig.10*

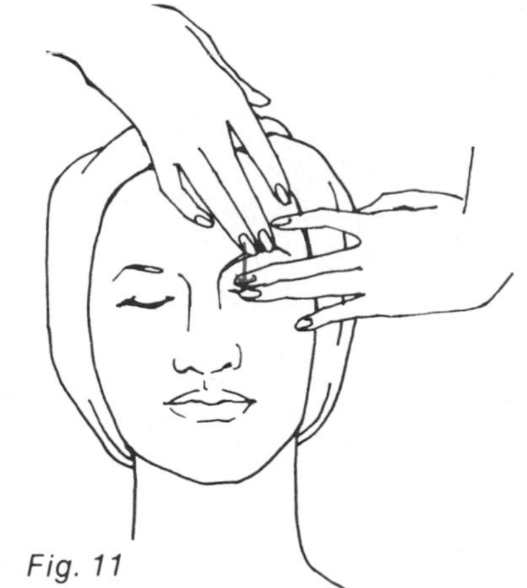

*Fig. 11*

*10. Bring the left hand over and lift the right eyebrow with the middle and ring fingers. With the middle and ring fingers of the right hand, apply the cleansing product to the eyelid with downward strokes.*

*11. Move the middle and ring fingers of the right hand over to the left side of the face, and lift the left eyebrow. With the middle fingers of the left hand, apply the cleansing product to the left lid with downward strokes.*

Repeat these movements until the cleansing product has been applied thoroughly to the client's face and neck.

***Removing Cleanser***

Some professional practitioners prefer to use wet cotton pads when cleansing and working on the face. Others prefer to use facial sponges. Both methods are correct and equally professional. Many practitioners use both methods. In some areas, the facial sponges are not readily available, whereas, cotton can be purchased at all drug and variety stores. Supply houses refer to cotton as "beautician's" cotton. Even when using sponges some cotton is needed during the treatment for eyepads, extracting blackheads, and applying products such as astringent.

***Procedure for Removing Lipcolor***

If the client is wearing lipcolor, fold a tissue into a square pad and apply a small amount of cleansing lotion to the tissue. Cleanse the lips at the outside corner of the lips, and slide the tissue to the center of the lips. Alternate the strokes on both sides of the mouth. Turn the tissue to the clean side, and repeat the procedure until all the cleanser is removed and the lips are clean.

***Procedure for Removing Cleanser with a Cotton Pad***

It is important that the client be comfortable and relaxed throughout the facial treatment. Moistened cotton pads should be kept at a comfortable temperature, as very cold pads can be shocking and uncomfortable. Excess water should be squeezed from a prepared cotton pad so that no water drips on the client during the cleansing procedure.

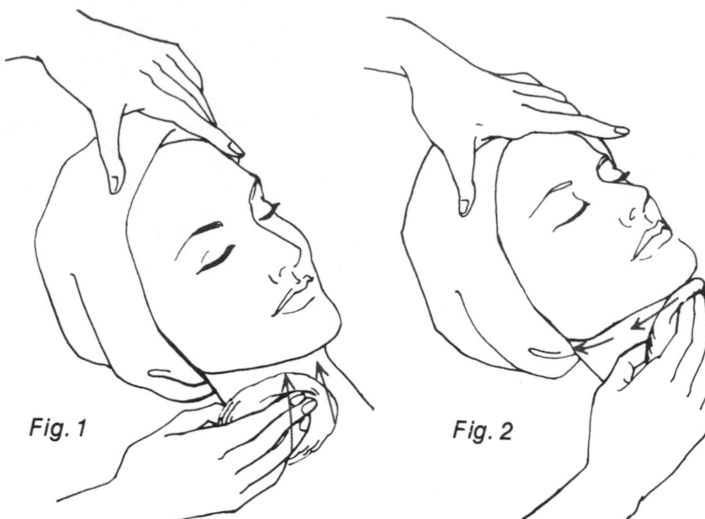

*Fig. 1* *Fig. 2*

*1. Begin the cleansing procedure at the base of the neck, using upward strokes. If you are cleansing a man's face do all the cleansing movements in the direction of the beard growth.*

*2. Place the pad directly under the chin and slide it upward along the jawline. Stop directly under the ear.*

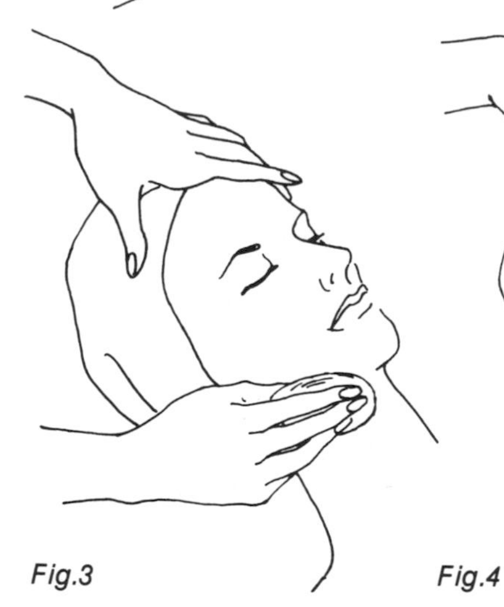

*Fig.3*

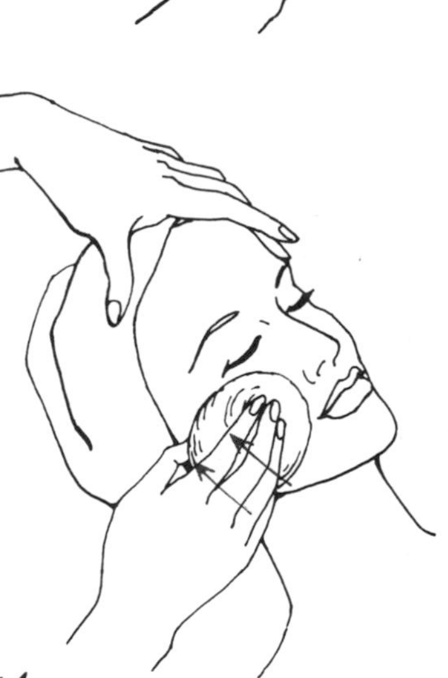

*Fig.4*

*3. Repeat the movement on the other side of the face.*

*4. Beginning at the jawline, use upward movements to cleanse the cheek.*

*Fig.5*

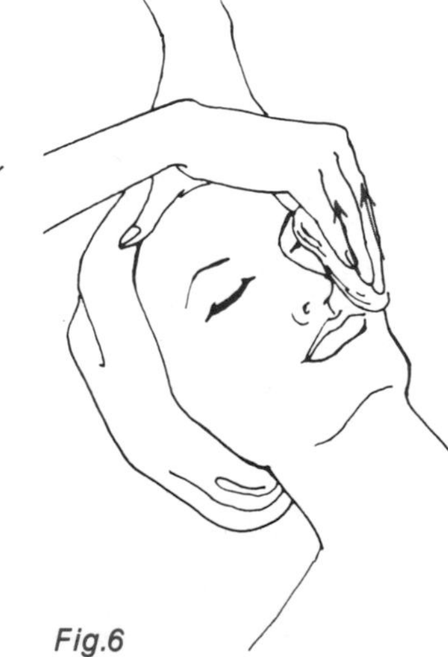

*Fig.6*

*5. Continue the upward movement, crossing over the chin.*

*6. Continue upward stroking movements to cleanse the cheeks.*

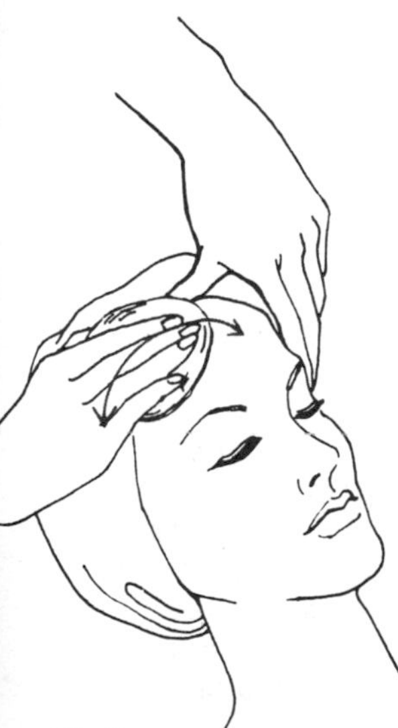

*Fig.7*

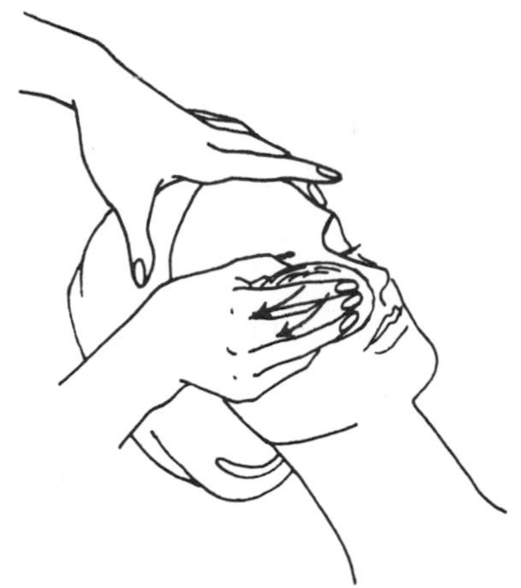

*Fig.8*

*7. Cleanse the area directly under the nose. Begin at the center, working outward toward the corners of the mouth. Alternate the movements back and forth three times on each side of the face.*

*8. Begin on the bridge of the nose, and cleanse the right side and the area directly beside the nose. Repeat on the left side.*

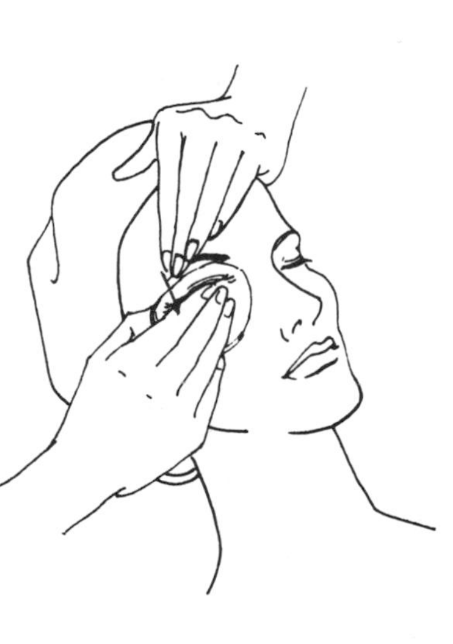

*Fig.9*

*Fig.10*

*9. Place the pad on the center of the forehead, and slide it to the right temple. Apply slight pressure to the temple. Repeat on the left side.*

*10. With the middle and ring fingers of the left hand, lift the eyebrow. Use downward movements with the cleansing pad to cleanse the eyelids and lashes. Repeat the movements until both eyes are cleansed. Finally, take a clean pad and go over the entire face gently. Blot the face dry with a tissue if necessary. You are now ready to apply massage cream or lotion for the massage procedure. Use the same techniques as for applying cleansing lotion.*

## Manipulations for Face Massage

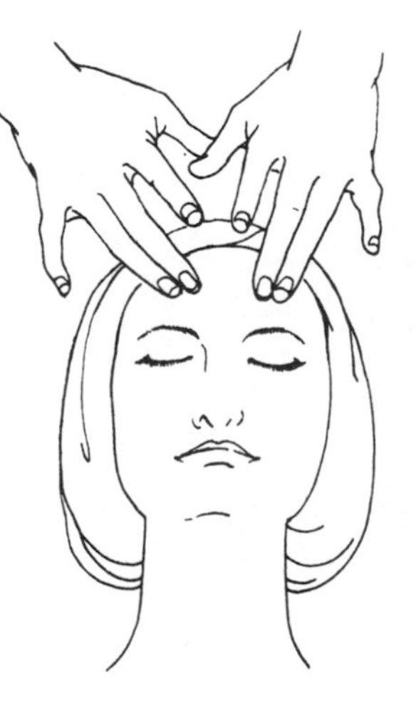

*Effleurage is a light continuous movement applied to the skin with the fingers and palms in a slow and rhythmic manner. Over large surfaces, the palm of the hand is used. Over small areas as on the face, the cushions of the fingertips are employed. Massage movements are generally directed toward the origin of the muscles in order to avoid damage to delicate muscular tissues.*

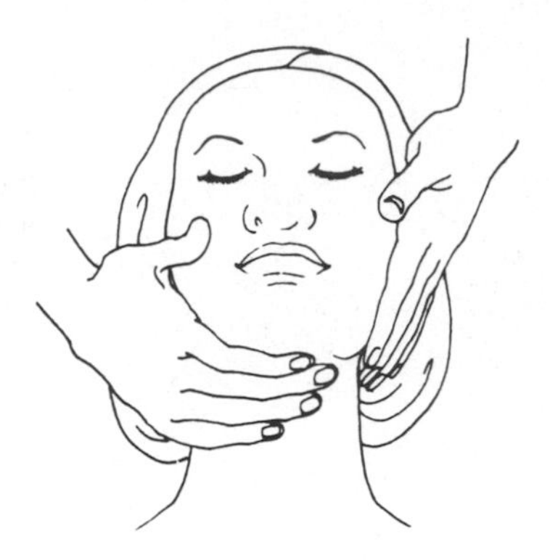

*Digital and palmar stroking of the face. For the correct position for stroking, the fingers should be slightly curved, with just the cushions of the fingertips (not the tips of the nails) touching the skin.*

*The correct position for palmar stroking is to keep the wrist and fingers flexible, curving the fingers to conform to the shape of the area being massaged.*

*Petrissage. This is a kneading movement whereby the skin and flesh are grasped gently between the thumb and the forefinger. As the tissues are lifted from their underlying structures, they are squeezed, rolled, or pinched with a gentle but firm pressure. When grasping and releasing the fleshy parts of the face, a smooth, rhythmic movement should be maintained. Kneading movements give deeper stimulation, improve circulation, and help to empty the oil ducts.*

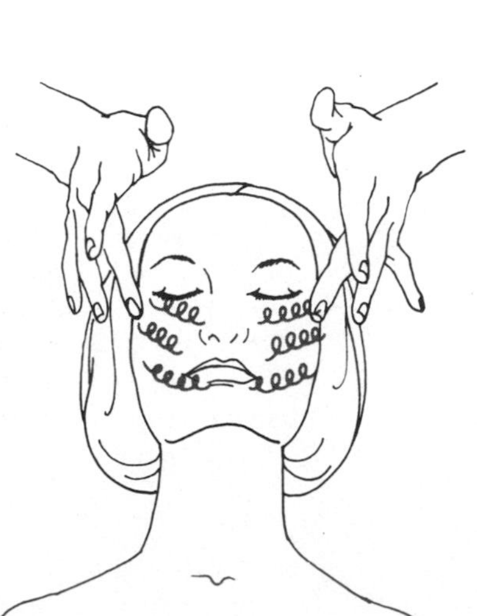

*Friction. This is a movement that requires light pressure on the skin while it is moved over the underlying structures. The fingers and palms are employed in this movement. Friction has a marked influence on the circulation and glandular activity of the skin.*

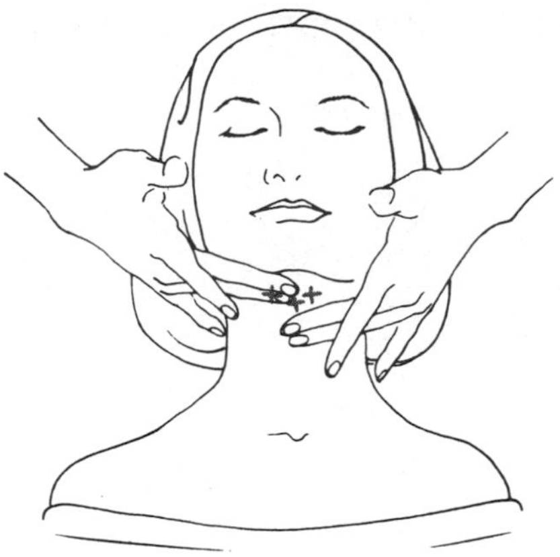

*Percussion or tapotement. This type of movement consists of tapping, slapping, and hacking movements. This is the most stimulating form of massage and should be performed with extreme care. In facial massage, only light digital tapping is used. In tapping, the fingertips are brought down against the skin in rapid succession. The fingers must be flexible to create an even force over the area being treated.*

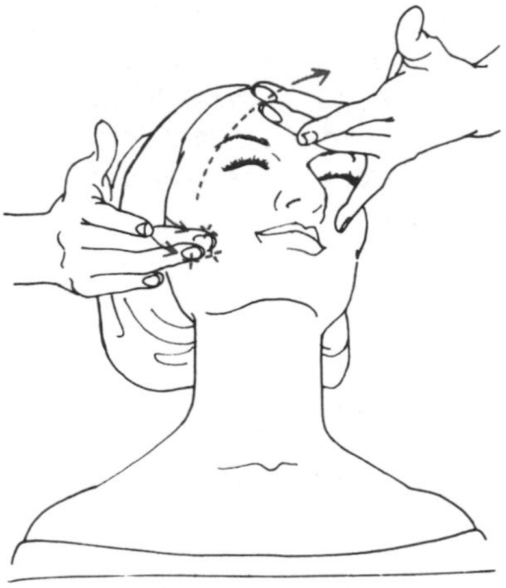

*Slapping movements. Slapping requires flexible wrists to permit the palms to come in contact with the skin in very light, firm, and rapid slapping movements. One hand follows the other in a rhythmic movement. When used in face massage, care must be taken to apply gentle movements only.*

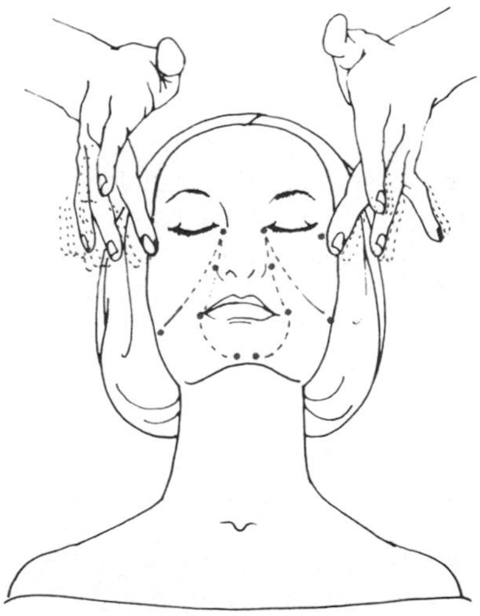

*Vibration or shaking movements. Vibration is a movement accomplished by rapid muscular contractions in the arms while pressing the fingertips firmly on the point of application. It is a highly stimulating movement and should be used sparingly. It should never exceed a few seconds duration on any one spot.*

Muscular contractions can also be produced by use of apparatus such as mechanical vibrators. To obtain proper results from face massage, you should have a thorough knowledge of anatomy, especially of muscles, nerves, and blood vessels affected by massage. Almost every muscle and nerve has a motor point. The position of motor points will vary in location in individuals due to differences in body structure. A few manipulations on the right motor points will induce relaxation at the beginning of the massage treatment.

**Massage Procedure** Spread the facial oil over the face and neck using the same
Apply Facial Oil movement as in applying cleansing lotion to the face.

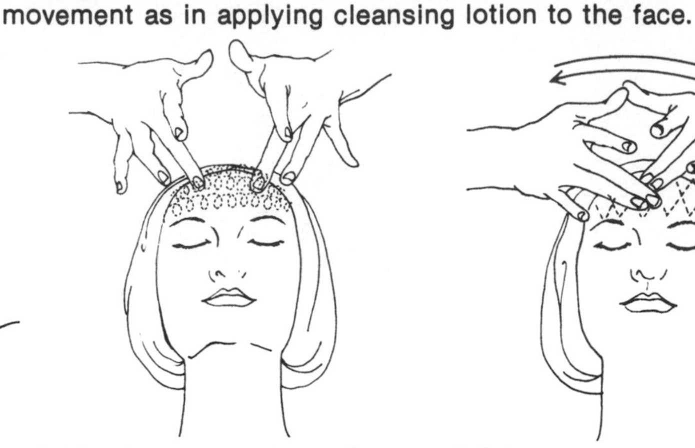

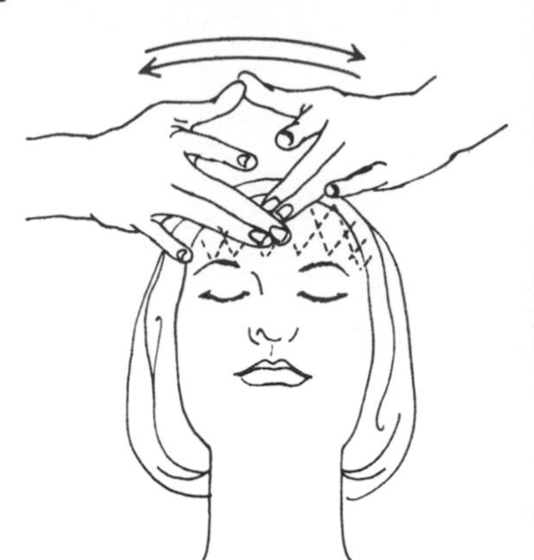

*1. Linear movement over forehead. Slide the fingers to the temples, rotate with pressure on an upward stroke, slide to left eyebrow; then stroke the forehead across and back.*

*2. Circular movement over the forehead. Begin at the eyebrow line, work across the middle of the forehead, and then toward the hairline.*

*3. Criss-cross movement. Begin at one side of the forehead making cross movements then working back.*

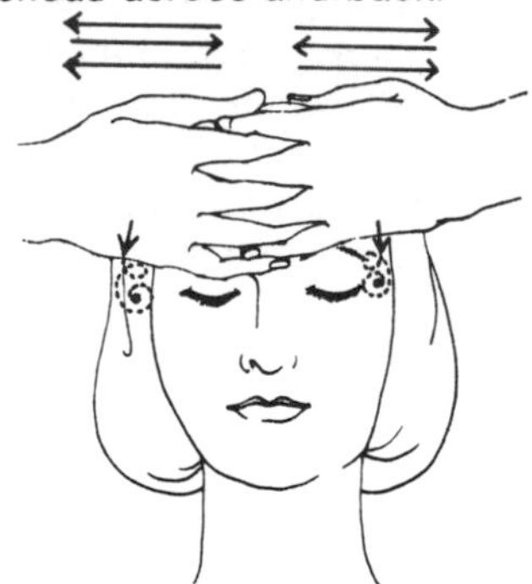

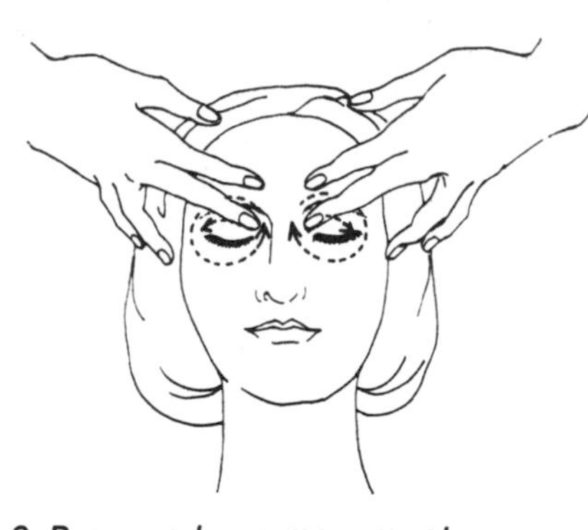

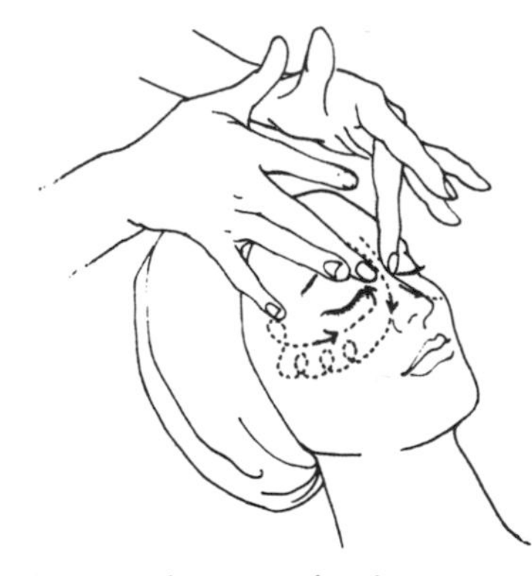

*7. Stroking movement. Slide the fingers to the center of the forehead then, with slight pressure, draw the fingers toward the temples and rotate.*

*8. Brow and eye movement. Place the middle finger at the inner corners of the eyes and the index finger over the brows. Slide the fingers to the outer corners of the eyes, under the eyes, and back.*

*9. Nose and upper cheek. Apply rotary movements across the cheeks to the temples, and rotate gently. Slide the fingers under the eyes and back to the bridge of the nose.*

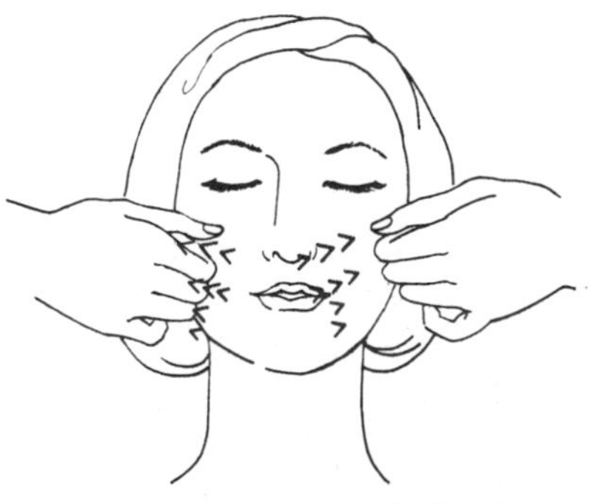

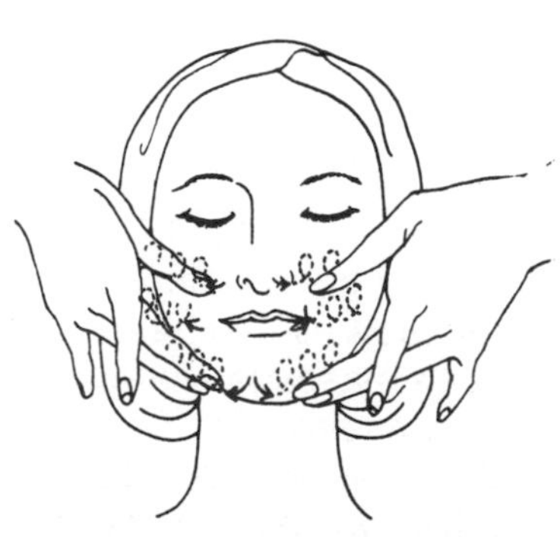

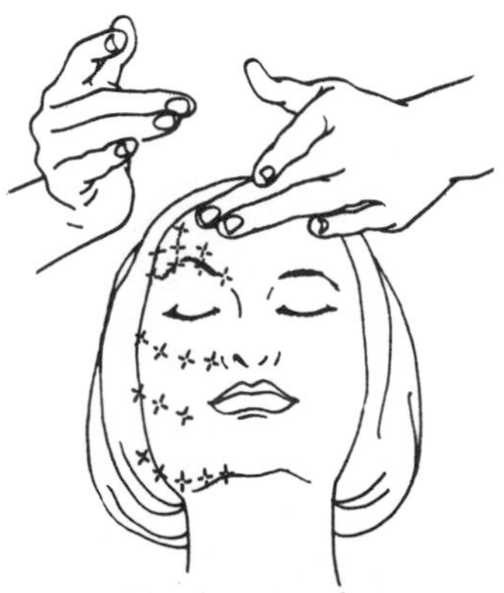

*13. Lifting movement of cheeks. Use knuckles to lift gently from mouth to ears, and then from nose to the top part of the ears.*

*14. Rotary movement of cheeks. Massage from chin to earlobes, and from the nose to the top of the ears.*

*15. Light tapping movement. Do light tapping movements from chin to earlobe, mouth to ear, and then across the forehead.*

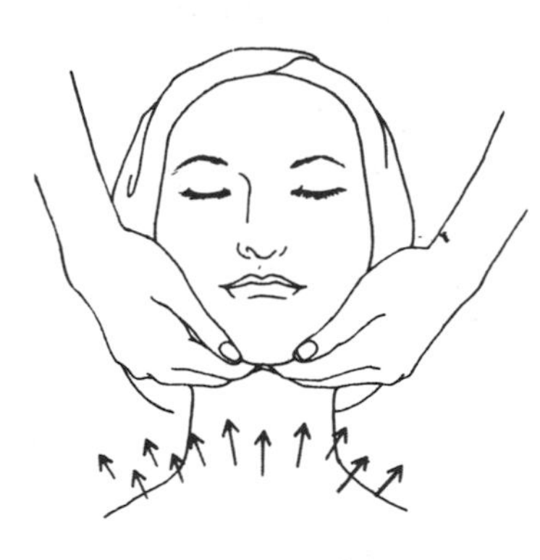

4. Chin movement. Use light pressure with fingertips to lift chin.

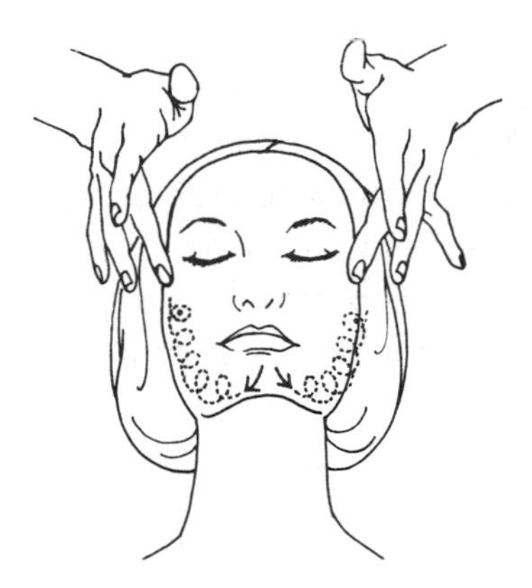

5. Lower cheek. Use circular movement from chin to ear and rotate.

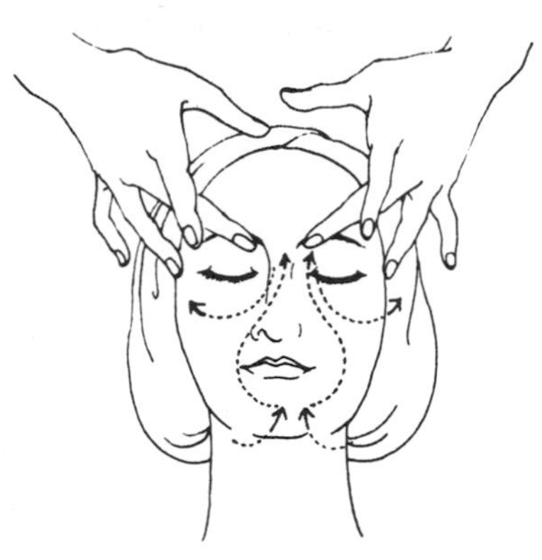

6. Mouth, nose, and cheek movement. Make light circular movements from the chin.

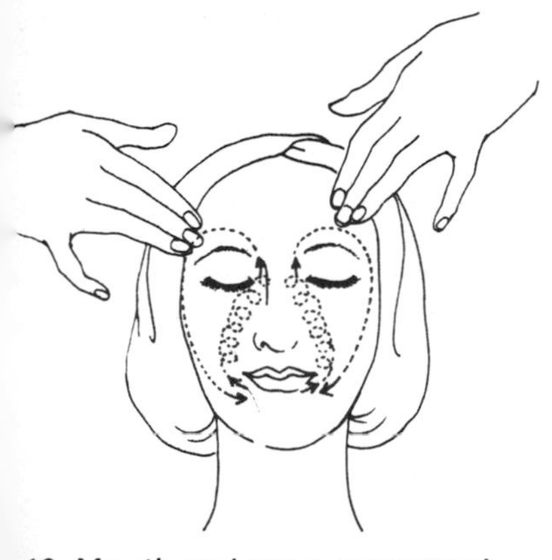

10. Mouth and nose movement. Apply circular movement from the corners of the mouth up the sides of the nose. Slide fingers over the brows and down to the corners of the mouth.

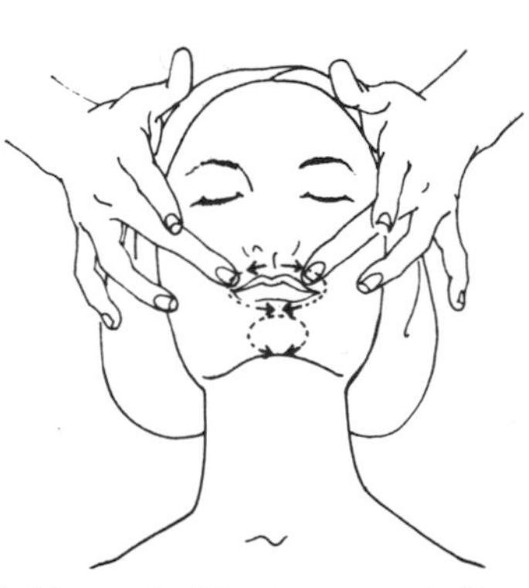

11. Lip and chin movement. Draw the fingers from the center of the upper lip, around the mouth, and under the lower lip and chin.

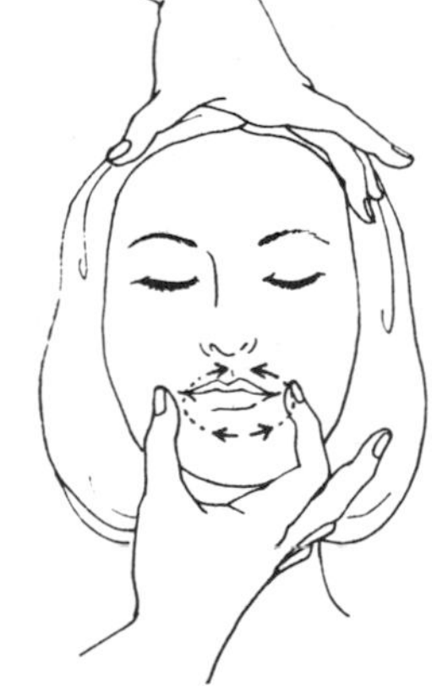

12. Optional movement. Hold the client's head with the left hand, draw the fingers of the right hand from under the lower lip, around mouth.

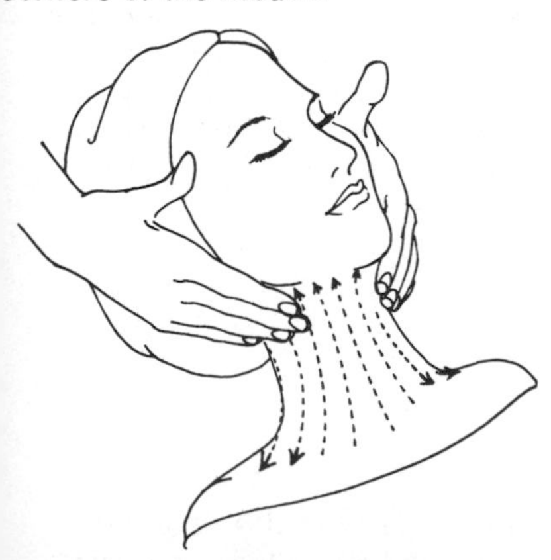

16. Stroking movement of the neck. Apply light upward strokes over the front of the neck. Use heavier pressure on the sides of the neck in downward strokes.

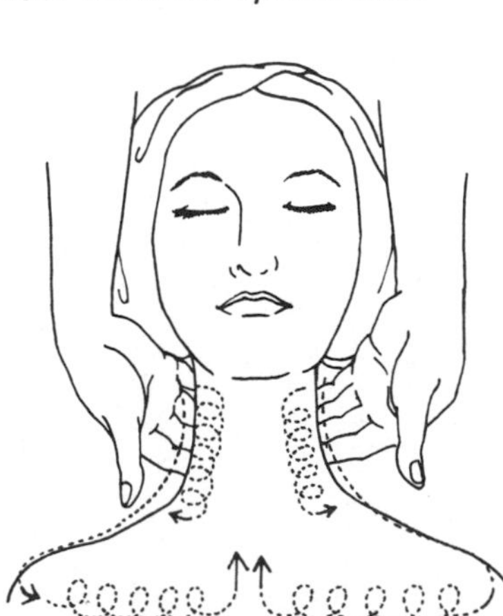

17. Circular movements over neck and chest. Beginning at the back of the ears, apply circular movement down the sides of the neck, over the shoulders, and across the neck.

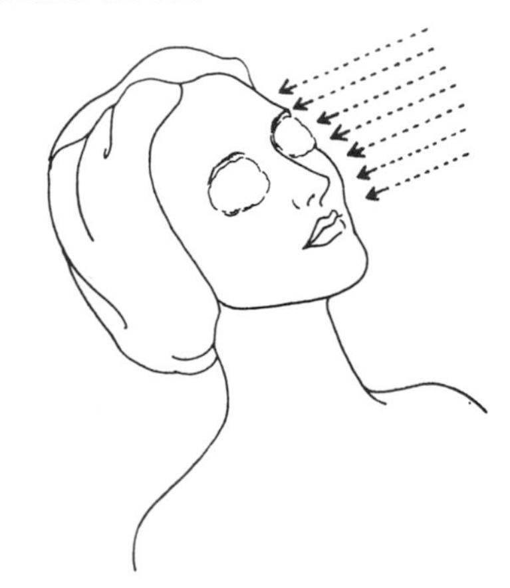

18. Infrared lamp (optional). Protect eyes with eyepads. Adjust the lamp over the client's face, and leave it on for about five minutes.

**CHEST AND BACK MASSAGE**

Chest, back, and neck manipulations (optional). Some practitioners prefer to treat these areas first before giving the facial. A suggested procedure is as follows:

1. Apply and remove cleansing cream or lotion.
2. Apply massage cream or oil.
3. Give manipulations.
4. Remove cream or lotion with tissues or warm moist towel.
5. Dust the back lightly with talcum powder.

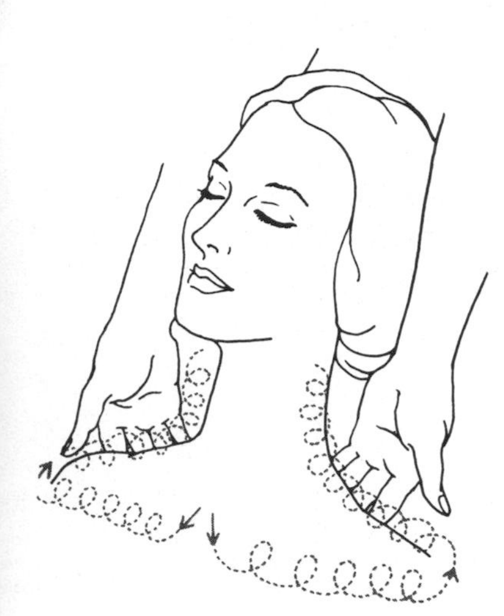

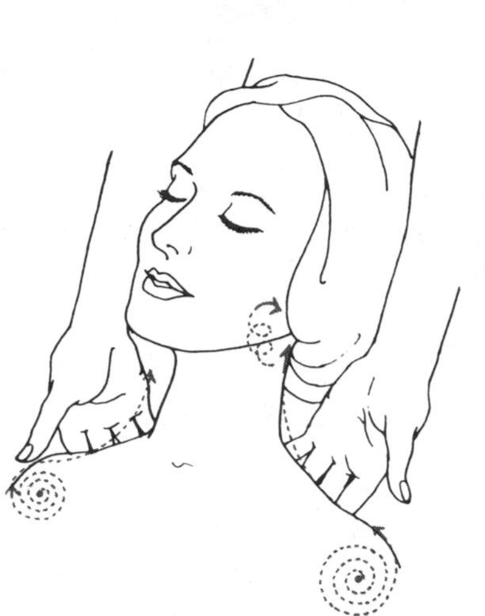

*1. Chest and back movements. Use rotary movements across the chest and shoulders and then the spine. Slide the fingers to base of the neck and rotate three times.*

*2. Shoulder and back movements. Rotate shoulders three times. Slide the fingers to the spine, then to the base of the neck. Apply circular movements up to the back of the ear, then slide the fingers to front of the earlobe and rotate three times.*

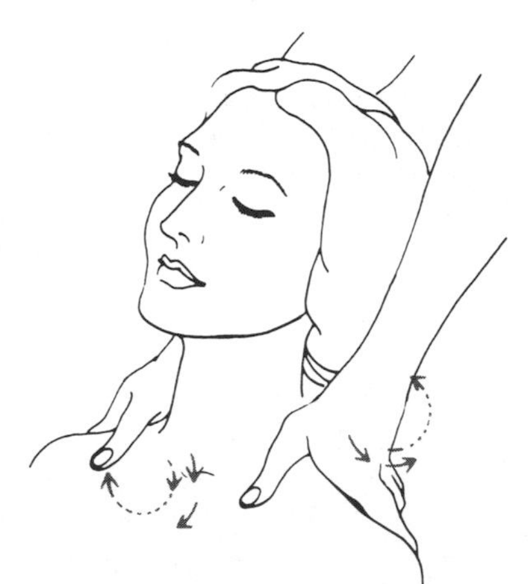

*3. Back massage (optional). To relax the client, use thumbs and bend index fingers to grasp the tissue at the back of the neck. Rotate six times. Repeat over the shoulders and back to the spine.*

Following the complete face massage, cleanse the face with a fresh, moist pad, apply astringent (for oily skin) or skin freshening lotion (for normal and dry skin). Finish with a light application of moisturizing cream or lotion, or a protective cream or lotion.

## SCALP MASSAGE

In scalp massage, apply firm pressure on upward strokes. Firm rotary movements are given to loosen scalp tissues. These movements improve the health of hair and scalp by increasing the circulation of blood to the scalp and hair papillae. When giving a scalp massage, care should be taken to give the manipulations slowly, without pulling the hair in any way.

The massage practitioner does not confuse the basic relaxing scalp massage with full treatments and massage of the scalp as given by a professional hair stylist or cosmetologist. The practitioner does not treat scalp disorders or massage the scalp if it is not in healthy condition. Basic manipulations are given by the massage practitioner as part of the massage treatment because they tend to promote relaxation. A good scalp massage can be beneficial in stimulating blood and lymph flow, in resting and soothing the nerves, and as an aid to keeping the scalp healthy and hair lustrous.

### A Guide to Massage and Its Influence on the Scalp

| MASSAGE MOVEMENTS | MUSCLES | NERVES | ARTERIES |
|---|---|---|---|
| Figure 1 | Auricularis superior | Posterior auricular | Frontal<br>Parietal |
| Figure 2 | Auricularis posterior<br>Occipitalis | Greater occipital | Occipital |
| Figure 3 | Frontalis | Supra-orbital | Frontal |
| Figure 4 | Frontalis | Supra-orbital | Frontal<br>Parietal |
| Figure 5 | Auricularis posterior<br>Occipitalis | Greater occipital | Posterior auricular<br>Parietal |
| Figure 6 | Auricularis anterior and superior | Temporal auricular | Frontal<br>Parietal |

### Procedure for Scalp Massage

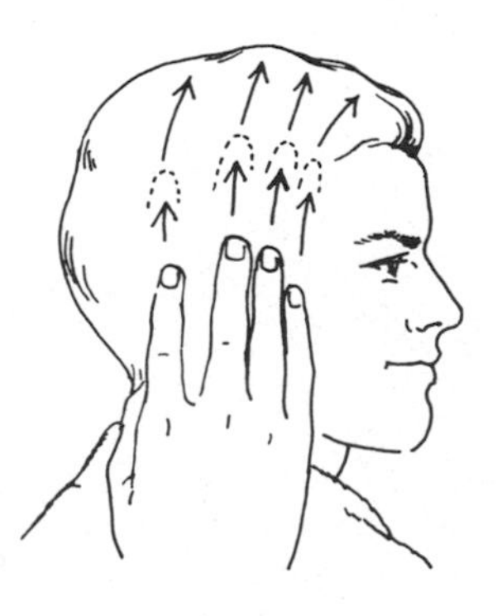

*Figure 1. Place the fingertips of each hand at the hairline on each side of the client's head, pointing the hands upward. Slide the fingers firmly upward spreading the fingertips. Continue until the fingers meet at the center or top of the scalp. Repeat three or four times.*

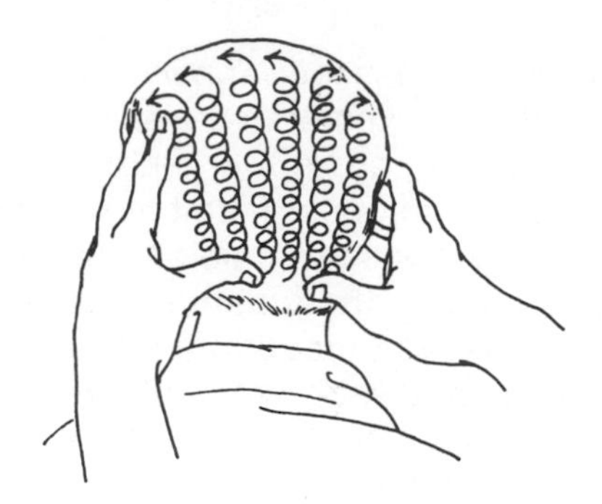

*Figure 2. Place the fingers of each hand on either side of the client's head behind the ears. Use the thumbs to massage from behind the ears toward the crown. Repeat four or five times. Move your fingers until both thumbs meet at the hairline at the back of the client's neck. Rotate your thumbs upward towards the crown.*

*Figure 3. Step to the right side of the client. Place the left hand at the back of the head. Place the thumb and fingers of the right hand over the forehead, just above the eyebrows. With the cushion tips of the right hand, thumb and fingers, massage slowly and firmly in an upward direction toward the crown while keeping the left hand in a fixed position at the back of the head. Repeat four or five times.*

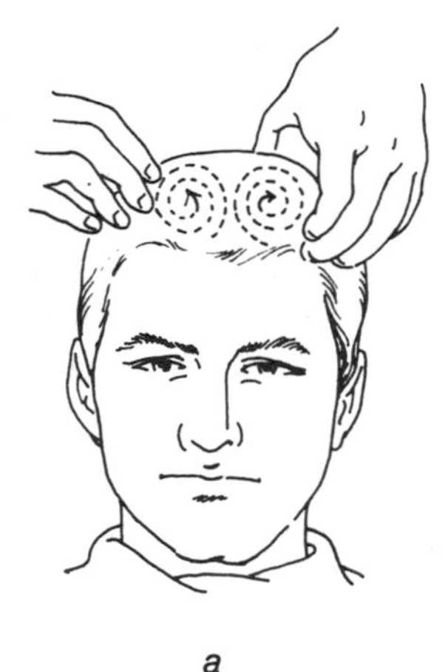

*a*

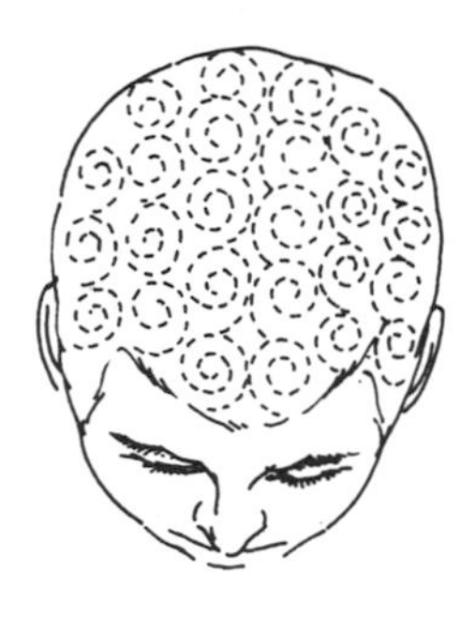

*b*

*Figure 4. Step to the back of the client. a) Place the hands on each side of the head, at the front hairline. Rotate the fingertips three times. On the fourth rotation, apply a quick, upward twist, firm enough to move the scalp. b) Continue this movement on the sides and tip of the scalp. Repeat three or four times.*

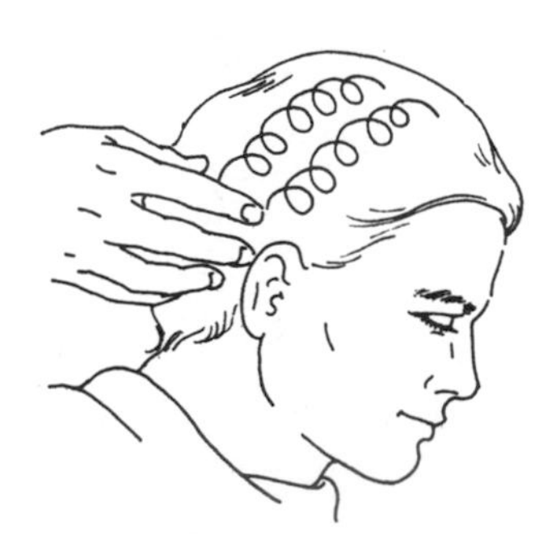

*Figure 5. Place the fingers (of each hand) below the back of each ear. Rotate the fingers upward from behind the ears to the crown. Repeat three or four times. Move the fingers toward the back of the head, and repeat the movement with both hands. Apply rotary movements in an upward direction toward the crown.*

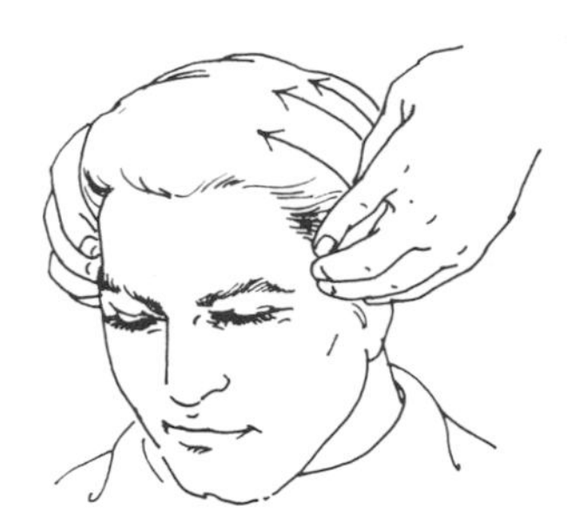

*Figure 6. Place both hands at the sides of the client's head. Keep the fingers close together, and hold the index fingers at hairline above the ears. Firmly move both hands directly upward to the top of the head. Repeat four times. Move the hands to above the ears and repeat the movement. Move hands again to back of the ears and repeat the movement.*

**QUESTIONS FOR DISCUSSION AND REVIEW**

1. When is a face massage not given?
2. What is the first important step in a face massage procedure?
3. How do movements in face massage differ from those used for body massage?
4. What are the main benefits of face massage?
5. Why is cleansing the face before massage so important?
6. What are the main benefits of scalp massage?
7. When does the practitioner avoid giving scalp massage?
8. What is the massage practitioner's main purpose in including face and scalp massages in his or her procedures?

**ANSWERS TO QUESTIONS FOR DISCUSSION AND REVIEW**

1. When the client does not want face massage or when there is some contraindication to face massage.
2. Cleansing the face.
3. In face massage, movements are very gentle. While movements such as hacking, twisting, or heavy strokes may be beneficial to parts of the body, they are not used on face muscles.
4. Face massage increases circulation of the blood, which nourishes the tissues. Face massage also helps to tone muscles and keeps sebaceous (oil) glands and sudoriferous (sweat) glands functioning properly.
5. Cleansing removes deeply embedded and surface soil. The cleansing procedure removes this debris and helps to prevent blackheads and infectious conditions.
6. Scalp massage stimulates the flow of blood to the tissues. Scalp massage soothes the nerves and is an aid to keeping the scalp healthy and hair lustrous.
7. When the client does not want it and when there are certain contraindications for scalp massage.
8. The massage practitioner gives face and scalp massage as an aid to relaxing and soothing the client, and as an aid to healthy functioning of the face and scalp tissues.

# Chapter 12 Hydrotherapy, Heat and Lamp Treatments

**LEARNING OBJECTIVES**

After you have mastered this chapter, you will be able to:

1. Explain the use of heat and light in body treatments.
2. Describe types of apparatus that may be approved for use by the massage practitioner.
3. Describe types of apparatus that may not be approved for use by the massage practitioner.
4. Explain contraindications for suntanning.
5. Explain hydrotherapy as a therapeutic aid.
6. Explain the effects of different water temperatures on the body.
7. Give a Swedish shampoo.
8. Give a salt rub.
9. Explain how to assist a client in various bath treatments.
10. Explain contraindications, safety rules, and time limits for various bath treatments.

## INTRODUCTION

Although body massage is generally done by hand, there is a wide range of treatments that combine manual massage and various equipment. These treatments are designed to encourage circulation, improve the body's efficiency in eliminating toxins, and promote relaxation. They are also used as an aid to toning and slimming the figure.

## THE USE OF ELECTRICAL APPARATUS

The practitioner must have sound knowledge of procedures involving electrical equipment and its benefits as well as any contraindications of its use. While no machine can replace the well-trained hands of the practitioner, machines can offer advantages when used in conjunction with manual massage. Mainly, the machine is used as a means to conserve the practitioner's energy and to increase the benefits of various treatments.

One of the most popular items used for body massage is the rotary and vibratory massager. It is used to produce either a relaxing or stimulating effect depending on the method of application and the desired results. These machines are usually free standing with an attachment for different kinds of applicator heads. The heads are designed to achieve different effects.

Vacuum massage units are used as an aid to toning and slimming the figure. They are designed with different size suction cups to pick up and release fatty tissue. There are also electronic muscle exercising machines that contract and relax the muscles to aid in toning and slimming the figure. It is important for the massage practitioner to understand how to use electrical equipment safely and for the right purposes. The manufacturer of a machine will usually provide instructions and an instruction booklet for reference.

## ELECTROTHERAPY

Treatments using electrical apparatus are used effectively in facial and body massage and are often called electrotherapy. These treatments are vibratory massage, high-frequency current treatment, and galvanic treatment. There are various types of vibratory equipment. Some of these have attachments to stimulate the action of manual massage including effleurage, tapotement, and petrissage. Generally, a larger floor model with attachments is used to massage larger areas of the body, while smaller hand models are used for smaller and more sensitive areas. Vibrators should not be used when contraindications exist. Examples are:

Areas where varicose or couperose veins (tiny broken veins) are present.

Areas exhibiting a skin condition, wound, or scar tissue.

When the client is being treated for internal problems.

### Procedure for Vibratory Treatment

Preparation is the same for a vibratory treatment as for any other massage procedure. The vibratory treatment may follow manual massage if desired.

Talc is applied to the part to be massaged.

The smooth-surfaced vibrator attachment is usually used first.

The vibrator is used in light, smooth, upward strokes toward the heart.

The applicator designed for kneading is used on the heavier muscles of the legs and buttocks.

The brush applicator can be used on any part of the body.

Manual movements that do not break contact with the skin are used throughout the treatment to reinforce the effects of the movements made with the attachments. It is important to know which applicator to use for specific effects and to be able to change the applicators when necessary without a long break in the continuity of the massage. The main benefits of vibratory massage are:

Stimulation of the circulatory system.

Toning of the skin by increasing blood supply to tissues.

Relaxing tension in muscles.

Relieving minor aches and pains.

Following the treatment, the equipment should be cleaned and sterilized. Records should be completed.

### *Safety Precautions*

The safety of the client is of primary concern when using any kind of electrical equipment. It is important to see that all electrical equipment is in good working order before it is used and that electrical outlets, cords, switches, and plugs are inspected regularly.

### High-Frequency Current

Of interest to the practitioner is the Tesla current, commonly called the violet ray. The primary action of this current is heat producing, or thermal. The electrodes for high-frequency current are made of glass or metal and are of various shapes. As the current passes through the glass electrode, tiny sparks are emitted. Treatments should begin with a mild current and increase gradually to the desired strength. The length of the treatment depends on the condition to be treated. It is important to follow the manufacturer's instructions for use of any Tesla equipment. Benefits derived from use of Tesla (high-frequency) current include:

Stimulation of blood circulation.

Increase in glandular activity.

Increase in the rate of metabolism.

A calming, soothing, and sedative effect.

### Galvanic Current

Galvanic current (also called a chemical current) is a direct and constant (DC) current rectified to a safe, low voltage level. Galvanic current is used to force chemicals through the unbroken skin by the process of phoresis or ionization. Cataphoresis is the use of the positive pole to introduce a positive charged substance such as acid pH astringent solution into the skin. Anaphoresis is the use of the negative pole to force a negatively charged substance such as an alkaline pH solution into the skin. These processes are often used when giving facial treatments.

Galvanic current is often used in the treatment of cellulite, a condition in which the fat cells of the body become massed underneath the skin.

Polarity means the opposite poles in an electric current. It is important for the practitioner to know which is the positive and which is the negative pole, and to follow the manufacturer's instruction for use. Most electrical appliances have a polarity indicator. The positive pole is called the anode and is identified by the letter "p" or the plus sign. The negative pole, the cathode, is identified by the letter "n" or the minus sign. Each pole produces an effect the opposite of the other.

### Faradic and Sinusoidal Current

In recent years some states have passed laws that prohibit the use of certain electrical apparatus, and particularly the use of faradic and sinusoidal current, except by a licensed physician. The owner or manager of a massage establishment should contact the state board in the state in which he or she plans to operate to inquire about local regulations. In the classroom the student should be guided by his or her instructor in the use of electrical apparatus.

## THE USE OF HEAT AND LIGHT

The rays used in body treatments are visible light, ultraviolet, and infrared rays. Some lamps are designed to provide more than one kind of ray.

### Visible Light

Visible light occurs as one of a spectrum of colors of different wave lengths. The decreasing order is red, orange, yellow, green, blue, and violet ranging from 7000 to 4000 Angstrom units. An Angstrom unit, or one hundred millionth of a centimeter, is used to measure the length of light waves. Below the range of visible light are the invisible rays such as ultraviolet, x-rays, gamma rays, and cosmic rays.

The lamp used to reproduce visible light is usually a dome-shaped reflector mounted on a pedestal with a flexible neck. The metal lining of the dome reflects the rays. The bulbs used with this lamp are available in white, red, and blue. Visible light is often used for scalp and facial treatments. White light is effective in the relief of minor aches and pains. Blue light has a tonic effect on the skin and a soothing effect on the nerves.

Red light has strong heat rays that provide a stimulating effect on the skin. Red light aids in the penetration of cosmetic products and is often recommended in the treatment of very dry skin. Creams, oils, and powders are not used with visible light.

### Ultraviolet Rays

Ultraviolet rays are invisible rays whose action is both chemical and germicidal. These rays are essential for healthy growth of the human body and in the maintenance of health metabolism. Ultraviolet rays increase resistance to disease by increasing the iron and vitamin D content and the number of red and white cells in the blood. They stimulate circulation and improve the flow of blood and lymph. Suntanning is the result of exposure of the skin to ultraviolet rays.

Ultraviolet rays have shorter wave lengths than visible light, but they are often used together either in radiant or duo-ray lamps, to provide an extra measure of safety. Ultraviolet rays are the shortest rays of the spectrum. The farther they are from the visible light region the shorter they become. If the lamp is placed 30 to 36 inches away, few of the shorter rays will reach the skin, and the action is limited to the effect of the longer rays. The shorter rays are utilized when the lamp is about 12 inches from the skin. It is important to follow the manufacturer's instructions for proper use of a lamp.

Skin can be easily overexposed. Generally, a short exposure of about 2 to 3 minutes will be enough for an initial treatment; later, exposure can be increased to 5 to 8 minutes.

Both the practitioner and the client must wear protective goggles during the use of ultraviolet lamp treatments. Ultraviolet light should not be used on sensitive skin or when conditions such as eczema or dermatitis are present. It is not advisable when the client has an allergy or is taking medication. When in doubt, it is best to consult the client's physician.

Records of all treatments should be kept including the effects of the treatment and any additional notes of importance.

**Infrared Rays**

Infrared rays (heat radiation) create a rosy glow. When absorbed by the skin, infrared rays have a calming effect on the nerves and tend to increase the activity of the sudoriferous (sweat) glands. For some clients, infrared treatments are effective in relief of pain and sore muscles. Infrared rays are not used when contraindications exist. This means any condition requiring medical treatment such as varicose veins, skin disease, diabetes, and respiratory problems.

The infrared lamp is operated at a safe distance of about 30 inches from the skin. The proper length of exposure is about three to five minutes. The client's eyes must be protected with cotton pads that have been moistened with a soothing solution such as witch hazel. No oil or cream is used on the skin. Following the treatment, a soothing oil or cream may be applied and a gentle massage given.

**Dispersion of Light Rays By a Prism**

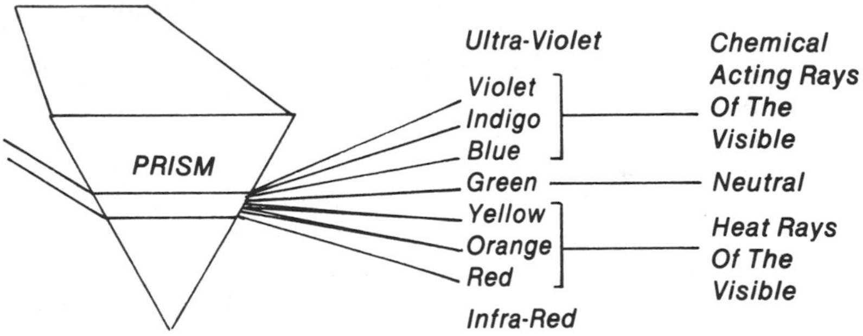

| | | | |
|---|---|---|---|
| *ULTRA-VIOLET RAYS (Cold Invisible Rays)* | *1847 AU to 3900 AU* | *Far 1847-2200*<br>*Middle 2200-2900*<br>*Near 2900-3900* | *Germicidal*<br>*Therapeutic*<br>*Tonic* |
| *SOLAR SPECTRUM (Visible Rays)* | *3900 AU to 7700 AU* | *Violet, Indigo, Blue, Green, Yellow, Orange, Red* | |
| *INFRA-RED RAYS (Invisible Heat Rays)* | *7700 AU to 14,000 AU* | *Penetrating* | *Analgesic* |

*NATURAL SUNSHINE IS COMPOSED OF:*
*8% ultra-violet rays; 12% visible light rays; 80% infra-red rays.*

*Properties of Infra-Red Rays:*

1. *Long wave length.*
2. *Low frequency.*
3. *Deep penetrating power.*

*Properties of Ultra-Violet Rays:*

1. *Short wave length.*
2. *High frequency.*
3. *Weak penetrating power.*

A *therapeutic lamp* is an electrical apparatus capable of producing certain light rays. There are separate lamps for infrared and for ultraviolet rays.

*Ultraviolet lamps*—There are three general types: the glass bulb, the hot quartz and the cold quartz.

The *glass bulb lamp* is used mainly for cosmetic or tanning purposes.

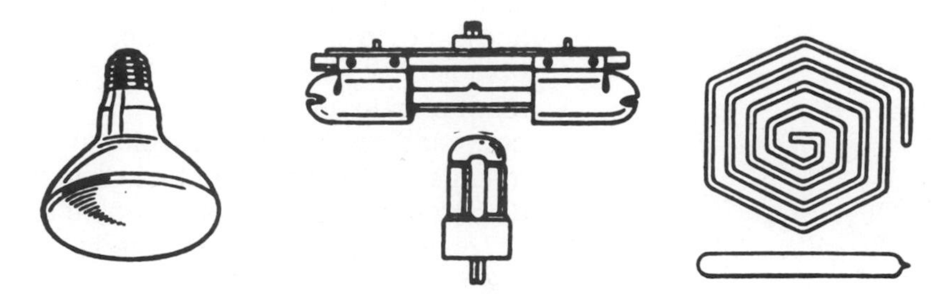

*Glass bulb type* *Hot quartz type* *Cold quartz type*

The *hot quartz lamp* is a general all-purpose lamp suitable for tanning, health, cosmetic or germicidal purposes.

The *cold quartz lamp* produces mostly short ultraviolet rays. It is used primarily in hospitals.

**SUNTANNING**

Overexposure to the sun can be harmful to the skin because the ultraviolet rays of the sun penetrate not only the epidermis but also the dermis where the living cells are affected. One of the skin's main defenses against too much sun is its ability to tan. Tanning is a shield set up by the skin to prevent damage to the underlying tissues. This is why it is so important to tan gradually and to apply a good suncreening product before exposing the skin to the sun. Excessive suntanning is considered to be the primary cause of skin cancer and premature aging of the skin. Dark skin, due to its pigmentation is not as affected by sun rays as light skin, which burns easily.

Burns are classified as first, second, and third degree burns according to the depth and extent of tissue damage.

In first-degree burns there is pain, redness, and edema. The damage is done only to the epidermis or outermost layer of the skin. Normal healing occurs within a few days. Second-degree burns result in blistering and deeper damage to tissue. Healing may take one to three weeks. Third-degree burns are the most severe and can result in destruction of the epidermis and its appendages. Nerve fibers are destroyed and scarring usually occurs. Healing may take many months, and corrective surgery may be required.

The massage practitioner, though not so concerned with whether the client has a suntan, must be very concerned with any suntanning equipment (suntanning cabinets or beds) for which he or she may be responsible. Tanning cabinets or beds have escalated in popularity since their introduction to the United States in 1979. Before that, sunlamps and tanning booths were in use. These items emitted B rays (ultraviolet B), which caused sunburn; consequently this equipment had to be used with much care. Today's tanning beds, cabinets, and booths utilize ultraviolet A rays (UVA), which provide radiation that tans without burning.

A tanning bed is usually made of aluminum with the upper and lower halves hinged so they can be moved up and down. The lamps are covered in acrylic, providing a cool surface for clients to lie on during the tanning session. The client must wear goggles (FDA mandatory) to avoid damage to the eyes. Most tanning beds also feature stereo headphones so the client can enjoy music while tanning. Suntanning cabinets or booths are similar except the client stands or sits. Some manufacturers declare suntanning beds and cabinets to have all the qualities of natural sunlight with none of the hazards. There are others who warn against use of tanning by such artificial methods.

We know that the sun has some healthful effects, such as acting on substances in the skin to manufacture vitamin D. Vitamin D is vitally important to healthy functioning of the nervous system and utilization of calcium for bone formation. UVA is also an accepted treatment for such skin conditions as psoriasis. However, the FDA (Food and Drug Administration) advises that all forms of tanning be avoided by people who want to minimize the risk of skin cancer or premature aging of the skin. Those who insist on using a tanning bed for cosmetic purposes should take the following precautions:

Always follow recommended instructions for use of the equipment.

Wear protective goggles.

Do not expect an instant tan. Begin with a shorter exposure time and build up to a longer (but safe) exposure.

Be sure an attendant or someone familiar with the equipment is nearby in case of emergency.

Report any injury from use of such equipment to the manufacturer and to the FDA.

The practitioner does not massage skin that is burned, peeling, or showing signs that it is too tender for the application of massage movements. However, the practitioner can do a valuable service by informing the client of the benefits and dangers of the sun and of suntanning equipment.

The client may not realize that when the skin is exposed to natural sunlight or to artificial ultraviolet radiation, the body's protective responses are generated so that the superficial layers of the skin begin to thicken and melanin (the coloring matter) begins to form in stages. People with very fair skin are more prone to spotting, freckling, and skin cancer. Premature aging of the skin is also accelerated, especially in thin, dry, sensitive skin. The client who insists on suntanning should be advised to use a good sunscreen product. Products are formulated for skins that tan easily and require minimum protection and for skins that require maximum protection.

The massage practitioner should be sure clients are advised about the use of any facilities or equipment in his or her place of business and should not allow the client to misuse equipment. Rules should be posted for the protection of both the client and owners.

## HYDROTHERAPY

Hydrotherapy is the science of water treatments for external application to the body. When properly used with body massage, hydrotherapy is an additional aid to the healthy functioning of the body.

Water has certain properties that make it a valuable therapeutic agent. In its solid form as ice it can be used as an effective cooling agent; in its vapor form it can be used for facials and steam baths, and in its liquid state it can be used for sprays and immersion baths.

The temperature of water affects the body, therefore it is important to understand how water temperature relates to body temperature. The normal temperature of the human body is 98.6 degrees Fahrenheit or 37 degrees Centigrade. The boiling point of water is 212 degrees Fahrenheit or 100 Centigrade. Obviously we must not use water of too high or too low a temperature because it would be injurious to body tissues. Water temperatures above that of the body (98.6 degrees Fahrenheit) are considered to be hot. Temperature of water that is slightly below that of normal body temperature is medium to warm (about 94 to 96 degrees Fahrenheit). The freezing point of water is 32 degrees Fahrenheit or 0 degrees Centigrade. Water that is about 70 to 80 degrees Fahrenheit is considered to be cool, and at 55 degrees Fahrenheit and below, it is considered cold.

Changes in the body as a result of hydrotherapy are classified as thermal, mechanical, and chemical. Thermal effects of water are produced by the application of water at temperatures above or below that of the body. This is done by way of baths, packs, wraps and the like that raise or lower the temperature of the body. Mechanical effects are produced by sprays, whirlpool baths, and friction. Chemical effects are produced by drinking water as an aid to digestion and elimination.

To use hydrotherapy effectively, the following supplies and equipment are needed:

Bath tubs and showers.

Running hot and cold water.

Spray attachments.

Bath thermometer.

Towels, bath blankets, bath brushes, sponges, loofahs, bath mitts, etc.

A slab usually of marble or simulated material.

A resting couch and blanket or other covering.

A robe and slippers for the client.

### Bath Accessories

Soap, bath salts, oils, powders, effervescent tablets, are preparations that may be used during the bath. Soap is used for its cleansing action on the body. Bath salts increase the cleansing action of soap, especially in hard water. Bath oils also tend to increase the cleansing action of soap. Effervescent tablets produce bubbles of carbon dioxide gas that have a mild stimulating effect on the body. Dusting powders, body oils and moisturizing lotions are used after the bath. Dusting powders impart fragrance and aid in drying the body. Body oils and moisturizing lotions help to lubricate the skin and replace natural oils lost during bathing. Following a hot bath or cabinet bath, a salt rub or Swedish shampoo may be given.

**Water Treatments**

The various procedures used in hydrotherapy may be classified as follows:

1. *Baths:* Practices whereby the body is surrounded by water, or vapor, such as in a whirlpool bath, cabinet bath, or Russian bath.
2. *Sprays:* The projection of one or more streams of water against the body, such as a shower bath or needle spray.
3. *Sponging:* The application of a liquid to the body by means of a sponge, a cloth, or the hand.
4. *Tonic friction:* The application of friction to the body with cold water so as to produce a stimulating or tonic effect.
5. *Shampoos:* Cleansing measures accomplished with water and soap, such as a Swedish shampoo.
6. *Whirlpool, jacuzzi, hot tubs:* These are usually large tubs equipped with apparatus that causes the water to flow in different directions. The main benefit derived from this type of bath or water treatment is relaxation.
7. *Special water treatments:* The use of compresses, water packs, and the like.

**Contraindications**

Water treatments should not be given when the client has cardiac impairment, diabetes, lung disease, kidney infection, extremely high or low blood pressure, acute Inflammation of joints, or an infectious skin condition. The client's physician should be consulted when any questionable condition exists.

**Body Reactions to Water Treatments**

Water treatments are based on the simple physical property of water; namely, that heat, cold, or pressure can be conveyed to many blood vessels and nerves in the skin. The effects of water on the body vary and whether the application is general or local in character. The circulation of the blood and the sensations produced by the many nerve endings in the skin can be greatly influenced by skillfully applied water treatments.

The average temperature of the skin surface is about 92 degrees Fahrenheit. Water approximating the temperature of the skin has no marked effect upon the body. If water at a temperature different from that of the skin is applied, it will either transfer heat or absorb heat from the body. The difference in temperature has a stimulating effect on the vast network of blood vessels and nerves in the skin. The greater the difference between the temperature of water and that of the skin, the greater is the stimulating effect of the treatment.

Each water application releases a series of definite reactions that are the result of the body accommodating itself to the new condition. The body reaction may be either stimulating or soothing to the circulatory system, the nervous system, and the eliminatory processes. The practitioner who uses hydrotherapy should be familiar with the specific effects of cold, hot, and warm applications on the body.

Cold applications are valuable in improving the circulation, stimulating the nerves, and awakening the functional activity of body cells. The prolonged use of cold applications is to be avoided, as they produce a depressing effect on the body.

***Effects of Cold Water***

The specific effects of water applications on the body are an immediate and temporary effect or a secondary and more lasting effect. The immediate effects of cold water applications are manifested in the following ways:

1. The skin is chilled.
2. Surface blood vessels contract and blood is driven to the interior of the body.
3. The flow of nerve force is partially interrupted.
4. The functional activity of body cells slows.

As soon as the cold application is discontinued, there occurs a secondary and more lasting effect in the body.

1. The skin becomes warmed and relaxed.
2. The surface blood vessels expand, bringing more blood to the skin.
3. The flow of nerve force is increased.
4. Adjacent body cells are stimulated in their functional activity.

***Effects of Hot Water***

The immediate effect of hot water applications is to draw the blood away from the interior and bring it to the surface temporarily. A secondary and more lasting effect occurs after the hot application is discontinued. Then the blood goes back to the interior of the body. Long and continued hot applications increase all skin functions and cause profuse sweating. Moderately warm applications have a relaxing effect on the blood vessels, muscles, and nerves, and promote the functional activity of body cells.

**Kinds of Baths**

All baths have for their aim the attainment of two objectives: external cleanliness and stimulation of skin functions.

Depending on the temperature of water, the following kinds of baths are available for use.

1. Cold bath (40 to 65 degrees Fahrenheit equal to 4.4 to 18.3 degrees Centigrade).
2. Cool bath (65 to 75 degrees Fahrenheit equal to 18.3 to 23.8 degrees Centigrade).
3. Tepid bath (85 to 95 degrees Fahrenheit equal to 29.4 to 35 degrees Centigrade).
4. Saline (salt) bath (90 to 94 degrees Fahrenheit equal to 32.2 to 35.5 degrees Centigrade).
5. Warm bath (95 to 100 degrees Fahrenheit equal to 35 to 37.7 degrees Centigrade).
6. Hot bath (100 to 110 degrees Fahrenheit equal to 37.7 to 43.3 degrees Centigrade).
7. Sitz or hip bath (either hot or cold).

Generally, the skin can tolerate hot water having a temperature of 110 degrees Fahrenheit. Above that temperature, water is injurious and may cause burns. However, the skin usually can tolerate steam vapor as high as 140 degrees Fahrenheit. It is important to consider the client's sensitivity and tolerance to heat or cold.

A reliable bath thermometer is required in order to judge water temperature accurately. The temperature reading is obtained by moving the thermometer about in the water.

**Cool Baths**

Whether a cold bath is beneficial depends on its duration and the state of vitality and reserve strength of the client. If after a cold bath or shower the client comes out chilly, shivering, blue-lipped, or goose-fleshed, it indicates that his or her body reaction is not good. For the client who experiences a pleasant reaction and a feeling of warmth, the cold bath may be safely continued. A short cold bath or cold sponging of the body may be better tolerated if it is accompanied by friction and gentle rubbing with a rough towel.

The average time exposure for a cold bath or shower should be limited from 3 to 5 minutes.

A cool bath provides a satisfactory temperature for all around bathing, particularly during warm weather. A tepid (slightly warm) bath exerts a soothing and relaxing effect on the body, and is recommended for nervous and excitable people.

**Saline (Salt) Bath**

A saline (salt) bath, at a temperature of 90 to 94 degrees Fahrenheit produces a marked tonic effect by stimulating the circulation. The effect is similar to natural bathing in sea water. The amount of common salt to use is 3 to 5 pounds to a tub of water. The client is left in the saline bath for 10 to 20 minutes.

**Hot or Warm Baths**

A warm or hot bath quiets tired nerves, soothes aching muscles, and helps to relieve insomnia. A cool shower should generally follow a warm bath because it forces some of the blood away from the skin, closes the pores, and leaves the body in a refreshed condition.

The warm or hot bath induces relaxation and relieves nervous tension. The hot bath is a popular method of weight reduction and should be used with caution. To accustom the body to the high temperature, first fill the tub with warm water then gradually add hot water until the desired temperature is reached. The average time for hot baths or showers should range from 5 to 10 minutes. The following safety precautions should also be observed by the practitioner:

Take the wrist pulse before and during the hot bath.

Give the client water to drink during the hot bath.

If the client complains of unpleasant reactions, place cold compresses over the forehead.

Very hot baths as well as very cold baths should be used only for clients who are in a healthy condition and who can withstand such treatments. For those clients whose health is not in the best condition, injurious effects may be produced. The hot bath or shower may give undue stimulation to the body and may overwork the heart. A cold bath or shower, on the other hand, is a tremendous shock to the nervous system.

### *Sitz Hip Bath*

The sitz or hip bath is applied only to the hips and pelvic region of the body, which is kept immersed in either hot, tepid, or cold water; or alternately hot and cold water. For a hot sitz bath, 5 to 10 minutes contact is usually sufficient. The time for a cold sitz bath varies from 3 to 5 minutes. The effects of a sitz bath depends primarily on the temperature of the water and its length of contact with the body. Generally, the sitz bath is given as a stimulant to the pelvic region. The temperature of the hot sitz is usually 105 to 115 degrees Fahrenheit.

Besides being effective in overcoming chronic constipation, sitz baths are also beneficial for the kidneys, bladder, and sex organs.

A large basin or bathtub is suitable for a sitz bath. The bath is prepared by filling the basin or tub with water (in the correct temperature) to about a depth of four inches or enough to immerse the client's buttocks comfortably. When using a basin (the feet outside) a blanket should be placed around the feet for warmth and a towel can be placed behind the knees for added comfort. The client sits in such a manner that the buttocks and upper thighs are immersed.

## SWEDISH SHAMPOO

A Swedish shampoo, or body shampoo, is really a cleansing bath applied over the entire body with the aid of a shampoo brush or bath mitt and soap and water. A good Swedish shampoo, when properly applied, does the following:

Loosens dead surface cells of the skin.

Promotes the growth of new skin cells.

Imparts a healthy radiance to the skin.

### Procedure for a Swedish Shampoo

#### *Preparation*

Apply warm water over the marble slab, then have the client lie down on his or her back on the slab. The practitioner begins with the arms, then proceeds to the fronts of the legs, chest, abdomen, backs of the legs, and back of the body.

1. Shampooing the Arm
   a. Apply sufficient soap to form a thick lather. Hold the client's left hand, and apply three long strokes over the entire surface of the arm.
   b. Using a brush, apply circular and frictional movements over the entire left arm, then use long strokes to brush the entire arm.
   c. Repeat the movements over the right arm.
2. Shampooing the Legs
   a. Apply sufficient soap on the brush to form a lather. Hold the client's leg just above the heel. Apply the brush in long strokes to the entire surface of the leg from foot to knee.
   b. Continuing with the brush, apply friction three times over the leg from foot to knee.

c. Lift the knee (by placing hand underneath bend of knee), and apply three strokes followed by friction over the entire surface from hip to knee.

d. Repeat the entire procedure on the other leg.

3. Shampooing the Chest and Abdomen

a. Apply soap by hand over the chest and abdomen (between and around the breasts).

b. With a brush apply gentle friction over the upper chest, between the breasts, and up the sides. Brush under the arm, down the side and across the abdomen to the other side. Brush up the side, under the arm, and down the side again.

c. Apply the brush in three long strokes over the center of the chest, down each side and across the abdomen.

d. Have the client change to a prone (face down) position.

4. Shampooing the Backs of the Legs

a. Apply sufficient soap to the brush to form a thick lather.

b. Lift the left foot at the ankle, and brush the sole of the foot, using three strokes over the entire surface.

c. Using the brush, apply friction over the same area.

d. Lift the knee by placing a hand underneath the kneecap. Apply the brush in three long strokes over the entire surface from heel to hip. Apply the brush with friction over the same area.

e. Apply three long strokes over the same area from heel to hip.

f. Repeat the same procedures over the back of the right leg.

5. Shampooing the Back of the Body

a. Apply soap with the hands over the entire back.

b. Apply the brush over the spine and down, then up the sides (three times) using long strokes.

c. Using the brush, apply friction three times over the same area of the back and sides of the body, then apply three long strokes over the lower part of the back.

6. Finishing the Body Shampoo

Apply warm or cool shower or spray to remove all traces of shampoo from the client's body. Dry the body thoroughly then apply dusting powder and body oil. Allow the client to rest on a comfortable surface (massage table) for about 30 minutes before leaving.

**SALT RUB**

A salt rub is a frictional application of wet salt over the client's body. It may be given as a separate treatment or after any hot bath or cabinet bath. The benefits of a salt rub are derived chiefly from its stimulation of the circulation and its tonic value to the body. This treatment should be recommended only to clients who can withstand a high degree of stimulation. The salt rub should not be given if there is any indication of skin disease or open wounds.

**Procedure for a Salt Rub**

Have two to three pounds of salt and all other supplies and equipment ready before the client arrives. Adjust the room to a comfortable temperature, and apply warm water over the slab just before having the client lie on it in a supine position.

The treatment begins with the arms then proceeds to the legs, chest, abdomen, and finally to the back of the body.

***Procedure***

1. Application to the Arm
   a. Moisten the salt slightly, and apply it over the client's arm from the hand to the shoulder.
   b. Using both hands, rub salt quickly into the skin going three times up and down over the entire surface of the arm.
   c. Apply three long strokes up and down over the same area.
   d. Repeat the entire procedure over the other arm.
2. Application to Legs
   a. Moisten the salt slightly then apply it from ankle to hip. Using both hands, rub the salt quickly into the skin, going three times up and down, covering the entire front surface of the leg.
   b. Apply three long strokes, over the same area.
   c. Repeat the procedure over the other leg.
3. Application to Chest and Abdomen
   a. Moisten the salt slightly, then apply it over chest and abdomen.
   b. Using both hands, rub salt quickly into the skin covering the entire surface of the chest (except the breasts) then the entire surface of the abdomen.
   c. Apply three long strokes from chest to abdomen.
4. Application to Back
   a. Have the client change to a prone position.
   b. Moisten the salt slightly then apply it over the entire back, from top of shoulders to buttocks.
   c. Using both hands, rub salt quickly into the skin over the entire surface.
   d. Apply three long strokes over the same area.
5. Final Steps
   a. Apply a warm then cool shower or spray to remove all traces of salt from the client's body, then dry the body thoroughly.
   b. Apply dusting powder and body oil.
   c. Allow the client to rest on a comfortable surface (massage table) for about 30 minutes before leaving.

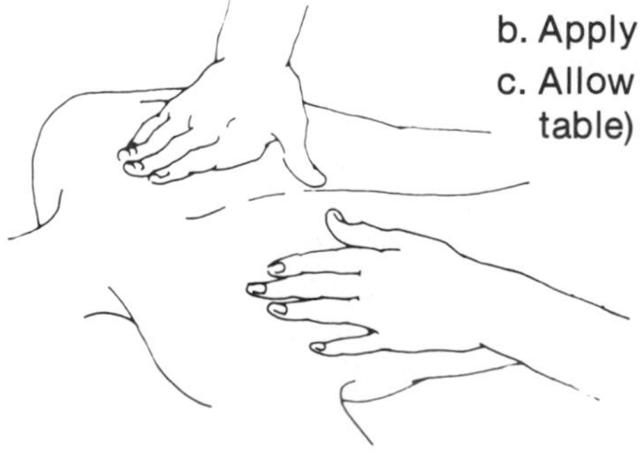

## CABINET BATHS

Bath cabinets are also known as vapor or steam cabinets, electric bath cabinets, and electric light cabinets. As used in body massage treatments, they are constructed in an upright or reclining position to accommodate the client's body while leaving the head exposed. When in operation, heat is generated and warm, moist air surrounds the client's body. The heat, besides having a relaxing effect on the client, induces profuse perspiration that contributes to weight reduction. The intensity and duration of the heat can be controlled by a switch for low, medium, or high heat, and by an automatic time clock. At the discretion of the practitioner, heat (dry, moist, or both) and therapeutic lights (ultraviolet or infrared rays) can be used separately or in conjuction. The manufacturer's instructions are the most reliable guide for the proper use and care of the bath cabinet.

Not all clients react the same way to the cabinet bath. Knowing the condition and tolerance of the client is of assistance in controlling the temperature and duration of this treatment. A client in a weakened or nervous condition should be given gentle treatments of short duration until improvement is shown. Always consult a physician before administering cabinet baths for a client with a systemic disorder such as heart trouble, high blood pressure, or any severe illness.

### Length of Treatment

The exposure time in a cabinet bath ranges from 10 to 15 minutes. During this time, the practitioner should attend to the comfort and safety of the client and not to his or her reactions to the heat treatment. The client's heat tolerance will be greater if there is a gradual rise in the temperature of the bath cabinet. Postpone treatment if the client is ill, has an abnormal pulse or body temperature, and reacts unfavorably to the treatment.

The heat treatment induces profuse perspiration. To replace the water lost and also to prevent body weakness, the practitioner should give mild saline drinks to the client at periodic intervals. If the client complains of a headache or a throbbing in the head during the treatment, cold compresses can be applied.

Following the cabinet bath, a mild tonic such as a tepid shower, a Swedish shampoo, or salt rub followed by a tepid shower may be given. After this treatment, keep the client warmly wrapped to prevent chilling of the body.

## WHIRLPOOL BATH

A whirlpool bath is a partial immersion bath in which the water is agitated to produce a slight pressure on the body. A whirlpool bath is beneficial to circulation, soothing to the muscles, and relaxing to the nerves. Whirlpool baths are often used by physicians as part of physical therapy for conditions such as arthritis, sprains, strained muscles, and relief of pain. List of supplies and equipment needed:

1. Whirlpool tub.
2. Bath mats and towels.

3. Robe and sandals (disposable paper sandals).
4. Lotion or oil.
5. Bath thermometer.
6. Ice bag (optional).
7. Material for cold compress, if needed.
8. Tank suits for women and trunks for men.

**Procedure**

1. Fill the whirlpool tub to the recommended depth and test the temperature. Generally, the most desirable temperature is about 105 to 110 degrees Fahrenheit, but the bath may be cooler.
2. Add the recommended antiseptic agents to the water.
3. Instruct the client in how to safely enter the tub.
4. The treatment time is usually about 15 to 30 minutes.
5. Instruct the client about rest period, showers, and drying off.
6. Complete the client's records noting benefits, reactions, effects, etc.
7. Be sure the tub is sanitized thoroughly before it is used again.

**FRICTION BATH**

The friction bath is given with terry towels, friction, or loofah mitts and applications of cold water. This treatment is beneficial in that it stimulates circulation and metabolism. List of supplies and equipment needed:

1. Bath towels.
2. Bath blankets.
3. Loofah or friction mitts.
4. Cold water and appropriate basin (temperature between 40 and 75 degrees Fahrenheit.

**Procedure**

1. Be sure the room is at a comfortable temperature.
2. Explain the procedure to the client. Have client lie face down on a bath blanket.
3. Keep the client's body covered except for the area being treated.
4. Apply friction movements first to the arms. Wring the towel or mitts out in the water then briskly rub the part for 5 to 10 seconds. Be aware of sensitivity of the client's skin, and do not apply excessive pressure that may cause pain.
5. Dry the part with a towel while applying light friction movements.
6. Cover the finished part and proceed to the next. Generally, you will do the arms and legs then the back and chest areas.
7. Following the treatment, be sure the client is warm and dry. Allow a short rest period following the friction bath.
8. Keep a complete record of the friction treatments, and note benefits or any adverse reactions.

**RELAXING NEUTRAL TUB BATH**

The neutral tub bath is basically for relaxation and has a sedative effect. The body is immersed in a tub of water at a neutral temperature (about 94 to 98 degrees Fahrenheit) for about 15 to 25 minutes. List of supplies and equipment needed:

1. Bath tub and bath thermometer.
2. Bath towels and mat.
3. Shower cap, robe, and slippers for client.
4. Bath oil and lotion.
5. Bath sheets.
6. Compress cloth and basin of cool water.
7. Air pillow and towel.

**Procedure**

1. Check the room temperature to be sure it is comfortable for the client.
2. Lubricate the client's skin with oil or lotion.
3. Fill the tub to the appropriate level.
4. Test the temperature of the water to be sure its comfortable. A recommended range is 94 to 98 degrees Fahrenheit.
5. Assist the client into the tub, and place an air pillow or towel underneath his or her head.
6. Cover the client's body with a large towel or bath sheet.
7. Allow the client to relax for 15 to 25 minutes. Warm water may be added if desired.
8. Assist the client out of the tub, and dry his or her body with a towel while applying light friction.
9. Supply the client with robe and slippers.
10. Allow the client time to rest. Complete the client's records noting benefits of the bath or any adverse reactions. Be sure the tub is sanitized thoroughly before the next bath.

**THE RUSSIAN BATH**

The Russian bath is a full body steam bath for the purpose of causing perspiration. The primary benefits are cleansing, relaxation, and improved metabolism. List of supplies and equipment needed:

1. Steam room with a slab or table for reclining.
2. Padding and bath sheet for slab.
3. Towels for neck and protection.
4. Air pillow with a towel to cover.
5. Shower cap to protect hair.
6. Robe and slippers.
7. Fomentation cloth for wrapping the feet and to place underneath the curve of the spine.
8. Compress cloth and basin of cool water.
9. Pitcher and glass of drinking water.
10. Appropriate product to add to the bath.

**Procedure**

1. Prepare the steam room for the desired temperature. Usually this is 110 to 120 degrees Fahrenheit.
2. Take and record the client's pulse and temperature.
3. Have the client lie on the slab, and place the fomentation cloth underneath the curve of the spine. Adjust the pillow underneath the client's head.
4. Wrap the feet with the fomentation cloth.
5. Cover the client with a large towel or bath sheet.
6. Apply a cool compress to the head if desired.
7. Check pulse as necessary.
8. Give client instructions about drinking water during treatment.
9. Allow the client to relax 5 to 15 minutes.
10. Assist the client in drying off following the steam bath.
11. Allow the client to rest following the treatment.
12. Complete the client's records. Record the pulse, temperature, reactions, etc.

**QUESTIONS FOR DISCUSSION AND REVIEW**

1. Name the three rays used in body treatments.
2. What basic effects do blue, white, or red lights produce?
3. When should light rays not be used?
4. What are the main benefits of vibratory massage?
5. What are the concerns of the practitioner when advising a client about suntanning?
6. Define hydrotherapy.
7. How are the effects of water treatments controlled?
8. In which three ways are cold applications beneficial?
9. When are cold applications undesirable?
10. What are the benefits of hot water applications?
11. How high a temperature can the skin safely tolerate?
12. What is the average duration of a cold bath, cold shower, or cold sitz bath?
13. What is the average duration of a hot saline or sitz bath?
14. What is a Swedish shampoo?
15. When is a salt rub usually given?
16. What is the purpose of the cabinet bath?
17. What safety precautions should be observed during the operation of a bath cabinet?
18. What are the main benefits of a whirlpool bath?

## ANSWERS TO QUESTIONS FOR DISCUSSION AND REVIEW

1. The three rays used in body treatments are visible light, ultraviolet, and infrared rays.
2. White light relieves minor aches and pain; red light is stimulating and penetrating; blue light is soothing to the nerves and has a tonic effect on the skin.
3. Light rays should not be used when any condition exists that requires medical attention. Examples are varicose veins, skin disease, diabetes, heart, or respiratory problems and the like.
4. The main benefits of vibratory massage are stimulation of the circulatory system, relaxation of muscular tension, toning of the skin, and relief of minor aches and pains.
5. The practitioner's main concern when advising a client about suntanning is that he or she acquires the suntan in the most safe and healthful manner. The practitioner must be concerned about his or her own responsibility when operating or supervising suntanning equipment.
6. Hydrotherapy is the science of water treatments for external application to the body.
7. Water treatments are controlled by regulating the temperature, duration, and intensity of treatment.
8. Cold applications are beneficial because they improve circulation, stimulate nerves, and increase the activity of body cells.
9. Cold applications are undesirable over prolonged periods as they may produce a depressing effect.
10. Hot water applications improve skin functions by promoting perspiration and by increasing the circulation of blood to the surface of the skin.
11. The skin can safely tolerate 110 degrees Fahrenheit of hot water and approximately 140 degrees Fahrenheit of steam vapor.
12. The average duration of a cold bath, shower or sitz bath is approximately 3 to 5 minutes.
13. The duration of a hot saline or sitz bath is approximately 10 to 20 minutes.
14. A Swedish shampoo is a cleansing body bath applied with the aid of a brush or bath mitt, and mild soap and warm water followed by rinsing and drying the body.
15. A salt rub is usually given following a hot bath or cabinet bath, or it may be given as a separate treatment.
16. The purpose of a cabinet bath is to induce perspiration that contributes to a weight reduction, and to induce relaxation. It is also considered to be a cleansing procedure.
17. Safety precautions to observe during the operation of a bath cabinet include following the manufacturer's instructions for use of the cabinet, observing the client's general reactions, state of health and tolerance to temperature.
18. The main benefits of a whirlpool bath are increased blood circulation, the soothing of muscles and relaxing of the nerves.

# Chapter 13 Massage for Nursing and Healthcare

**LEARNING OBJECTIVES**

After you have mastered this chapter you will be able to:

1. Explain the benefits of massage as given by nurses and other healthcare professionals.
2. Explain why a patient's physician is consulted before massage is included in a patient's care.
3. Explain how massage aids in healing and convalescence.
4. Give a brief review of Swedish massage movements and the benefits of the various movements.
5. Explain the main contraindications for massage.
6. Demonstrate basic massage movements.
7. Demonstrate joint movements used in conjunction with massage.
8. Explain the difference between centripetal and centrifugal movements.
9. Demonstrate a step-by-step massage.
10. Demonstrate an alcohol or oil rubdown.
11. Demonstrate how to take a client's or patient's medical history.
12. Explain when and why a mini-massage might be recommended.

**INTRODUCTION**

Health education is an essential component of nursing. Nurses and other healthcare professionals are involved not only in helping to restore their patients to health but also in teaching them how to live as healthy and productive a life as possible. In addition to assisting the physician, nurses and other healthcare assistants provide many other invaluable services in hospitals and healthcare facilities.

Nurses are employed in industry, research, education, private practices and in hospitals. Although nurses work under the supervision of physicians, they are called upon to assess the daily needs of their patients and to encourage them to participate in their own recovery. The mental attitude of the patient has a great deal to do with the individual's successful recovery and rehabilitation.

Patients need the healing touch of their physicians and nurses as much as they may need the right medication. Touching an area of the patient's body can help the nurse to note changes in body temperature and pick up other clues to the patient's state of health.

A good rubdown or massage does much to help the patient, both physically and mentally.

## MASSAGE AS A THERAPEUTIC AID IN NURSING PRACTICE

Massage is one of the most beneficial services for patients during convalescence. Exercise and massage are often prescribed as a means of restoring the patient's fitness and sense of well-being. Swedish massage movements are most frequently used by nurses. The basic movements (manipulations) are effleurage, petrissage, and friction.

*Effleurage,* the light or heavy rubbing or stroking of the skin surface helps to stimulate the circulation of blood, relieves tension and tones muscles.

*Petrissage* is the squeezing and deep kneading of the superficial fascia and underlying muscles. Compression movements require a squeezing and rubbing action over the skin and its underlying structures. *Friction* and *vibration* are also included in this classification and are particularly useful in stimulating the flow of blood and lymph and in preventing sore, stiff muscles. The nurse may use chucking, rolling, and wringing movements (variations of friction) when appropriate. *Wringing* requires the flesh to be grasped firmly and squeezed gently as one would squeeze moisture from a cloth. *Rolling* is done by compressing the tissues against the bone and moving back and forth.

*Percussion* (tapping with fingertips or hands) is done gently on the back, shoulders, arms, and legs to bring blood to the surface and to tone muscles.

In nursing, general massage consisting of basic movements or manipulations to increase the psychological and physiological wellbeing of the patient may be recommended. There are also specialized treatments in which the nurse is called upon to deal with some abnormal condition affecting the patient's body systems. In the case of specialized massage, the patient's physician may assign therapy procedures to a physiotherapist who is trained to work with nurses and physicians. The use of exercise, massage, electrotherapy, hydrotherapy, and related techniques that may be used in the treatment of specific diseases and injuries. For example, a sprained ankle may require special care, such as a heat or ice treatment, before massage.

Massage is valuable in the treatment of injuries to bones and joints and is prescribed in a wide range of conditions. Massage is used in some cases to treat nervous fatigue, insomnia, headache, tension, stress, and other disorders.

The nurse or healthcare practitioner should have a thorough understanding of anatomy and physiology in order to determine the effects of various massage manipulations on the functions of the body's organs and systems. It is important to know when the patient will benefit from massage and when there are contraindications.

Nurses and other healthcare professionals are expected to practice the same code of ethics as other massage practitioners. They must have the same concern for the patient's comfort, privacy, and self-esteem. The main difference between nurses and massage practitioners is that nurses deal with patients who have a health problem or injury that requires hospital and physician care. The massage practitioner may also work under the supervision of a physician but may be employed in a salon, health facility, or sports complex. Many athletic organizations employ massage practitioners to travel with a team of professional athletes. Many industrial or business organizations employ a doctor, nurse, and massage practitioner as part of their staff. The massage practitioner usually works in an environment where massage is part of a client's regimen for keeping fit and healthy rather than as an aid to recovery from disease or injury.

In nursing and healthcare, massage is used as part of the physiological and psychological rehabilitation process. When a person becomes ill or is injured, it is common to feel a sense of apprehension, insecurity, and anxiety, which often leads to restlessness and insomnia. A good massage will increase the patient's comfort, induce relaxation, and help to relieve anxiety. When a patient is confined to bed for a period of convalescence, muscles lose their tone, joints become stiff, and skin develops sensitivity. Unless a patient is turned or is able to move, bedsores may develop. Massage helps to prevent these problems.

In addition to increasing the patient's comfort, massage aids healing by increasing the number of white and red blood cells and by improving circulation, which in turn nourishes the tissues. Massage, when done correctly, improves the action of lymph so that toxins are carried away. It also helps to promote blood supply to the brain and nerves so that the patient feels more in control of his or her faculties. Massage is used as an aid to preventing constipation by improving the peristaltic action of the small intestines and colon. There are numerous ways in which massage has been found to benefit patients of all ages, and many doctors recommend it as an aid to a speedier recovery.

Massage also has a place in the maintenance of good health. It acts as a stimulant or as a sedative for the nervous system and aids in the metabolic process and glandular activity. Because the skin is an organ of respiration and elimination, massage improves these functions. As the vascomotor system becomes more active, the skin is better nourished and both tone and elasticity are improved. The following is a brief review of some of the therapeutic benefits of massage to body systems.

**Benefits of Massage**

Massage benefits the circulatory system by:
Helping to develop a stronger heart.
Improving oxygen supply to cells.
Improving the supply of nutrients to cells.
Elimination of metabolic wastes.
Decreasing blood pressure.
Increasing circulation of lymph.

Massage benefits the digestive system by:
Relaxing the abdominal and intestinal muscles.
Relieving tension.
Stimulating activity of liver and kidneys.
Elimination of waste material.

Massage benefits the muscular system by:
Relaxing or stimulating muscles.
Strengthening muscles and connective tissue.
Helping to keep muscles flexible and pliable.
Relieving soreness, tension, and stiffness.

Massage benefits the nervous system by:
Stimulating motor nerve points.
Relieving restlessness and insomnia.
Promoting a sense of well-being.
Relieving pain.

Massage benefits the respiratory system by:
Developing respiratory muscles.
Assisting in proper breathing.

Massage benefits the lymph system by:
Cleansing the body of metabolic wastes.
Draining sluggish lymph nodes.

Massage benefits the integumentary system (the skin) by:
Stimulating blood to better nourish skin.
Improving tone and elasticity of skin.
Helping to normalize glandular functions.

Massage benefits the skeletal system by:
Improving body alignment.
Relieving stiff joints.
Relieving tired, aching feet.

**Contraindications**

The nurse or healthcare assistant does not apply massage in cases of illness or injury without the supervision or permission of the patient's physician.

## REVIEW OF SWEDISH MASSAGE MOVEMENTS USED IN NURSING

Effleurage or stroking movements are done with slow, even pressure toward the heart. This increases lymph flow and circulation of the blood, thus increasing capillary and arterial circulation. Effleurage is called centripetal stroking because the movement is given in the direction of the lymph and venous blood stream. When effleurage is applied to reflex areas of the body, related organs are stimulated. It is important to understand which organs are principally affected by massage.

The better the circulation of blood to the extremities, the more oxygen is made available to tissues and the more efficiently wastes are removed from the cells.

Effleurage over muscles can assist in dilating blood vessels, allowing more blood to flow into the area. After surgery when movement is limited to a specific area or where there has been prolonged muscle strain, massage is beneficial in loosening tight muscle fibers and restoring motion to the affected part.

Petrissage or kneading movements are done on the muscles by wringing, squeezing, pressing, and lifting. These movements are never done so firmly as to cause pain. The hands are used to manipulate large areas and the fingers and thumbs for small areas. Petrissage is primarily used to stimulate action of sebaceous (oil) glands and sudoriferous (sweat) glands.

Friction movements are achieved by applying pressure and making straight or circular movements with the hands or just the fingertips. Friction is used to warm tissues and is done over bony areas as well as larger groups of muscles. It is especially valuable in improving functioning of muscles and nerves. Circular friction is used to stimulate blood to the surface of the skin to nourish tissues. Gentle circular movements are used on bony areas.

Tapotement or percussion movements include tapping, slapping, hacking, patting, and beating. These movements should not be done so firmly as to cause pain. The movements are done on large, muscular and fleshy areas of the body to stimulate nerves and reflex areas.

Shaking, vibrating, and trembling movements are done with a degree of pressure on the area of the body to be massaged. For example, when light pressure and vibration are applied to the abdominal region, the internal organs are affected by reflex action.

## CONTRAINDICATIONS FOR MASSAGE IN NURSING AND HEALTHCARE

Unlike the practitioner who deals with healthy clients, the nurse or other healthcare professional deals with people who are ill or injured, or recovering. The stage of the person's illness or injury will often determine the extent that massage might be given beneficially, or if it should be given at all. It is important to be sure massage is approved by the patient's physician.

The use of external heat and stimulation of the tissues by massage bring more fluid, blood, nutrients, and oxygen to affected areas of the body, but there are times when massage must not be given to or near an affected part. The patient's physician will note deterioration of muscles or skin that could be benefitted by massage and will also be aware of contraindications for massage. The following is a general review of contraindications:

Bleeding—internal or external.

Skin problems such as rashes, growths, lesions.

Newly formed scar tissue, scabs, wounds and burns.

Infections, swollen areas, pain, inflammation, heat in the area.

Nausea, vomiting, and fever.

Edema—Excessive lymph fluid often causes swelling in feet and legs, particularly in elderly people. Sometimes the physician will recommend gentle effleurage in the direction of the lymphatic flow to help relieve this condition.

Varicose veins—High blood pressure and being on the feet for many hours (as in some occupations) are the main reasons a person develops varicose veins. Veins in the legs become dilated and lengthen due to increased blood pressure. In mild cases, massage may be done on nearby areas but not directly on the affected part.

Inflammed joints such as arthritis and bursitis—Massage is not done on the area when it is painful and inflamed.

Cancer—When any symptom of cancer is detected or if any condition is suspicious of cancer, massage is avoided on or near the area.

The following are a few symptoms that are associated with cancer and are contraindications for massage:

Any sore that has not healed normally.

A mole or skin tag.

Lumps underneath the arms or in the breasts.

Persistent hoarseness, coughing, or sore throat.

Abnormal functioning of any internal organ, such as changes in the bladder or bowels.

Discharge or bleeding from any part of the body.

## Basic Massage Procedures

### *Effleurage—Stroking Movements*

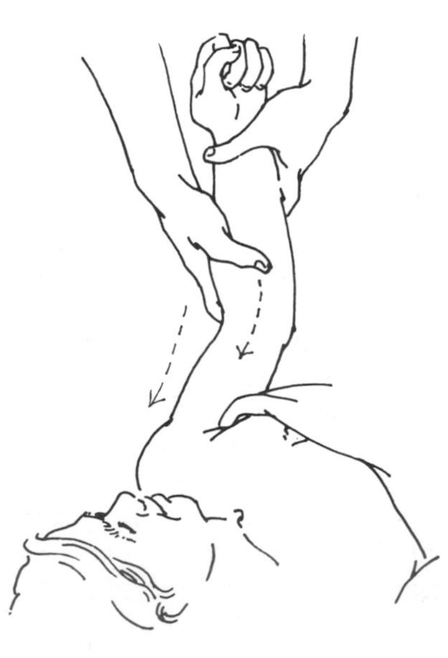

*Direction of effleurage and position of arm. The same upward movement is applied when massaging the back of the arm.*

*Direction of effleurage to inner thigh and position of the hands. The same upward movements are applied when massaging the back of the leg.*

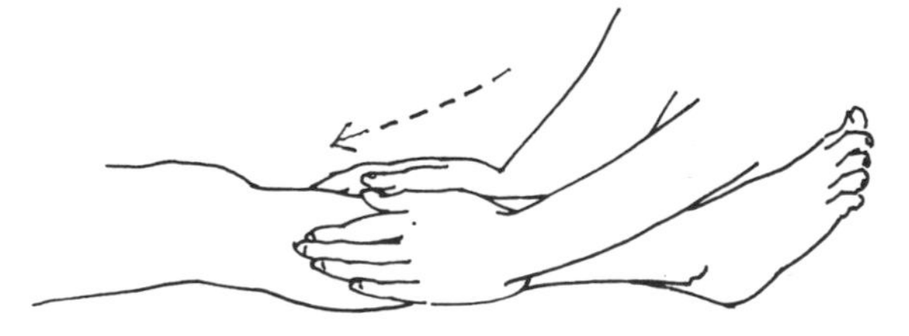

*Direction of effleurage on the lower leg. The same upward movements are applied when massaging the back of the lower leg.*

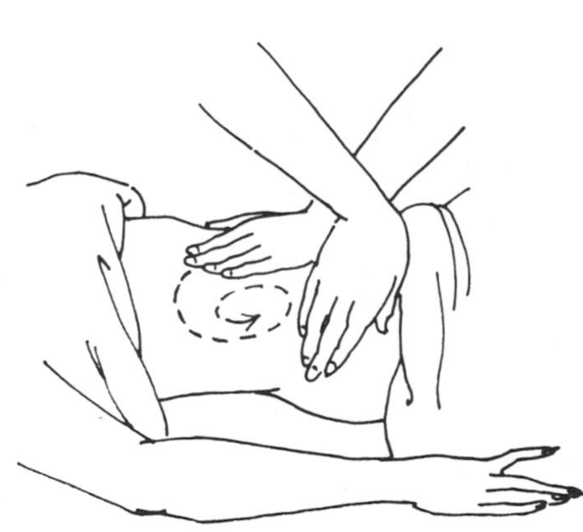

*Deep circular movements are applied to the abdomen.*

*Effleurage is applied to the center of the chest, and underarms in upward then downward strokes.*

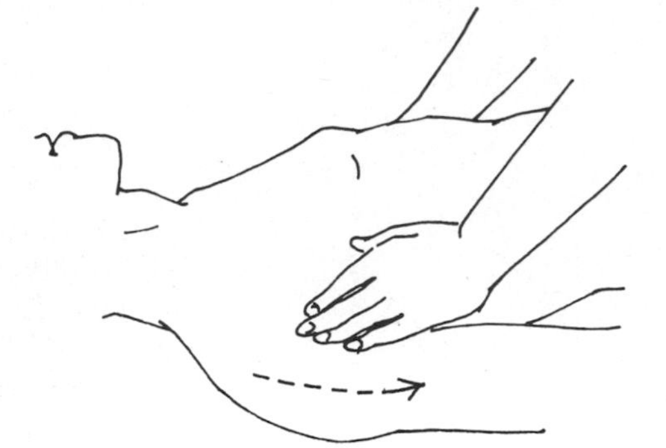

*Effleurage is applied to the shoulders moving upward on the sides of the neck and back down the back of the shoulders and across the chest.*

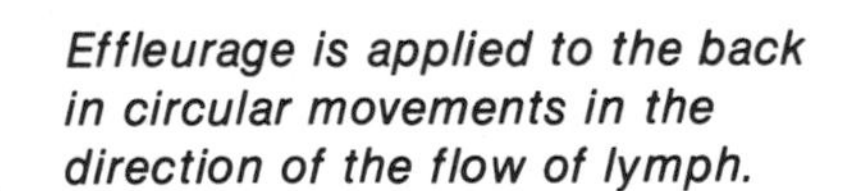

*Effleurage is applied to the back in circular movements in the direction of the flow of lymph.*

Effleurage movements may be done in the sequence most suitable for the individual.

**Petrissage—Kneading**

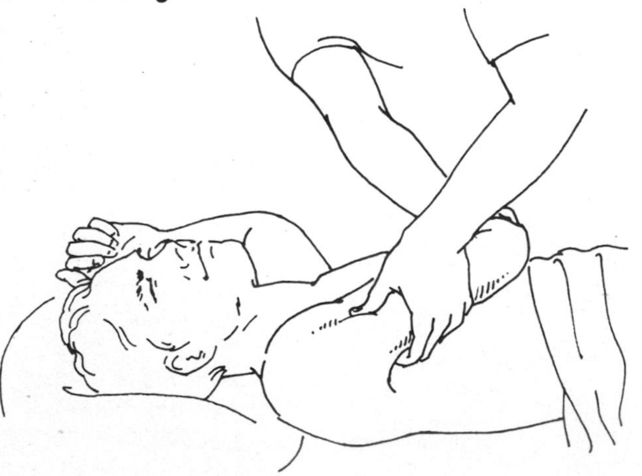

*Petrissage to the triceps.*

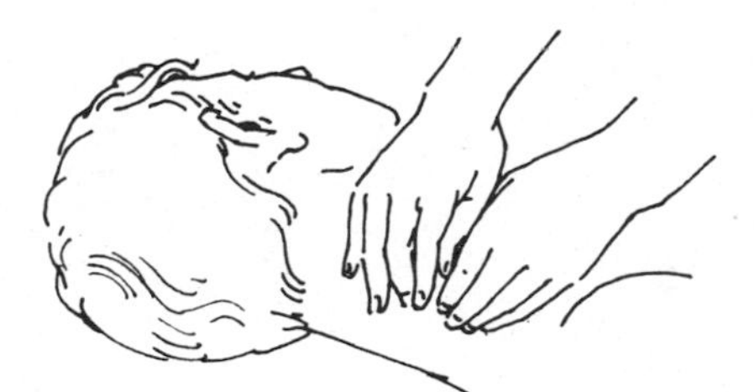

*Petrissage to back of neck and shoulder region.*

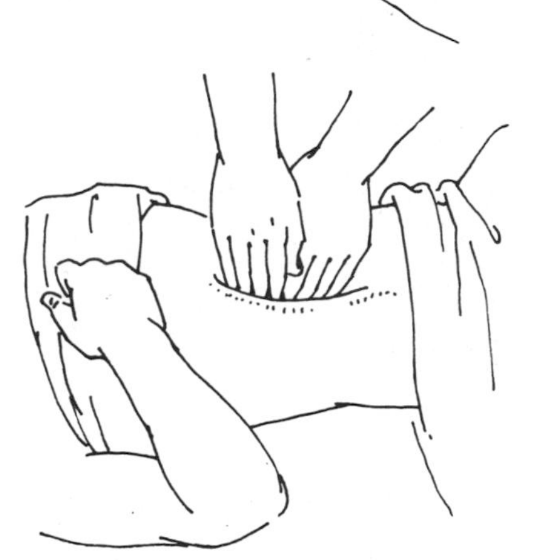

*Petrissage to the abdomen applying downward kneading movements.*

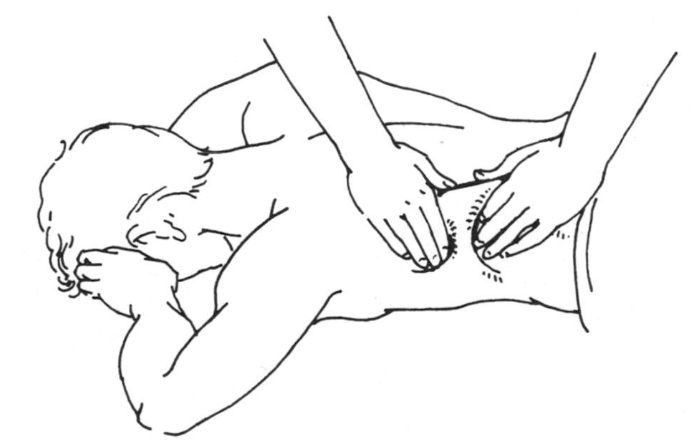

*Petrissage to muscles of the back.*

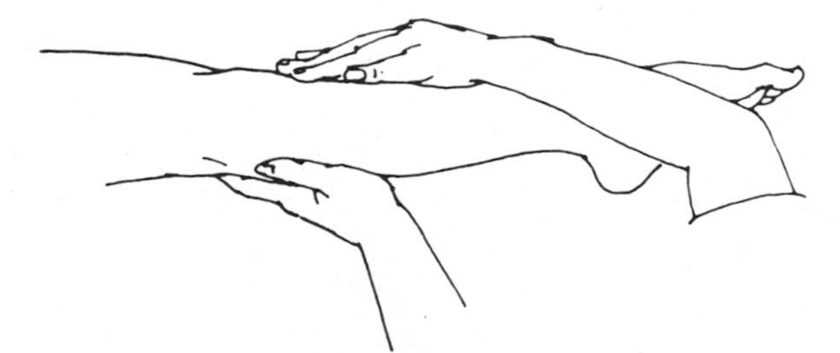

*Circular kneading of muscles of the leg and thigh.*

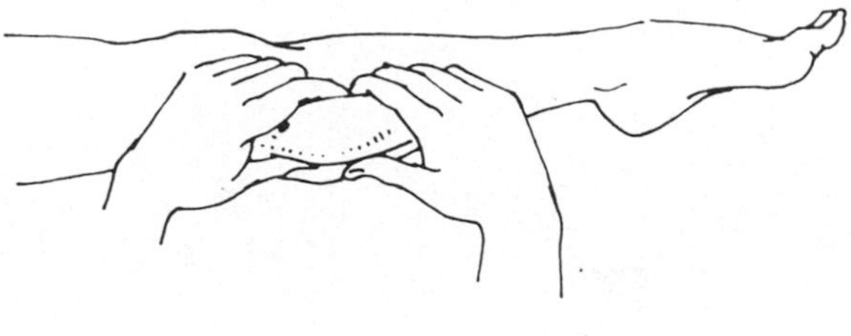

*Kneading of calf muscles.*

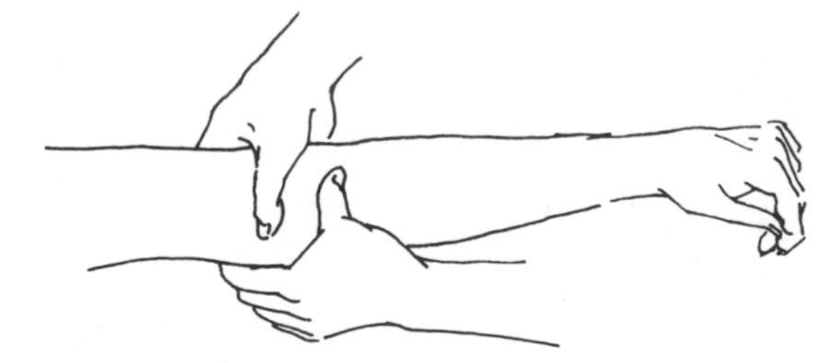

*Wringing the arm.*

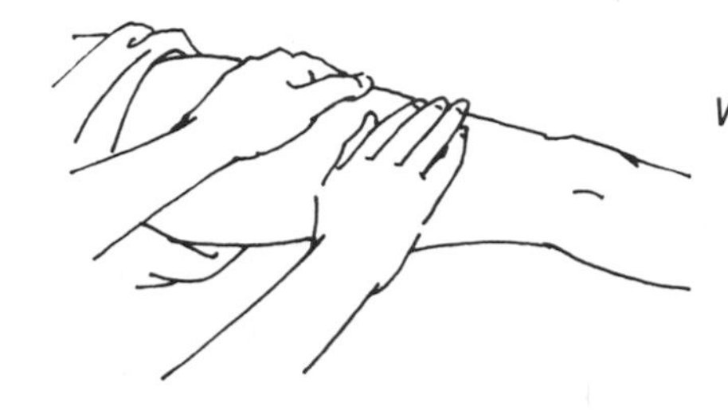

*Wringing muscles of thigh.*

Petrissage should be done carefully. Adjust pressure to the patient's needs. Petrissage should be done in the most suitable sequence. Painful areas of the body should be avoided.

***Friction—Circular***

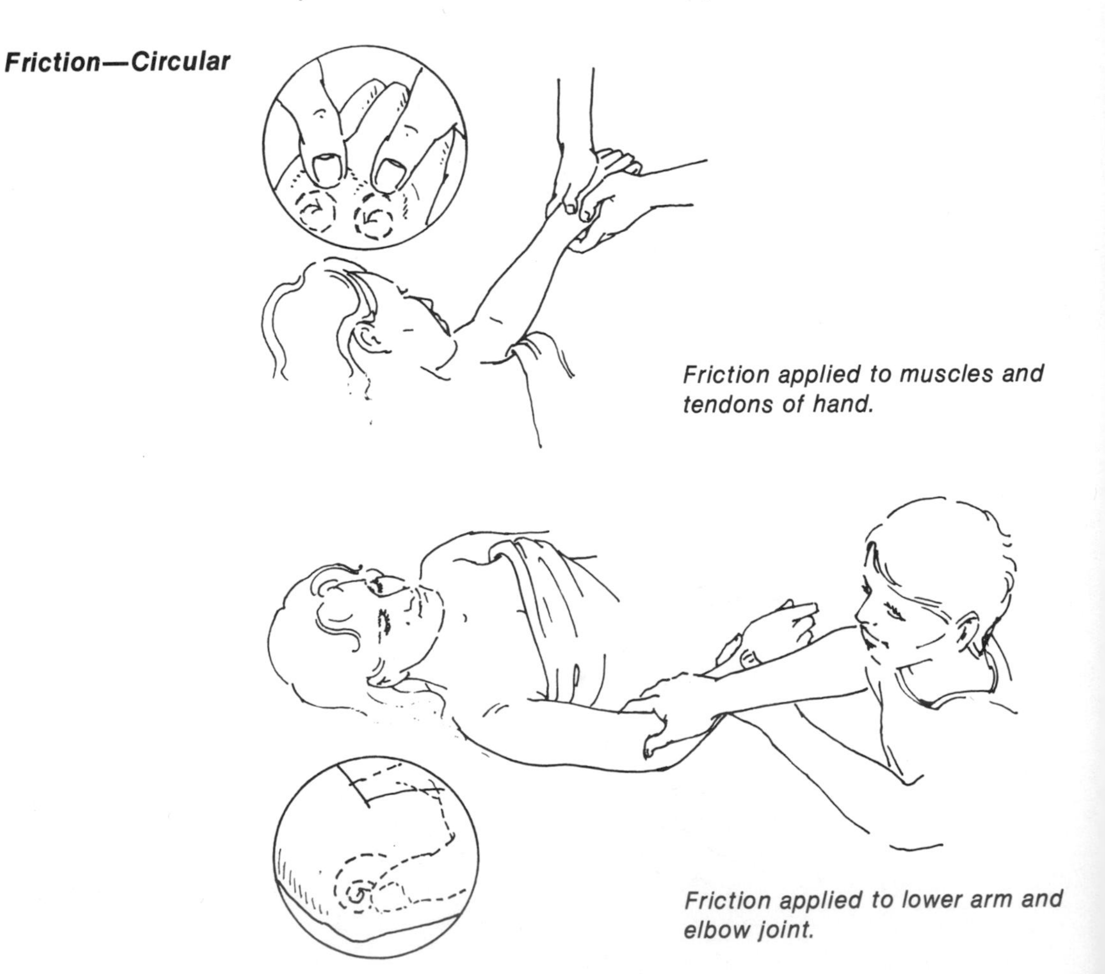

*Friction applied to muscles and tendons of hand.*

*Friction applied to lower arm and elbow joint.*

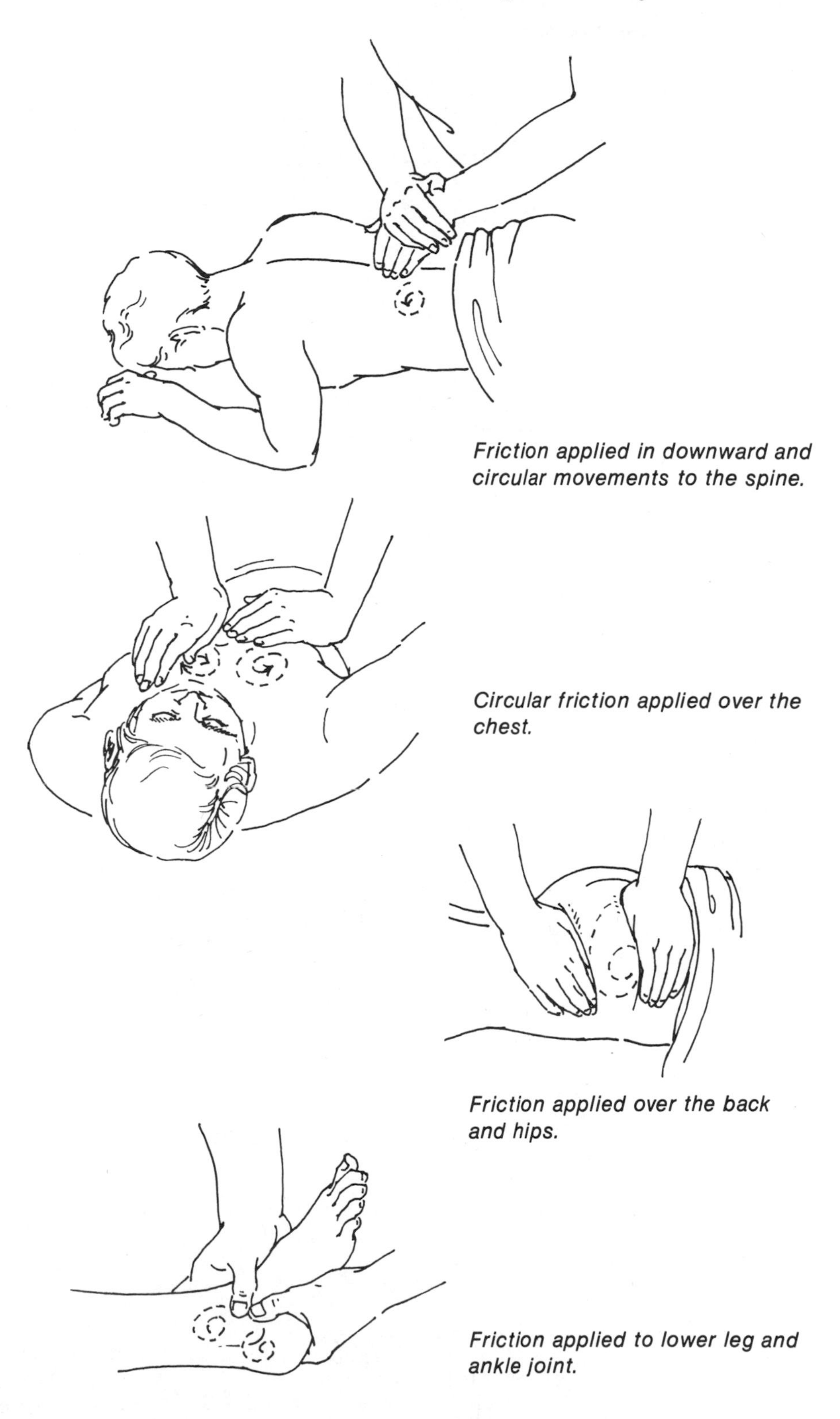

*Friction applied in downward and circular movements to the spine.*

*Circular friction applied over the chest.*

*Friction applied over the back and hips.*

*Friction applied to lower leg and ankle joint.*

Circular friction may be applied in the sequence most appropriate for the patient's needs.

### *Percussion*

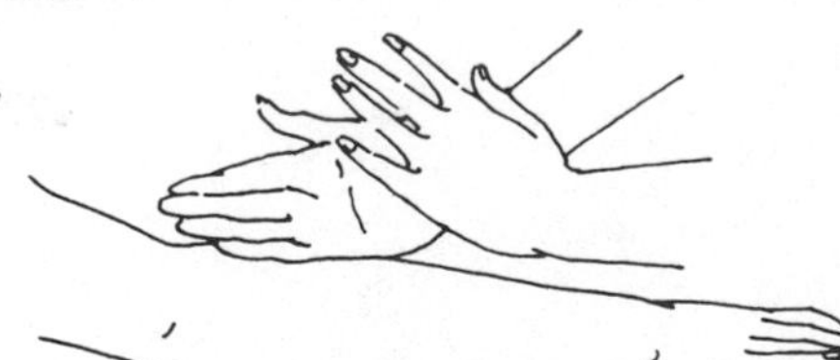

*Hacking movements are applied to the arm muscles with alternating (little finger) sides of the hands.*

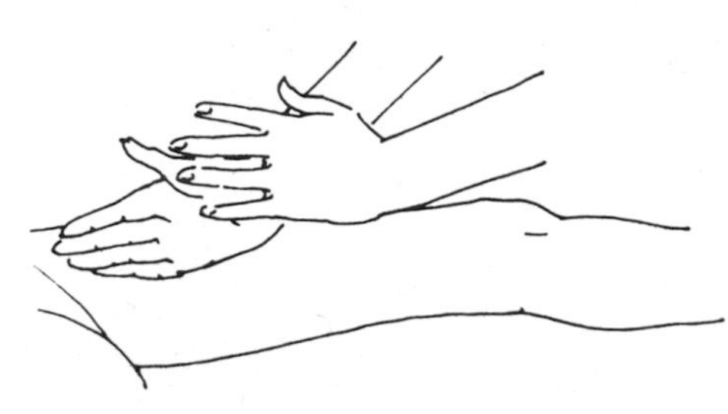

*Hacking movements are applied to thigh muscles with alternating sides of the hands.*

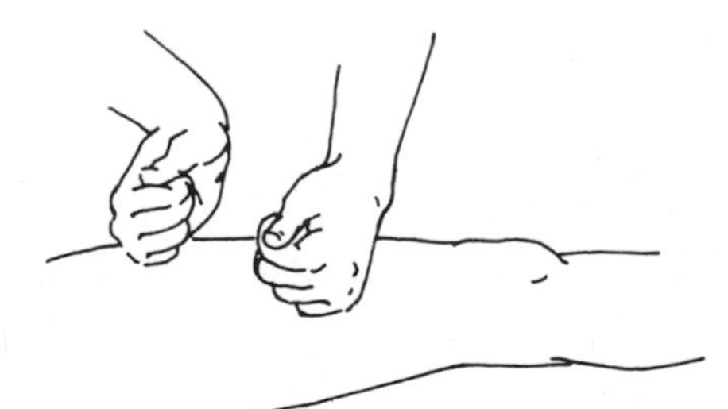

*Beating movements are applied to the thigh muscles with hands alternating in a loose fist position.*

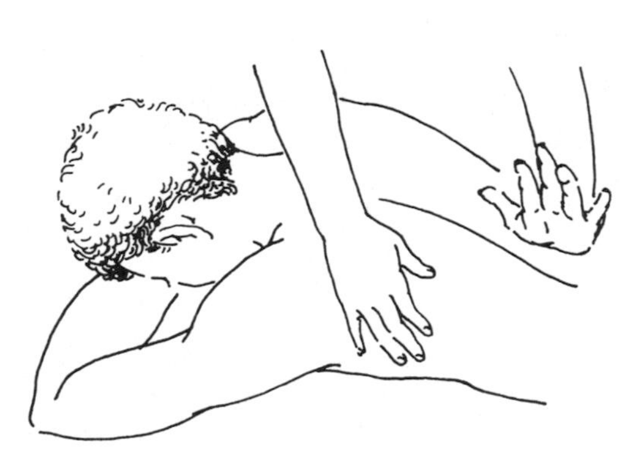

*Hacking movements are appied to the back muscles with alternating sides of the hands.*

*Beating movements are applied to the back muscles with the closed fist of one hand moving against the other hand that is held flat against the patient's back.*

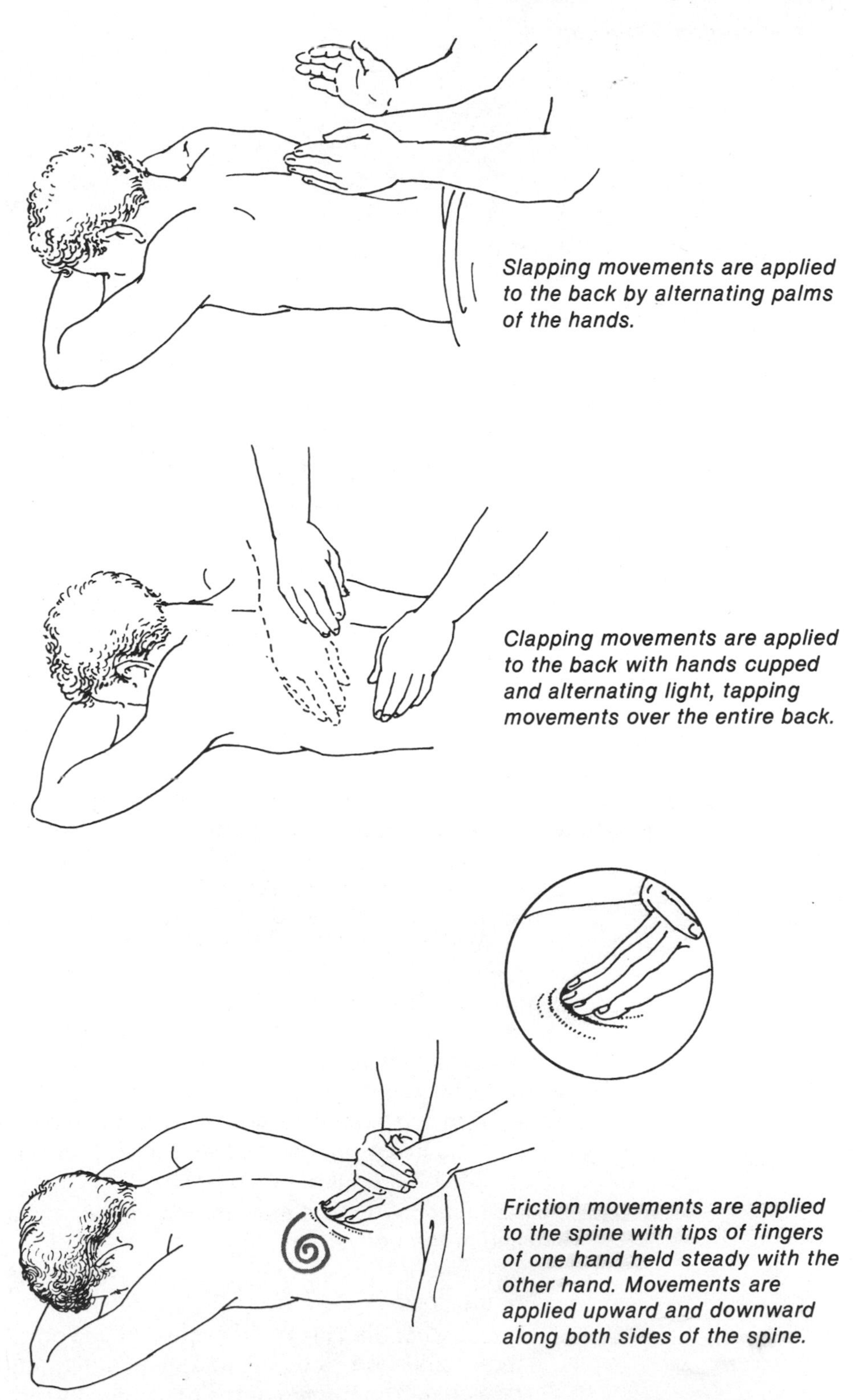

*Slapping movements are applied to the back by alternating palms of the hands.*

*Clapping movements are applied to the back with hands cupped and alternating light, tapping movements over the entire back.*

*Friction movements are applied to the spine with tips of fingers of one hand held steady with the other hand. Movements are applied upward and downward along both sides of the spine.*

Tapping, slapping, hacking, beating, cupping, friction or like movements should be applied according to individual needs and when they will be of specific benefit to the patient.

***Vibration—Shaking***

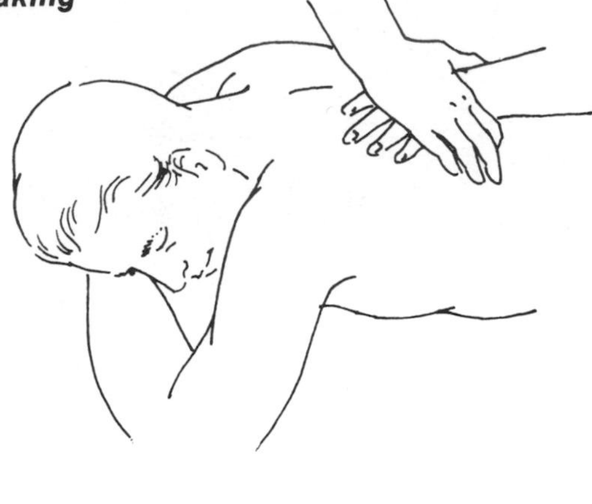

*Vibration movements are applied over each vertebrae by placing one hand flat on the client's back then the other hand on top.*

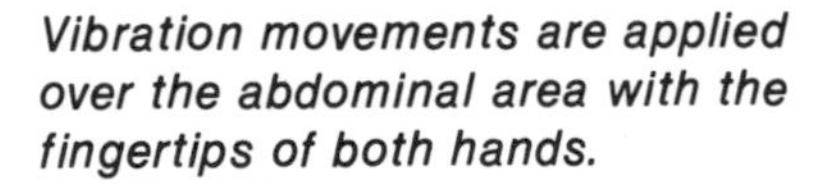

*Vibration movements are applied over the abdominal area with the fingertips of both hands.*

**Joint Movements in Massage**

Joint movements can be either active or passive. In active movement, the patient participates by moving joints and contracting muscles. The patient's participation can be either assistive or resistive. When the patient works with the nurse's movement it is called assistive movement. In passive movement, the patient relaxes while the nurse moves the joint. When the patient moves the joint without assistance or resistance, it is called free movement.

The terms used to describe the movements of the joints are flexion, extension, abduction, adduction, circumduction, pronation and supination.

*Flexion and extension:* Movements used to develop movements in joints that move on one axis such as the knee joint, elbow and joints of the fingers (phalanges).

*Abduction:* This is a movement of a part away from the median line of the body.

*Adduction:* This is a movement of a part toward the median line of the body.

*Circumduction:* This is a movement used on all joints moving on three axis such as the shoulders and hip joints.

*Pronation:* The turning of the palm of the hand downward during a movement.

*Supination:* The turning of the palm upward during a movement. Also turning of the sole of the foot inward.

**Joint Movements in Massage**

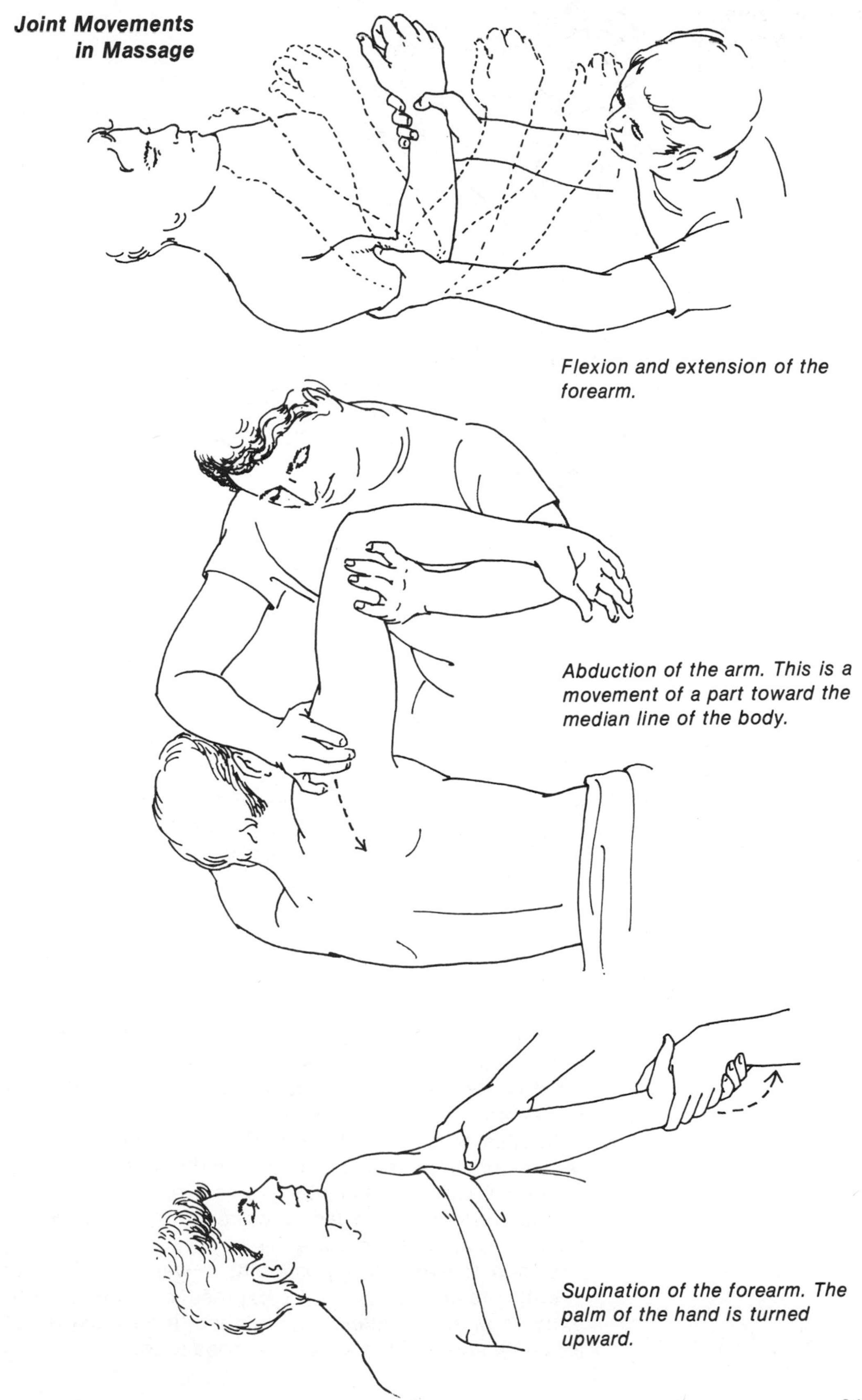

Flexion and extension of the forearm.

Abduction of the arm. This is a movement of a part toward the median line of the body.

Supination of the forearm. The palm of the hand is turned upward.

**Joint Movements in Massage**
*(Continued)*

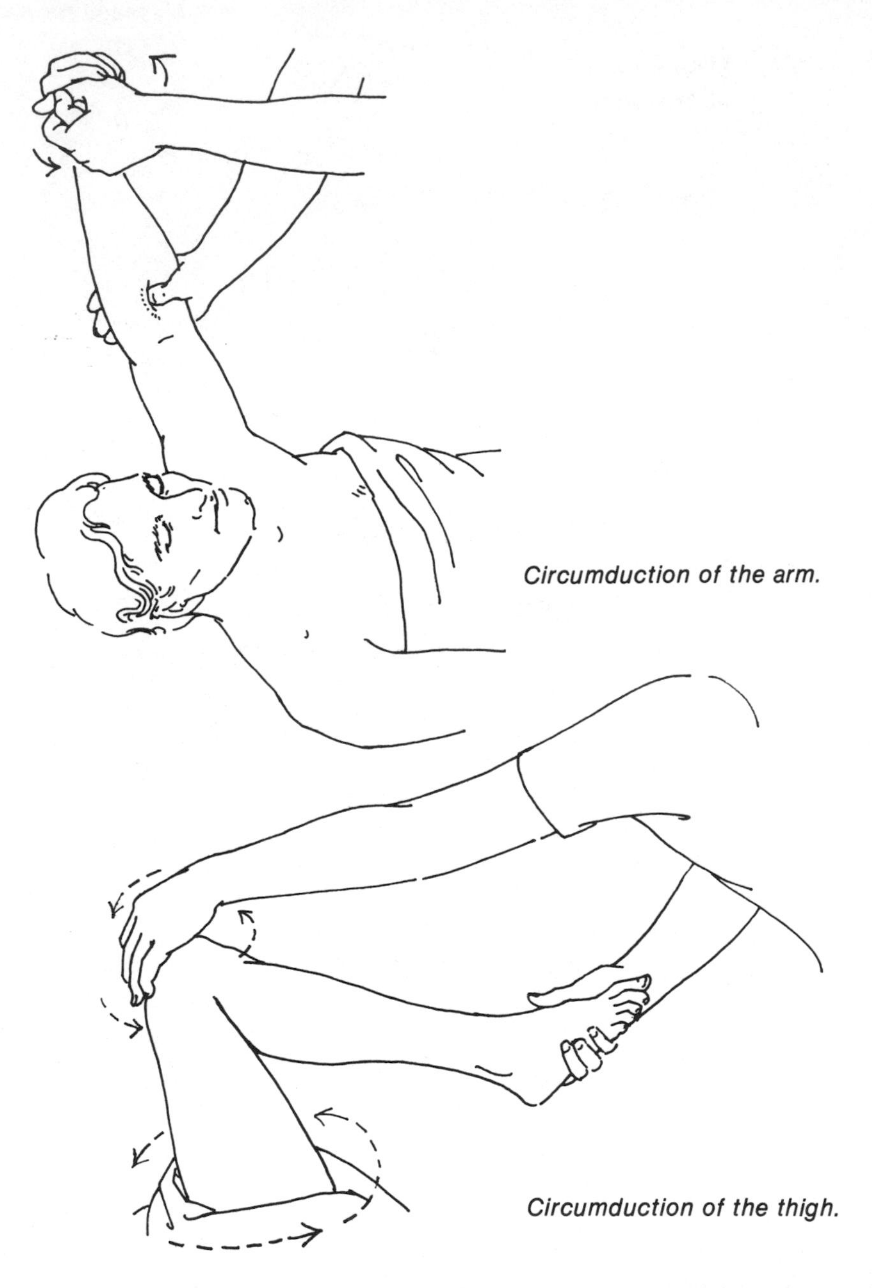

*Circumduction of the arm.*

*Circumduction of the thigh.*

Joint movements can be active or passive. In active movements the patient (or client) participates by moving as directed by the nurse or practitioner. This is called assisting movement.

In passive movement (without assistance or resistance) the patient (or client) relaxes and allows the nurse or practitioner to move the joint. This is called free movement.

It is important to understand the various movements and to be able to apply them correctly.

During the application of joint movements the patient (or client) should be asked to express any discomfort. When extreme pain or a questionable condition exists, the patient's (or client's) physician should be consulted.

**Joint Movements in Massage**
*(Continued)*

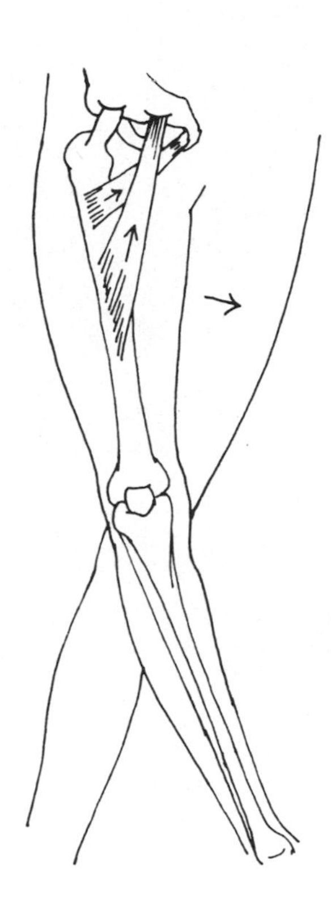

*Adduction Movement—This movement (toward median line) involves the adductor muscles, femur (long) bone, pubic bone and hip joint (ball and socket).*

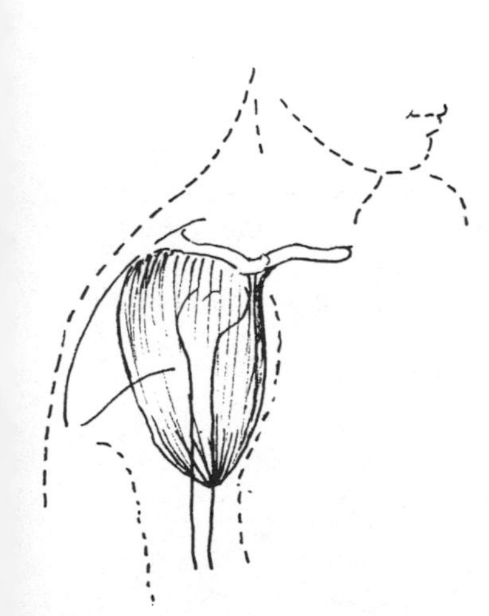

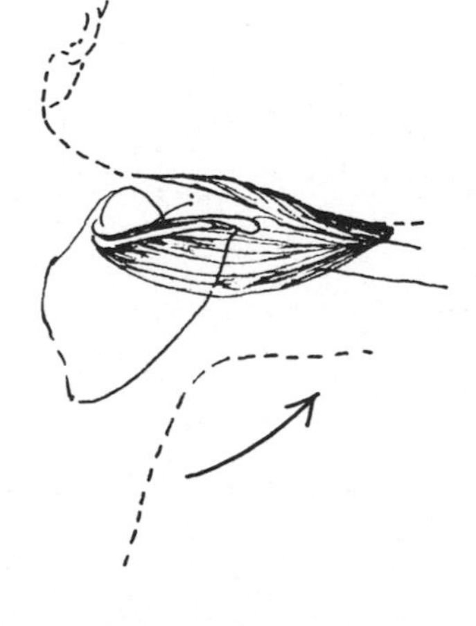

*Abduction movement: This movement (away from median line) involves the deltoid muscle, the scapula bone, clavicle bone and humerus bone and shoulder joint (ball and socket).*

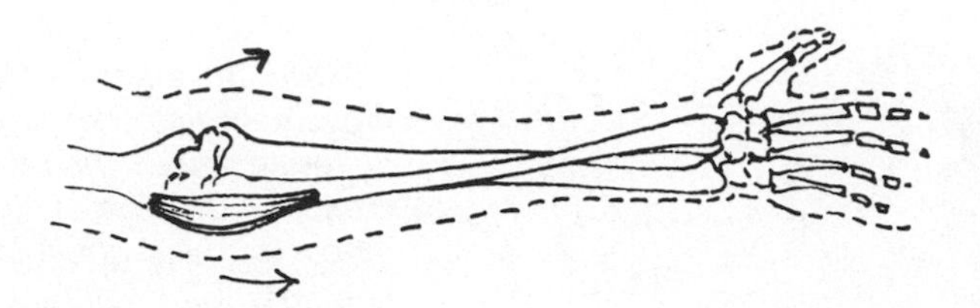

*Rotation Movement: This movement (rotating forward and back) involves the supinator muscle, humerus, ulna, and elbow (hinge joint).*

**Joint Movements in Massage**
*(Continued)*

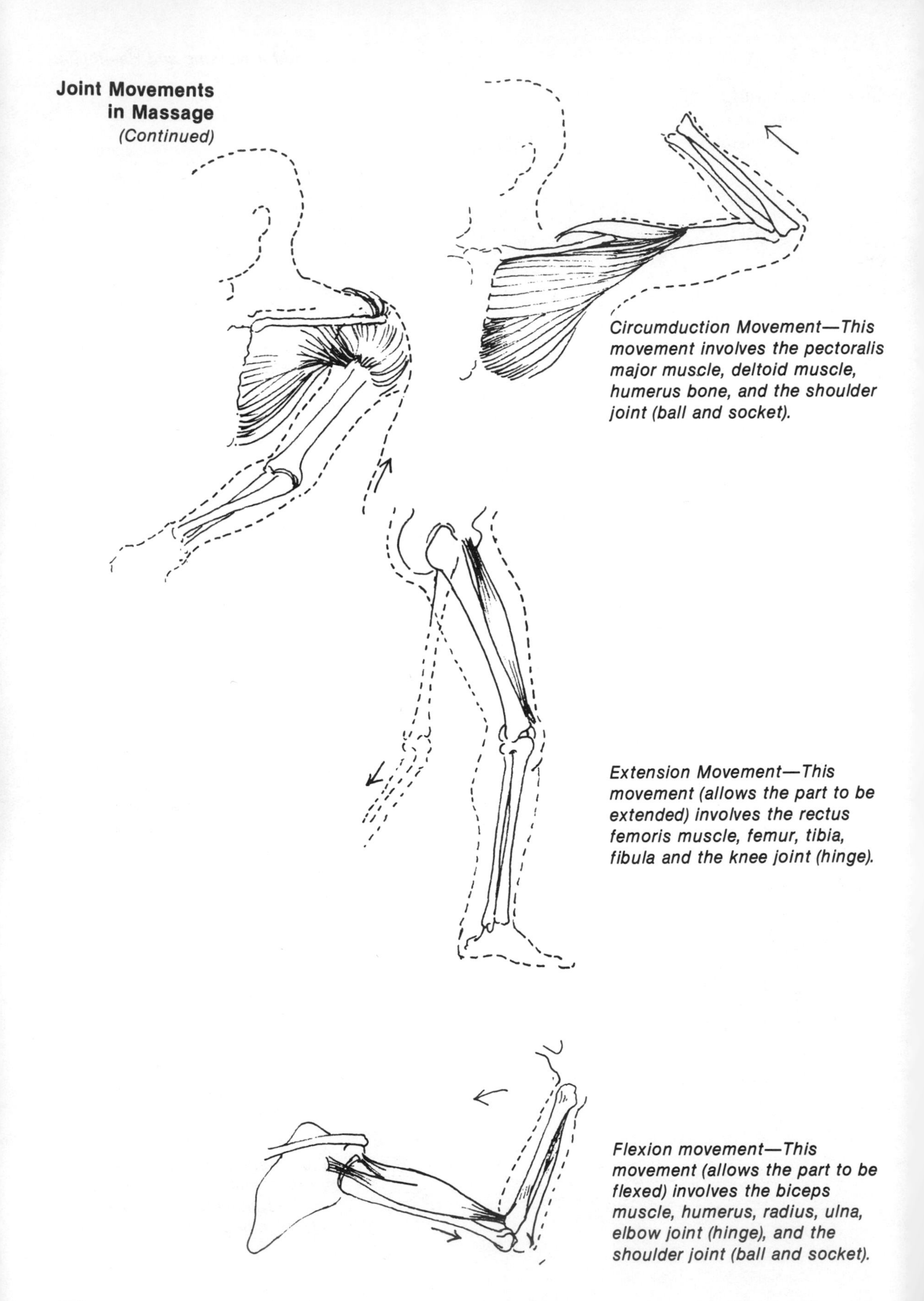

*Circumduction Movement—This movement involves the pectoralis major muscle, deltoid muscle, humerus bone, and the shoulder joint (ball and socket).*

*Extension Movement—This movement (allows the part to be extended) involves the rectus femoris muscle, femur, tibia, fibula and the knee joint (hinge).*

*Flexion movement—This movement (allows the part to be flexed) involves the biceps muscle, humerus, radius, ulna, elbow joint (hinge), and the shoulder joint (ball and socket).*

In order to control joint movement, the nurse places one hand above the joint to be moved and the other below the joint. This helps to control the degree of resistance or assistance on the part of the patient. Both passive and active movements improve circulation to the joints and help to prevent stiffness.

Active movements of the muscles help to prevent loss of muscle tone and strength. The following is a general guide:

1. The Arm
   a. Begin with fingers and the thumb. Use flexion and extension, both passive and active. Follow with abduction and adduction, both passive and active.
   b. Exercise the wrist. Use circumduction, passive; and radial and ulner flexion, passive. Follow with dorsal flexion, passive.
   c. Exercise the elbow. Use flexion and extension, both passive and active. Follow by both supination and pronation, passive and active.
   d. Exercise the shoulder. Begin with circumduction, passive. Follow with anteflexion and retroflexion, passive and active.
2. The Leg
   a. Begin with the toes. Exercise with flexion and extension, passive and active; and circumduction, passive.
   b. Exercise the ankle. Use dorsal and plantar flexion, passive and active.
   c. Exercise the knee. Use flexion and extension, passive and active.
   d. Exercise the hip. Begin with circumduction, passive. Continue with extension and flexion, both passive and active. Do abduction and adduction, passive and active. Repeat exercise on upper and lower extremities.
3. Movements for the Head and Neck

   The patient should be sitting comfortably with arms relaxed at sides.
   a. Begin with flexion forward, backward, and to the right and left, with passive response.
   b. Use rotation to the right and left, passive.
   c. Continue with flexion forward, backward, then to the right and left, with resistance.
   d. Continue with rotation to the right and left, with active resistance.
   e. Follow with circumduction to the right and left, passive.
   f. Complete the exercise with stretching of the neck, passive.

## CLIENT (PATIENT) INFORMATION FORM

The following is a basic form used to obtain information about a client or patient. Generally, this type of form would be useful in a clinic. A hospital or other healthcare facility might provide a more extensive form tailored to the records needed by the physician and the facility.

---

Name ________________________________

Address ________________________________

City ____________ State ____________ Zip ____________

Phone:
Home ____________ Business ____________

Referred by ________________________________

Medication(s) Taken ________________________________

Major medical problems? Please explain:

1. Back problems ____________________________
2. Cancer ____________________________
3. Heart ____________________________
4. Broken bones or fractures ____________________________
5. Nervous disorder (tension, stress, anxiety) ____________
6. Weight normal? ____________________________
7. Skin problems ____________________________
8. Other ____________________________

Are you under the care of a physician? ____________

Name ____________ Address ____________ Phone ____________
(contacted only by permission)

____________________
Please sign

I understand that ____________ does *not* diagnose or treat illnesses or injuries. I am solely responsible for my physical condition and for seeking medical treatment when I feel it is necessary for my well-being.

---

## STEP-BY-STEP GENERAL BODY MASSAGE

The following step-by-step procedure for general body massage is the one preferred by most nurses and other healthcare professionals because it can be adjusted to meet the needs of the patient. It is gentle, yet thorough. The order of movements can be easily adjusted to combine or delete movements.

Authorities in the art of massage suggest beginning the general massage with the extremities. Massaging the extremities first tends to relax tension and helps to prepare the patient for the rest of the massage. This is particularly helpful when giving massage to the patient for the first time or to patients who are shy and withdrawn.

The use of passive and active joint movements are not described in detail in the following general massage procedures; however, they may be used where appropriate. Flexion, circumduction and extension movements may also be included in general massage and are given before centrifugal (finishing) strokes.

**Preparation**

1. Check the temperature of the room to be sure it will be comfortable for the patient during the massage.
2. Assemble all the products and materials you will need.
3. Prepare the patient.

When possible, it is desirable to have the patient bathe, empty the bladder, and evacuate the bowels.

**Procedure**

Place a small amount of massage oil or cream into the palm of the hand then rub the hands together to distribute the product evenly. Use oil or cream sparingly because too much lubrication will make it difficult to perform some massage movements efficiently. Use only enough of the lubricating product to allow the hands to glide smoothly across the skin.

***Massage for the Arms***

1. Begin the massage with the patient's arm (either the right or left). Use both hands to apply light effleurage from the hand to the shoulder, returning with rotary movements back to the hand. Repeat the movements several times.
2. Press the metacarpals (bones of the hand) then knead each finger from tip to knuckles. Rotate each finger.
3. Use the palm and heel of your hand to apply effleurage to the palm of the patient's hand, extending the movements several inches above the wrist. Repeat the movement on the back (dorsal surface) of the hand and wrist.
4. Bend the patient's arm so that it is resting on the elbow. Rotate the arm several times. Follow with effleurage to the forearm.
5. With palms of both hands, apply effleurage to the patient's upper arm with sweeping movements up and over the shoulder. Apply light petrissage movements to the upper arm. Repeat effleurage.
6. Use circular friction movements on the upper arm following the direction of the muscles from insertion to origin.
7. Apply circular friction to the joints of each finger, beginning with the forefinger and moving to the middle finger, the ring finger, the little finger, then back to the thumb. Alternate these movements with light effleurage to the hand and fingers.
8. Apply digital friction to elbow joints followed by effleurage. Repeat the movements several times.
9. Apply petrissage to the biceps, triceps, and deltoids. Alternate with effleurage.
10. Use both hands to apply firm, rhythmic effleurage and gentle centrifugal movements from hand to shoulder. Follow with tapotement (percussion) movements from the hand to the shoulder and back to the hand. Rotate the arm and finish this part of the massage with light centrifugal (stroking) movements.

Repeat the massage on the other arm and hand.

### *Massage for the Legs*

1. Begin with either the right or left leg. Use the palms of both hands to apply effleurage from the upper (dorsal) surface of the foot to the knee joint, returning with large rotary movements to the foot. Repeat the effleurage movements of the feet, alternating with circular friction over the tarsals (ankle bones) and the metatarsals (bones of instep).
2. Apply effleurage to the back of the leg, followed by effleurage to the foot. Apply effleurage to the front (over the tibia) of the leg, and repeat effleurage to the foot.
3. Use both hands to apply effleurage from inner to outer thigh. Repeat the movements on the thighs, then stroke downward to the foot.
4. Use both hands to apply circular movements from foot to hip joint, covering both the inner and outer surfaces of the leg.
5. Apply circular friction to the foot, followed by light petrissage movements. Apply circular friction to the ankle joint, followed by effleurage.
6. Use both hands to apply petrissage to calf of the leg. Follow with effleurage. Apply circular friction along the sides of the tibia, followed by effleurage
7. Use both hands to apply petrissage to the inner surface of the thigh, followed by light effleurage. Repeat the movements on the outer surface of the thigh.
8. Use both hands to apply effleurage from the foot to the top of the thigh.
9. Apply light percussion movements such as clapping, slapping, and hacking to the thighs, moving around and down to the calf and the foot.
10. Use both hands to finish this part of the massage with light centrifugal stroking from the hip joint, down the thigh, to the foot. Repeat the movements several times with a light feathering or tapering off of movements.

### *Massage for the Chest*

1. Use both hands to apply effleurge to the chest, sweeping from the base of the sternum, up to the median line of the chest, and outward to the shoulders. Finish the movement with rotary movements downward on the chest. Repeat the effleurage movements from back of ears and base of neck (in direction of lymph flow), downward and outward around the breast. Repeat the movements several times.
2. Use fingers and palms of hand to apply circular friction from shoulder to sternum, circulating around the breast. Alternate the movement with effleurage several times.
3. Apply petrissage movements with thumb and fingers from neck to shoulders, alternating with effleurage.
4. Apply percussion movements (clapping, hacking, slapping) from neck and shoulders to chest, alternating with light effleurage. Do not apply movements over the breast.

**Massage for the Abdomen**

1. The patient should flex the knees slightly with the feet flat on the bed. Use the palms of both hands to apply circular, clockwise (downward and outward) movements over the abdomen. Follow by light effleurage (in direction of lymph flow) to the abdomen.
2. Apply petrissage over the entire abdominal area, alternating with effleurage.
3. Place one hand flat on the abdominal area below the navel. Place the other hand on top to assist in applying pressure. With hands in place one on top of the other, apply several vibrating movements, then relax the pressure.
4. Apply effleurage (upwards in direction of lymph flow) to the abdomen.
5. Apply light percussion movements followed by gentle effleurage.

**Massage for the Back**

Have the patient lie in prone position.

1. With palms of hands begin the stroking movements from below the waistline, sweeping up the sides of the spine, and back down in large circles. Do this several times, followed by effleurage downward over the back muscles.
2. Apply petrissage to neck and upper portion of the back, working down the spine. Use your thumbs and fingers to massage as you feel the vertebrae.
3. Apply petrissage to the gluteus maximus (buttocks), alternating the movements with effleurage.
4. Apply circular (friction) movements with the tips of your fingers working down each side of the spine.
5. Apply kneading movements with the heel of your hands to each side of the spine, beginning at the scapula and ending at the coccyx (tail bone). Follow with effleurage to the the entire back.
6. Apply percussion movements along the sides of the spine moving downward; follow the movements with light effleurage.
7. Use the palms of both hands to apply effleurage to buttocks, followed by petrissage and additional effleurage movements.
8. Apply percussion movements over the entire gluteus maximus, followed by effleurage.

Following the completion of the general massage, a brief centripetal rub is recommended. This is a light over-all massage using effleurage movements in one direction and light percussion followed by very light centrifugal strokes to finish. Follow the same order as the general massage—arms, legs, chest, abdomen, and back. This is also called mini-massage and may be recommended in place of a more extensive massage. A mini-massage is particularly helpful when the patient is convalescing.

## THE THERAPEUTIC RUBDOWN

A rubdown using oil or alcohol is often a part of patient care. It is usually not as long of duration as the general body massage.

### Oil Rubdown

The oil rubdown is especially good for dry skin. A mild massage oil, baby oil, cocoa butter, or other mild lotion or oil can be used. The oil is applied with light effleurage (stroking) and light, circular friction movements. The oil rubdown is usually given in the following order:

1. Upper extremities.
2. Lower extremities.
3. Neck, chest, and shoulders.
4. Abdominal region.
5. Hips and back.

***Preparation***

The patient should be bathed and prepared with proper draping.

A bath blanket is placed under the patient.

The oil should be warmed by placing the container in a basin of hot water for a few minutes. (Do not use highly scented oil. It may be offensive or irritating to sensitive skin.)

Towels should be available to wipe away excess oil.

***Procedure***

Use effleurage and friction movements.

1. Put about a teaspoonful of oil in your cupped hand. Apply oil, then massage the hands, arms, and shoulders.
2. Apply oil to the chest and follow with massage.
3. Apply oil to the posterior surface of thighs and lower legs. Apply massage.
4. Have the patient turn over. Apply oil to shoulders, back, and buttocks. Apply appropriate massage.
5. Stroke the spine from neck to waist using the back of the hand in sweeping movements.

### Alcohol Rubdown

The alcohol rubdown is often used to refresh the patient when a bath cannot be given, to lower body temperature when fever is present, to create a cooling effect after applications of heat, and to tone the skin.

***Preparation***

The patient should be prepared with proper draping. A bath blanket is placed on the bed. The bottle of alcohol can be warmed by placing it in a basin of warm water. Caution: Do not use pure grain alcohol unless it has been properly diluted. Read the label to be sure it is safe for use on the skin. Alcohol can be diluted to a 70% solution or a solution of two parts alcohol to one part water.

***Procedure***

1. The patient's body should be dry.
2. Drape the patient and explain what you will do and why.
3. Place a small amount of alcohol into your cupped hand.
4. Apply the alcohol to the upper extremities first. Use light, upward strokes, returning with small, rotary movements until all the parts have been covered. Repeat if necessary. Finish with several unbroken strokes from shoulder to hand. Be sure there is no excess alcohol left on the patient's skin.

5. Apply alcohol to the chest. Use long strokes from rib cage to shoulders. Return with rotary movements to the lateral part of the chest. Repeat the movement several times.
6. Apply alcohol to both hands, and stroke the shoulder on one side with long sweeping strokes. Repeat on the other side.
7. Apply alcohol to both hands, and use long sweeping strokes to the posterior surface of the thigh and lower leg. Repeat on the other side.
8. Turn the patient over, and apply alcohol to the shoulders, back, and buttocks. Use long, sweeping strokes from buttocks to shoulders. Follow with light rotary movements over the shoulders, back, and buttocks.
9. Stroke the spine from neck to waist, using both hands to alternate the sweeping movements.
10. Be sure no excess alcohol is left on patient's skin. Indicate that you have finished the alcohol rub, and assist the patient to assume a comfortable position.

**QUESTIONS FOR DISCUSSION AND REVIEW**

1. In addition to having technical skills that help to restore the patient's health, what is an important task of the nurse or healthcare professional?
2. How do the jobs of the general massage practitioner and the nurse differ as related to massage treatments?
3. Why do massage practitioners use the Swedish massage method along with other therapeutic aids to help restore the patient to health?
4. Why must the nurse be particularly aware of contraindications for massage?
5. Why are active movements so beneficial to muscles when the patient is convalescing?
6. What is the difference between centripetal and centrifugal movements?
7. When are centrifugal movements usually done in massage?
8. Why is it necessary to obtain a medical history of a client or patient before giving a massage treatment?
9. Why is the alcohol rubdown used so frequently in patient care?
10. Why is an oil rubdown often used in patient care?

**ANSWERS TO QUESTIONS FOR DISCUSSION AND REVIEW**

1. To teach a patient to maintain his or her health and to live a healthy and productive life.
2. The general practitioner deals with healthy clients or those sent by a physician. The nurse deals with patients under a physician's care who are ill, injured, or recovering.
3. The Swedish method is made up of movements that have been recognized by the medical profession as being beneficial.
4. While massage may not affect a healthy person adversely, the same movements could be detrimental to someone who is ill or has been injured.

5. Active movements help to prevent loss of muscle strength and tone.
6. Centripetal movements are stronger strokes directed toward a center, such as the heart, and following the direction of the blood current. Centrifugal movements are done by moving away from the center, thus decreasing the flow of blood and lessoning pressure to the heart.
7. Centrifugal movements usually conclude the massage and are used to decrease the heartbeat and blood flow.
8. It is important to know the client's or the patient's physical condition in order to determine if massage will be beneficial or harmful. Also, the medical history form signed by the patient or client serves as protection for the massage practitioner or healthcare professional.
9. The alcohol rubdown refreshes the patient when a bath cannot be given. It tends to lower temperature when fever is present, creates a soothing and cooling effect after applications of heat, and has a beneficial astringent effect on the skin.
10. The oil rubdown is particularly beneficial in relieving dry skin and skin sensitivity caused by the patient having to lie in bed for long periods of time.

# Chapter 14 Athletic Massage

**LEARNING OBJECTIVES**

After you have mastered this chapter you will be able to:

1. Explain the purposes of athletic massage.
2. Explain the causes of muscle fatigue.
3. Explain the major benefits of athletic massage.
4. Explain contraindications for athletic massage.
5. Locate the major stress points of the body.
6. Explain the importance of warm-up exercises and massage to the athlete's performance.
7. Explain the relationship of certain athletic or sports activities to possible injuries.
8. Demonstrate the basic applications of athletic massage and the general procedures for each.

## INTRODUCTION

As far back as antiquity, massage was used to restore and to rejuvenate war-torn and weary soldiers as they returned to Rome. The Roman athletes enjoyed the benefits of restorative massage and baths.

For many years the great athletes of the European and Soviet countries have included massage as part of their intensive and continuous training schedules. Much research has been done to determine what types of massage work best in different sports and what the best form of massage is for each phase of training as well as in the rehabilitation of injuries.

In the United States, massage is recognized as a valuable asset to improve the athlete's ability to perform better with fewer physical ill effects from maximum effort. In 1984 for the first time, massage was made available for all athletes competing in the Summer Olympic Games in Los Angeles. Since then, massage areas have become a common sight at many athletic events across the country. Many athletes participate in regular massage as part of their training regimen, and massage has become the therapy of choice in the rehabilitation of minor sports injuries.

## PURPOSE OF ATHLETIC MASSAGE

Athletic, also called sport massage enables athletes to attain their highest potential by enhancing their capabilities to participate more often in rigorous physical training and conditioning. Massage helps to reduce the chance of injury by identifying and eliminating potential risk of injury. In cases where injury has occurred, massage helps to restore mobility and flexibility to injured muscle tissue, while reducing recovery time. Athletic massage, when done correctly, can improve the athlete's ability to perform while reducing the incidence of lost time due to injury and fatigue.

## The Athletic-Sport Massage Therapist

In order to be an effective athletic (sport) massage therapist, a person should have a thorough understanding of anatomy, physiology, kinesiology, biomechanics, and massage technique. The massage therapist should have a sound knowledge of anatomy and be familiar with the various structures of the body. Of particular interest are the skeletal system, and the muscular system. It is important to also understand the circulatory system and the nervous sytem, especially the neuro-muscular functions. An understanding of kinesiology, which is the study of body movement, helps the therapist recognize what structures are involved in the movements of particular sports especially when pain is present.

Physiology is important in understanding the role each system plays in supporting the others so they function as a whole organism.

Biomechanics refer to the integrated movement of the entire body. For instance, the manner in which the foot is placed affects what the knees, hip, back, shoulders, and head do. Tension in a particular body area also indicates tension of misalignment in other areas of the body. Because the body is used in a particular way, specific areas are going to be stressed. A deviation in the structure of one area of the body will be reflected throughout the body. Deviations often appear as patterns of structural imbalances. These deviations when stressed, often result in injury. The more severe the deviation, the sooner an injury may occur.

## Techniques of Athletic Massage

A thorough knowledge of the various massage techniques and their proper application makes the difference between an effective or ineffective sport massage therapist. Many of the techniques of athletic massage are identical with those of classical Swedish massage such as effleurage, petrissage, kneading, passive joint movements, compression, and friction. There are some therapeutic techniques in sports massage that bear special consideration.

### *Compression Strokes*

Compression strokes cause increased amounts of blood to remain in the muscle over an extended period of time. This (hyperemia) is of value in pre-event, restorative, and rehabilitive massage. When applied with short transverse movement, at the deepest pressure of the compression, it also acts to broaden and separate muscle fascia adhesions that result from post-edemic gluing of the muscle fibers and fascicles.

### *Transverse or Cross-Fiber Friction*

Transverse or cross-fiber friction, which is generally done with the tips of the fingers or thumb, is effective at breaking down adhesions as well as crystalline roughness that forms on tendon sheaths often resulting in painful tendonitis.

### *Active Joint Movements*

A form of active joint movements is called strain/counter strain. A more sophisticated form of this is proprioceptor neuromuscular facilitation or PNF which helps to counteract muscle spasm, improve flexibility, and restore muscle strength. This is performed by moving a body part involving the affected muscle into a flexed or stretched position to a point of pain or discomfort, then moving it back out of that position to a point where there is no discomfort. The therapist then supports the body part in this position while the client contracts the muscles for five to thirty seconds, then relaxes. The process is then repeated several times through the entire range of motion of the affected muscle or articulation until flexibility is restored and spasm reduced. Caution: the extent of these techniques is regulated by the level of pain experienced by the client. If any movement caues the client to tense due to pain, that movement is contraindicated.

## Athletic Injuries

Most injuries are either the result of traumatic contact (with another athlete or in a fall) or the result of excessive and/or repeated stress to an area of the body due to muscular exertion. Injuries of the traumatic sort are often in the form of broken bones, dislocated joints, and torn ligaments. Such injuries are generally accidental and nonpreventable. Injuries of the second type are far more common and generally affect the soft tissue in the form of muscle strains, pulls and tears, or inflammation of tendons and ligaments. These are usually the result of fatigue, poor tissue integrity, muscular weakness, imbalance, or biomechanical deviation. The majority of these injuries are preventable and treatable by massage and proper training.

### *Fascia*

Fascia is connective tissue that surrounds muscle tissue. There are many layers and forms of fascia in the body. Each muscle fiber is surrounded by a delicate covering called the endomysium. Groups of muscle fibers are held together in muscle bundles called fascicles by perimysium (connective tissue) that penetrates into the muscle and its covering, the epimysium.

Deep fascia covers muscle groups somewhat like envelopes in that it allows muscle groups such as the flexors and extensors to work individually. Superficial fascia in the subcutaneous area connects deeper layers with the skin and contains adipose (fatty) tissue. Fascia supports various structures in the body such as nerves, muscles, and organs, while at the same time allowing movement of individual parts within that structure.

Athletic injuries often result in the tearing of one or more layers of fascia. As a result of the healing process, a binding together of one layer of fascia with another or to other tissue such as bone or muscle may occur. When the cell walls in tissue are injured, the body responds by increasing the amount of interstitial fluid in the area. These injuries may be as small as microtrauma to individual muscle fibers or as severe as torn tendons, ligaments, or broken bones. Often this swelling is accompanied by pain. The positive effects of swelling is to immobilize the area so the natural healing process of the body can start to repair the injury.

The cells that mend the connective tissue are called fibroblasts, which produce collagen fibers. These are the same as the fibers in fibrous connective tissue such as fascia and tendons.

When tissue is injured, swelling takes place and creates space between the edges of the damaged tissue. It also creates space between the layers of fascia. Because of the distance between the edges of the injury, the fibroblasts create collagen fibers, much like cobwebs, that bind together several layers of fascia. The resulting fibrosis reduces flexability and pliability of the areas. It also reduces circulation to the area and creates the potential for further injury.

As swelling is reduced, a crystalline residue is left behind that sticks or glues the adjoining layers of fascia together. The gluing may also be the result of stressed and confined muscle movement over a long period of time. The resulting adhesions reduce stretch and flexability with reduction of power and greater chance of injury. Both of these conditions can be greatly reduced with proper first aid and athletic massage therapy.

**Injuries to Joints**

Bones are classified as long, short, flat, and irregular. Long bones as in the arms and legs serve as levers of action in running, swimming, and other active sports.

Short bones as in the feet, ankles, and kneecaps serve as shock absorbers. Flat bones as the sternum (breastbone), scapula (shoulder blade), and pelvis provide the bases to which the muscles and limbs are attached. Irregular bones include bones of the skull, face, and spine.

An articulation, or joint, is the place of union between two separate bones, especially where one permits some freedom of movement. The ends of movable bones are held in place by ligaments forming joint capsules. Ligaments are bands of very dense fibrous tissue that connect bones or support organs of the body. Cartilage is the tough, elastic form of connective tissue composed of cells embedded in a translucent matrix where it originates. Cartilage is either homogenous (having the same characteristics or composition) or it is fibrous. The cartilage around the ends of bones also serve as shock absorbers.

In active sports there is always a chance that muscular ligaments will be torn, cartilage damaged, and bones fractured or broken. Injury to shoulder and knee joints (the largest joints in the body) is particularly common in sports such as football, baseball, hockey, polo, and other sports that require turning and twisting movements. The femor (upper leg bone) is attached to the tibia (lower leg bone) by ligaments and the patella or kneecap. The two crescent-shaped cartilages of the knee are situated between the upper and lower leg bones. There are four major ligaments of the knee called the outside (medial and lateral collateral) ligaments that serve to protect the knee from side to side movement and the anterior and posterior cruciate ligaments that keep the joint from moving from forward to backward when the leg is in motion. These ligaments also hold the joint together. The kneecap is a protective shield for the joint and provides greater mobility. The bursae (fibrous sacs containing synovial fluid placed between ligaments and bones) provide a lubricant that allows the joints to move smoothly and freely.

Proper exercise of the knee joints strengthens associated muscles and helps to prevent injuries. Such exercises as fast deep-knee bends, as done in weight lifting or jumping, tend to place too much stress on the joints and should be avoided until the legs have been properly conditioned

***Shoulder Joints***

Shoulder joint injuries are due to such sports as baseball, bowling, basketball, and other sports requiring exertion of the arm and shoulder. These usually result in injury to the rotator cuff or associated muscles

**Review of Muscles**

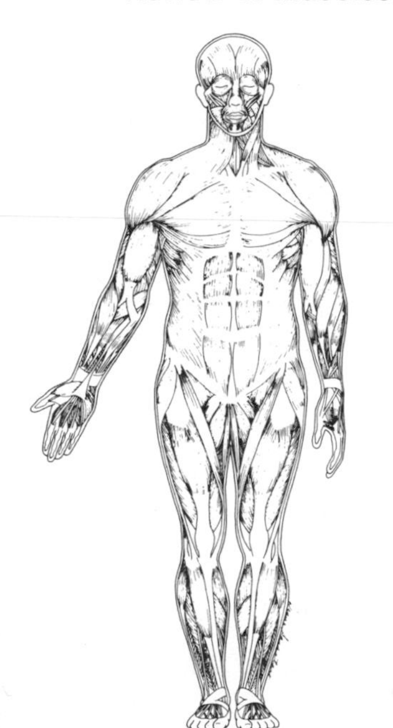

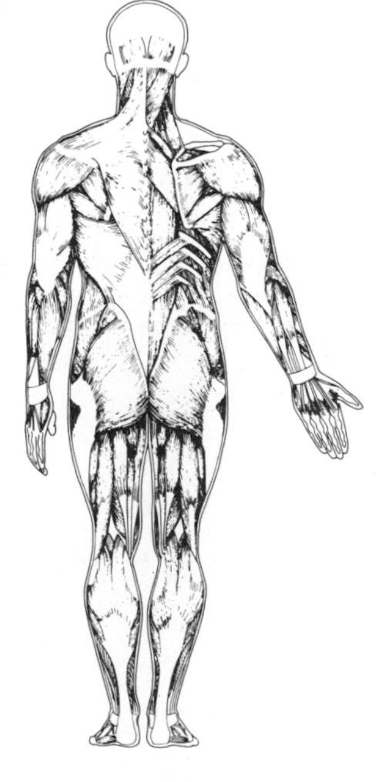

In Chapter 5, the anatomy chapter of this book, you learned that striated (striped) muscles or skeletal muscles are those that function voluntarily, or at will. Nonstriated muscles (smooth) are those muscles associated with organs. Such muscles function involuntary or without a person having to think about movement of that particular muscle. There are muscles called voluntary-involuntary because they work both independently and at will. Skeletal muscles have two ends; the end featuring a fixed or stationary attachment of a muscle is called the origin, and the more movable attachment is called the insertion.

The thicker part of a muscle is called the belly. The viscosity of a muscle refers to the thickness or thinness of its fibers. These fibers can be built up by exercises, or they can atrophy (waste) due to certain diseases, injuries, or lack of use. Hypertrophy of muscle fiber results when muscles are forcefully worked as in weight lifting.

In sports, specialized training and conditioning methods increase the lung's ability to oxygenate and the heart's ability to pump more blood into the muscles so that they will be capable of increased activity. Adequate oxygen is important to muscular activity and is called the fuel of combustion. When there is insufficient oxygen, cellular respiration is hampered, causing fatigue. Nutrients and oxygen are taken in and delivered to the muscles by different body systems and a network of blood vessels.

Muscle tone refers to the readiness of muscles to respond. Muscle tone is improved by an increased supply of nutrients and oxygen and consistant exercise. This can be enhanced by massage and physical activity. Full muscle contractions improve the strength of muscle fibers and can generate or restrict muscle motion. As a muscle contracts, it pulls the bone to which it is attached in the direction of the contraction. As the muscle relaxes and its opposite muscle pulls the bone the other way, motion is generated.

Muscles pull, they do not push. The strength of a muscle is dependent on its size and ability to contract. Muscle has a higher density than fat, and fat does not have the ability to contract. Muscle is vascular tissue, while fat has no blood vessels of its own. Fat in and around muscle fibers increases resistance to motion and restricts oxygen supply to tissues. This reduces the ability of the muscles to perform. Therefore, the athlete with less fat is in better condition.

Approximately 40 percent of an adult's body weight is skeletal muscle, which is made up of numerous fibers. Most fibers extend the entire length of a muscle and have a nerve ending. Each of these fibers contains thousands of myofibrils. When a muscle contracts, this fiber folds over into itself. When this contraction is prolonged, it causes fatigue. Action of the muscle becomes weaker due to the depletion of ATP (adenosinetriphosphate) in the muscle fiber. When oxygenation of glucose takes place, the main supply of energy is inhibited; the muscles lose their ability to respond.

The power of a muscle is the product of synergetic action of groups of muscles responding to nerve impulses. As some muscles contract in a smooth, wavelike action, opposing muscles freely release and stretch with the least amount of resistance.

**Beneficial Effects of Athletic Massage**

1. Massage causes hyperemia, making more oxygen and nutrients available to the body area being massaged.
2. Massage flushes out metabolic wastes of exertion quickly and is three to five times more effective in combating fatigue than resting.
3. Massage breaks down the "gluing" between fascial sheaths.
4. Massage separates fibrositis, breaks up adhesions, and helps to realign collagen fibers formed as a result of injury.
5. Massage identifies possible trouble areas and helps to eliminate them.

***Special Benefits of Massage to Athletes***

1. Massage allows the athlete to reach peak performance sooner and sustain it longer.
2. Massage eliminates muscle stiffness due to excess lactic acid build-up. It rejuvenates muscles quicker after intense workouts or events.
3. With massage, muscles improve in flexibility and are able to respond more quickly and powerfully.
4. With massage, injuries heal more quickly without loss of power due to transverse fibrosis.
5. Massage encourages better performance and reduces the chance of injury.

**Applications for Athletic Massage**

There are four basic applications for athletic massage, and each may require a different approach. The basic applications are:

1. Massage previous to an event
2. Massage after an event.
3. Massage during training.
4. Massage during rehabilitation.

Another possible application is massage during or between events or training sessions.

***Pre-Event Massage***

Massage prior to an event prepares the body for intense activity. Therefore, the massage should be short and stimulating, and aimed at the parts of the body that will be involved in the exertion. This is not the time for relaxing movements. Pre-event massage warms up the muscles causing increased blood supply (hyperemia) in specific muscle areas. This enables the athlete to reach his or her peak performance earlier in the event and to maintain that performance longer. This pre-event massage is not a replacement for proper warm-up before a performance, but is an aid to warming up the muscles. Nor is this a good time for the athlete to receive his or her first massage because the effects of the massage may "throw off" an athlete's timing and interfere with performance. The main objective of the pre-event massage is to wake up the muscles and to increase blood circulation in the areas of the body about to be used. Specific techniques are compression, shaking, jostling, rolling, and kneading. Light centrifugal movements are used to pull blood away from the heart and into the needed areas.

***Post-Event Massage***

Post-event massage is used within the first hour or two after participating in an event. The aim of this treatment is to clean out metabolic residue caused by the intense effort of the body. Research shows that massage of this type promotes rapid removal of metabolic wastes and is three to four times as effective as rest in recovery from muscle fatigue. These techniques enhance the movement of blood and lymph out of the most intensely worked muscles and back toward the heart and center of the body. Lactic and pyruvic acids formed as a result of oxygen depletion are flushed from the muscles. This prevents soreness and reduces the time it takes for the body to recover from exertion.

The most effective techniques for post-event massage are light and deep effleurage, petrissage, kneading, compression, fibrilation, and generalized friction movements. All movements are aimed at "stripping out" the areas of the body that have been used during the event. The post-event massage varies from 15 to 30 minutes.

***Massage During Training***

Massage during training is the most beneficial form of massage for the athlete. Massage is usually on the athlete's training schedule and is considered a regular and valuable part of his or her training.

Regular massage during training can locate and relieve areas of stress that carry high risk of injury. Massage reduces minor cross-fiber adhesions resulting from microtrauma, thereby increasing muscle response. Massage also alleviates muscle boundness (by breaking down muscle bundles) so that muscle contractions and relaxation are more efficient. This allows finer-tuned muscle response.

Massage during training increases blood and lymph circulation, which allows more efficient oxygen and nutrient supply as well as more efficient removal of metabolic waste. All of these benefits make more intense and frequent workouts possible, thereby improving overall performance.

Another benefit of massage is the breaking down of any transverse adhesions that may have resulted from previous injuries, thus promoting more muscle power, better circulation, less chance of reinjury, increased mobility and flexibility, and better performance. The athlete is able to achieve maximum effort sooner, more often, and maintain it longer with fewer, if any, ill effects.

The massage process systematically involves every part of the athlete's body, including not only those muscles or body parts specifically involved in the sport but also other areas that are indirectly involved.

***Massage During Rehabilitation***

After trouble areas are mapped out, massages may deal with target areas. When there are several indications of trouble, it is beneficial to have frequent treatments well in advance of the next competition in order to build the system back to its maximum state. Also the athlete will have plenty of practice time to adjust to his or her new or regained ability.

Rehabilitation massage tends to be deep and intense. The athlete must understand that a great deal of pain may be a part of a treatment and be willing to work with the therapist on deep breathing and relaxation techniques. The practitioner must not persist if in the process of working the muscle becomes tighter. If muscle tightening occurs and the practitioner continues to "dig," there is a chance of actual injury; the condition could worsen instead of improve. The athlete and practitioner should work together for the improvement of the athlete's ability to train and condition his or her body.

The primary techniques in this aspect of athletic massage include: compression, deep pressure, cross-fiber and trans-fiber frictions, deep longitudinal strokings, and a variety of shaking and vibrating movements. Effleurage and petrissage are also used, but to a lesser degree. There are also a number of therapist-assisted joint movements that are very effective in this stage of massage. They include position release (or preferred position) strain/counter strain and PNF (proprioceptor neuro-muscular facilitation).

There is no standard or set procedure for athletic massage due to the variety of sports situations to which it is applicable. However, there is a process to follow in order to choose an effective treatment plan. When interviewing the client it is important to find out the following:

The sport or sports in which he or she is involved.

The location and extent of present trouble areas.

The location and extent of previous injuries.

The workout schedule and planned events.

The extent to which the athletic massage is to be incorporated in the athlete's training.

By learning the client's regular sports, the practitioner can give special consideration to related muscle areas. Trouble areas can point to particular muscle groups on which to concentrate.

Previous injuries can also target trouble areas. Often an injury occurs as a result of a muscle not being flexible enough or not being able to let go. Trouble areas may also indicate fascia that is stuck or bound together. Injuries, especially when muscle spasm or tears exist, also point to synergistic, or opposing muscle as being primary or potential problems.

Workout schedules indicate how serious a person is about a particular sport and can also reveal injury prone week-end warriors. How much or how often the athlete wants to include massage in his or her training program helps the practitioner to determine the frequency and intensity of treatments. If the plan is to include only one or two sessions, then the massage should be limited. However, if several regular sessions are planned, a thorough preliminary massage can be given. Work can then be done systematically on troubled areas or areas that receive continuous and intense use.

The first massage is primarily a hunt-and-search process using compression and deep pressure to seek out muscle bundles and spasms as well as constrictions and areas of fibrosis. These bands or bundles of muscles usually feel like cords or lumpy growths that roll around or snap under the skin. Healthy, pliable muscle is smooth and evenly textured across its whole breadth and length. To the client such trouble areas generally show up as pain.

Muscles also have alarm (stress) points that are generally located where muscle ends and where it joins tendon or tendon sheath. This is where fascia and connective tissue are more prevalent. Because many muscle fibers terminate here, the area is vulnerable to trauma and microtrauma. This is also where the ratio of blood vessels to tissue is less and, therefore, where fatigue occurs first. Often when a muscle is headed for trouble, the first indication appears in this area.

Deep pressure on the alarm points gives the first clue to future problems. Early treatment on the muscles associated with the alarm points can stop an injury long before it begins to adversely affect the athlete's performance. Once the trouble areas have been located, the procedures for working on them should stretch, broaden, and soften the muscle while encouraging the increase of blood and lymph capabilities. Initial circulation is enhanced by effleurage movements that work venous blood and lymph toward the heart.

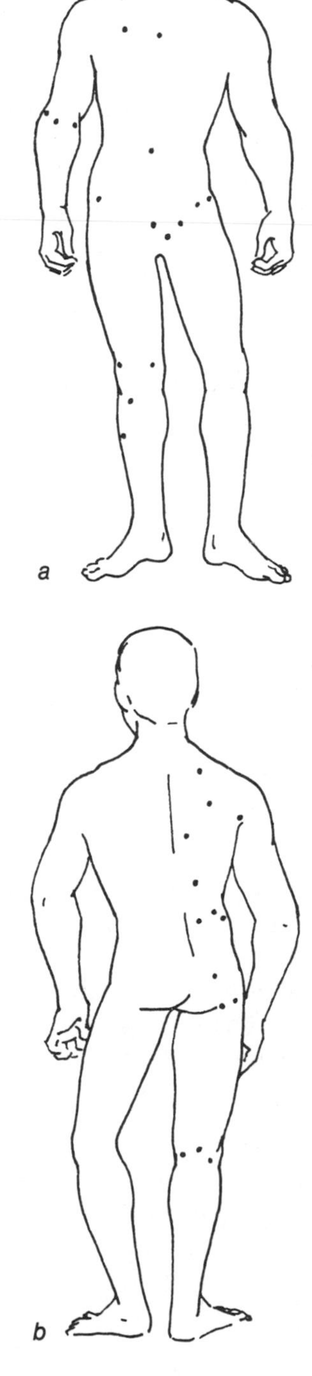


*Major alarm (stress) points of the body; (a) Anterior and (b) Posterior views.*

## Compression Strokes for Athletic Massage

The heel, palm, or broad part of the hand or fist can be used to repeatedly press the muscle against the bone. At the deepest part of the compression, the tissue is slightly stretched, either along or across the line of muscle fibers. This promotes increased circulation deep in the muscle at the same time that the fibers are stretched out and separated. The proper way to apply compression is to start at the origin of the muscle (part nearest the torso) and proceed to the insertion of the muscle in one-half-inch to one-inch steps. This procedure may be repeated three or more times along each part of the muscle, with special attention given to the ends of the muscle. Large, broad muscles require several passes to adequately cover the entire muscle.

Usually in the process of applying compressions, specific areas of the muscle are identified as the source of the problem. The stroke can be changed to a cross-fiber movement to mash and separate the muscle fibers. When done correctly this stroke broadens the tissue and slightly stretches it, causing a broadening of the muscle and a breaking up of the binding fascia surrounding the fibers.

### *Cross-Fiber Friction*

Beginning at the origin of the muscle, the thumb, fingertips, or fist can be used to apply deep pressure. As much pressure as the person can tolerate may be applied, released, and reapplied. This movement may be followed by cross-fiber friction, which consists of oscillating laterally across the tied-up tendons (being careful not to bounce across it), working into the fibers, and spreading them apart while working deeper into the tissue. These movements along the entire length of the affected area should be followed by a deep-tissue stretch stroke from either the insertion or origin of the muscle. The fingertips, thumbs, heel of hand, or even the elbow can be used to achieve results.

Beginning at the tendon of the muscle insertion, the practitioner may apply deep, firm pressure and work the muscles along the length of the fibers with slow, deep, gliding strokes. The thumbs, heel of the hand, or elbow can be used to stretch the fibers and iron them out. These last two procedures can be intensely painful, so it is important to only work as deep as can be tolerated by the athlete without causing tension. These two processes may be repeated three or more times.

Another effective technique for breaking down fibrosis at the site of old injuries or areas where fascia is bound together is to apply deep pressure, using the thumbs or heel of the hand, just beside the affected area. The tissue is then stretched along the line of the tissue fibers and away from the lesion. The fibers should be stretched as far as they will move without the hand or the thumb sliding across the client's skin. It is important that the hand and skin move as a unit in order to stretch the deeper tissue. No oil should be used. The movement is repeated several times for each lesion and is followed by light cross-fiber friction.

A good way to relieve the intensity of deep work on the muscle is to shake or jostle the entire muscle mass or limb vigorously. This not only releases the tension that may result from the manipulations but also works to loosen fascia and to improve lymph movement.

When shaking a limb, it is important not to hyperextend any joint, especially the elbow or knee. The proper way to shake a muscle is to place the massaging hand across the muscle at the origin, then lightly grasp and vigorously move the muscle laterally across the axis, working from origin to insertion.

Rolling is done by placing one hand on either side of the limb and rhythmically rolling the flesh around the bone. The massage routine may be completed with passive stretching and effleurage to clear the area. This procedure may be repeated on all affected body areas.

The massage just described is like an intense workout and should be done on days when training is light or on days the athlete is off training. The massage should not be given just before a competition. It is preferable to allow at least a couple of practice days (usually no more) between a deep massage and an event so that the athlete can become familiar with how his or her newly released muscles respond.

A great number of therapeutic techniques are valuable in treating injuries in any of their progressive stages and/or degrees of severity. The application of proper techniques to the type of injury is important. Improper use of movement and pressure can aggravate a condition and possibly cause more permanent damage. This could result in a liability sult.

The massage practitioner should practice therapy at this level only after receiving proper training under the supervision of a qualified instructor who is familiar with sports injuries and the practice of therapeutic athletic massage.

The advantages of massage therapy are numerous. Prompt application of the appropriate therapy can reduce much swelling and pain caused by an injury. Proper therapy allows the injured tissues to remain in close proximity so that healing progresses faster and with less need for the body to produce excess scar tissue. When massage is administered, the quality of healed tissue is far superior than if an injury is left to heal on its own.

Proper therapy improves circulation, enabling excess fluid and damaged tissue to be carried away. With improved circulation, more nutrients are brought to the rebuilding tissue so that it becomes strong and pliable, and heals more quickly. Research has also shown that with massage therapy fibrositis (excess fibrous tissue) caused by muscle injury is much reduced, and the presence of transverse adhesions is almost nonexistent.

Proper therapy and more rapid healing of injuries means that the athlete's "down time" is cut to a minimum. With continued treatment during the rehabilitation period, there will also be fewer ill effects on performance.

Therapy may be given at the rate of once or twice a day during the time the athlete is out of training and every other day or every third day until he or she is back to a full training schedule. Massage for new or fresh injuries should only be given by properly trained therapists in conjunction with a physician's approval.

## CONTRAINDICATIONS

The athlete's physician (employed by the organization or school) takes case histories and is responsible for pre-season evaluations and for advising the athlete on health care and care of injuries. The physician treats illnesses and injuries and is responsible for rehabilitation of the athlete. The massage practitioner or trainer works under the direction of the physician and follows his or her guidelines when massage is to be a part of treatment or rehabilitation of injuries.

It should be kept in mind that the physician or practitioner avoids doing anything that might make him or her liable or subject to malpractice. Negligence is defined as imprudent action or failure to act properly or failure to take reasonable precautions. Athletes understand that there are always some risks involved and that a physician or therapist is not held liable for poor judgment on the part of the athlete. Athletic massage is contraindicated in any abnormal condition, injury, illness, or disease except as advised by the athlete's physician.

There are times when an amateur or school athlete will request the services of the massage practitioner. The same contraindications for massage applies for this client as for the professional. The client must take responsibility for his or her own health and provide a physician's report if deemed necessary. Any heart condition, anemia, diabetes, thyroid disorders, liver and lung conditions, cancer, skin disease, varicose veins, hypertension, internal injuries, wounds, or like conditions are contraindications for massage. In these cases, massage would be only done upon the recommendation of the client's physician and at the request of the client.

## GENERAL PROBLEM AREAS AND SUGGESTED MASSAGE

### The Foot and Ankle

The heels take a lot of shock in sports such as jogging and running and muscles can become painful to pressure.

*Massage:* To apply general massage to the foot, have the athlete lie face down with feet over the edge of the table, you may sit on a stool if you are more comfortable. Use your finger or thumb to apply deep friction to sore spots. Apply cross-fiber friction for about 10 counts, pause then repeat the movement.

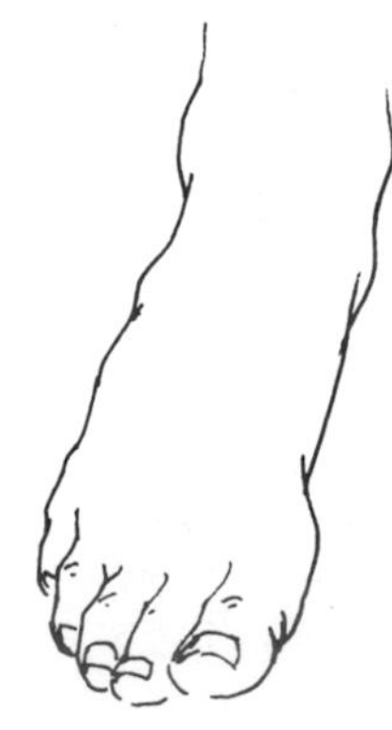

*The foot and ankle.*

***Achilles Tendon***

The Achilles tendon, located just above the heel, may become swollen and painful if the ankle has been strained or if the tendon has been pulled at its attachment to the heel. Tendonitis also may have formed at the attachment to the calf muscle.

*Massage:* Use your thumbs to apply 10 or more direct pressure movements, followed by cross-fiber friction. Repeat direct pressure to the tendon, followed by compression with your thumb. Search the calf muscle for related fibrosis or knots. Caution: It is contraindicated to do deep strokes along a fibrous tendon like the Achilles tendon because it tends to aggrevate abnormal conditions such as pulls and tears.

***Metatarsal Cramp or Fatigue***

An athlete often suffers muscle cramps, tightening and spasms of the muscles in the foot.

*Massage:* Hold the foot steady as you use the tip of your thumb to apply pressure to the stress point near the big toe. Follow pressure with deep cross-fiber friction for 10 to 20 counts, then release and repeat the movement. Move your thumb to the stress point near the little toe, and repeat the same movements. Check for stress points near the heel. Apply deep strokes from toes to heel, and gently stretch the plantar tendon.

***Ankle Strains and Twists***

The feet and ankles play an important part in sports and due to the varied and stressful movements, are prime targets for injury and fatigue.

*Massage:* Use your thumb and forefinger to apply pressure and cross-fiber friction to the stress points near the ankle bone. Continue for 20 counts. Release and repeat. This must be done gently, as the area may be painful. Apply friction to the instep, working gently and from the toes to the heel. Move to the stress point of the outer ankle, and apply direct pressure for 10 counts. Release and repeat the movement. Shake and rotate the foot, then gently stretch it in every direction. Finish the massage with friction.

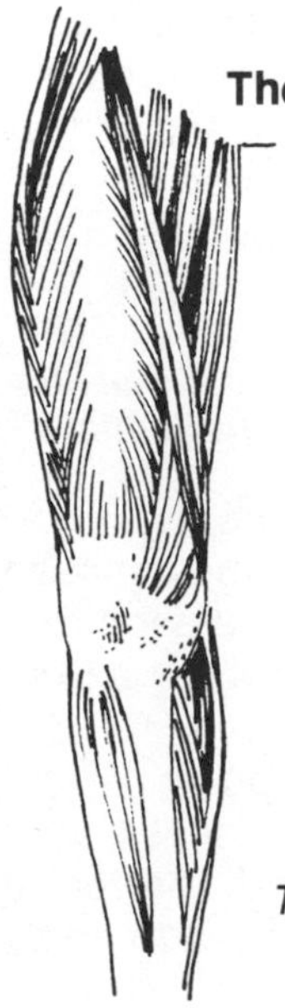

**The Thigh, Calf and Knee**

Sports such as skiing, skating, ice hockey, surfing, horseback riding, and cycling all require quick reflexes and muscle power. While the neck, shoulders, and back are under stress in these sports, the muscles of the lower back and hips also undergo stress and strain. Often there is pain in the knee area and thigh after a day of heavy exertion.

*Massage:* Use the tips of your fingers to apply direct pressure to the stress points of the knee, then follow with cross-fiber friction. Repeat the sequence several times. Use your fingertips to apply circular friction over the knee. Use your fist to finish with circular friction movements. Locate the stress areas in the thighs above the knee and in the groin and inguinal fold. With your thumb apply pressure for 10 counts; release and repeat the movement several times. Apply cross-fiber friction for 10 counts. Release and repeat several times. Finish the massage by applying deep strokes from knee to hip, and shaking and rolling the thigh.

*The thigh, calf and knee*

**Golf Knee**

In golf the twisting movements of the torso cause the knee to rotate until the ligaments are sometime strained. Golf appears to be a mild enough game, but injuries to the knees (and back) do occur.

*Massage:* Locate the stress points. Use the middle or thumb finger to apply direct pressure. Hold for 20 counts. Release and repeat the movement. Apply cross-fiber friction for 20 counts; release and repeat the movement. Apply friction around the patella. Movements should be gentle.

**Calf**

Tennis and similar games place stress on the muscles of the calves and ankles, often causing spasms.

*Massage:* Have the athlete lie face down. Bend the knee and flex the ankle several times. Locate the stress points at the outside of the knee joint. Use your thumbs to apply direct pressure, holding for 10 counts. Release and repeat the movement. Follow with cross-fiber friction on the stress points. Repeat the direct pressure and friction on the lower stress points of the ankle. Use the palm of your hand to apply deep compression all over the calf muscles. Follow with compression, then finish the massage with cross-fiber friction along fibrous bands in the muscle. Apply deep strokes from heel to knee, followed with shaking of the muscle and effleurage.

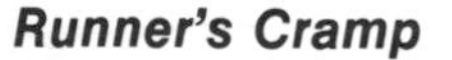

**Runner's Cramp**

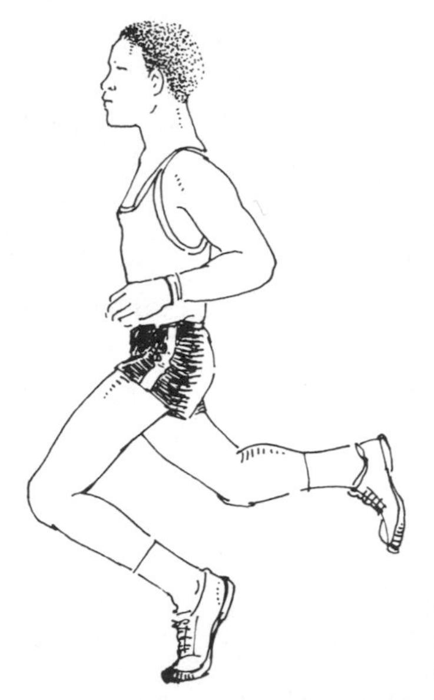

The runner will often suffer muscle cramps, spasm, muscle tightening, and calf pull. Ice may be applied to the spasmed area. Have the athlete tighten and relax the antagonist muscle to the one in spasm several times while slightly stretching the spasmed muscles between contractions.

*Massage:* To massage the leg, have the athlete lie face down on the table. After the spasm subsides, bend and flex the knee several times. Flex the ankle, and rotate it several times. Locate the stress points below the knee joint, then with your thumb, apply pressure for 10 counts, release, and repeat the movements. Find the stress point on the ankle, and repeat the same movements. Apply steady, firm compression movements to the calf. Compress stress points for 10 counts, release, and follow with cross-fiber friction. Repeat the compression. Apply several deep strokes from heel to knee. Shake and jostle the calf muscle from knee to ankle, and apply effleurage to the area.

*Sports or athletic massage is useful in preventing tight, sore muscles, to relieve muscle strain, fatigue and to promote healing of affected or injured muscles.*

**Strain to Hamstrings**

Sports requiring sustained leg tension for some time can lead to strain. Examples of such sports are dance and distance running. Generally, the strain will be in the back mid-thigh extending to the back of the knee.

*Massage:* Use your thumb to locate the stress point behind the knee and in the gluteal crease, and apply direct pressure for 10 counts. Release and repeat. Apply cross-fiber friction for 10 counts. Release and repeat. Use the palm of your hand to apply compression over the entire back of the thigh from the buttock to the knee. Slightly flex the knee while supporting the ankle. Release and repeat. Use your knuckles to do deep compression to the thigh gently from buttock to knee. Finish the massage with deep strokes along the hamstring from knee to hip for 10 counts.

This basic outline of movements can serve as a guideline to massage for other parts of the body. Adapt the massage movements to the location and to the extent of the muscle strain or condition needing relief.

### The Elbow and Arm

The muscles in the arm and shoulder may be weakened by overuse or strain from an activity such as tennis. Muscles can become stiff and sore. Generally, the extensor muscles of the forearm will be affected. In the acute state this condition is characterized by inflammation, swelling, and intense pain.

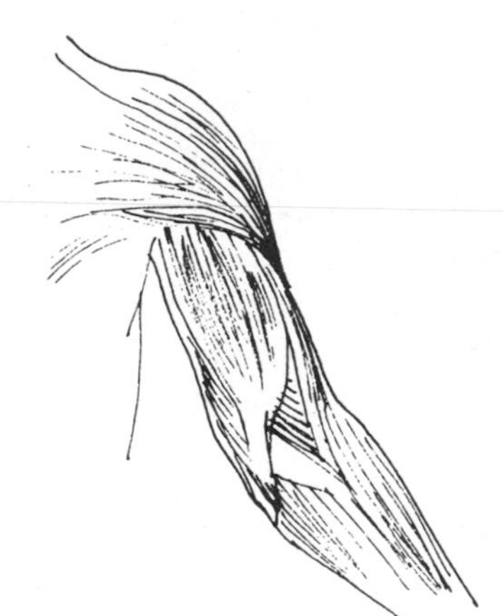

*The elbow and arm*

*Massage:* Using the heel of your hand, apply compression to the wrist for 10 counts. From the wrist work up to the elbow, the shoulder, then back down to the wrist so that the entire arm is covered. Find the pressure point at the inner side of the elbow, and with your thumb apply direct pressure for about 10 counts. Release and repeat the pressure three or more times. Using cross-fiber friction, move to the next pressure point. Follow along the length of the muscle repeating the cross-fiber friction where the muscle fibers seem stuck together. Follow this with several more compressions along the muscle. Apply deep stroking movements along the muscle from insertion to origin, and follow these with shaking and jostling movements. Repeat the same procedure to other stress points, and finish with general compression on the entire arm, gentle passive-joint movements, stretching and soothing effleurage. Instruct the athlete to rest the arm, and repeat the treatment daily until all symptoms are gone.

### The Wrist

The ligament, tendons, and muscles of the wrist can be affected by tension caused by grasping and tensing for long periods of time. Examples are grasping the handle bars of a bicycle and lifting weights.

*Massage:* Find the pressure point. Use your fingertips to apply direct pressure to the stress point, holding for 10 counts. Release then repeat the movements several times. Apply cross-fiber friction for 10 counts; release and repeat. Use your thumb to apply cross-fiber friction all around the wrist and back again. Do this for about 15 to 20 counts; release and repeat the movement. Follow with a series of compressions using the heel of your hand. Apply compression up the forearm from wrist to elbow going all around the arm. Repeat these movements several times. Finish the massage by applying direct pressure to the stress points for 10 to 20 counts; release and repeat the movement.

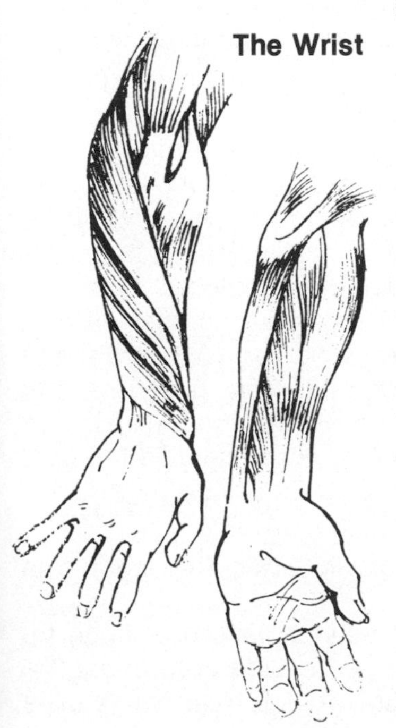

*The wrist*

**Back, Shoulder and Neck**

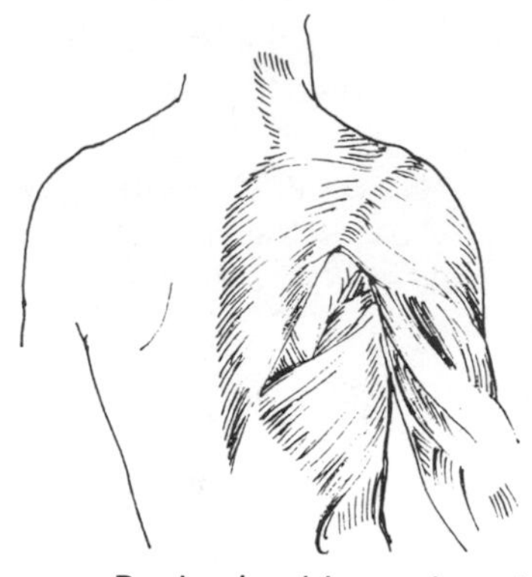

*Back, shoulder and neck*

The back and shoulder muscles are often strained during weight lifting, bowling, golf and other sports.

*Massage:* Have the athlete lie face down on the table. Use the thumb to apply deep pressure and cross-fiber friction at high stress areas for 10 counts. Release and repeat the movement. Do this sequence about 4 times. Apply cross-fiber friction to the side of the neck and downward on the shoulder. Apply for 10 counts; release and repeat until the area has been covered. Find the stress points on the shoulder blade. Apply direct pressure for 10 counts; release and repeat the action. Apply cross-fiber friction for 10 counts; release and repeat the movement. Do this sequence several times. Find the stress points around the shoulder blade and repeat the direct prèssure for 10 counts. Release and repeat the cross-fiber movements for 10 counts. Finish the massage with compression done with the palm.

**Mid-Back and Lower Back**

*Massage:* Have the athlete lie on the table face down. Find the stress points in the muscular bands along each side of the spine. With your thumb, apply direct pressure for 10 counts. Release and repeat the movement all the way down the back. Do the sequence down the back several times. Work with the client's breathing. Apply pressure on the exhale and release on the inhale. Apply cross-fiber friction with your thumb for 10 counts. Release and repeat the movement moving an inch or so down the back. Use the palm of your hand to apply several compressions on the muscle. Use your thumb to apply cross-fiber friction on the outerside of the muscle. Return to cross-fiber friction with your thumbs for 10 counts. Release and repeat the movement. Do this sequence several times. Apply deep strokes with the thumbs from the top of the shoulders down to the tailbone, then shake and vibrate the muscles back up to the shoulders. Apply compressions to the buttock with the heel of your hand, and finish by flushing out the area with effleurage.

**Raquetball Shoulder**

This is somewhat like tennis elbow, but can be more severe. It affects the trapezius and deltoid muscles.

*Massage:* Begin with direct pressure on the stress points, holding for 10 counts. Apply friction over the back including the neck for about 20 counts. Use compression movement on the shoulders. Release and repeat the movements. Massage the entire back from the waist upward over the shoulders. Massage over the deltoid muscle. Find the pressure points of the shoulders, and apply deep compression for 10 counts and release. Continue with cross-fiber friction for 10 counts and release, then finish with compression, using deep stroking to stretch the fibers. Shake the involved areas to release tension. Apply repeated pressure to the stress points once more, then apply effleurage to th entire area.

**Triceps Strain**

This is a condition usually occurring when the muscle is overused and stressed.

*Massage:* Find the stress point. Use your thumb or fingertip to apply direct pressure for 10 counts. Release and repeat the movements. Apply cross-fiber friction for 10 counts. Release and repeat the movements. Do this sequence (gently) several times. Apply deep strokes from elbow to shoulder, then shake and flush out the area.

**Hip, Leg, Buttock and Groin**

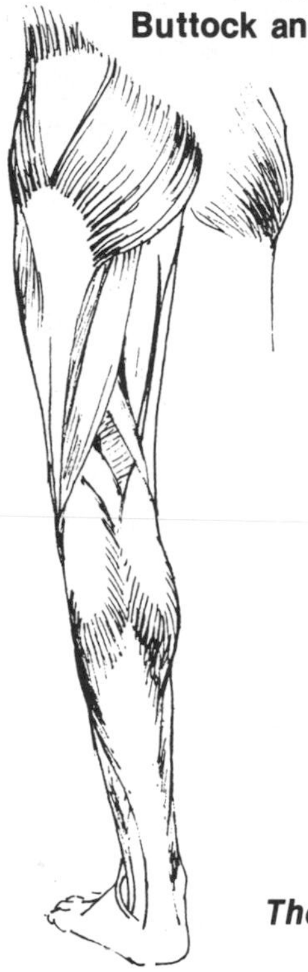

Sports such as golf cause strain to the back because of the twisting and swinging motions.

In the hip area there are four main stress points with which you need to be concerned: The side of the hip, the leg, the buttock, and the groin area.

*Massage:* Have the athlete lie face down on the table. Use the point of your thumb to apply direct pressure all over the buttock area. Locate tight stress areas. Apply pressure for 10 counts, release, and repeat the movement several times. Controlled use of the elbow is very effective in this area. Apply cross-fiber friction for 20 counts. Release and repeat the movement. Use the thumb to apply direct pressure to the lateral side of the leg to 10 counts. Release and repeat. Apply direct pressure to the lateral side of the mid-calf. Find the pressure point in the buttock and along the iliac crest. Apply deep direct pressure for 10 counts; release and repeat the movement. Apply cross-fiber friction for 10 counts to each affected area; release and repeat the movement. Repeat the cross-fiber friction for 10 counts; release and repeat the movement. Apply direct pressure again using the thumb or elbow. Apply for 10 counts; release and repeat the movement. Repeat the cross-fiber friction, and finish with deep shaking and vibration movements.

***The Groin***

The groin is more likely to be pulled in sports such as horseback riding, gymnastics and soccer. This is a painful condition caused by overstretching of the gracilis and adductor muscle located high on the inner thigh.

*Hip, leg, buttock, groin and hamstrings*

*Massage:* Have the athlete lie on his back with the knee of the affected leg bent and turned outward. Use your thumb to apply pressure and cross-fiber friction for 20 counts. Release and repeat the movement. This area will be quite tender, so it is necessary to be gentle. Find the spasm area, and apply compression with your fingertips. Release and repeat the movement.

**The Chest and Abdomen**

During some sports and especially weight lifting, the pectorals and the intercostal muscles may be strained. There may be spasm, soreness, and tenderness.

*Massage:* The athlete should lie on his back with the body relaxed. Apply circular compressions using the palm of your hand to the pectoral muscles moving from the breastbone to collarbone across the chest and shoulders. Avoid doing movements over or near the nipples because this is a sensitive area. Follow compression movements with effleurage. Apply light percussion (hacking movements) with the little finger sides of your hand over the pectoral muscles only. Finish with a few light strokes over the entire chest area.

**The Abdomen**

The rectus abdominis is often affected by sports that involve bending and twisting movements. Tension, soreness and spasm may develop in the area around the navel. Keep in mind that the abdominal region of the body is sensitive to pressure. The athlete should lie on his back with knees slightly raised and feet flat on the table. Raising the knees helps to relax the abdominal area. Use gentle movements and direct pressure downward (never upward) from the waistline toward the pubic bone.

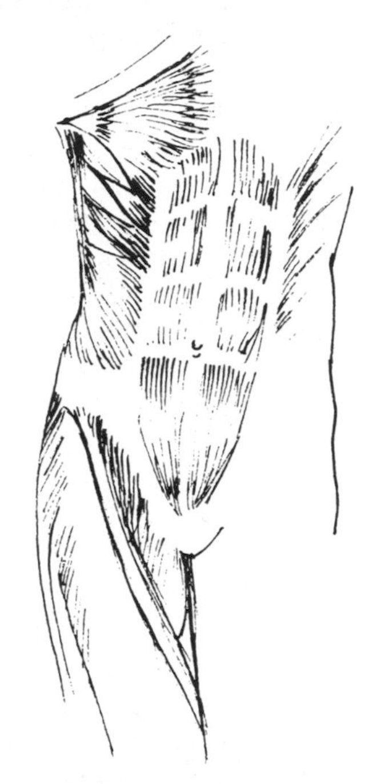

*The Chest and Abdomen*

**STEP BY STEP PROCEDURE FOR ATHLETIC MASSAGE**

Preparation and draping for athletic massage is the same as for regular massage. The athlete lies face down on the table, and a slight amount of oil is applied to the part to be massaged first. Some therapists use no oil. The following routine may be varied as necessary or desirable. However, this is the sequence usually preferred.

1. Foot Massage
   a. Grasp the foot so that your fingers are on the sole and your thumb is on top of the foot to hold it firmly.
   b. Use deep strokes with the tips of your fingers from toes across the instep and to the heel and back again. Apply about 10 strokes.
   c. Hold the foot firmly around the toes while pressing the knuckles of the other hand into the ball of the foot moving down to the instep and heel. Repeat the movements several times.
   d. Apply compression with the tips of your thumbs over the sole of the foot, moving across and down the foot.
   e. Rotate the ankle clockwise and counterclockwise.
   f. Rotate each toe.

   g. Use circular friction movements with the fingers and thumbs to massage tendons and ligaments and to massage over the foot and the ankle bone.
   h. Repeat rotation and combine with flexing.
2. Lower Leg Massage
   a. With the heel of your hand apply deep compression movements from the outside of the knee to the ankle, concentrating on the muscle mass. This movement is done by making a dozen or so compressive movements to a pass and about three to five passes. Finish this part of the massage by using the palm of your hand or fingers in circular friction movements across the front of the leg. Apply deep strokes from ankle to knee. Massage the other leg.
3. Thigh Massage
   a. Use your palms to apply firm compression movements to the front of the leg, beginning with the knee. Make about five or six passes applying compression movements over the thigh from the hip area to the knee joint.
   b. Apply circular friction to the knee joint.
   c. Apply kneading movements, working up to the knee and to the groin then down again.
   d. Apply compression movements.
   e. Apply percussion movements to the entire thigh area (use hacking and beating movements).
   f. Finish with deep effleurage strokes and flexing of the knee and hip.
   g. Bend the knee toward the chest and extend it several times. Rotate the femur in its socket, then make circles with the knee while flexing it.
   h. Massage the other thigh.
4. Arm Massage
   a. Use the fingers, pad of your thumb, or the heel of your hand to apply compression to the entire length of the arm, from wrist to shoulder.
   b. Apply circular friction to the back of the hand.
   c. Use the tips of your fingers to make deep thrusting movements to the palm of the hand and around the wrists.
   d. Finish with deep effleurage and flexing of the elbow.
   e. Shake the arm vigorously.
   f. Massage the other arm.
5. Abdominal Massage

   For massage of the abdomen, the athlete should raise his knees slightly keeping the feet flat on the table. This tends to relax the abdominals.

   a. Begin with kneading movements over the entire abdominal area, graduating from gentle to stronger movements.

b. Use the thumbs to apply direct pressure to stress areas along the pubic and ribs.

6. Chest Massage

a. Use the palm of your hand to apply circular compression to the pectoral muscles of the chest, over the breastbone, collarbone, and shoulders. Avoid any movement over the sensitive area of the nipples.

b. With the palm of your hand, apply circular friction movements over the rib cage.

c. Use the outer edge of your hands to apply percussion (hacking) movements to the pectorals. This should not be so brisk as to cause discomfort.

7. Back Massage

The athlete turns over to a prone position. It is advisable to place a bolster or support under the ankles.

a. Use your palm to apply petrissage movements, beginning with the shoulder blades and covering the entire back to the knees. Make six or eight circles in the same place then move on to another area. Do three to four passes.

b. Use your fist to apply pressure (not heavy) to both sides of the spine.

c. Apply direct compression (with palms) to the shoulders about 20 to 50 compressions.

d. Use thumbs to apply pressure to stress points across shoulders, around the scapula, along spine above, and below the iliac crest.

e. Apply cross-fiber friction to "tight" areas.

f. Apply deep compression to the buttock.

g. Use the thumbs or heel of the hand to apply gentle circular friction movements along the spine.

h. Apply slow compression with the heel of the hand to the sides of the spine moving upward from the waistline to the neck.

i. Apply compression with the tips of your fingers to the entire upper back and across the shoulder blades to the base of the neck.

j. Apply kneading movements to the trapezius and base of the neck.

k. Apply percussion with your fist using hacking and beating movements over the shoulders.

l. To finish the massage do light percussion over the entire back.

8. Back of the Leg Massage

a. Use the palm of your hand to apply compression to the entire calf and posterior thigh.

b. Use kneading movement from the ankle, up the thigh, and over the buttock.

c. Use your fist or the heel of your hand to apply compressions down to the inner side of the leg to the knee, then repeat the movements to the middle and outside portions of the leg. Do three to six passes for each section.

d. Use the fist or palm to apply compression movements to the buttock. Begin with the gluteus maximus, and move upward to cover the entire areas of both buttocks. The number of compressions depend on the size of the person being massaged. Generally, 50 compressions for each section will be sufficient.

e. Use your thumbs to apply direct pressure to stress points.

f. Apply percussion movements from the knee to the buttocks.

g. Finish the massage by bending the knee several times. Grasp the foot and bend the knee by pushing the foot toward the buttocks.

9. Neck Massage

   Have the athlete fold his hands palms down and rest his forehead on them.

   a. Apply compression movements from the base of the neck to the base of the skull. Cover the entire area of the back of the neck.

   b. Apply compression movements to shoulders with the palms of the hands.

   c. Apply effleurage to the shoulders and neck.

10. Revisit areas and repeat massage movements as necessary especially in heavily used or tight areas of the body.

**QUESTIONS FOR DISCUSSION AND REVIEW**

1. In addition to thorough understanding of human anatomy and physiology, which four major body systems and their functions must the therapist know?
2. Approximately what percent of an adult's body weight is made of skeletal muscle?
3. When is athletic massage contraindicated?
4. What are the four basic applications for athletic massage?
5. When is massage considered to be the most beneficial to the athlete?
6. Why must the therapist be sure to apply proper techniques at all times?
7. How does massage therapy affect the healing time of injuries?
8. Who is qualified to give athletic massage to new or fresh injuries?
9. Although golf is considered to be a fairly mild form of exercise, what parts of the body are most likely to sustain injuries?
10. Where is the Achilles tendon located?

## ANSWERS TO QUESTIONS FOR DISCUSSION AND REVIEW

1. The therapist must know the functions of the circulatory, skeletal, muscular, and nervous systems of the body.
2. Approximately 40 percent of an adult's body weight is skeletal muscle.
3. Athletic massage is contraindicated in any abnormal condition, injury, illness, or disease except as advised by the athlete's physician.
4. The four basic applications for athletic massage are massage previous to an event, massage after an event, massage during training, and massage during rehabilitation.
5. Massage is considered to be most beneficial to the athlete during his or her scheduled training.
6. The therapist must be sure to apply proper techniques in order to avoid aggravating a condition or causing permanent damage to the area. Proper techniques also help prevent possibility of a liability suit.
7. Proper massage therapy improves circulation, enabling damaged tissue to be carried away while making rebuilding nutrients available so that healing time is reduced.
8. Massage for new or fresh injuries should only be given by properly trained therapists in conjunction with a physician's approval.
9. While golf is a fairly mild form of exercise, the athlete may sustain injuries to his or her wrists, ankles, back, legs, knees or hips.
10. The Achilles tendon is located just above the heel.

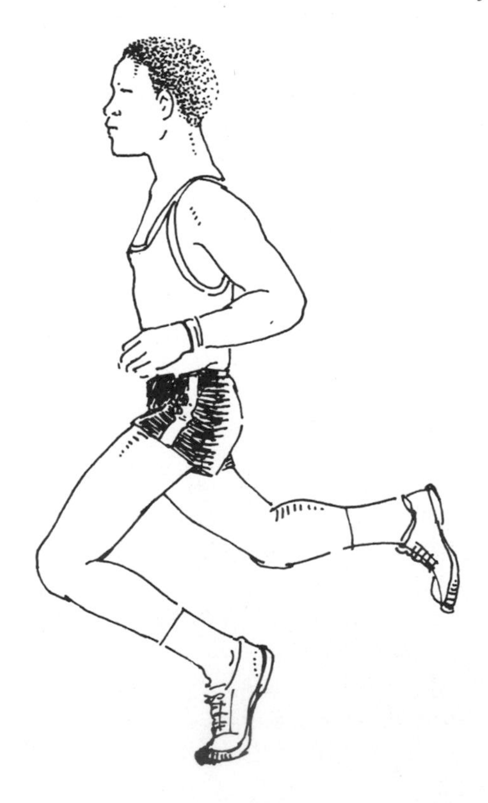

# Chapter 15 Specialized Massage

**LEARNING OBJECTIVES**

After you have mastered this chapter, you will be able to:

1. Explain the benefits of prenatal massage.
2. Explain contraindications for prenatal massage.
3. Explain the benefits of lymph massage.
4. Describe the basic functions of the lymphatic system.
5. Explain the purpose of structural integration.
6. Explain the basic philosophy of acupressure and acupuncture.
7. Describe shiatsu as related to pressure points of the body.
8. Explain the benefits of stress therapy massage.
9. Define reflexology.
10. Demonstrate a basic arm and hand massage.
11. Demonstrate a basic foot massage.
12. Explain the benefits of hand and foot massage.

## INTRODUCTION

In recent years there has been a resurgence of interest in various massage therapies that relate to the maintenance of physical, mental, and emotional health. Many of these techniques are related to or are descendants of Swedish massage in that they encourage relaxation, increase the movement of body fluids, and soothe the nervous system. Some of these touch techniques are referred to as bodywork.

## DEEP TISSUE MASSAGE

In most deep tissue massage techniques the aim is to affect the various layers of fascia that support muscle tissues and loosen bonds between the layers of connective tissues. Some of these deep tissue massage techniques are named after the person who developed or specialized in them.

It is not within the scope of this book to cover in detail all of the therapies. However, the serious student or practitioner will find a wealth of reference material listed in the massage reference list. The brief outlines included in this chapter will serve to acquaint the beginner with some of the basic concepts of the various philosophies from which the techniques have grown.

## PRENATAL MASSAGE

In normal, healthy pregnancies, massage has proven to be beneficial to both mother and unborn child. Properly applied massage can aid relaxation, benefit circulation, and soothe nerves. Prenatal massage is applied like any regular massage except for the following consideration:

*Positioning:* The client may take any of several positions depending on which is more comfortable. If the client takes a supine position, a small pillow or a folded towel is placed under her lower back. A pillow or a small (six or eight inch) bolster can also be placed under the bend of her knees to take the strain off her abdominal muscles. If the client would be more comfortable, she may lie on her side or try a prone position. During the first two to three months of pregnancy, there is no problem with the prone position. However, as the abdomen becomes larger, pillows placed underneath the client's head, chest, abdomen and legs will add to her comfort. She may prefer lying on her side or on her back especially during the final months of pregnancy. The client should be asked to indicate if at anytime during the treatment she becomes uncomfortable.

**Body Areas Subject to Discomfort**

The lower back is a common area of strain during pregnancy due to the extra weight of the growing fetus. Lateral and abdominal muscles are also under strain from carrying the extra weight, and from stretching to accommodate the growing fetus. Effleurage and light petrissage are soothing and will relieve tension in the muscles. The main aim of prenatal massage is to help the expectant mother to relax.

Before beginning a prenatal massage, it is important to ask the expectant mother if there is any reason why massage over the abdominal area would not be advisable.

Strokes should be done in a clockwise manner the same as for any abdominal massage. However, the strokes must be light, and only very gentle pressure is used. Women often comment on how pleasant and soothing they find massage to be during pregnancy because of its calming and reassuring effects.

**Positions for Prenatal Massage**

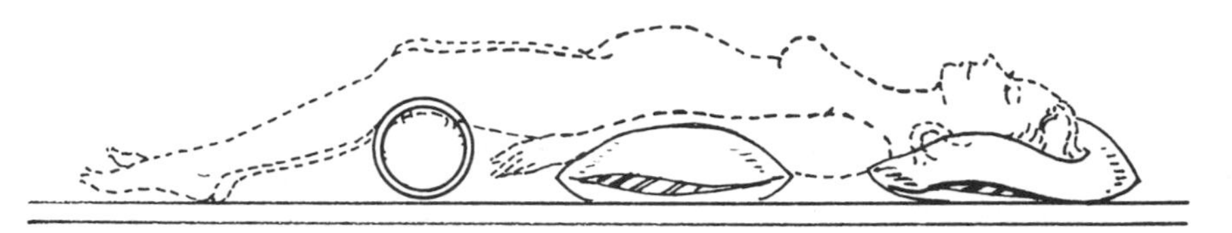

*Lying in a supine position, a small pillow or a folded towel is placed in the small of the client's lower back for added comfort. A small bolster is placed under the bend of her knees.*

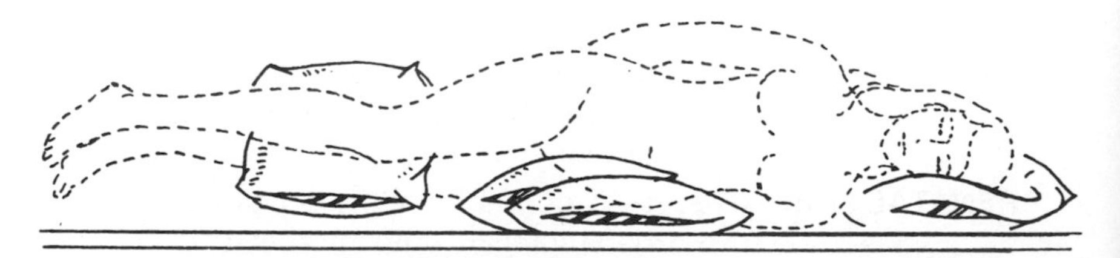

*Lying on side, a small pillow is placed between her knees and another pillow placed under her abdomen for additional support. A pillow is provided for her head.*

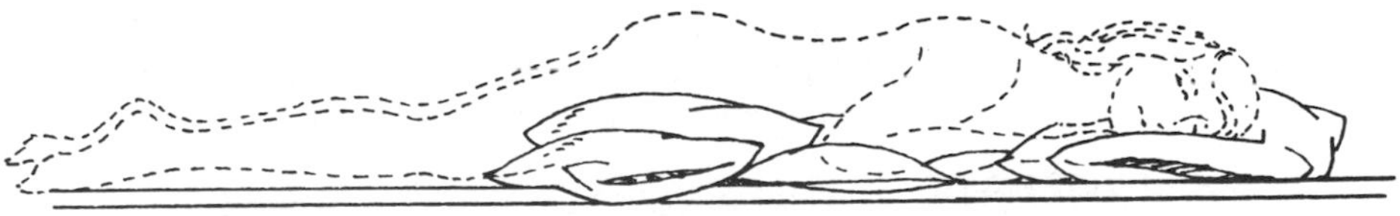

*Lying in a prone position, the client will be more comfortable if support is provided beneath her body. Small pillows may be placed beneath her legs, abdomen, breasts, and her head.*

### Contraindications for Prenatal Massage

During pregnancy, massage is not given when contraindications are present. Problems can occur during pregnancy and the expectant mother should be under her physician's care regarding diet, exercise, and massage. However, many physicians recommend massage for its therapeutic effects.

#### *Conditions Associated With Pregnancy*

Preclampsia, a type of toxemia, is a condition sometimes occurring in the latter half of pregnancy and is characterized by high blood pressure, edema (swelling of hands, feet, and face), and sodium retention. This condition can be brought about by excessive weight gain or protein in the urine. The expectant mother may suffer headaches and dizziness, and in serious cases, convulsions. When toxemia is suspected, the expectant mother should see her physician without delay.

If edema is minimal, it is acceptable to massage (effleurage) the legs and arms. If the edema is serious, massage should not be done and the client should be referred to her physician.

Varicose veins are often a problem during pregnancy due to the effects of progesterone on the blood vessels and to the increased pressure on the main blood vessels that return blood from the legs. Light effleurage can be done around, but not on, affected areas.

## MASSAGE DURING LABOR

A physician may recommend light effleurage on the patient's abdomen and upper legs as a means of obtaining relief during contractions. Lower back pains can also be relieved by the application of firm continuous counterpressure. During a contraction, counterpressure can be applied to both sides of the spine in the area of the sacrum.

## MASSAGE FOLLOWING BIRTH

Many times a mother will request massage throughout her pregnancy and after the child is born. Massage helps to relieve neck, shoulder, and lower back discomfort and is an aid in the relief of tension. When combined with proper exercise and diet, massage will be of value in regaining normal weight and firming slack muscles.

## LYMPH MASSAGE

Lymph or lymphatic massage is a descendent of Swedish massage. Dr. Emile Vodder of Copenhagen, Denmark, pioneered the practice of lymph drainage massage. He is credited with having discovered the benefits of lymphatic massage and for the development of massage techniques widely used today.

Before beginning the study of lymph massage, the practitioner or student must have a thorough knowledge of anatomy and particularly of the lymphatic system. Lymph drainage massage requires careful training procedures, therefore the student must be guided by the instructor at all times.

The following overview will be helpful to understanding the basic functions of the lymphatic system and the principles of the lymph drainage massage.

## THE LYMPHATIC SYSTEM

The lymphatic system is a system of vessels and nodes (glands) supplementary to the blood vascular system. The spleen, tonsils and thymus are related organs. Lymph capillaries are small, thin-walled tubes that collect lymph from interstitial fluid in the tissues and from other lymphatic vessels. In structure the larger vessels are like veins but have thinner walls and more numerous valves. The larger vessels converge to form the right lymphatic duct, which carries the lymph from the right arm, the right side of the thorax, the right side of the head and neck, and empties into the right brachiocephalic vein. Though smaller than the lymphatic duct, the thoracic duct is an important lymphatic channel because it collects lymph that flows from other parts of the body.

Lymph is the portion of the interstitial fluid that is absorbed into the lymphatic system. It is composed of proteins, salts, water, and other substances derived from blood plasma. It is through this fluid that tissues receive their nourishment and building materials. Without lymph, tissues would soon dry out and degenerate. Lymph is also the means by which unwanted cellular debris, excess protein, and cell waste are flushed away.

Lymph circulation is vital to life; when it slows down, waste products can accumulate and stagnate. This produces a feeling of fatigue, and normal metabolism is affected. The movement of lymph is maintained by the difference in the pressure within the lymphatic system, by normal respiration, and by muscular movements of the body in general.

The immune system, of which the lymphatic system is an important part, produces lymphocytes and other cells in response to the presence of inflammation, antigens, bacteria, and other cellular debris in the body. Specialized lymph vessels called lacteals carry away fat that is absorbed in the digestive tract.

A lymphocyte, or leukocyte, is a white blood corpuscle found in the lymphatic tissue, blood, and lymph. Lymphocytes are active in the immune responses of the body and play a major role in the healing of wounds and fighting of infections. They penetrate all tissues and are abundant in lymph tissue, blood, bone marrow, mucous membranes, connective tissue, skin, and all body organs.

### Lymph Nodes or Glands

Lymph nodes or glands, are small masses of lymphatic tissue. They vary in size and shape but are usually less than 1 inch (2.5 cm) in length. They are often bead-like or bean shaped compact structures that lie in groups along the course of lymphatic vessels. When inflamed, lymph can be felt beneath the skin. The chief function of lymph nodes is to produce lymphocytes and serve as a filtering system.

Lymph enter the lymph nodes by way of the afferent (inward) lymph vessels. Contaminants that may be harmful if left to circulate freely through the vascular system, are carried by the lymph and deposited in the nodes. Here, antigens, broken down cells, and toxins are acted upon, broken down, or devoured by the lymphocytes and turned into harmless substances, then are passed out of the lymph nodes through efferent (outward) vessels and back into the blood system to be eliminated.

Lymph nodes are usually distributed in groups. Regional lymph nodes include:

Submaxillary nodes, located beneath the mandible.

Preauricular nodes, located in front of the ear.

Postauricular nodes, located behind the ear in the region of the mastoid process.

Occipital nodes, located at the base of the skull.

Superficial cervical nodes, located at the side of and over the sternocleidal mastoid muscle. Axillary nodes are located in the armpit. Constituting the main group of the upper extremity, axillary nodes receive lymph from vessels that drain the wall of the thorax, mammary glands, and upper wall of the abdomen.

Supratrochlear nodes, located in the elbows.

Inguinal nodes, located in the groin constituting the most important group of the lower extremity, inguinal nodes, receive lymph from the leg, external genitalia, and lower abdominal wall.

Deep cervical nodes, located along the carotid artery and internal jugular vein.

Popliteal nodes, located behind the knee.

Abdominal and pelvic cavities also have lymph nodes.

## INFLUENCE OF MASSAGE ON BODY FLUIDS

It is important to understand the influence of massage on circulation of fluids in the human body, because both the lymphatic and venous circulations are accelerated by massage movements. These movements are applied from the extremities toward the heart stimulating lymphatic circulation. The capillaries, which end in the tissues, absorb lymph and assist its flow into the lymphatic vessels. Lymphatic chains can be compared to pumping stations. While blood is being returned to the heart by way of the veins, the lymphatics are draining the tissues of interstitial fluid needed for nourishment and growth. Lymph drainage stimulates the activity of the lymph centers, increases the production of lymphocytes and lymph corpuscles, and improves body metabolism. The natural movements of the body such as walking, standing, and exercising aids this process, but correct massage more fully augments the working of the lymph system.

Correct lymph massage accelerates the flow of lymph, helping to rid the body of toxins and waste materials. Lymph drainage massage promotes balance of the body's internal chemistry, purifies and regenerates tissues, helps to normalize the functions of organs, and promotes the function of the immune system.

## Techniques of Lymph Drainage Massage

The techniques of lymph drainage massage are based on alternate pressure and release movements. Decreased pressure opens lymph valves, while increased pressure closes them.

Lymphatic massage is a pumping motion done with the palm of the hand pressing toward the center of the body. Attention should be paid to muscle tissue, with concentration on the proximal areas of the limb where there is a higher concentration of lymph tissue. Successful lymph drainage massage depends on the expertise of the practitioner. He or she must consider the effects to be achieved by various movements. For example, body fluids can be displaced intravascularly (within vessels) or extravascularly (in the interstitial spaces). This displacement of fluid is achieved by manual strokes.

Lymph movement is also increased in the muscles and organs by stimulation of neuro-lymphatic reflexes located primarily on the front and back of the trunk and on the medial and lateral aspects of the thigh. Affected points may be massaged with strong, deep friction massage for 20 to 30 seconds. These points may be quite tender and more evident on the front of the body.

Before attempting lymph massage, the practitioner should be thoroughly familiar with the functions of the lymphatic system. An illustration of the lymphatic system is included in the anatomy section of this book. See Chapter 5.

Lymph massage is done to encourage, but not force, the movement of lymph through the lymphatic system. The procedure begins at the junction of the right thoracic lymph duct and vein adjacent to the junction of the jugular veins, and just behind the cervical near its articulation to the sternum. This is where the lymph and blood systems dump their waste into the venous blood.

The practitioner uses a pumping action in this area of the neck first on one side and then on the other side. Pressure should not be applied to both sides at once because the junction of the thoracic ducts are very near the brachiocephalic vein, the jugular vein, and the junction of the carotid artery and the aorta. Stimulation and/or pressure to both sides could adversely affect the blood flow to the brain. The practitioner may want to do one side of the lymph drainage area before proceeding to the other. For example, beginning with the right lymphatic duct then proceeding to the thoracic duct and the area drained by it, then the rest of the body.

### *Procedure for a Lymph Massage*

The following procedure should be done only under the supervision of an instructor.

1. *Base of neck:* Begin with the right side of the neck just superior to the clavical. Apply direct compression movements toward the clavicular-sternal sinus, then proceed up the side of the neck to include the entire area from the occiput to the submandibular area and to the cervicospinal process. Continue to the sternalcleidol mastoid. Finish with effleurage in a downard direction on the entire side of the head and neck.

2. *Pectoral and axillary area:* Right side compression begins along the sternal and clavicular borders and is directed toward the center of the body proceeding down and out to cover the entire chest area. If the client is a woman, pressure is not put directly on the mammary, or breast, tissue.
3. *Right arm:* Support the arm abducted and elevated to expose the underside of the arm and axillary area. Do compression movements to the entire arm beginning in the axillary area (proceeding distally) while directing the compressions toward the bone and up the arm toward the shoulder. Finish with effleurage. Left side: Proceed in a similar manner on the left side of the body.
4. *Head and neck:* Apply gentle compression movements followed by effleurage.
5. *Axillary area:* Apply gentle downward and outward compression. Finish with light effleurage.
6. *Left arm:* Repeat the procedure used for the right arm.
7. *Abdomen:* The lymph from the abdomen, lower extremities, and the digestive system empty into the cisterna chyli located at the inferior end of the thoracic duct, at a level just inferior to the umbilicus (the navel). All compressions are directed towards this area. Begin compressions on the upper abdomen near the costal border, directing the compression upward and toward the center while proceeding down the inguinal crease in the groin area. Movements are more effective if the knees are elevated so the feet remain flat on the table. Finish with deep effleurage. Repeat the movements on the other side of the abdomen.
8. *Legs:* Begin in the groin area of the right leg, and continue compression movements on down the leg. Direct force into the leg and upward. Pay special attention to the medial portion of the thigh, making sure not to be so forceful as to cause the client discomfort. Finish the massage with effleurage, continuing up to the abdomen. Repeat the massage on the left leg.
9. *Back of legs:* The client should assume a prone position. Begin in the gluteal area around the iliac crest, and apply compression movements covering the entire buttock and leg, proceeding from the hip to the heel. Do not use heavy pressure in the popliteal space behind the knee. Finish the massage with deep effleurage. Do the other leg and buttock.
10. *Back:* In lymph massage little effect is achieved over a large portion of the back. However, there are neuro-lymphatic reflexes along both sides of the spine that may be stimulated with deep circular friction. Compression massage may be continued in the area of the latisimus dorsi, teres, and upper trapezius area. Deep effleurage over the entire back concludes the massage.

Lymphatic massage is very stimulating and invigorating, so the client should be encouraged to rest for a few minutes before getting off the massage table.

**Lymphatic Pump Manipulation**

The lymphatic pump manipulation enhances the flow of lymph through the entire system and may be done in conjunction with a lymph drainage massage at the beginning or end of the massage or as a separate manipulation.

***Procedure***

The client lies supine. The practitioner stands at the head of the massage table and places his or her hands to cover as much of the client's rib cage as possible. This enables the practitioner to press his or her weight into the client's ribs. The client is encouraged to breathe deeply for five or more deep breaths, forcing the ribs up under the pressure of the practitioner's hands. As the client breathes deeply, the practitioner begins to bounce at the rate of about 150 bounces per minute using the weight of his or her upper body. Pressure should be sufficient to force complete expulsion of the breath but not so heavy as to prevent inhalation. The client should lie quietly for a few minutes following this procedure.

This process is contraindicated for persons with high blood pressure, heart condition, or broken or cracked ribs.

**Deep Tissue Technique**

The term deep tissue refers to various regimens or massage styles that affect the deeper tissue structures of the body. Some of the techniques focus just on the physiological release of tension or bonds in the tissues, while others use bodywork in conjunction with or as a means of psychological release. Some of the deep tissue techniques include rolfing, acupressure, shiatsu, and reflexology. Athletic massage is also included in this category and has been covered in more depth in Chapter 14 of this book. The following are brief explanations of some of these techniques.

**Structural Integration**

As the name implies, structural integration attempts to bring the physical structure of the body into alignment around a central axis. This is done by affecting the fascia of the structural muscles. After structural integrations both physical and psychological balance are often experienced by the client.

Throughout life, traumas, both physical and emotional, may cause a reduction of movement that results in a shortening or binding together of the connective tissue surrounding muscles. Restriction may affect fibers, bundles, and whole muscles. This condition can also come about as a result of habitual postures while sitting, walking, and standing. Poor posture can be learned by imitating parents or from environmental factors or as a reaction to some forms of punishment and emotionally charged situations. Structural integration can be beneficial when given by a practitioner who knows the methods and understands how to achieve the desired results.

***Rolfing***

Rolfing, a method of structural integration, is a deep connective tissue massage originated by Dr. Ida Rolf, a biochemist and massage practitioner. Dr. Rolf discovered that in a normal, healthy body the spine is correctly aligned, allowing the organs to function properly. However, during childhood and in early adult formative years, poor posture habits are often formed and the body is thrown off center or out of its normal, healthy alignment. This in turn can cause structural problems. Incorrect body alignment can also cause tension in muscles and connective tissues and may interfere with normal functioning of internal organs. Dr. Rolf originated a series of treatments called "Rolfing" to bring the body into proper structural integration.

The goal of Rolfing treatments is to reshape the body's physical posture and to realign the muscular and connective tissue. The benefits of Rolfing also include increased suppleness of the muscles, improved appearance and a renewed sense of well being.

Rolfing techniques involve the use of heavy pressure applied carefully to the client's body with the fingers, a knuckle, a fist, or sometimes an elbow. Rolfing is usually done in a series of 10 treatments of one hour duration each. During this time, the practitioner (Rolfer) works on various portions of the body.

Contraindications for Rolfing are the same as for any other type of massage. When in doubt about the use of this type of treatment, the client's physician should be consulted. The practitioner who wishes to pursue Rolfing techniques should study under the supervision of a qualified instructor.

**Energetic Manipulation**

Throughout the philosophies of Eastern countries is the premise that there is a force, or vibration common to all living matter. It is believed that the smooth flow of this force is the predeterminator of good health.

When this flow is out of balance in the body, the person experiences physical illness and a sense of uneasiness. Techniques have been developed that in some cases detect imbalances in the flow of the force in the body and affect it in such a way as to bring it back into balance, or homeostasis.

Some techniques based on these theories are acupuncture (a medical procedure rather than a massage technique), acupressure, shiatsu, polarity, and reflexology. The following is a brief explanation of these techniques.

**Acupuncture**

Acupuncture is said to have originated in China more than 5,000 years ago. It is recognized around the world today as a remedial and medical technique. Throughout history, more people have been treated with acupuncture than all other therapies combined. Acupuncture is not an exact massage technique, however. The basic philosophy underlies to some degree many of the energetic massage techniques. Touch is an integral part of acupuncture treatment. Acupuncture is summed up as a medical practice whereby the skin is punctured with needles at specific points for therapeutic purposes. Acupuncture must be done only by highly trained practitioners.

It is not within the scope of this book to cover the philosophy that support such therapies as acupuncture and shiatsu but the following information will help the beginning practitioner or student to gain a better understanding of the therapies that originated in the ancient cultures of China and Japan.

**Buddhist Thought**

Buddhist thought speaks of "Tao" or "the way" and refers to the law of the universe or "that which is all there is." The belief is that Tao was split into two parts and those two parts became opposed and dynamically in motion, thus creating the energy that sustains the whole. These two parts are represented by Yin and Yang.

***Symbol for Yin and Yang***

The yin and yang theory demonstrates the natural process of continuous change where nothing is of itself, but is seen as aspects of the whole or as two opposites, yet complementary, aspects of existence. Therefore, yin and yang are seen as opposites of the same phenomena and exist only in relation to one another. The following list of words will show yin and yang contrasts:

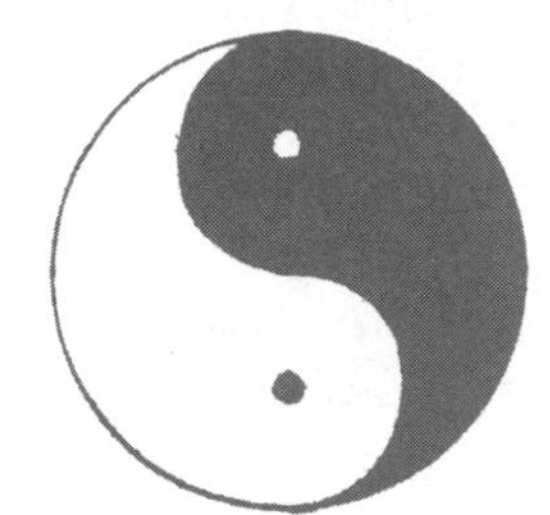

***Opposites***

| YIN | YANG |
|---|---|
| dark or night | light or day |
| low | high |
| cold | hot |
| inside | outside |
| contracting | expanding |
| passive | active |
| deficient | excessive |

***For the Body***

| YIN | YANG |
|---|---|
| front of the body | back of the body |
| inner body | outer body |
| lower body | upper body |
| underactive | overactive |
| coldness | hotness |
| weak | forceful |

Although yin and yang are diametrically opposed, one has no meaning without the other. There is continuous and constant vying as one creates and transforms into the other while at the same time holding the other in check. It is said that when yin and yang are in balance there is harmony and well being. The outcome of long-term disharmony is disease. If yang is too strong or excessive, yin will appear to be too weak. If yang is weak, yin will be overbearing. If the imbalance becomes too severe, yin and yang will separate, and the result is death of the organism. Breathing, digestion, metabolic rest and activity, even the seasons are examples of this interaction. It is this relationship that is considered to be the source of all change and movement.

**Ki or Bioforce**

In the constant interplay of yin and yang, there is created a subtle vibratory substance or a force or energy existing in all life forms and recognized by many philosophers as the vital force of growth and change. *Chi* (China) and *ki* (Japan) are two of the words used to describe this concept, while *bioenergy* and *bioforce* are terms in current usage that reflect similar ideas. There is no one word in English that adequately translates the yin and yang concept of chi (ki).

In discussing ki as it relates to health, it is much clearer to speak in terms of function. Ki in the body comes from three major sources: heredity from parents, the food we eat, and the air we breath. These three sources combine and permeate our beings. According to ancient philosophy, ki (or chi) manifests itself as five interrelated aspects of energy, which are as five elements. These are fire, earth, metal, water, and wood. Everything is created from one or more of these elements. Humans are said to be combinations of all five.

Meridian ki refers to the ki that circulates in a network of meridians, channels, and collaterals in the body. Channels and meridians are like rivers of ki (energy) that course along the extremities into the body and through related organs. Collaterals flow from meridian to meridian and allow for regulation and hormonization of ki. Along these meridians are small areas of high conductivity called acupoints (acupuncture points), where ki can be affected by a number of modalities such as pressure, heat, electricity, needles, and touch.

There are 12 meridians, or channels, that are associated with bilateral organs, and eight that have regulatory effect. A number of extra acupoints are not located on a specific meridian. Along the meridians are 395 points where the ki (or chi) flow can most easily be influenced. It is at these points that the acupuncturist will insert needles or apply pressure.

Meridians have been mapped on the body very specifically in terms of location and direction of energy flow. The practitioner who is seriously interested in pursuing the mastery of the subject must learn the location of each meridian, the direction of ki flow within the meridian, and the commonly used meridian points. The eight meridians that have a regulatory effect are:

| | |
|---|---|
| Conception vessel | Governing vessel |
| Regulatory channel of yin | Regulatory channel of yang |
| Connecting channel of yin | Connecting channel of yang |
| Belt channel | Vital or penetrating channel |

It is this balance of yin and yang that is the aim of most "energy therapists." Imbalance in the body is recognized by a number of signs and symptoms. Various therapists have differing means of recognizing imbalances and differing techniques for affecting and regulating energy flow so that a more healthful condition might be achieved.

**Organ Meridians According to Yin and Yang**

| ORGAN MERIDIAN | YIN or YANG | ELEMENT | LOCATION |
|---|---|---|---|
| Lung | Yin | Metal | Chest to end of thumb. |
| Large intestine | Yang | Metal | Index finger to face. |
| Stomach | Yang | Earth | Face to front of body to end of second toe. |
| Spleen | Yin | Earth | Middle side of large toe to inside of leg to chest. |
| Heart | Yin | Fire | Chest to inside of arm to end of little finger. |
| Small intestine | Yang | Fire | Small finger to back of arm to side of face. |
| Bladder | Yang | Water | Medial side of eye, over the head, and down the back and back of leg to little toe. |
| Kidney | Yin | Water | Bottom of foot and along inside of leg to upper chest. |
| Pericardium | Yin | Fire | Chest to end of middle finger. |
| Triple heater | Yang | Fire | End of ring finger back to side of head. |
| Gall bladder | Yang | Wood | Side of head and body and along side of leg to the fourth toe. |
| Liver | Yin | Wood | Big toe and along inside of leg to chest. |
| Governing vessel | Yang | | Tip of tailbone, up midline of back, and over the heart to upper lip. |
| Conception vessel | Yin | | Perineum and up front of midline to bottom lip and chin. |

**The Meridians**

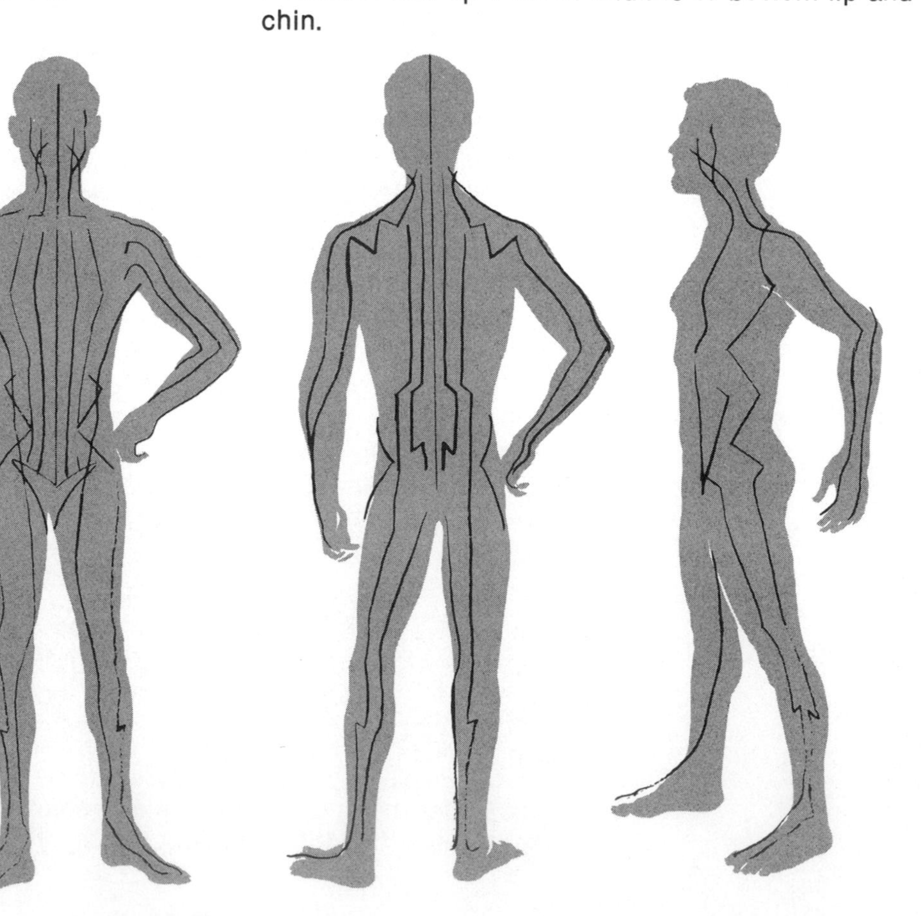

**Acupressure**

Acupressure refers to any of a number of treatment systems that incorporate various manipulations of acupoints. Although the basic philosophy comes from the traditional Chinese, most Eastern societies incorporate some touch pressure in their traditional touch remedies, and a number of acupressure techniques have been developed in Western societies.

Acupressure is often used to facilitate better circulation of blood to an affected area and to relieve pain. Techniques usually include touching, pressing or rubbing one or more points, depending on what is to be achieved. Acupressure as well as many of the health practices of oriental origin are used in conjunction with diet, exercise, and meditation. The goal is to balance the physical and psychological aspects of a person's being into a holistic (wholesome) way of life.

**Shiatsu**

The Japanese word *shiatsu* (composed of shi, finger, and atsu pressure), means pressure of the fingers or digits. In a sense it is like acupuncture without the use of needles. The purpose of shiatsu is to increase circulation and prevent imbalances in the body. It is also an aid to soothing the nervous system and is said to be particularly effective in relieving headache, fatigue, insomnia, nervous tension, sore and stiff muscles, and such disorders as constipation and high blood pressure.

Like acupuncture, shiatsu follows strategic points or energy pathways (called tsubo) situated on the meridians, but which do not correspond entirely to the Chinese method. Instead of using needles, the shiatsu expert uses the ball of the thumb to apply pressure. The treatment can be given to the entire body to restore complete harmony or according to specific needs. By applying pressure to the points, the natural recuperative powers of the body are generated, toxins are dispersed, muscles are relaxed, circulation of blood and lymph are improved and the entire body is revitalized.

To be effective, the practitioner must practice to build strength and dexterity of the fingers, thumb, and entire hand. Three fingers held together may be used generally for the face, abdomen, and adjacent areas. Pressure is applied with only the tips of the fingers pointing straight down. One finger with another finger placed over it as a brace is also used. The palm of the hand is sometimes used. However, the thumbs are used most often in shiatsu, and only the ball and thumb is used to press straight down (no rubbing motions) on the pressure points. Pressure is exerted perpendicularly to the surface of the skin with the pads of the fingers or thumb, for 2 to 5 seconds or more, depending on the area being treated.

## PRESSURE POINTS

To become better acquainted with pressure points, study the illustrations then note the basic benefits attributed to pressure points on specific areas of the body. The practitioner who wishes to become proficient in the art and science of shiatsu must learn basic physiology and anatomy and study the techniques under the direction of a skilled teacher. Shiatsu is not exceptionally difficult to learn, but it is an art that cannot be learned correctly by hit-or miss methods or experimentation. Certain contraindications, as with other massage techniques, must be observed.

Shiatsu need not be applied in the order listed below. Judge the area to be treated, then determine the duration of pressure and procedure to follow for maximum benefit to the individual.

**Anterior View of Pressure Points**

Reading clockwise, the following will correspond to the illustration of pressure points:

1. Frontal crown of the head, forehead, temple, and mastoid process. Use the thumbs on pressure points to relieve headache and tension.
2. Sides and front of the neck. Use the thumbs to press first the right and then the left carotid artery. Pressure here relieves stiff neck and fatigue.
3. Intercostal area. Gentle pressure with thumbs encourages relaxation.
4. Upper arm, cubital fossa forearm, elbow joint. People who use their arms a lot enjoy relief from fatigue when this technique is used. Apply pressure to points using the thumbs.
5. Descending colon and sigmoid flexure. Use the palms of the hands and the fingertips on pressure points. Pressure here relaxes tension, improves metabolism.
6. Outside of thigh and outside of lower leg. Use the fingers on the pressure points to relieve fatigue and sore muscles.
7. Toes, metatarsus, and ankle. Use the thumbs to press the toes several times each. Repeat on the metatarsus, and ankle. This relieves fatigue, tension, and soreness.
8. Knee joint, front, and inside of the thigh. Use the thumbs to work down the front and inside of the thigh. Apply pressure above and below the kneecap. Relieves strained muscles and prevents soreness.
9. Palm of the hand. Use the thumbs on the pressure points to relieve strained muscles, stiffness and soreness.
10. Bladder, small intestines, ascending mesocolon. Use fingertips to apply pressure to the points, and use the palm of the hand to apply pressure to the abdomen. This stimulates the flow of blood to the area and relieves constipation.
11. Gastric region and liver. Use the tips of the fingers to apply pressure. This relaxes nerves and promotes good digestion.
12. Inside upper arm and axilla. Use the thumbs on the pressure points to relieve strain and soreness.
13. Breastbone. Use the fingertips to apply pressure. This stimulates the endocrine gland.
14. Shoulder. Use the fingertips on pressure points to relieve soreness, strain and fatigue of muscles.

## Anterior View of Pressure Points

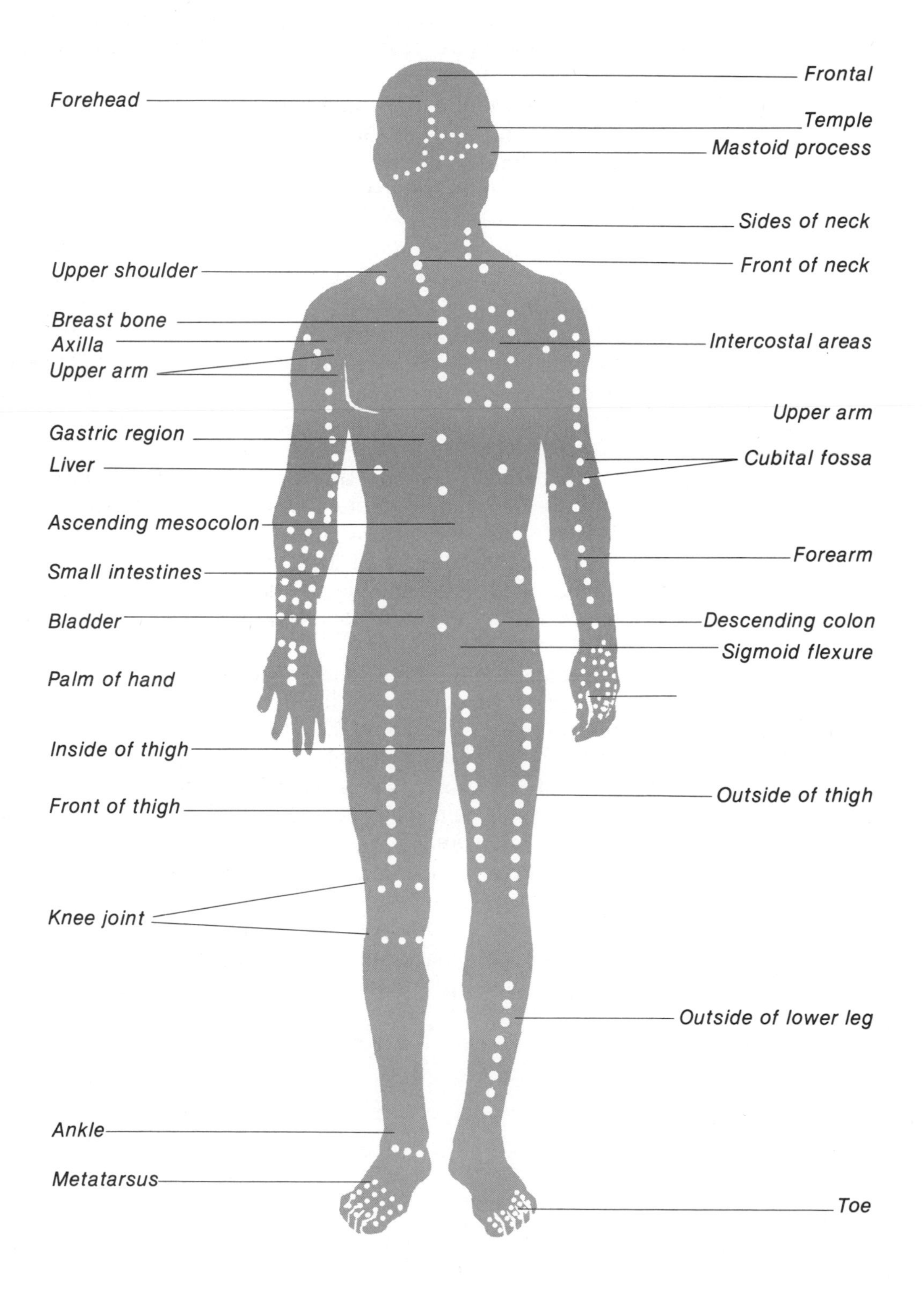

**Posterior View of Pressure Points**

Reading clockwise, the following will correspond to the illustration of pressure points:

1. Medulla oblongata. Use the fingertips on the pressure points to relieve fatigue, restore energy, soothe headaches, and promote alertness.
2. Back of upper arm. Use the thumbs on the pressure points to relieve fatigue, soreness, and stiffness.
3. Dorsum (back). Use thumbs on pressure points to increase circulation, relieve tension, relax muscles, and soothe anxieties.
4. Lumbar vertebrae and upper end of thigh bone. Use thumbs on the pressure points to stimulate circulation to the area, relieve fatigue and impart a sense of well-being.
5. Buttocks and sacrum. Use thumbs on the pressure points to relieve aching lower back, fatigue, and feelings of anxiety.
6. Back of thigh, lower back of thigh and the back of knee. Use the tips of the fingers on pressure points to relieve soreness, fatigue, and strain in muscles.
7. Calf and Achilles tendon. Use the fingers to pinch the calves, and use the thumbs to press the points from calf to ankle. This relieves soreness, strain, and fatigue in muscles.
8. Heel and sole of the foot. Use the thumbs on the pressure points of the instep and the plantar arch (sole). Pressure here relieves strain and soreness, relaxes nerves and strengthens muscles of the foot.
9. Metacarpal bones, hand, and fingers. Press the tips of all the fingers on the surfaces of the hand. Move pressure until all fingers have been treated. This technique adds strength and flexibility and improves general well-being.
10. Back of forearm. Use the thumbs on the pressure points from wrist to elbow to relieve muscles that are fatigued, strained and sore.
11. Shoulder blade and interscapular region. Use the thumbs on the pressure points to improve circulation to the area, soothe nerves and relieve anxieties.
12. Occipital. Use the thumbs on the pressure points to help regulate blood pressure and relieve fatigue, insomnia, and headache.

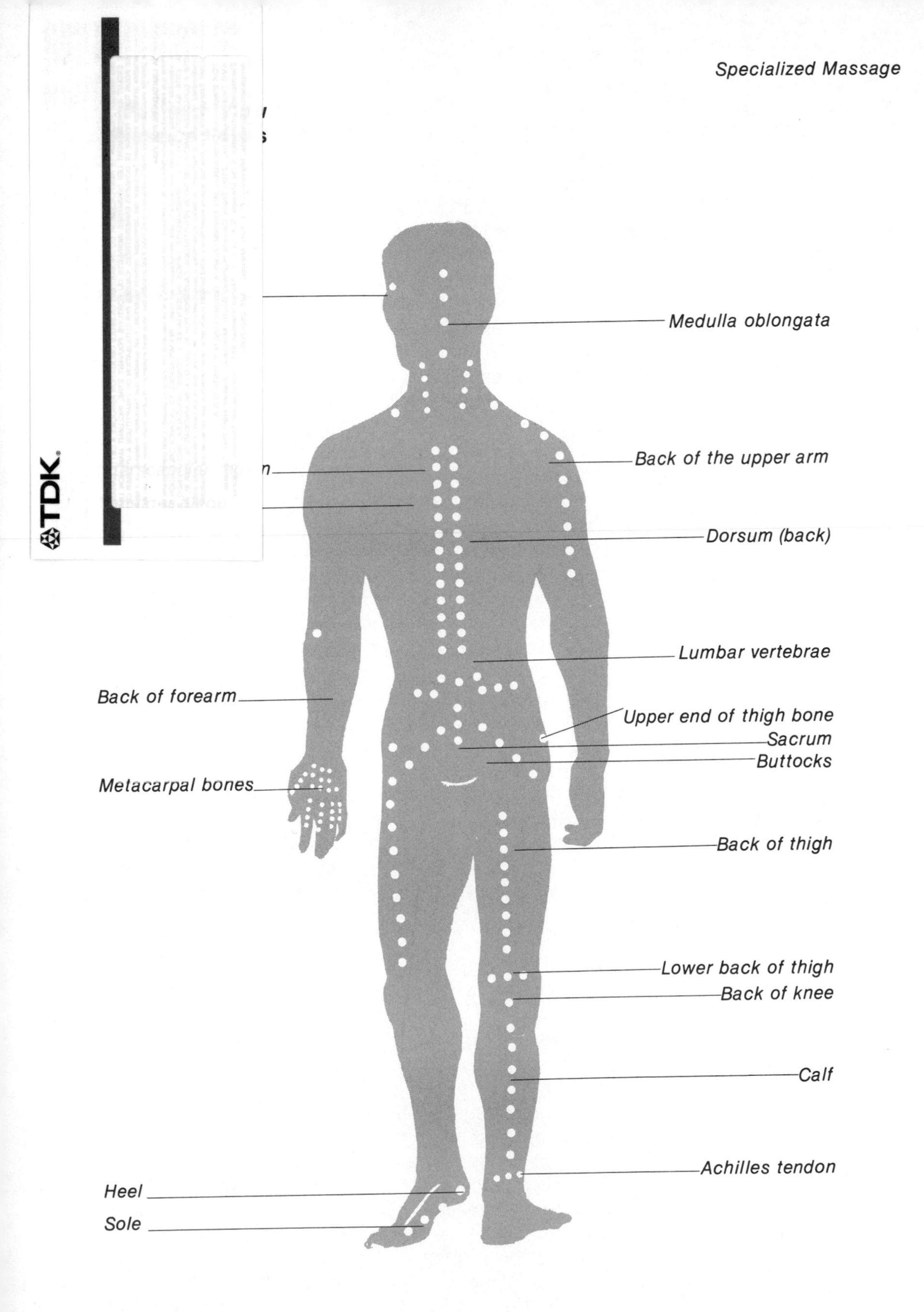
Medulla oblongata
Back of the upper arm
Dorsum (back)
Lumbar vertebrae
Back of forearm
Upper end of thigh bone
Sacrum
Buttocks
Metacarpal bones
Back of thigh
Lower back of thigh
Back of knee
Calf
Achilles tendon
Heel
Sole

## STRESS THERAPY AND RELAXATION MASSAGE

Stress is a condition that affects both the body and the mind. Originally it was caused by certain physical reactions in humans and animals that served as life-saving signals to enable the organism to react quickly when danger threatened. This became known as the "flight or fight" response. Today, we face different kinds of stress situations, but the body still reacts in somewhat the same manner. To prepare the body to flee or to confront a problem, the sympathetic nervous system increases blood pressure and elevates the pulse rate. Hormones (adrenalin and noradrenalin) are released, and energy reserves are mobilized.

In cases of extreme fright or certain forms of nervous tension, a person may perspire profusely. The skin may become affected by the contraction of the arrector pilorum muscles around a hair follicle. This condition, resembling a profusion of small bumps with erect hairs is referred to as "gooseflesh."

A certain amount of stress is normal and desirable, but there is a difference between positive and negative stress. Stress is an involuntary response. Whether it is positive or negative, the body deals with it in the same way. Positive stress expels excess energy, stimulates motivation, and is advantageous, while negative stress can cause adverse responses. For example, when under stress the body's metabolism changes, and if prolonged, body systems begin to react. A person may develop internal problems such as ulcers, or skin problems such as psoriasis, hives, and problem blemishes. The great danger of stress is that when it becomes a chronic condition rather than an occasional reaction, it can eventually lead to serious health problems. Continued anxiety, tension, or hypertension can lead to allergies, arthritis, indigestion, constipation, high blood pressure, heart disease, insomnia, and many other conditions.

Stress related illnesses account for most of the reasons for nonproductivity on the job as well as for problems that affect people personally and socially. When a person is suffering from negative stress, incidents that are normally accepted as minor or inconvenient are blown out of proportion as to their actual seriousness. Many times the affected person will react by exhibiting excessive anger and frustration. Stress tends to deplete the body's supply of vitamins and minerals, therefore, people under stress should pay attention to their dietary habits. When under stress, there is a tendency to eat too fast and to eat meals lacking essential nutrients. Sometimes stress stimulates a craving for food or causes a feeling of fullness without satisfaction. Also it is not uncommon for the stressed individual to lose his or her appetite altogether.

A sense of hopelessness is often associated with stress. When depression sets in, a person may turn to drugs or alcohol or both hoping to find relief. However, alcohol and drugs only compound the problem. The most effective way to deal with stress when it becomes unmanageable is to seek counseling and treatment. It is important to identify causes and look for a solution. For example, when stress is work related, making a list of daily, weekly, and monthly activities may be helpful in pinpointing stress-producing activities that can be rescheduled or eliminated.

Individuals respond differently to the same stressful situations. For example, major life changes, a new job, illness, or financial setback may be devastating to one person while another will be able to handle such events with less distress. Those individuals who have stressful life experiences should make an effort to balance their lives with some type of enjoyable recreation such as a hobby or special interest. A good balance of work and relaxation helps to combat stress.

Doctors often recommend massage for the relief of tension, anxiety, worry, and anger—all causes of stress. Many practitioners create a restful environment with relaxing background music for clients who are experiencing stress and for those who want to prevent stress-related illnesses. The goal is to induce complete mental and physical relaxation. When working with clients who are highly stressed, the practitioner should be aware of the affects of pressure, rhythm, and duration of each movement as well as the client's response. In some cases the client may experience deep relaxation that is somewhat like a hypnotic state.

A great deal can be determined during the consultation, so the client should be encouraged to express his or her feelings. Also the practitioner will want to know how long the beneficial effects of the massage lasted; clients often experience renewed energy and relief from stress for several days or longer.

When giving relaxation massage the practitioner's hands are much better than any machine. In stress therapy and relaxation massage, human contact is most important. The massage practitioner is not expected to serve as the client's personal psychologist or counselor, but he or she should have an instinct for what is right for the client and an understanding of human feelings in order to apply a therapeutic "healing touch."

## REFLEXOLOGY DEFINED

Reflexology is defined as the art and science of stimulating the body's own healing forces through special massage techniques. A form of compression massage, reflexology is based on the principles that reflex points in the hands and feet are related to every organ in the body. By applying pressure to a reflex point, the practitioner can effect certain beneficial changes. For example, when reflex massage is given on the big toe, it is said to relieve headache and tension. Various parts of the hands and feet are linked with specific glands, organs, and muscles. Activating these links through reflex massage can relieve tension, improve the blood supply to certain regions of the body, and help to normalize body functions.

In recent years public interest in reflexology has been aroused. Some people are skeptical as to whether this form of massage is beneficial while others credit the method with remarkable success.

Practitioners do not claim reflexology to be a "major cure all." They encourage those who are interested to be sure to master the techniques well before attempting to put them to use.

For further sources of study in the art and science of body, hand and foot reflexology, see the massage reference list.

**Reflexology Foot Chart**

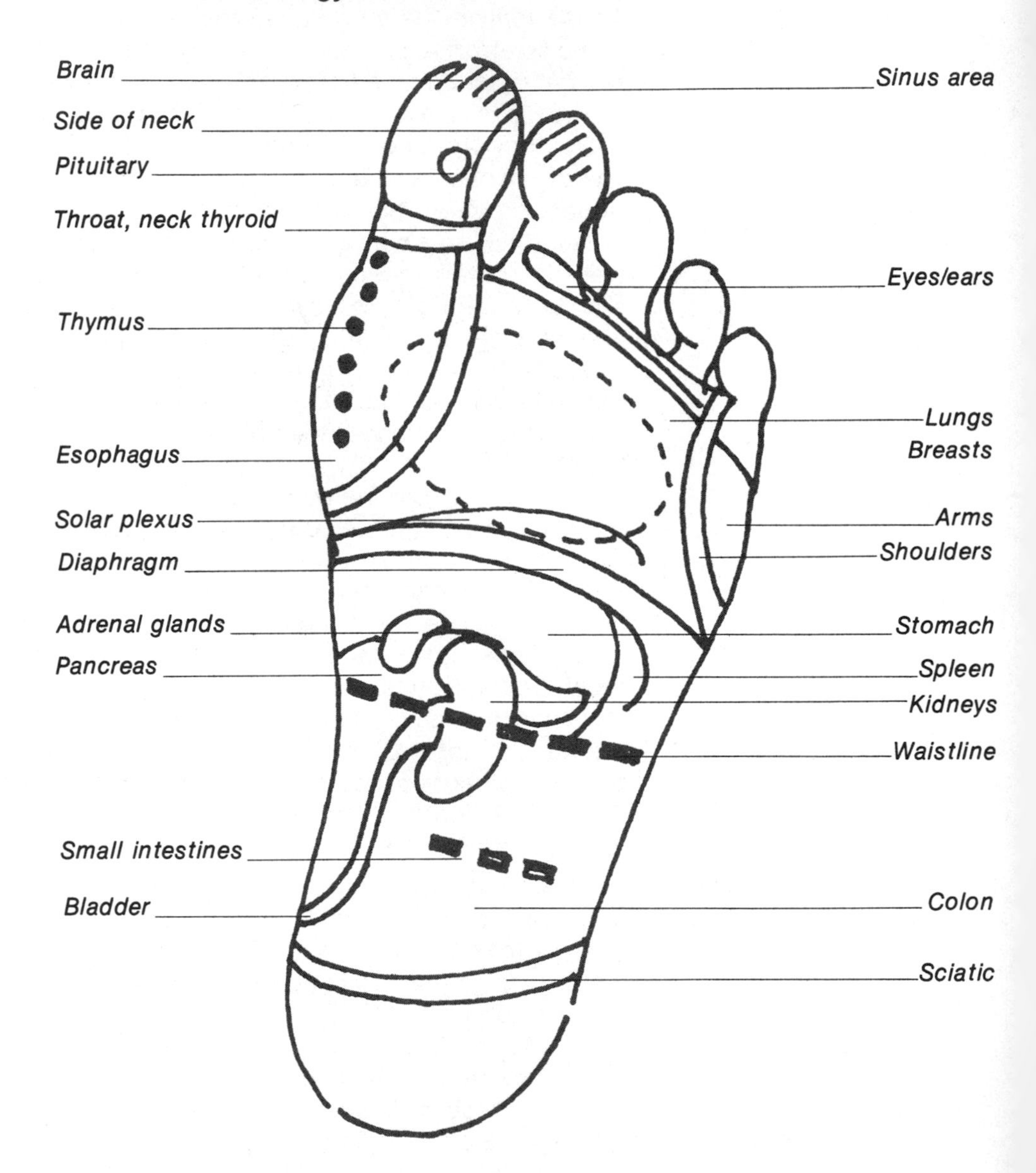

**Massage for the Hand and Arm**

A manicurist will usually give a basic hand massage as part of a manicure. However, the practitioner may wish to give a more thorough hand massage as part of the regular massage procedure. The female client is especially conscious of the appearance of her hands and appreciates this extra attention to keeping her hands supple and strong. Massage increases the flow of blood to the hands to nourish the skin. Massage oil or cream relieves dryness as it softens the skin of the hands, arms and elbows.

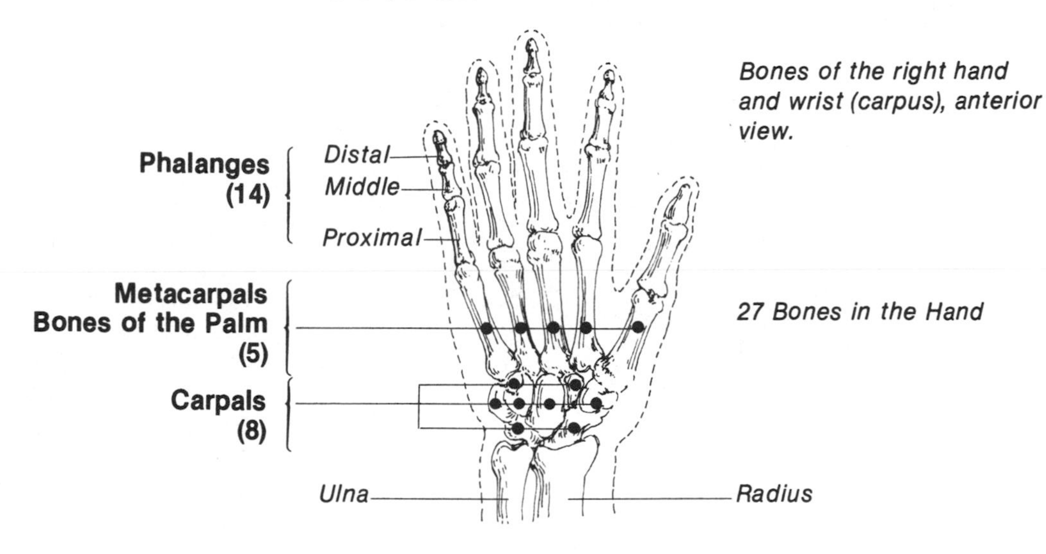


*Bones of the right hand and wrist (carpus), anterior view.*

***Procedure for Hand Massage***

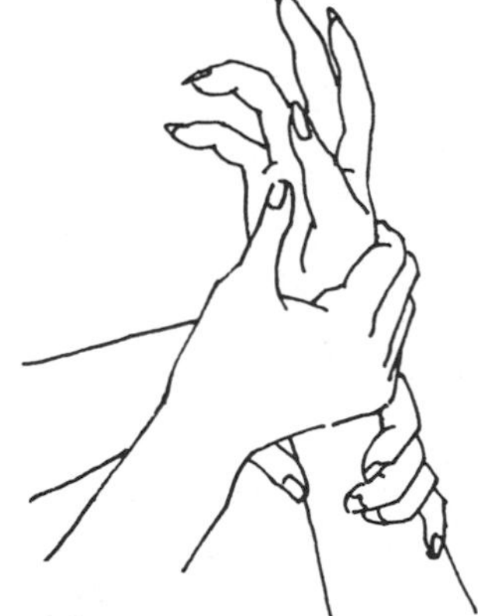

*Figure 1*

1. While holding the client's hand, place a dab of massage cream or lotion on the back of the hand and spread it over the metacarpals and fingers and upward over the wrist. Repeat three times (see figure 1).

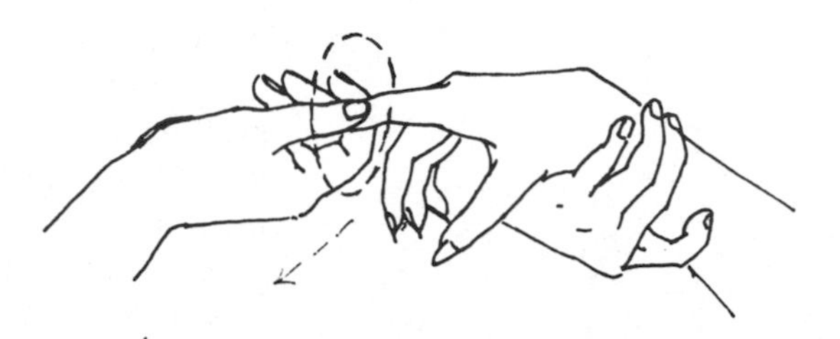

*Figure 2*

2. Hold the client's hand firmly then bend it forward and backward to limber the wrist. Grasp each finger and bend it forward and backward until it has been exercised (see figure 2). As the fingers are bent, slide your thumb down toward the fingertips.

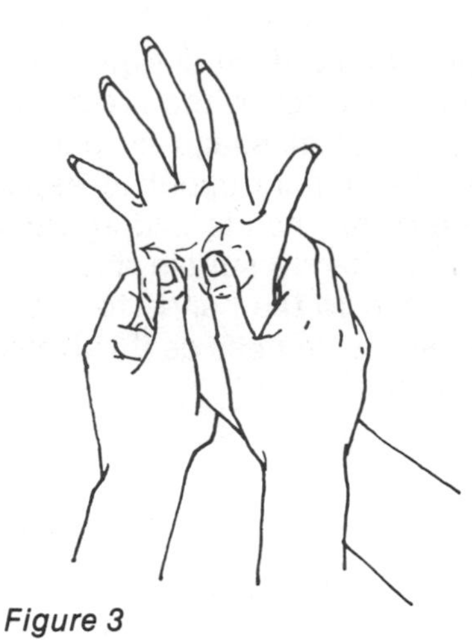

Figure 3

3. With the client's elbow resting on the table, hold the hand upright and massage the palm of the hand with the cushions of your thumbs, using circular movements in alternate direction (see figure 3). This relaxes the hand.

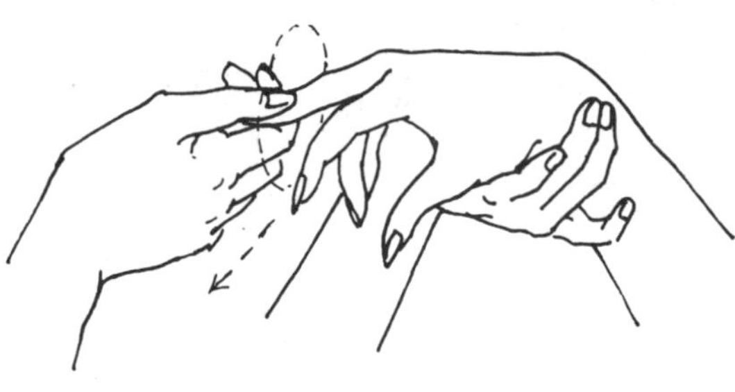

Figure 4

4. Rest the client's elbow on the table. Massage each finger from the base then rotate the finger in large circles. Finish with a gentle squeeze of the fingertip (see figure 4). Repeat on each finger.

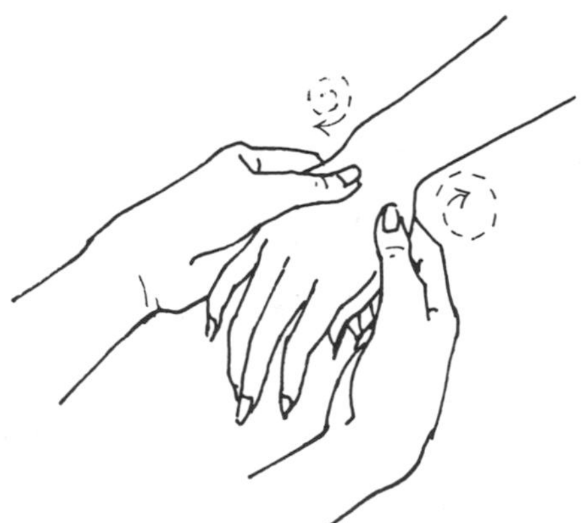

Figure 5

5. Use your thumbs to massage the client's wrists and the top of the hand. Use circular movements clockwise then counterclockwise (see figure 5). Repeat three times.

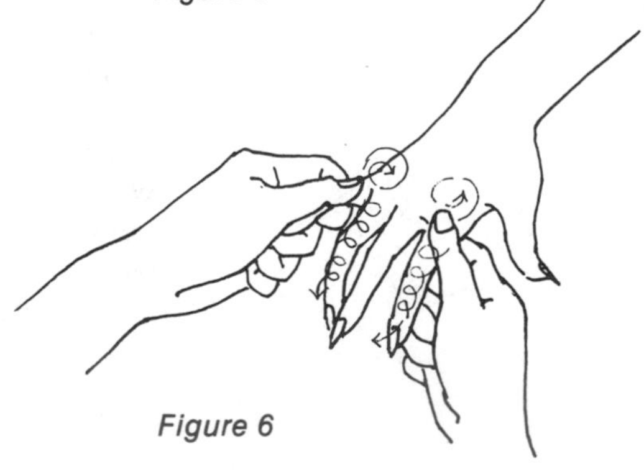

Figure 6

6. Finish the massage by tapering each finger. Beginning at the base of each finger, rotate, pause, and squeeze with gentle pressure. Pull lightly downward until the tip of the finger is reached (see figure 6). Repeat three times. Repeat the entire procedure on the other hand.

**Massage for the Arm**

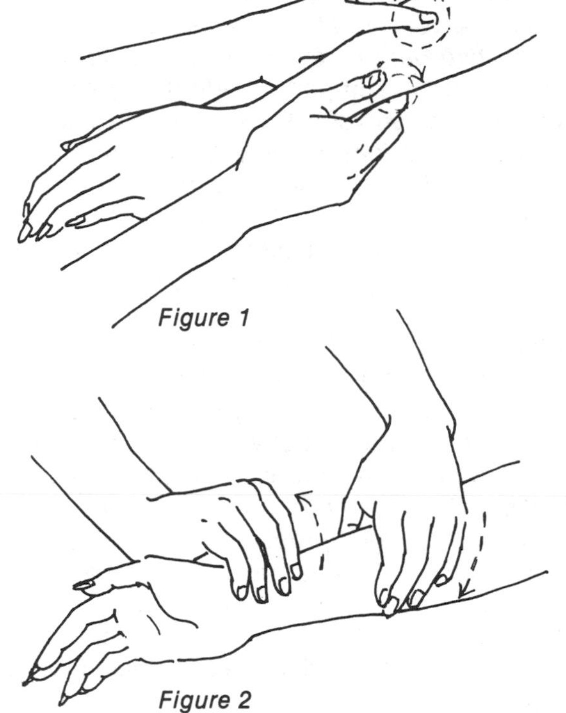

*Figure 1*

*Figure 2*

1. After completing the hand massage, place the client's arm on the table, palm turned upward. Massage the arm from wrist to elbow, using slow, circular motions in alternate directions (see figure 1). Turn the client's palm upward, and repeat the same movements three times.

2. Place your fingers on the client's arm, and firmly massage the underpart of the arm to the elbow, using the fingers of each hand in alternate crosswise directions (see figure 2). Repeat three times.

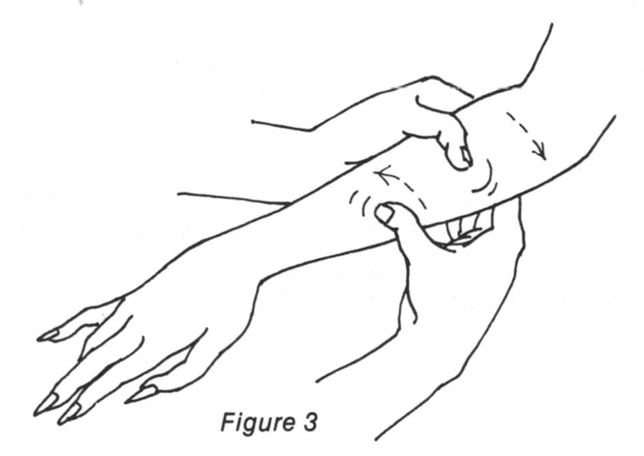

*Figure 3*

3. Massage the outer part of the arm from the wrist including the elbow. Apply thumbs in opposite directions with a squeezing motion (see figure 3). Repeat three times. Cup the elbow in your hand and massage it with a circular motion. Repeat three times.

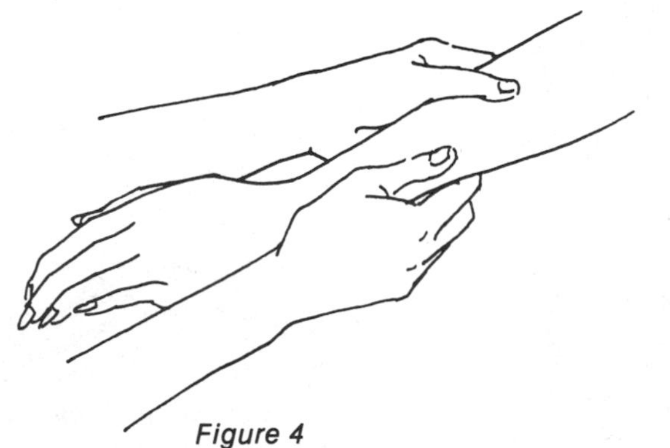

*Figure 4*

4. Stroke the arm, firmly moving the thumbs in opposite directions. Finish the massage by stroking each finger and ending with a gentle squeeze of the fingertips (see figure 4). Following the massage, blot the hands and arms with a clean dry towel to remove excess lotion.

**Massage for the Feet**

The human foot is designed for locomotion (walking) and is composed of intricate bones, joints, ligaments, tendons, muscles, nerves, blood vessels, skin, and nails. The foot acts as a shock absorber to prevent excessive jarring of the spinal cord, nervous system, and particularly the brain and internal organs.

According to surveys, there is an extremely high incidence of foot trouble and foot disease. Common foot troubles are those caused by ill-fitting shoes that pinch the feet, causing corns, calluses, and bunions. The wrong shoes can contribute to aching back, fatigue, headache, and foot and leg pains. Poor posture and improper walking throw the body out of alignment, causing problems that affect the entire body.

Athlete's foot, epidermophytosis, is a dermatitis caused by fungus germs that thrive in dark, moist interiors of shoes. Severe itching is the main symptom of athlete's foot. In some cases scales will form between the toes. The vesicular type of athlete's foot is characterized by small, vesicles (small itching red blisters). When rubbed, these blisters break open and spread the infection. Simple cases of athlete's foot can usually be corrected by keeping the feet clean and dry, and by use of medicated powder. However, if the condition persists, a chiropodist or podiatrist should be consulted. Today, many foot problems can be treated in the specialist's office. Laser surgery is now used successfully for a number of foot disorders.

Because the feet are located farthest from the heart, many people experience poor circulation in their feet. Foot massage stimulates circulation, relieves tension, and helps to keep the feet flexible. Good foot hygiene includes washing and drying the feet thoroughly, using foot powder as necessary, keeping the toenails trimmed correctly, and wearing correctly fitted shoes. Regular exercise of the feet is also important to foot health. Walking, stretching, and bending of the toes and rotating of the ankles are beneficial exercises.

There are 26 bones in each foot.

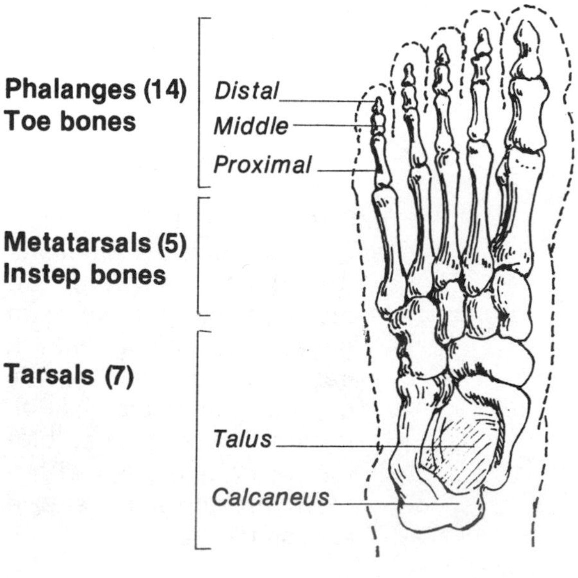

**Phalanges (14)**
**Toe bones**

*Distal*
*Middle*
*Proximal*

**Metatarsals (5)**
**Instep bones**

**Tarsals (7)**

*Talus*
*Calcaneus*

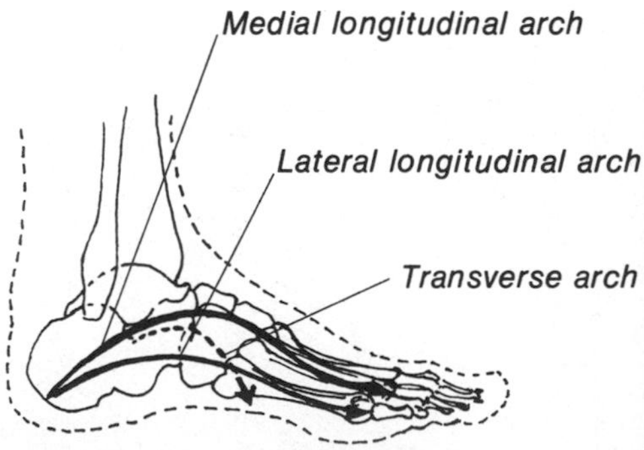

*Medial longitudinal arch*
*Lateral longitudinal arch*
*Transverse arch*

*Bones of the right ankle and foot, superior view.*

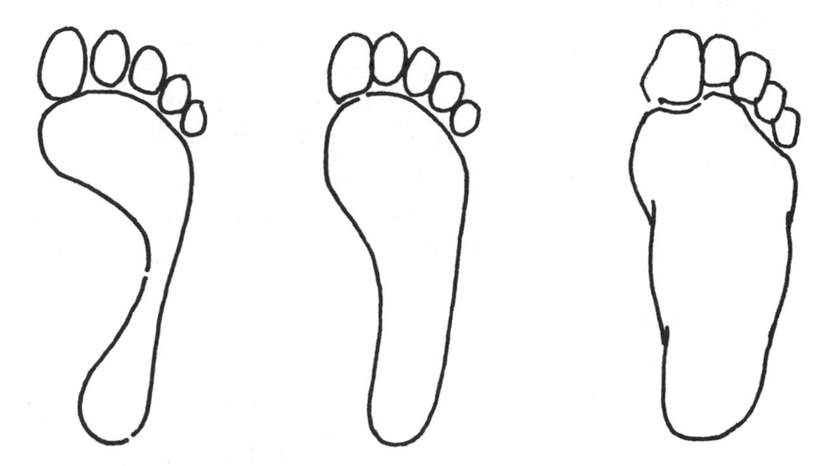

*Footprints showing from left to right, a high arch, a weak arch and a flat foot with no arch.*

***Procedure for Foot Massage***

Apply massage cream or lotion over both feet.

1. Apply effleurage to both the top and bottom of the foot, working from the toes upward toward the heart.
2. Apply friction with the fingers and thumbs between the tendons and bones and on all surfaces of the foot.
3. Do knuckle stroking down the plantar surface (sole) of the foot.
4. Massage and rotate each toe. Slide the fingers to the tip of the toe, and finish with light pressure.
5. Rotate the foot, and stretch the tarsus (instep).
6. Stretch the dorsal aspect (back) of the foot and the toes.
7. Grasp the heel in one hand, holding the toes with the other, then move the foot back and forth. This is called the Achilles stretch. (Note the practitioner's posture and stance.)
8. Repeat the Achilles stretch.

This completes the massage of one foot. Repeat the entire procedure on the other foot. Use a clean towel to remove any excess lotion or massage cream from the feet.

**QUESTIONS FOR DISCUSSION AND REVIEW**

1. What are the main benefits of deep tissue massage?
2. How does prenatal massage benefit the expectant mother?
3. What are the major benefits of lymph massage?
4. What are lymphocytes?
5. What is the lymphatic pump?
6. What is the purpose of structural integration?
7. Where is acupuncture said to have originated?
8. In Buddhist thought there are two parts that contrast or exist as opposites of the same phenomena. What are these two parts called?
9. What are the three main techniques used in acupressure?

10. What is the meaning of the Japanese word *shiatsu*?
11. Why do doctors often recommend massage to people who are suffering from stressful life experiences?
12. What is the main purpose of reflexology?
13. Of what benefit is hand massage?
14. What are the main causes of common foot problems?
15. What are the three main benefits of foot massage?

**ANSWERS TO QUESTIONS FOR DISCUSSION AND REVIEW**

1. Related to Swedish massage, deep tissue massage encourages relaxation, increases movement of body fluids, and soothes the nervous system.
2. Properly applied, prenatal massage can foster relaxation, benefit circulation, and soothe the nerves.
3. Correct lymph massage helps to stimulate the flow of lymph, which rids the body of toxins and waste materials. It promotes the balance of the body's internal chemistry, purifies and regenerates tissues, and helps to normalize the functions of all body organs and the immune system.
4. Lymphocytes (leucocytes) or white corpuscles are found in lymphatic tissue, blood, and lymph. They are active in the immune responses of the body and play a major part in healing wounds and fighting infections.
5. The lymphatic pump is a manipulation that enhances the flow of lymph through the entire system.
6. Structural integration attempts to bring the physical structure of the body into balance and alignment around a central axis.
7. Acupuncture is said to have originated in China more than 5000 years ago.
8. Yin and yang are the two parts that contrast or exist as opposites of the same phenomenon.
9. Acupressure techniques include rubbing, touching, and pressing of pressure points.
10. The Japanese word *shiatsu* (shi, finger, and atsu, pressure) means pressure of the fingers.
11. Doctors often recommend massage for the relief of tension, anxiety, and stress.
12. Reflexology is used to stimulate the body's own healing forces through special massage techniques.
13. Hand massage is beneficial in keeping the hands strong and supple.
14. Common foot problems are often caused by ill-fitting shoes.
15. Foot massage stimulates circulation, relieves tension, and helps to keep the feet flexible.

# PART VI KEEPING FIT

# Chapter 16 Nutrition and Weight Control

## LEARNING OBJECTIVES

After you have mastered this chapter you will be able to:

1. Explain the importance of good nutrition to the maintenance of health.
2. Explain the difference between proteins, carbohydrates, and fats.
3. Explain why a well-balanced diet is essential to health.
4. Explain how calories are the factors in gaining or losing weight.
5. Explain the importance of vitamins and minerals in the daily diet.
6. Name the basic four food groups that make up balanced meals.
7. Name the better-known vitamins and their best sources.
8. Explain how vitamin deficiencies lead to health problems.
9. Explain how food tables are used in planning diets.
10. Explain the causes of obesity and how weight may be lost safely.
11. Read a weight chart to determine approximate normal weights for men and women.
12. Fill out a client's progress chart.
13. Fill out a client's measurement chart.
14. Explain the causes of cellulite.

## INTRODUCTION

Because the massage practitioner is dedicated to the maintenance of the client's physical and psychological health, it is important to understand the role nutrition plays in body metabolism. Numerous medical studies have revealed that many disorders and diseases are related to lack of essential vitamins and minerals in the diet. While the massage practitioner does not attempt to diagnose or treat dietary deficiencies, he or she should be knowledgeable enough to detect some of the more obvious dietary problems and recommend that a client see a physician.

The massage practitioner can suggest that certain discomforts can be relieved by attention to proper diet. Many people have allergies caused by substances to which they are highly sensitive. Some symptoms are nausea, skin irritations (such as hives), headache, diarrhea, and constipation. Stress, hypertension, emotional problems, and anxiety are often the underlying causes of other physical problems. A well-balanced diet and soothing massages will do much to alleviate these conditions.

## THE ROLE OF NUTRITION IN KEEPING FIT

Scientists have known for decades that a well-balanced diet is one of the best defenses against many diseases. A healthy diet consists of varying amounts of fats, carbohydrates, and proteins.

### Fats

The body needs some fats to keep the sebaceous glands functioning properly. These glands produce sebum, the natural lubricating oil of the skin. Some fat is also necessary for the body's retention of heat. People who need to lose weight often think they should have no fat at all in the diet. Some fat, however, is recommended. It is now possible to have low-fat milk and other dairy products. Reduction in fat to control cholesterol and weight is more sensible if saturated fats such as butter, cream, and heavy oils are limited. Meat is less fatty if broiled or baked, and excess fat should be trimmed off before cooking. Most doctors do not suggest that all fat be cut out of the diet because many foods that contain fat and cholesterol also provide many of the essential vitamins and minerals as well as high-quality protein the body needs.

### Carbohydrates

Carbohydrates are foods that give the body most of its energy. The most important carbohydrate is glucose, which is stored in the muscles and liver as glycogen (animal starch). When the muscles are used, the glycogen stored in them is broken down to provide the energy they need to do their work. Fats and carbohydrates are major sources of energy and also of calories. The diet should include some starch and fiber, both of which are found in carbohydrate foods. Fruits, cereals, whole-grain bread, vegetables, beans and nuts are good sources of fiber, which is essential to healthy digestion and elimination. When selecting carbohydrate foods, it is best to avoid foods containing an unusual amount of sugar. Also salt and highly salted foods should be used in moderation, especially by people with hypertension (high blood pressure).

### Proteins

Collagen is the chief protein that makes up connective tissue and is considered the essential staff of life. Proteins are made from millions of small residues called amino acids. There are approximately 20 types of amino acids that are joined with peptide either lengthwise or by end bonds to form long chains of polypeptides. These chains may be spiral or round and are called simple chains. There are also complex chains that are bound together by cystine or sulphur cross-bonds. Protein foods are classifeid as A and B proteins. A proteins are such foods as fish, meat, eggs, milk, and the like. These are foods that contain high levels of sulphur amino acids (cystine and cysteine). B proteins are such foods as beans, peas, nuts and grains, which contain low levels of sulphur amino acids.

When the body does not get the protein it requires, there can be serious complications. The body can lose its resistance to infection, skin disorders may develop, and internal organs can become impaired. Proteins are the materials the body utilizes to build and repair tissues. It is more important to body health than carbohydrates and fats.

*Protein Deficiency:* When the body does not get the protein it requires, a child's growth can be retarded and an adult will lose weight. A few of the consequences of protein deficiency are: anemia, loss of resistance to infection, and impairment of internal and external organs.

**Simple Protein (Highly Magnified)**

**Complex Protein (Section)**

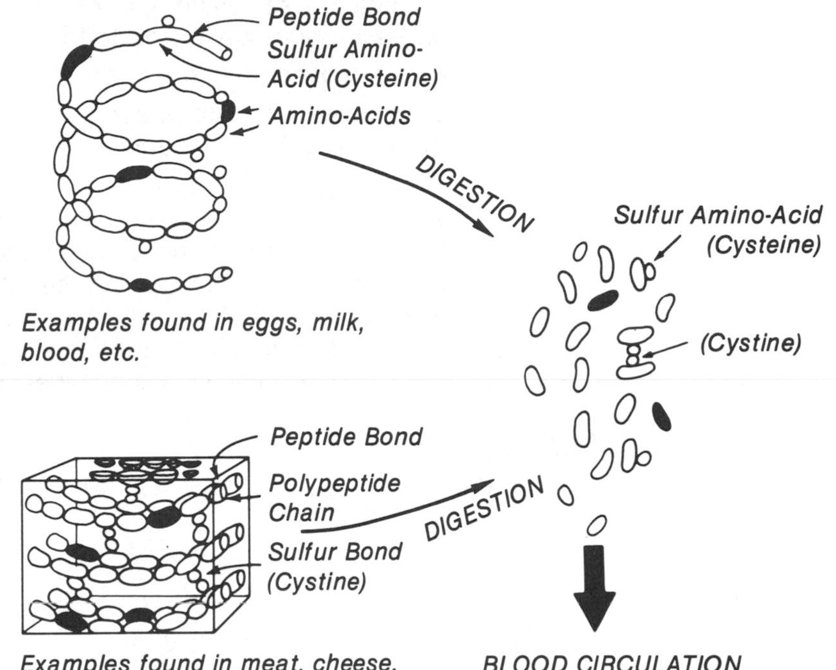


*Examples found in eggs, milk, blood, etc.*

*Examples found in meat, cheese, fish, etc.*

*Summary:* Proteins are made from millions of small residues called amino acids (approximately 20 types). The amino-acids are joined lengthwise by peptide or end bonds to form long chains of polypeptides. Polypeptide chains may be:

1. Simple spiral or round chains. These are easily digested, releasing contained amino-acids.
2. Complex chains bound together by cystine or sulfur cross bonds.

**Calories**

It takes energy for a person to live and to accomplish daily activities. This energy is measured in terms of calories, which are units of heat. A calorie is defined as one of two recognized units used to express the heat or energy-producing contents of foods. The larger kilogram calorie is the amount of heat required to raise the temperature of one kilogram of water one degree centigrade. The lesser or gram calorie is the amount of heat required to raise one gram of water one degree centigrade. The larger calorie is the measure of the energy value of foods or the heat output of living organisms.

All foods contribute calories, however, some foods such as butter, sugar-laden desserts, and sauces generally are high in calorie content. The person who wants to lose weight or to maintain normal weight should realize that it is the grand total of calories from all forms of food measured against the grand total of energy the body uses that determines whether the dieter will gain, lose, or maintain normal weight.

## THE HUMAN DIGESTIVE SYSTEM

Faulty elimination (constipation) is one of the most frequent causes of poor health. This is a condition that is associated with other ailments; some of the unpleasant symptoms are: irritability, fatigue, skin blemishes, offensive breath, headaches, and general sluggishness. Faulty elimination develops when the elimination of waste matter from the intestinal tract is unsatisfactory in any of the following ways:

Bowel movements are incomplete, irregular, or difficult.

Elimination of stool is accompanied by pain, excess gas, and extremely offensive odor.

When the bowel is not emptied regularly and normally, the waste matter begins to decay, forming poisonous substances that are harmful to the body. Occasional variations in elimination may not be cause for concern, but if constipation is severe and persists, a physician should be consulted without delay. Usually, the condition is caused by lack of exercise, stress or emotional problems, lack of variety in the diet (especially lack of

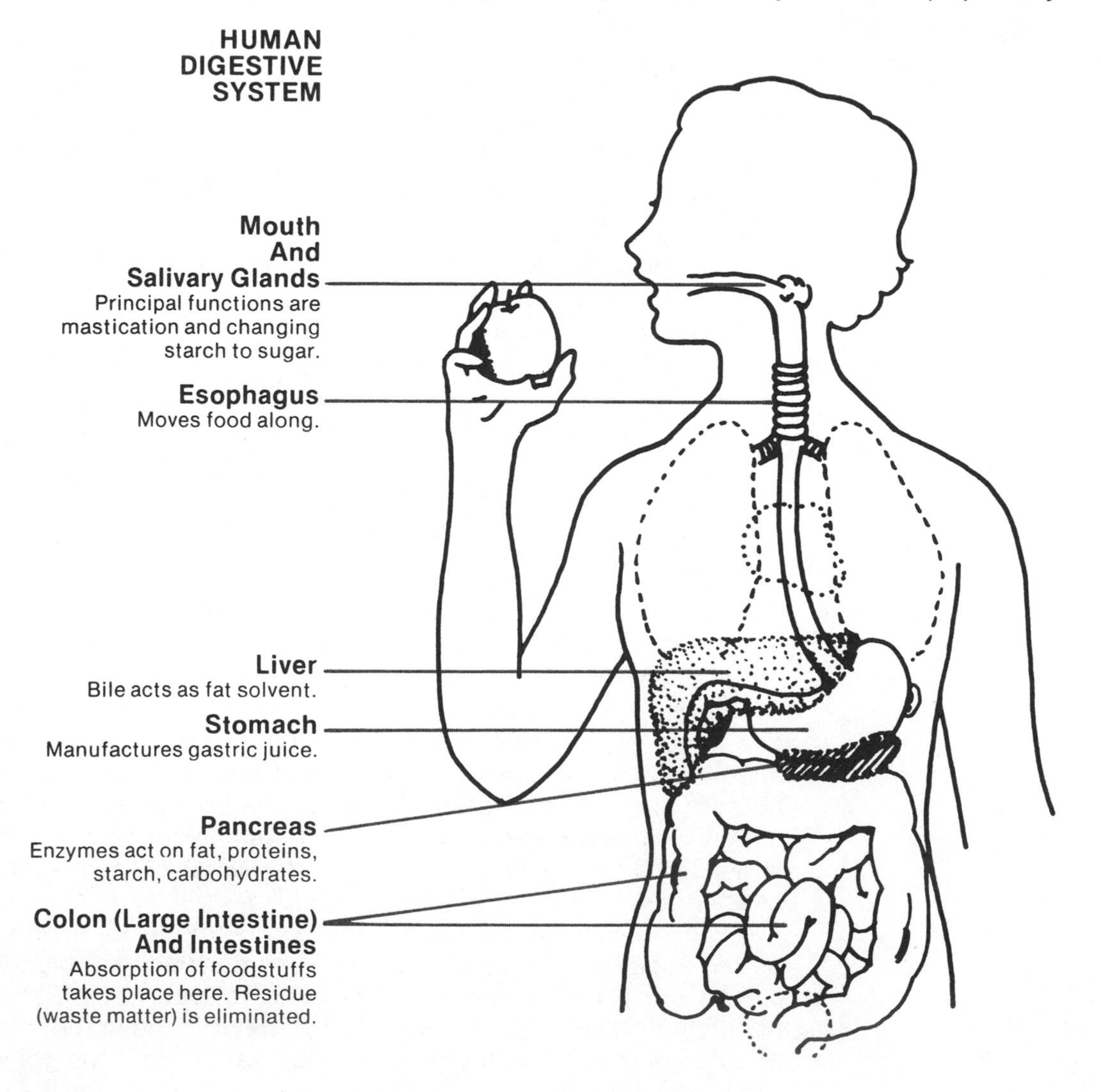

fruits and vegetables), and general poor health. Organic constipation is often due to ulcers, tumors, or inflammation of the intestines. Functional constipation is due to repeated errors in diet, health habits, and often habitual use of laxatives. Functional constipation may be spastic or atonic in nature. In spastic constipation, pains generally occur in the lower bowel. In atonic constipation, the bowel is sluggish and has lost much of its tone and power of contraction. Correcting diet, regular exercise, massage, and relaxation are the most effective remedies.

When any abnormal or irregular condition of the bowels persists, a physician should be consulted without delay. Self-treatment with possibly the wrong kind of laxative may cause the condition to worsen.

## Metabolism

Metabolism is the sum total of all the body processes whereby the living body utilizes oxygen and food in the building up and breaking down of its tissues. When food is utilized in the body, energy is extracted. This breakdown of complex molecules into simpler forms releases the energy required to hold the large, complex molecules together. It is a complicated process, but it is in this break-down of larger molecules into smaller ones that vitamins and enzymes play their important roles.

### *Enzymes*

Enzymes are often called biological catalysts. They are protein in nature, the protein being a special one for each different kind of enzyme. The job of enzymes is to initiate or accelerate specific chemical reactions in the metabolism.

## Vitamins and Minerals

The vitamins and minerals that are important to health are small and relatively simple structures that give the whole protein vitamin complex its special importance in human nutrition. The breakdown of the foods we eat provide the energy and the building blocks on which our lives depend and can only be achieved by the action of hundreds of enzymes. Since these enzymes are comprised, in part, of those relatively simple structures known as vitamins, we can see why they are so essential to healthy bodily functions.

By studying the Vitamin and Mineral Chart in this chapter, you will be able to see the relationship between vitamins, minerals, and the maintenance of health. It is to your advantage as a massage practitioner to learn the names of vitamins and minerals, their best sources, how they function as aids to health, and general symptoms of vitamin deficiency. While the practitioner does not prescribe special diets and megadoses of vitamins and minerals, he or she may suggest to a client that a balanced diet containing adequate vitamins and minerals will do much to assure good health. When a vitamin deficiency is suspected, the client can be encouraged to have a physician prescribe vitamin supplements. Generally, a daily all-purpose vitamin or vitamin-mineral supplement is a good idea unless a person is allergic to a particular substance or vitamin.

## VITAMIN INFORMATION CHART

Courtesy *Body Forum Magazine*

| Vitamin | Name | Need In Human Nutrition | U.S. RDA | Deficiency Disease | Subclinical Symptoms | Natural/Food Sources | Antagonists | Toxicity Level |
|---|---|---|---|---|---|---|---|---|
| **A** | Retinol | Essential for growth and maintenance of body tissue, strong bones and teeth, and good eyesight. (Helps to form and maintain healthy function of eyes, skin, hair, teeth, gums, various glands and mucous membranes. Also involved in fat metabolism.*) | 5,000I.U., for adults and children four or more years of age, except pregnant and lactating women, for whom the RDA is 8,000I.U. | Xerophthalmia; Night Blindness | Eyes—Inability to adjust to darkness; dry and inflamed eyeball; sties. Face and/or Skin Blemishes—rough, dry, prematurely aged skin. General—Loss of smell; loss of appetite; frequent fatigue; diarrhea. | Fish liver oil; carrots; green and yellow vegetables; liver; whole milk and dairy products; egg yolk, yellow fruits. | Excessive consumption of alcoholic beverages; mineral oil; cortisone (and other drugs); polyunsaturated fatty acids with carotene (unless anti-oxidants are present). | More than 50,000 I.U. daily could produce some toxic effects. |
| **B Complex** | Thiamine ($B_1$) | Essential for utilization of carbohydrates in energy production. Promotes healthy central nervous system and mental attitude, and improvement of food assimilation and digestion. | 1.5 mg. | Beriberi | Muscles—Cramps; general weakness; tenderness in calf. General—Loss of appetite; fatigue; loss of weight; burning sensation in soles of feet. | Brewer's yeast; wheat germ;bran; liver. | Cooking heat, air, water; caffeine; food processing techniques; sulfa drugs; sleeping pills; estrogen; alcohol. | No known toxic effects. |
| **B Complex** | Riboflavin ($B_2$) | Essential for good vision and healthy skin, nails and hair. Functions with other substances to breakdown and utilize carbohydrates, fats and proteins. | 1.7 mg. | Ariboflavinosis—lesions of the mouth, lips, skin and genitalia. | Eyes—burning sensation; bloodshot. | Milk; liver; enriched cereals; brewer's yeast; leafy green vegetables; fish; eggs. | Water; cooking; sunlight; food processing techniques; sulfa drugs; sleeping pills; estrogen; alcohol. | No known toxic effects. |
| **B Complex** | Niacin (Niacinamide or Nicotinic Acid) | Essential for healthy brain functions, nervous system, and skin. Important in tissue respiration. Essential for synthesis of sex hormones. | 20mg. | Pellagra. | Nervous System—hostility; suspicion; insomnia; loss of memory; irritability; anxiety. General—Abdominal pain; burning sensation in tongue; dry and scaly patches of skin. | Liver; brewer's yeast; kidney; wheat germ; whole grains; fish eggs; lean meat; nuts. | Water; food processing techniques; sulfa drugs; sleeping pills; estrogen; alcohol. | Nontoxic, except some side effects may result from more than 100 mg. daily. |
| **B Complex** | Cobalamin, Cyanocobalamin ($B_{12}$) | Essential for maintenance of healthy nervous system, and for utilization of carbohydrates, fats and proteins. | 6mcg. | Pernicious anemia; brain damage. | Nervousness; heart palpitations; inflamed tongue. | Liver; kidney; milk and dairy products; some types of meat. | Water; sunlight; acids; alkalis; food processing techniques; sulfa drugs; sleeping pills; estrogen; alcohol. | No known toxic effects. |
| **B Complex** | Para-Aminobenzoic Acid (PABA) | Helps to form folic acid, and in utilization of proteins. | Not established. | Depression; headache; eczema. | Fatigue; irritability; constipation; nervousness; graying hair. | Liver; kidney; whole grains. | Water; food processing techniques; sulfa drugs; sleeping pills; estrogen; alcohol. | No known toxic effects. |
| **B Complex** | Folacin, or Folic Acid | Essential for division of body cells, for production of nucleic acids (RNA and DNA) and for utilization of sugar and amino acids. | 0.4 mg. (400 mcg.) | Anemia | Gastrointestinal disorders. | Liver; Tortula yeast; green vegetables. | Water; food processing techniques; sulfa drugs; sleeping pills; estrogen; alcohol; sunlight. | No known toxic effects. |
| **B Complex** | Inositol | Combines with choline to form lecithin, which in turn metabolizes fats and cholesterol. Important for healthy hair. | Not established. | Eczema | Loss of hair; constipation. | Liver; brewer's yeast, whole grains; wheat germ; unrefined molasses; corn; citrus fruits. | Water; food processing techniques, sulfa drugs; sleeping pills; estrogen; alcohol. | No known toxic effects. |
| **B Complex** | Choline | Combines with inositol to form lecithin, which in turn metabolizes fat and cholesterol. Essential for healthy liver and kidneys. | Not established. | Kidney damage. | Deteriorating kidneys, abnormally high blood pressure. | Brewer's yeast; liver; kidney; wheat germ; egg yolk. | Water; food processing techniques; sulfa drugs; sleeping pills; estrogen; alcohol. | No known toxic effects. |

| | | | | | | | | |
|---|---|---|---|---|---|---|---|---|
| Complex | nol; Calcium Pantothenate | and sugar to energy, for use of PABA and choline, and vital to proper function of adrenal glands. | | mia; other blood disorders; duodenal ulcers; skin disorders. | dominal pains; muscle cramps; burning sensation in feet. | germ; bran; kidney; liver; heart; green vegetables; brewer's yeast. | caffeine; food processing techniques; sulfa drugs; sleeping pills; estrogen; alcohol. | No known toxic effects. |
| **B Complex** | Pyridoxine ($B_6$) | Essential for metabolism of amino acids. Aids in blood building, utilization of fats, and normal functioning of brain, nervous system and muscles. | 2 mg. | Anemia | Loss of hair; water retention during pregnancy; nervous system disorder; cracks around mouth and eyes; increase in urination. | Brewer's yeast; wheat bran; rice bran; wheat germ; liver; kidney; heart; blackstrap molasses; milk; eggs; cabbage; beef. | Canning; long storage; roasting or stewing (meat); water; food processing techniques; sulfa drugs; sleeping pills; estrogen; alcohol. | No known toxic effects. |
| **B Complex** | Biotin (Also called Coenzyme R or Vitamin H) | Essential for utilization of proteins, carbohydrates and fats, and for healthy hair and skin. Aids in the maintenance of the thyroid and adrenal glands, reproductive tract, and the nervous system. | 0.3 mg. (300 mcg.) | Dermatitis, depression; anemia; anorexia. | Mental depression; dry, peeling skin; muscular pains; poor appetite; lack of energy. | Brewer's yeast; egg yolk; liver; milk; kidney. | Water; food processing techniques; sulfa drugs; sleeping pills; estrogen; alcohol. | No known toxic effects. |
| **C** | Ascorbic Acid | Principal function is to maintain collagen, which is necessary for the connective tissue that holds body cells together. It is involved in wound healing, the formation of red blood cells and believed to be involved in disease resistance. | 60 mg. | Scurvy | Slow wound healing; loss of appetite; bleeding gums; muscular weakness; shortness of breath. | Fresh fruits and vegetables. | Heat; light; oxygen; water. Much Vitamin C is destroyed when vegetables are overwashed or cooked, and when fruit is overwashed. | No known toxic effect. Although not proven, excessive use of Vita min C has been associated with kidney stones in some persons, and has a diuretic and/or laxative effect on some people. |
| **D** | Calciferol | Essential for utilization of calcium and phosphorus. Necessary for strong teeth and bones. | 400 I.U. | Rickets; osteomalacia; senile osteoporosis. | Weakening bones, including teeth; weakening muscles. | Fish liver oils; milk and dairy products; sunlight. | Mineral Oil. | 25,000 I.U. daily over a long period of time could produce a toxic effect in adults. |
| **E** | Tocopherol | Protects from oxidation Vitamin A, selenium, two sulphur amino acids, polyunsaturated fatty acids, and some Vitamin C. | 30 I.U. | Kidney and liver damage; anemia | Muscle degeneration; enlarged prostate; red blood cell damage. | Vegetable oils; whole raw seeds and nuts; soybeans. | Food processing techniques; heat; freezing temperatures; oxygen; iron; mineral oil. | Nontoxic, except for persons with high blood pressure or chronic rheumatic heart disease. |
| **K** | Menadione | Essential for formation of prothrombin, a blood clotting chemical. Important to proper liver function and longevity. | Not established. | Celiac disease; sprue; colitis; hemorrhage. | Diarrhea; bleeding nose. | Yogurt; egg yolk; safflower oil; fish liver oils; kelp; alfalfa; leafy green vegetables. | Aspirin; x-rays and radiation; frozen foods; industrial air pollution. | Natural Vitamin K is considered nontoxic but more than 500 mcg. per day of synthetic Vitamin K is not recommended. |
| **P** | Bioflavonoids | Essential for proper use of Vitamin C. | Not established. | With Vit. C, rheumatism and rheumatic fever. | High tendency to bleed easily. | White pigments of citrus fruits; rutin. | Same as Vitamin C. | No known toxicity. |

Sources for the chart were: Raj Chopra, Private Formulations, Hempstead, N.Y.; *Dictionary of Nutrition*, by Richard Ashley and Heidi Duggal. *Remington's Pharmaceutical Sciences*, Managing Editor John E. Hoover; *Nutrition Almanac*, Nutrition Search, Inc.

## A WELL-BALANCED DIET

Unless an individual has a health problem that prohibits the ingestion of certain foods, it is important to try to include a variety of foods in the daily diet. In addition to eating vitamin- and mineral-rich foods, it is important to drink plenty of fresh water and other healthful liquids. Water and other body fluids make up approximately one-half to two thirds of the body. Fluids are needed to sustain the health of the cells, regulate body temperature, aid digestion, and many other bodily functions.

Coffee, tea, carbonated beverages, artificially flavored drinks and alcoholic beverages should not be used as a substitute for water. The following is a brief explanation of the four major food groups that make up a healthy, well-balanced diet.

1. *Dairy Group:* Milk and dairy products such as milk, yogurt, cheese, and butter. Unless a physician recommends the elimination of milk from the diet, it is a good source of calcium and should be included in the diet of children and adults.
2. *Meat and Protein Alternative Group:* Good sources of protein are meat (beef, pork, lamb, organ meats, etc.); fish and poultry are also high protein foods. Alternative sources are nuts, peas, beans, and eggs. Two or more servings are recommended daily.
3. *Vegetable-Fruit Group:* Fruits and vegetables are important sources of vitamins A and C. Fruits and vegetables, raw and cooked, should be eaten every day. Generally two or more servings are recommended.
4. *Bread-Cereal Group:* Whole grain cereal is best. When selecting breads and cereals, read the labels to compare nutritional information. Two or more servings are recommended daily.

The amount of food (number of servings) or amount of each food group varies with individuals. A person's age, activities, and body metabolism must be considered. For example, an active teenager may require more food than a moderately active older person. It is better to eat enough food to maintain good health, but many people eat far more than is necessary. This places stress on the entire system.

### Vegetarian Diet

The person on a vegetarian diet (no meat) should be sure to include high protein foods such as nuts, beans, and tofu. Dairy products are also a good source of protein.

### Sample Balanced Menus

Once you know which foods are low and high in calorie content and which foods to combine in a well-balanced diet, it will be easy to plan meals that contain carbohydrates, proteins, and fats in the desired amounts. People who need to lose weight are concerned with meals that provide a healthy low-calorie diet. People who maintain their normal weight within a range of a few pounds need to be concerned with planning meals that provide all the essential vitamins and minerals without overloading calories. People who tend to be underweight and would like to add a few pounds still need to be concerned that meals are well balanced, however. They can add calories by selecting foods carefully and adding higher-caloric foods to their daily diet.

The following examples of balanced menus can be used as a guide to planning meals for the individual's specific needs. Foods in the four food groups can be exchanged for others as desired as long as quality and caloric content are considered.

**Low-Calorie Menu**

| BREAKFAST | CALORIES (approximate) |
|---|---|
| 1 small glass orange juice or 1 large orange | 100 |
| 1 poached egg | 70 |
| 1 teaspoon butter (or margarine) | 30 |
| 1 slice whole wheat toast (½ inch thick) | 65 |
| 1 cup plain coffee or tea | 0 |
| 1 teaspoon sugar (add 50 calories) | |
| 1 teaspoon cream (add 50 calories) | |
| 1 8-oz. glass whole milk | 170 |
| Total calories without cream and sugar | 435 |

| LUNCH | CALORIES (approximate) |
|---|---|
| 1 cup mixed vegetable soup | 100 |
| 2 slices whole wheat bread (½ inch thick) | 130 |
| ½ cup tuna salad (with bread as sandwich) | 200 |
| Tea with lemon | 0 |
| Total | 430 |

| AFTERNOON SNACK | CALORIES (approximate) |
|---|---|
| 1 large pear | 100 |

| DINNER | CALORIES (approximate) |
|---|---|
| 1 medium lamb chop | 250 |
| 1 baked potato (medium) | 100 |
| With butter (add 50) | |
| 1 cup steamed carrots | 50 |
| 1 cup steamed spinach | 50 |
| With butter (add 50) | |
| 1 cup Waldorf salad | 200 |
| Dessert: 1-inch slice fudge cake | 100 |
| Plain coffee or tea | 0 |
| Total | 850 |

| EVENING SNACK | CALORIES (approximate) |
|---|---|
| ½ cup ice cream | 200 |
| 1 medium fresh apple | 60 |
| Total for the day | 1540 |

Note: It is not advisable to attempt crash diets, fasting, or going on less-than-1000-calorie diets without first having the diet supervised and approved by a physician. This diet provides vitamins, minerals, and the four food groups.

**High-Calorie Menu**

| BREAKFAST | CALORIES (approximate) |
|---|---|
| Bacon (2 slices) | 100 |
| Eggs (2 medium poached) | 150 |
| 2 slices whole-wheat toast | 130 |
| 2 teaspoons butter or margarine | 60 |
| 1 teaspoon fruit jam | 55 |
| 1 8-oz. glass whole milk | 170 |
| 1 8-oz. glass orange juice | 125 |
| 1 cup coffee with 1 teaspoon cream | 50 |
| Total calories | 840 |

| LUNCH | CALORIES (approximate) |
|---|---|
| 1 cup creamed tomato soup | 250 |
| 1 sandwich meat, 2 slices whole-wheat bread, 1 teaspoon salad dressing | 450 |
| 1 oz. peanuts | 200 |
| 1 6-oz. carbonated drink | 75 |
| Total calories | 975 |

| AFTERNOON SNACK | CALORIES (approximate) |
|---|---|
| 8 large potato chips | 90 |
| 1 chocolate chip cookie | 55 |
| Total calories | 145 |

| DINNER | CALORIES (approximate) |
|---|---|
| 1 serving lean beef, 2-½" slices | 400 |
| 1 medium baked potato | 100 |
| With 2 teaspoons butter | 120 |
| 1 large (2 cups) salad (suggested vegetables: tomato, lettuce, green pepper) | 150 |
| With 2 tablespoons salad dressing) | 300 |
| 1 cup custard | 300 |
| 1 8-oz. glass whole milk | 170 |
| Total calories | 1540 |
| Total calories for all meals and snacks | 3500 |

This menu represents hearty meals and snacks. When excess calories are not used (burned up) they are stored as fat.

**Daily Meal Check Chart**

The following is an example of a daily meal check chart that is useful when the client is trying to balance meals and count calories. Recommend that all foods and beverages be listed and calories totaled for each day. This helps the client to see if meals are balanced and if meals are too high or too low in calories.

| Monday | Food | Calories |
|---|---|---|
| Breakfast | | |
| Mid-am snack | | |
| Lunch | | |
| Mid-pm snack | | |
| Dinner | | |
| Snack | | |
| TOTAL | | |

| Tuesday | Food | Calories |
|---|---|---|
| Breakfast | | |
| Mid-am snack | | |
| Lunch | | |
| Mid-pm snack | | |
| Dinner | | |
| Snack | | |
| TOTAL | | |

| Wednesday | Food | Calories |
|---|---|---|
| Breakfast | | |
| Mid-am snack | | |
| Lunch | | |
| Mid-pm snack | | |
| Dinner | | |
| Snack | | |
| TOTAL | | |

| Thursday | Food | Calories |
|---|---|---|
| Breakfast | | |
| Mid-am snack | | |
| Lunch | | |
| Mid-pm snack | | |
| Dinner | | |
| Snack | | |
| TOTAL | | |

| Friday | Food | Calories |
|---|---|---|
| Breakfast | | |
| Mid-am snack | | |
| Lunch | | |
| Mid-pm snack | | |
| Dinner | | |
| Snack | | |
| TOTAL | | |

| Saturday | Food | Calories |
|---|---|---|
| Breakfast | | |
| Mid-am snack | | |
| Lunch | | |
| Mid-pm snack | | |
| Dinner | | |
| Snack | | |
| TOTAL | | |

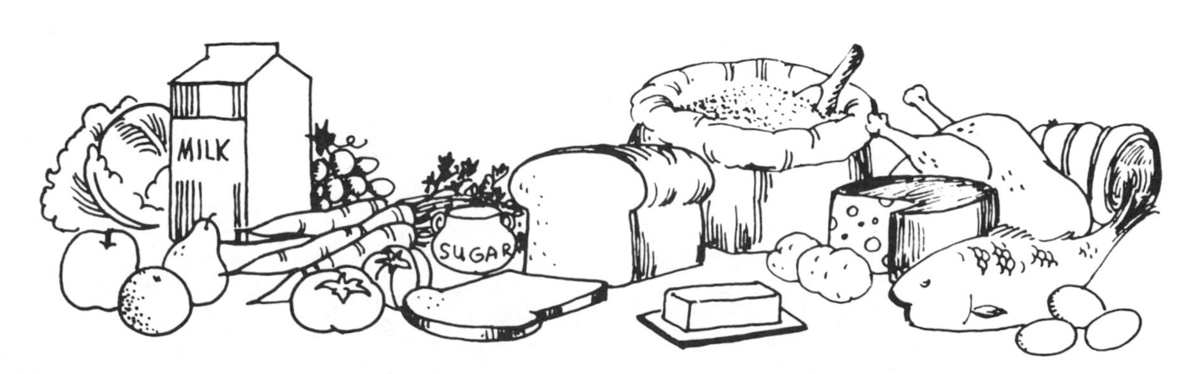


*Protective Foods* *Energy Foods* *Body Builders*

**Food Tables** Food tables provide a simple guide to understanding the calorie contents of various foods. If you do not see a particular food listed, find its equivalent. For example, a large apple or pear will contain approximately 100 calories. 1 cup of white beans or 1 cup of red beans contains approximately 100 calories. However, when you add butter, gravies, or sauces to these basic foods, the calorie count increases. Foods listed are fresh or cooked plain without seasonings.

| FOOD | AMOUNT OF SERVING | CALORIES |
|---|---|---|
| **Butter, Eggs, and Cheese** | | |
| Cheese, American or Swiss | 1-oz. slice | 110 |
| Butter | 1 tablespoon | 120 |
| Cottage cheese | 1 oz. | 30 |
| Creamed cheese | 1 oz. | 110 |
| Egg | 1 fried | 110 |
| Egg | 1 poached | 75 |
| **Vegetables** | | |
| Broccoli | ½ cup | 40 |
| Beets | ½ cup | 45 |
| Beans, red or white | 1 cup | 100 |
| Cabbage | 1 cup, shredded | 25 |
| Carrots | ½ cup | 50 |
| Celery | 2 stalks (7") | 10 |
| Corn | 1 medium ear or 1 cup | 60 |
| Green beans | ½ cup | 15 |
| Peas (green) | ½ cup canned or cooked | 75 |
| Potato, baked | 1 medium | 100 |
| Spinach | ½ cup | 50 |
| Tomato | 1 medium | 25 |
| Lettuce | ¼ small head | 10 |
| Mixed salad (tomato, lettuce, green pepper) | 2 large cups | 150 |
| **Breads** | | |
| Corn Meal Muffin | 1 medium | 100 |
| Frosted sweet roll | 1 medium | 350 |
| Graham cracker | 1 medium | 40 |
| Pancake | 1 medium | 100 |
| Rye | 1 slice | 75 |
| Rye crisp cracker | each | 25 |
| Soda cracker | each | 25 |
| Waffles | 1 medium | 225 |
| White enriched | 1 slice | 100 |
| Whole wheat | 1 slice | 65 |
| White bun | 1 medium | 200 |

| FOOD | AMOUNT OF SERVING | CALORIES |
|---|---|---|
| **Desserts** | | |
| Brownie | 1 serving (2 x 2 3/4") | 140 |
| Angel cake | 1½" wedge serving | 150 |
| Chocolate candy bar | 1 small | 125 |
| Cream puff | 1 regular | 250 |
| Fruit gelatin | ½ cup | 60 |
| Ice cream, vanilla | ½ cup | 200 |
| Marshmallows | 1 medium | 60 |
| Iced layer cake | 1½" wedge serving | 350 |
| Plain doughnut | 1 medium | 135 |
| Sherbet | ½ cup | 145 |
| Custard | 1 cup | 300 |
| **Meat, Fish, and Chicken** | | |
| Bacon | 4 lean slices | 200 |
| Beef roast | lean ½" slice | 200 |
| Broiled chicken | 1 medium lean piece | 200 |
| Clams | 6 medium | 35 |
| Frankfurter | 1 medium | 125 |
| Fresh fish | 3½ oz. broiled | 75 |
| Baked ham | 1 oz. slice | 250 |
| Broiled lamb chop | 1 oz. | 250 |
| Broiled lean steak | 2 oz. | 100 |
| Liver | ½ slice | 100 |
| Lobster | 4 oz. | 130 |
| Luncheon meat | 1 medium slice | 100 |
| Pork chop | 1 lean loin | 200 |
| Tuna fish | ½ cup | 125 |
| Veal roast | 1 medium slice | 100 |
| **Extras That Add Calories** | | |
| Bean soup | 1 cup, thick | 200 |
| Catsup | 1 tablespoon | 20 |
| Gravy (creamy) | 2 tablespoons | 100 |
| Mayonnaise | 1 tablespoon | 110 |
| Meat or chicken pie | 3¾" portion | 460 |
| Mustard | 1 tablespoon | 15 |
| Salad dressing | 2 tablespoons | 300 |
| Soup, creamed | 1 cup | 250 |
| Spaghetti with sauce | 2 cup serving | 420 |
| Tartar sauce | 1 tablespoon | 100 |
| Mixed vegetable soup | 1 cup | 100 |

If you don't find a particular food listed here, try to find the equivalent food and the caloric count. Half of a medium cantaloupe is about the same as one medium fresh peach, therefore, both would equal approximately 50 calories.

**Basic Calorie Values of Various Foods**

Remember these are approximate figures. A hamburger, as listed will be the average three-inch patty, not a jumbo size. This is a practical list that will serve to guide you in determining how much is "too" much.

| FOOD | AMOUNT OF SERVING | CALORIES |
|---|---|---|
| **Sandwiches** | | |
| Luncheon meats | 1 medium slice on whole-wheat bread | 250 |
| Cheese | 3½" square on rye bread | 400 |
| Hamburger on bun | 3" patty on 3" bun | 300 |
| Hot dog on long bun | | 325 |
| Peanut butter | 2 tablespoons on white bread | 400 |
| Roast beef | 1½ oz. on rye bread | 325 |

(Remember to add calories for extras such as mayonnaise, mustard, catsup, etc.)

| FOOD | AMOUNT OF SERVING | CALORIES |
|---|---|---|
| **Beverages** | | |
| Carbonated drinks, flavors and root beer | 8 oz. | 100 |
| Cocoa | 6 oz. | 180 |
| Cola drinks | 8 oz. | 100 |
| Ginger ale | 8 oz. can or bottle | 75 |
| Ice cream malted milk | 8 oz. | 400 |
| Ice cream sodas | 10 oz. | 350 |
| Skimmed milk | 8 oz. | 85 |
| Tea or coffee, plain | | 0 |
| with cream and sugar | | 100 |
| Whole milk | 8 oz. | 170 |
| **Fruits** | | |
| Apple | 1 medium size | 60 |
| Banana | 1 medium size | 90 |
| Prunes | 3 regular size | 70 |
| Grapes | 30 medium size | 90 |
| Orange | 1 large | 100 |
| Cherries | 20 fresh | 90 |
| **Nuts and Snack Foods** | | |
| Almonds | 10 | 130 |
| Cashews | 10 | 75 |
| Peanuts | 1 oz. bag | 200 |
| Pecans | 5 whole | 150 |
| Pizza | 4" serving | 185 |
| Popcorn, lightly buttered | 1 cup | 150 |
| Potato chips | 8 large | 90 |
| Pretzels | 5 medium | 25 |
| Cookie, chocolate chip | 1 medium | 55 |

## HARMFUL HABITS THAT AFFECT HEALTH

In order to obtain the most nutritional value from the food we eat, it is necessary to avoid habits that impair digestion.

A person's emotional state (anger, frustration, depression) can inhibit the digestive process. The "hurry habit" is the chief offender. It is better to make time for meals than to get in the habit of bolting down snack foods and always eating on the run. This puts a burden on the digestive system. Habitual overeating, smoking, chronic fatigue, and lack of exercise can also interfere with good digestion.

It is advisable not to exercise immediately after eating a large meal because activity takes the blood away from the stomach to the muscles and slows down the digestive processes.

**Rules for Clients Who Wish to Maintain Normal Weight:**

1. Eat well-balanced meals.
2. Eat a good breakfast.
3. Regulate the time of meals so that the largest meal is not eaten late at night.
4. Relax at mealtime. This should be a pleasant, unhurried time.
5. Exercise regularly.
6. Get adequate sleep and relaxation.
7. Avoid irregularity (constipation) by eating sufficient amounts of fiber foods such as found in a balanced diet.
8. Avoid stress by setting priorities and managing time effectively.

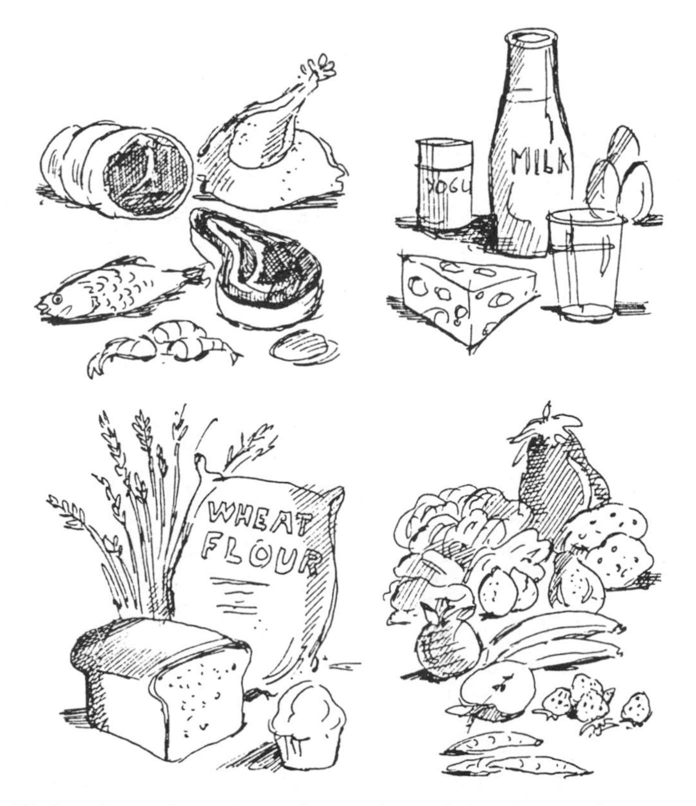


*Well balanced meals made up of a variety of nourishing foods, daily exercise and relaxation are the keys to maintaining your ideal weight.*

**Instant Weight Finder (Women)**

Your Ideal Weight in Pounds, According to Age, Height and Frame*

*N = Normal frame    H = Heavy frame    L = Light frame*

| Height in Feet and Inches | 21-24 | | | 25-29 | | | 30-34 | | | 35-39 | | | 40-44 | | |
|---|---|---|---|---|---|---|---|---|---|---|---|---|---|---|---|
| | N | H | L | N | H | L | N | H | L | N | H | L | N | H | L |
| 4' 9" | 108 | 121 | 99 | 110 | 123 | 101 | 112 | 125 | 103 | 112 | 125 | 103 | 111 | 124 | 103 |
| 4' 10" | 110 | 123 | 101 | 112 | 125 | 103 | 114 | 127 | 105 | 114 | 127 | 105 | 113 | 126 | 105 |
| 4' 11" | 112 | 125 | 103 | 114 | 127 | 105 | 116 | 129 | 107 | 116 | 129 | 107 | 115 | 128 | 107 |
| 5' 0" | 114 | 127 | 105 | 116 | 129 | 107 | 118 | 131 | 109 | 118 | 131 | 109 | 117 | 130 | 109 |
| 5' 1" | 116 | 128 | 107 | 118 | 130 | 109 | 120 | 132 | 111 | 120 | 132 | 111 | 119 | 131 | 111 |
| 5' 2" | 119 | 133 | 110 | 121 | 135 | 112 | 123 | 137 | 114 | 123 | 137 | 114 | 122 | 136 | 114 |
| 5' 3" | 123 | 134 | 112 | 125 | 136 | 114 | 127 | 138 | 116 | 127 | 138 | 116 | 126 | 137 | 116 |
| 5' 4" | 126 | 141 | 116 | 128 | 143 | 118 | 130 | 145 | 120 | 130 | 145 | 120 | 129 | 144 | 120 |
| 5' 5" | 130 | 142 | 119 | 132 | 144 | 121 | 134 | 146 | 123 | 134 | 146 | 123 | 133 | 145 | 123 |
| 5' 6" | 134 | 150 | 123 | 136 | 152 | 125 | 138 | 154 | 127 | 138 | 154 | 127 | 137 | 153 | 127 |
| 5' 7" | 138 | 152 | 127 | 140 | 154 | 129 | 142 | 156 | 131 | 142 | 156 | 131 | 141 | 155 | 131 |
| 5' 8" | 142 | 158 | 131 | 144 | 160 | 133 | 146 | 162 | 135 | 146 | 162 | 135 | 145 | 161 | 135 |
| 5' 9" | 146 | 161 | 134 | 148 | 163 | 136 | 150 | 165 | 138 | 150 | 165 | 138 | 149 | 164 | 138 |
| 5' 10" | 149 | 167 | 138 | 151 | 169 | 140 | 153 | 171 | 142 | 153 | 171 | 142 | 152 | 170 | 142 |
| 5' 11" | 153 | 170 | 141 | 155 | 172 | 143 | 158 | 175 | 146 | 158 | 175 | 146 | 157 | 174 | 146 |

| Height in Feet and Inches | 45-49 | | | 50-54 | | | 55-59 | | | 60-64 | | | 65-69 | | |
|---|---|---|---|---|---|---|---|---|---|---|---|---|---|---|---|
| | N | H | L | N | H | L | N | H | L | N | H | L | N | H | L |
| 4' 9" | 110 | 123 | 103 | 109 | 122 | 102 | 108 | 121 | 101 | 105 | 117 | 98 | 104 | 116 | 97 |
| 4' 10" | 112 | 125 | 105 | 111 | 124 | 104 | 110 | 123 | 103 | 107 | 119 | 100 | 106 | 118 | 99 |
| 4' 11" | 114 | 127 | 107 | 113 | 126 | 106 | 112 | 125 | 105 | 109 | 121 | 102 | 108 | 120 | 101 |
| 5' 0" | 116 | 129 | 109 | 115 | 128 | 108 | 114 | 127 | 107 | 111 | 123 | 104 | 110 | 122 | 103 |
| 5' 1" | 118 | 130 | 111 | 117 | 129 | 110 | 116 | 128 | 109 | 113 | 124 | 106 | 112 | 123 | 105 |
| 5' 2" | 121 | 135 | 114 | 120 | 134 | 113 | 119 | 133 | 112 | 116 | 129 | 109 | 115 | 128 | 108 |
| 5' 3" | 125 | 136 | 116 | 124 | 135 | 115 | 123 | 134 | 114 | 120 | 130 | 111 | 119 | 129 | 110 |
| 5' 4" | 128 | 143 | 120 | 127 | 142 | 119 | 126 | 141 | 118 | 123 | 137 | 115 | 122 | 136 | 114 |
| 5' 5" | 132 | 144 | 123 | 131 | 143 | 122 | 130 | 142 | 121 | 127 | 138 | 118 | 126 | 137 | 117 |
| 5' 6" | 136 | 152 | 127 | 135 | 151 | 126 | 134 | 150 | 125 | 131 | 146 | 122 | 130 | 145 | 121 |
| 5' 7" | 140 | 154 | 131 | 139 | 153 | 130 | 138 | 152 | 129 | 135 | 148 | 126 | 134 | 147 | 125 |
| 5' 8" | 144 | 160 | 135 | 143 | 159 | 134 | 142 | 158 | 133 | 139 | 154 | 130 | 138 | 153 | 129 |
| 5' 9" | 148 | 163 | 138 | 147 | 162 | 137 | 146 | 161 | 136 | 143 | 157 | 133 | 142 | 156 | 132 |
| 5' 10" | 151 | 169 | 142 | 150 | 168 | 141 | 149 | 167 | 140 | 146 | 163 | 137 | 145 | 162 | 136 |
| 5' 11" | 156 | 173 | 146 | 155 | 172 | 145 | 154 | 171 | 144 | 151 | 167 | 141 | 150 | 166 | 140 |

**Undressed. For clothing and shoes, allow 4 lbs.*

**Instant Weight Finder (Men)**

Your Ideal Weight in Pounds, According to Age, Height and Frame*

*N = Normal frame H = Heavy frame L = Light frame*

| Height in Feet and Inches | AGE GROUPS 21-24 | | | 25-29 | | | 30-34 | | | 35-39 | | | 40-44 | | |
|---|---|---|---|---|---|---|---|---|---|---|---|---|---|---|---|
| | N | H | L | N | H | L | N | H | L | N | H | L | N | H | L |
| 4' 9" | | | | | | | | | | | | | | | |
| 4' 10" | | | | | | | | | | | | | | | |
| 4' 11" | 112 | 134 | 106 | 116 | 138 | 110 | 118 | 140 | 112 | 118 | 140 | 112 | 117 | 139 | 112 |
| 5' 0" | 114 | 136 | 108 | 118 | 140 | 112 | 120 | 142 | 114 | 120 | 142 | 114 | 119 | 141 | 114 |
| 5' 1" | 116 | 138 | 110 | 120 | 142 | 114 | 122 | 144 | 116 | 122 | 144 | 116 | 121 | 143 | 116 |
| 5' 2" | 120 | 140 | 112 | 123 | 143 | 115 | 125 | 145 | 117 | 125 | 145 | 117 | 124 | 144 | 117 |
| 5' 3" | 124 | 144 | 116 | 126 | 146 | 118 | 128 | 148 | 120 | 128 | 148 | 120 | 127 | 147 | 120 |
| 5' 4" | 128 | 148 | 120 | 130 | 150 | 122 | 132 | 152 | 124 | 132 | 152 | 124 | 131 | 151 | 124 |
| 5' 5" | 132 | 152 | 123 | 134 | 154 | 125 | 136 | 156 | 127 | 136 | 156 | 127 | 135 | 155 | 127 |
| 5' 6" | 135 | 156 | 127 | 138 | 159 | 130 | 140 | 161 | 132 | 140 | 161 | 132 | 139 | 160 | 132 |
| 5' 7" | 139 | 160 | 130 | 142 | 163 | 133 | 144 | 165 | 135 | 144 | 165 | 135 | 143 | 164 | 135 |
| 5' 8" | 143 | 164 | 133 | 146 | 167 | 136 | 148 | 169 | 138 | 148 | 169 | 138 | 147 | 168 | 138 |
| 5' 9" | 147 | 170 | 137 | 150 | 173 | 140 | 153 | 176 | 143 | 153 | 176 | 143 | 152 | 175 | 143 |
| 5' 10" | 152 | 175 | 140 | 155 | 178 | 143 | 158 | 181 | 146 | 158 | 181 | 146 | 157 | 180 | 146 |
| 5' 11" | 156 | 180 | 144 | 161 | 185 | 149 | 164 | 188 | 152 | 164 | 188 | 152 | 163 | 187 | 152 |
| 6' 0" | 161 | 184 | 148 | 167 | 190 | 154 | 170 | 193 | 157 | 170 | 193 | 157 | 169 | 192 | 157 |
| 6' 1" | 167 | 187 | 153 | 173 | 193 | 159 | 176 | 196 | 162 | 176 | 196 | 162 | 175 | 195 | 162 |
| 6' 2" | 171 | 192 | 157 | 178 | 199 | 164 | 182 | 203 | 168 | 182 | 203 | 168 | 181 | 202 | 168 |

| Height in Feet and Inches | AGE GROUPS 45-49 | | | 50-54 | | | 55-59 | | | 60-64 | | | 65-69 | | |
|---|---|---|---|---|---|---|---|---|---|---|---|---|---|---|---|
| | N | H | L | N | H | L | N | H | L | N | H | L | N | H | L |
| 4' 9" | | | | | | | | | | | | | | | |
| 4' 10" | | | | | | | | | | | | | | | |
| 4' 11" | 116 | 138 | 112 | 115 | 137 | 111 | 114 | 136 | 110 | 111 | 132 | 107 | 110 | 131 | 106 |
| 5' 0" | 118 | 140 | 114 | 117 | 139 | 113 | 116 | 138 | 112 | 113 | 134 | 109 | 112 | 133 | 108 |
| 5' 1" | 120 | 142 | 116 | 119 | 141 | 115 | 118 | 140 | 114 | 115 | 136 | 111 | 114 | 135 | 110 |
| 5' 2" | 123 | 143 | 117 | 122 | 142 | 116 | 121 | 141 | 115 | 118 | 137 | 112 | 117 | 136 | 111 |
| 5' 3" | 126 | 146 | 120 | 125 | 145 | 119 | 124 | 144 | 118 | 121 | 140 | 115 | 120 | 139 | 114 |
| 5' 4" | 130 | 150 | 124 | 129 | 149 | 123 | 128 | 148 | 122 | 125 | 144 | 119 | 124 | 143 | 118 |
| 5' 5" | 134 | 154 | 127 | 133 | 153 | 126 | 132 | 152 | 125 | 129 | 148 | 122 | 128 | 147 | 121 |
| 5' 6" | 138 | 159 | 132 | 137 | 158 | 131 | 136 | 157 | 130 | 133 | 153 | 127 | 132 | 152 | 126 |
| 5' 7" | 142 | 163 | 135 | 141 | 162 | 134 | 140 | 161 | 133 | 137 | 157 | 130 | 136 | 156 | 129 |
| 5' 8" | 146 | 167 | 138 | 145 | 166 | 137 | 144 | 165 | 136 | 141 | 161 | 133 | 140 | 160 | 132 |
| 5' 9" | 151 | 174 | 143 | 150 | 173 | 142 | 149 | 172 | 141 | 146 | 168 | 138 | 145 | 167 | 137 |
| 5' 10" | 156 | 179 | 146 | 155 | 178 | 145 | 154 | 177 | 144 | 151 | 173 | 141 | 150 | 172 | 140 |
| 5' 11" | 162 | 186 | 152 | 161 | 185 | 151 | 160 | 184 | 150 | 157 | 180 | 147 | 156 | 179 | 146 |
| 6' 0" | 168 | 191 | 157 | 167 | 190 | 156 | 166 | 189 | 155 | 163 | 185 | 152 | 162 | 184 | 151 |
| 6' 1" | 174 | 194 | 162 | 173 | 193 | 161 | 172 | 192 | 160 | 169 | 188 | 157 | 168 | 187 | 156 |
| 6' 2" | 180 | 201 | 168 | 179 | 200 | 167 | 178 | 199 | 166 | 175 | 195 | 163 | 174 | 194 | 162 |

**Undressed. For clothing and shoes, allow 8 lbs.*

## FIGURE IMPROVEMENT THROUGH WEIGHT CONTROL

During a weight-reduction or weight-gain program, the client will usually be interested in any changes in the contours of his or her body. Therefore, measurements are taken at the beginning of the program, recorded, and compared each week. People of various ages differ in height, weight, and body structures, so it is difficult to determine ideal measurements. In some fields general requirements for weights and measurements are necessary. For instance, professional models are required to maintain specific measurements to model ready-to-wear clothes. Also, designers need some standards to follow when designing for the general population. Average figure measurements for men's, women's, and children's clothing can be found in pattern books, catalogs, and design books. Generally, when the body is at its normal weight, it will be fairly well proportioned. Eating fewer calories will cause one to lose weight, but it is exercise that helps to contour the body and keep the muscles firm.

## TIPS FOR THE CLIENT WHO IS TRYING TO GAIN WEIGHT

The practitioner will occasionally have a client who wants to gain weight. This may be for health reasons but generally, it is to improve the contours of the body. Today, both men and women are participating in weight-lifting and body-building programs to build both strength and attractiveness. Good nutrition is a must if optimum results are to be achieved.

The procedure for gaining weight is almost the opposite as that for weight reducing. The object in gaining weight is to develop the muscular parts of the body and to permit the even distribution of fat to fill out contours.

The important rules are:

1. To achieve a gain of about one pound a week, a person weighing 150 pounds requires 18 calories for each pound of body weight, thereby yielding a total of 18 x150, or 2700 calories daily. Adding calories (unless burned up by extra activity) will result in weight gain. So when possible, caloric intake should be increased, but not beyond the digestive capacity of the individual.
2. Eat frequently between meals rather than increase the amount of food eaten at regular meals. Be sure meals are balanced to assure adequate vitamins and minerals.
3. Get plenty of rest and relaxation.
4. Do exercises that tend to build muscle.
5. Eat slowly and chew food thoroughly to aid digestion.
6. Pay attention to grooming and dress. Wear clothes that detract from extremely thin parts of the body.

**MEASUREMENT CHART**

Name of Advisor ____________________ Date ____________

Name of Client ____________________ Age ____________

Height ____________ Weight ____________ Build: ☐ Small ☐ Medium ☐ Large

| Beginning date ______ | Weekly check | 1st | 2nd | 3rd | 4th | 5th | 6th | NOTES |
|---|---|---|---|---|---|---|---|---|
| Chest (men | | | | | | | | |
| Bustline (women) | | | | | | | | |
| Upper arm | | | | | | | | |
| Wrist | | | | | | | | |
| Waistline | | | | | | | | |
| Abdomen | | | | | | | | |
| Hips | | | | | | | | |
| Thigh | | | | | | | | |
| Above kneecap | | | | | | | | |
| Calf | | | | | | | | |
| Ankle | | | | | | | | |
| Other | | | | | | | | |
| | | | | | | | | |

**FIGURE MEASUREMENTS**

**Location of Main Points for Figure Measurement**

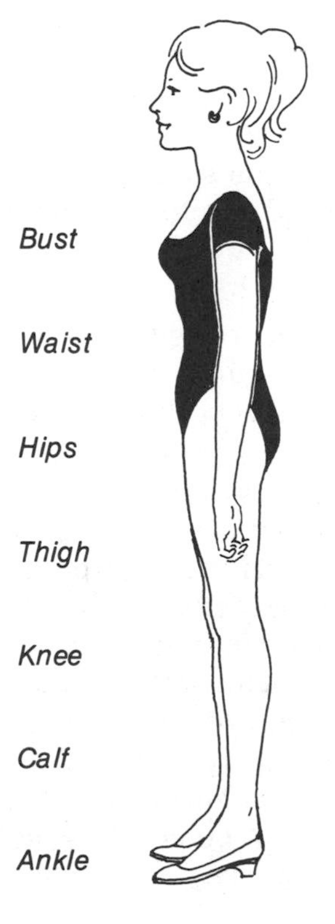


When taking figure measurements:

1. Measure without shoes.
2. Measure largest part of the chest (men) bust (women).
3. Measure the smallest part of the waistline with the tape measure snug.
4. The hips are measured at the largest projections of the buttocks.
5. Measure the largest part of the thigh.
6. Always measure the knee just above the kneecap.
7. Measure the largest portion of the calf.
8. The ankle is measured just above the anklebone.

## OBESITY AND WEIGHT LOSS

Obesity (overweight) affects millions of people and is considered dangerous to health. Doctors have found that being 10 to 20 percent or more overweight can contribute to cardiovascular disease, diabetes, high blood pressure, and a number of other serious health conditions. In addition, a person may become self-conscious about his or her appearance. An overweight person should be advised to see a physician who can prescribe a gradual weight-loss diet and recommend safe exercises.

Generally, obesity is due to eating more food than the body uses as energy, and this overload is stored as fat. On the other hand, this is not always the case. Obesity can be due to some glandular malfunction (e.g. malfunction of the thyroid). Some people have a predisposition to becoming overweight. This is why the client must have a thorough physical checkup by his or her physician before beginning a weight-loss program.

The massage practitioner may be employed in a place of business that offers a weight-control program or may work in some capacity with physicians who recommend massage therapy as an aid to losing weight. Knowledge of nutrition and how to help clients with their diet and exercise regimens can be a plus for the practitioner who may prefer working in a health-spa environment.

Many clients will not understand that to lose weight it is necessary to use more calories than the body needs to retain its present weight. The calories the body does not use are stored in fat cells. It is important to combine good nutrition (well balanced meals) with exercise in any weight-loss plan. Hydrotherapy, massage, exercise, and diet can all work together to reduce excess weight. The object is to draw upon the fat deposits of the body and prevent the accumulation of additional fat. The client should be advised not to go on any type of fad or crash diet. While some of these diets may take off pounds fast, the dieter tends to gain them back.

### Tips for the Client Who is Trying to Lose Weight

The client who is trying to lose weight may need to be reminded that disciplining the appetite is important if results are to be achieved. The following tips may be helpful:

1. Snack foods are more tempting when they are readily available. The best way to avoid eating high-calorie snacks is to keep them out of sight or unavailable. When dining out, a person who tends to be tempted too easily should remember to eat some low-calorie "fill-up" foods beforehand. Apples, celery, whole-grain bread, sliced carrots or a small piece of cheese will usually help to satisfy the appetite.
2. The person who is trying to lose weight will often have friends who will try to tempt them to eat more than they should. A simple, "no thank you," backed up by will power will do the trick. A person on a diet should not allow others to undo their progress.

3. The person on a diet to lose weight should be familiar with foods that are high and low in calories in order to judge caloric content of portions. The ability to count calories mentally before preparing meals and when eating in restaurants is well worth the effort.
4. Eating slowly helps the dieter to feel full faster, and he or she will enjoy the food more.
5. A tall glass of water or low-caloric beverage will also help to dull the appetite if drank just before the meal.
6. Meals should always be balanced to provide adequate vitamins and minerals—no fad diets without a physician's supervision.
7. The person who wants to lose weight should keep a mental picture of how he or she wants to look and feel.
8. It is important to learn to like low-calorie (food-for-you) foods. Taste buds can be retrained.
9. When dieting, increase the amount and variety of exercise and sports in accordance with the strength and capacity of the body.
10. When losing weight pay attention to grooming and dress and wear clothing that gives a slenderizing effect.

Generally, the proper amount of weight to lose each week should range between 1½ to 3½ pounds. Such a standard permits a gradual and uniform loss of weight over the entire body. To lose weight more rapidly may show itself mainly on the face, besides undermining the body's resistance and causing a strain on the heart.

The daily energy requirements for an adult are estimated to be 15 calories for each pound of body weight. For weight maintenance, a person weighing 150 pounds would need 15 x 150, or 2250 calories daily. To bring about a loss of about one pound a week, the number of calories can be safely reduced from 15 to 12 for each pound of body weight, thereby allowing 12 x 150, or 1800 calories daily.

In general, fruits, vegetables, lean meats, skim milk, and clear soups are not only low in calories but are also high in vitamins and minerals. On the other hand, dairy products, nuts, fats, fried foods, confections, and desserts are relatively high in calories and therefore should be eaten sparingly in a weight-reducing diet, but can be eaten freely in a weight-gaining diet.

**Finding Approximate Normal Weight**

A weight scale (professional type) should be part of the practitioner's equipment. Also, a device for measuring the client's height (without shoes) should be available. The client's height and weight should be recorded on the first day of the reducing program and his or her normal weight range determined. A weight chart can be used to record progress. Use the weight progress chart in this chapter as a guide. At the top of the chart record the client's high, ideal, and low weight. This represents the weight range. At the center, record the client's present weight. By using this chart as a graph you can follow any gain or loss of weight, week by week, until the goal is reached. For example, the sample chart shows the ideal weight for a young woman (height 5' 2", medium-to-large frame) as 110 pounds. Her actual weight is 140. If during the first week she gains 5 pounds, the chart will show that she is not making progress in her weight loss. If, by the fourth week she has lost this weight plus another 10 pounds, the graph will show progress.

**Weight Control Progress Chart**

Name of advisor ______________________ Date ______________

Name (client) ______________________ Age ______________

Height ______________ Build: ☐ Large ☐ Medium ☐ Small

Present weight ______________________

High weight ______________ Low weight ______________ Ideal weight ______________

| Date Weekly Check | 1st | 2nd | 3rd | 4th | 5th | 6th | NOTES |
|---|---|---|---|---|---|---|---|
| | 175 | | | | | | |
| | 170 | | | | | | |
| | 165 | | | | | | |
| | 160 | | | | | | |
| | 155 | | | | | | |
| | 150 | | | | | | |
| Weight Gain | 145 | 145 | | | | | |
| Beginning Weight | 140 | | | | | | |
| Weight Loss | 135 | | | | | | |
| | 130 | | | 130 | | | |
| | 125 | | | | | | |
| | 120 | | | | | | |
| | 115 | | | | | | |
| Goal | 110 | | | | | | |
| | | | | | | | |
| | | | | | | | |
| | | | | | | | |
| | | | | | | | |
| | | | | | | | |

## THE PROBLEM OF CELLULITE

Cellulite should not be confused with cellulitis, which is an acute inflammation of the tissues. Cellulite is an anatomical and functional condition of the connective (interstitial) tissue. Also, cellulite should not be confused with normal fat. Normal fat can be eliminated by diet and exercise, but cellulite does not burn up as fat does. Cellulite is a gel-like substance made up of wastes, water, and some fat and is located between the muscles. Lumps of this substance become trapped beneath the skin, causing a ripple effect and unsightly bulges. Cellulite appears more prominently on the upper and midback, upper arms, waistline, buttocks, inner thighs, and inside the leg near the knee.

Nutrition and the body's waste removal processes are partially responsible for the formation of cellulite. It is often described as a poisoning of connective tissues brought about by improper diet, insufficient liquid intake, faulty elimination, stress, fatigue, and circulatory problems.

There are three types of cellulite: edemous, hard, or soft. Cellulite is not a condition that is limited only to women who are overweight; thin women also develop cellulite areas. However, cellulite is considered to be a condition that affects primarily women because of the specialized functioning of their reproductive organs, primarily the ovaries and the pituitary gland, known as the master gland of the body. Cellulite may begin to affect young girls at puberty. It is also associated with pregnancy, and sometimes becomes prominent during menopause.

### Exercise

While exercise will not remove cellulite, it does much to stimulate circulation, tone the muscles, and improve the removal of body wastes. Exercises, such as swimming, that require movement of the entire body are recommended. Exercises should not be done to the point of fatigue.

### Massage

Regular manual massage can be adapted to cellulite areas, or a hand vibrator (with circular movement) will be effective. Massage improves circulation, relaxes tension, and helps to eliminate muscular fatigue.

### Body Therapy

In recent years more full-service salons and spas have begun offering body care programs to contour and reshape the figure. Before treatments are given, the client's measurements are taken, the health history is recorded, and the treatment is selected. Some of the methods used are as follows:

#### Baths

Mineral salts or sea salts are added to a hot tub to draw out toxic wastes and impurities from the tissues. This type of bath is more effective if taken twice a week. Steam baths, jacuzzi, hydrotherapy, saunas, pariffin treatment, herbal baths, and mud packs are given to increase circulation and induce relaxation.

#### Friction Rubs

Friction or surface rubs (also salt rubs) stimulate and draw the blood to the surface of the skin. They also soothe nerves and help to flush out waste from the cellulite deposits.

**Electrical Apparatus**

In addition to the hand vibrator, there are devices that are considered helpful in treating cellulite. Some use galvanic current to provide better penetration of products. Some use faradic current to exercise muscles and to increase circulation. Other techniques include use of suction, brushing, and jets of air or water. The practitioner should be sure to learn to use such devices correctly and according to safety rules.

**Body Wrapping**

There are various types of wraps used in the treatment of cellulite, but the three most popular ones are the wet wrap, the dry wrap, and the plastic wrap.

***Wet Wrap***

Wide cotton (usually 100 percent cotton) bandages are presoaked in tepid water or a specially prepared (such as herbal) solution and applied. Because the client is wet and there may be a drop in temperature during the treatment, a blanket or plastic cover should be used to keep the client warm and comfortable. Care must be taken to be sure bandages are not wrapped too tightly. This method helps to tone and firm the muscles.

***Dry Wrap***

The dry wrap is often preferred because it enables the client to move around and is less messy than the wet wrap. A product (usually a gel) containing ingredients that tone and firm muscles is applied with a brush or the practitioner's hands. Tapes (wrapping) are applied, and the client relaxes as the muscles are toned, tightened, and some of the cellulite reduced. These treatments are approximately one hour.

***Plastic Wrap***

A cream or oil is applied to the skin and a heavy plastic wrap (the kind used for wrapping foods) is firmly wrapped around the legs and torso. The client relaxes for an hour or so. Following the wrap, the client showers then measures the parts of the body that were treated and records the results. Some clients lose inches in one to six treatments, but the success of the body wrap treatments depends on the extent of the problem.

**QUESTIONS FOR DISCUSSION AND REVIEW**

1. Why should the massage practitioner be concerned with nutrition?
2. What are the three types of foods needed in a well-balanced diet?
3. Define a calorie.
4. Define metabolism.
5. What is the main job of enzymes?
6. What are the four basic food groups said to be essential to a well balanced diet?
7. What are the four most effective natural (nonlaxative) remedies for correcting faulty elimination?
8. How can studying a vitamin chart be of help to the massage practitioner?
9. What can be learned from studying food tables that show general caloric content and serving sizes of most foods?
10. Why should the massage practitioner understand how to deal with obesity?

11. What are the dangers of obesity?
12. What is the first step an obese person should take before starting a drastic weight loss program?
13. What instructions should an obese person receive concerning caloric intake?
14. What is the proper procedure for determining a client's weight, height, and ideal weight?
15. What are the three types of body frames?
16. What is the purpose of the weight-progress chart?
17. When helping a client to gain weight, what is the main goal?
18. What is the purpose of a figure measurement chart?
19. What is cellulite?
20. Why is cellulite a condition that primarily affects women?
21. Why should the massage practitioner have some knowledge of cellulite treatments?
22. What are the three types of wraps used in the treatment of cellulite?

## ANSWERS TO QUESTIONS FOR DISCUSSION AND REVIEW

1. Nutrition plays an important role in healthy body metabolism, and the massage practitioner is dedicated to the preservation and maintenance of the client's health.
2. The three types of foods needed in a well-balanced diet are: proteins, fats, and carbohydrates.
3. A calorie is defined as a unit of heat or energy.
4. Metabolism is the sum total of all the body processes whereby the living body utilizes oxygen and food in the building up and breaking down of its tissues.
5. The job of enzymes is to initiate or accelerate specific chemical reactions in the metabolism.
6. The four groups are dairy, meat (protein), vegetable and fruit, and bread and cereal.
7. Correcting the diet, regular exercise, massage, and proper relaxation are the most effective remedies for correcting faulty elimination.
8. Studying vitamin and mineral charts helps the practitioner to understand the importance of good nutrition to health. It is also valuable when discussing health and nutrition with clients.
9. Food tables showing general caloric content of common foods and serving sizes help the practitioner to learn how to work with clients in achieving health and weight goals. Such tables help to suggest meals that contain carbohydrates, fats, and proteins in the desired amounts.
10. The massage practitioner may be employed in a place of business that offers a weight-control program or may work in some capacity with physicians who recommend massage therapy as an aid to losing weight. The practitioner who knows how to deal with the problem of obesity will be a more valuable counselor and more understanding of client's needs.

11. Obesity can contribute to cardiovascular disease, diabetes, high blood pressure, and a number of other conditions.
12. An obese person should see a physician before beginning a weight-loss program. Weight loss should be gradual in order to avoid wrinkles and sagging skin.
13. The client should be advised not to go on any kind of crash or fad diet but to follow his or her physician's advice concerning caloric intake.
14. A weight scale and chart should be used to record the client's weight and ideal weight according to his or her age and bone structure. A doctor's scale or other device can be used for checking the client's height. Measuring the wrist above the wristbone is useful in determining bone structure.
15. Body frames are classified as light, normal, and heavy.
16. The weight-loss project chart enables the practitioner and client to keep a record that shows whether or not the weight-loss goal is being achieved.
17. The main goal in weight loss is to develop the muscular parts of the body and to permit even distribution of the fat to fill out contours of the body properly.
18. The figure measurement chart helps the client to see his or her weekly progress (or lack of progress).
19. Cellulite is an anatomical and functional condition of the tissues of certain parts of the body. Cellulite, unlike fat, does not burn up.
20. Cellulite is a condition that primarily affects women due to the specialized functioning of their reproductive organs, mainly the ovaries and the pituitary gland.
21. The massage practitioner should understand cellulite because massage can be used to improve the condition.
22. The wet wrap, dry wrap, and plastic wrap.

# Chapter 17 Therapeutic Exercise

**LEARNING OBJECTIVES**

After you have mastered this chapter you will be able to:

1. Explain the benefits of a regular exercise program.
2. Explain why exercise is important.
3. Describe warm-up and cooling-off exercises.
4. Instruct the client in proper breathing techniques.
5. Demonstrate good posture as part of a fitness program.
6. Explain basic posture problems.
7. Instruct the client in exercising to improve posture.
8. Instruct the client in general exercises.
9. Instruct the client in stress-reducing exercises.
10. Instruct the client in basic yogi poses for relaxation.
11. Plan a personal fitness program.
12. Complete a daily exercise record card.

**INTRODUCTION**

Since ancient times, physical fitness has gone hand in hand with concepts of mental alertness; a strong, healthy, well-proportioned body; and personal pride. The ancient Greeks were known for their athletic contests, which are still a part of modern athletics. The Olympic Games were named after Mount Olympus, thought to be the dwelling place of the gods.

In recent decades there has been an increased interest in physical fitness. Millions of people of all ages have made some type of sport or other workout a part of their daily lives. Many businesses and industrial firms have encouraged exercise by providing facilities where workers can swim, jog, play tennis, and use various machines and apparatus to keep themselves fit. Exercises set to dance rhythms (generally called dance exercise or aerobics) have become popular. *Aerobics* is a modern word meaning cardiorespiratory exercise. This type of exercise has been the answer for millions of business people who are unable to participate in regular sports, but who can join an exercise class or do the exercises at home using an instructional cassette tape or video.

**BENEFITS OF THERAPEUTIC EXERCISE**

While exercise is a must for optimum health, it can be harmful if done improperly. A person may decide to trim, slim, and develop a well-muscled body and enthusiastically may begin workouts with weights and various kinds of apparatus without understanding either the benefits or dangers. At first there may be some improvement, but unsupervised exercise can lead to strain upon the muscles, nerves, the heart, and other organs of the body. Also, improper exercise can cause muscles to become hard, stiff, and unattractive.

Ingesting fewer calories than the body needs will result in a loss of weight. However, dieting alone does not achieve the desired results because the proportions of the body tend to remain the same, only smaller. Proper diet combined with exercise will help to firm muscles, so as weight is lost, the body becomes better proportioned. The major benefits of exercise are:

Improvement in appearance.

Improvement in body functions.

Maintenance of normal weight.

Relief of tension and stress.

Prevention of fatigue.

Improvement of coordination.

Increased mental alertness.

Increased endurance.

Improved posture.

Enhanced sense of well-being.

## CONSULTATION FOR AN EXERCISE PROGRAM

Before beginning an exercise program, the client should confirm that he or she is in good health. Some salons, spas, dance schools, and exercise clubs require the client to have a physical checkup by a physician as a precautionary step. No one wants a person to be injured or become ill, and practitioners and owners of businesses do not want to be involved in a malpractice suit. Clients understand this, and few will object to giving relevant information and signing a statement releasing the business and its employees from responsibility.

### Consultation Card

Name ______________________ Telephone ____________

Address ________________________________________

City ____________ State ____________ Zip ____________

Birthdate ____________ Height ____________ Weight ____________

Posture: ☐ good ☐ fair ☐ poor

Exercise recommended ____________________________

Results desired ________________________________

Exercises recommended ___________________________

1. ____________________________________________
2. ____________________________________________
3. ____________________________________________
4. ____________________________________________

Restrictions (the client should not do certain exercises)

________________________________________________

General goals __________________________________

________________________________________________

Date (to begin program) __________________________

Statement of health

Client's signature ______________________________

I have no health problems that prevent normal exercising with or without machines or apparatus. I hereby release (name of business) and its employees from responsibility for injuries I may incur as the result of participation in a program of health-related exercises.

**Beginning An Exercise Program**

Exercising gradually and building up to more strenuous routines will help to prevent sore, stiff muscles. Each exercise should be done correctly, and it is best to have the exercise routine supervised by a trained instructor. It is better to exercise every day to promote the elimination of toxins from the system. Some people enjoy a brisk workout both morning and evening, others prefer different times. The individual can choose the time that is most suitable to his or her daily schedule.

**Types of Exercises**

It is important to begin the exercise routine with specific exercises that warm up the muscles and speed up the action of the heart and lungs. This is done to prepare the body for more strenuous exercises. Ballet dancers warm muscles gradually and wear leg warmers when the room is cool. Likewise, for any type of exercise program, it is important to wear appropriate exercise clothing and to prime the muscles before a workout.

Following warm-up exercises, conditioning exercises may be done to tone the abdomen, back, leg, and other major muscles. Conditioning exercises are those that contract muscles for longer periods of time. They are usually done slowly as in isometric (equal pressure) exercises or presses and lifts.

Circulatory exercises are those that stimulate and strengthen the circulatory and respiratory systems. They are done at a fairly fast pace and include such exercises as running, dancing, jumping, and skipping rope. Cooling down exercises are important in preventing sore, stiff muscles. Such exercises might include walking, bending over to touch the toes, stretching, and slow dancing exercises.

Basic rules for exercise instructors:

1. All machines and apparatus used in the exercise program should be in safe condition and the client should be instructed in how to use them correctly.
2. A clean towel or mat should be provided if the client is to sit or lie on the floor for exercises.
3. The client should wear the appropriate clothing and shoes.
4. The instructor should question the client about his or her health before determining a specific exercise routine.
5. The client should be told not to eat a heavy meal directly before exercising.
6. The client should be instructed in proper breathing techniques.
7. Types of exercises and benefits should be explained before the client begins the exercise routine.
8. The client should be allowed short rest periods between exercises.
9. The client should be instructed in how to warm up before strenuous exercises and how to cool down following them.
10. The client should not be allowed to exercise to the point of fatigue.
11. The exercise period should be regulated according to the client's strength and endurance.

12. The exercise record card should be explained to the client, completed, and filed by the instructor. The client should be given a card for at-home use.

**A Typical Weekly Exercise Record Card**

Week of ________________

Number of times I was able to do exercise on:

| No. and Name of Exercise | 1st day | 2nd | 3rd | 4th | 5th | 6th | 7th | Measurements at Beginning of week: |
|---|---|---|---|---|---|---|---|---|
| Warm-up | | | | | | | | Wt.____________ |
| etc. | | | | | | | | Bust ___________ |
| | | | | | | | | Waist _________ |
| | | | | | | | | Hips ___________ |
| | | | | | | | | End of Week: |
| | | | | | | | | Wt.____________ |
| | | | | | | | | Bust ___________ |
| | | | | | | | | Waist _________ |
| | | | | | | | | Hips ___________ |

### Breathing Exercises

By means of respiration, oxygen, which is essential to life, is taken into the system, and carbon dioxide is given off. A healthy person breathes approximately 20,000 to 30,000 times in a 24-hour period. The following is a brief description of the respiratory forces.

Inspiration is the act of inhaling, or breathing inward, while expiration is the act of exhaling, or breathing outward. Ordinary inspiration takes place because of the contraction of a muscle called the diaphragm. When the diaphragm contracts, its sides collapse and it becomes flatter towards the thorax. This contracting motion causes the thorax to enlarge downward and the abdominal walls to expand. Because of its attachment to the sternum and false ribs, the diaphragm tends to pull downward and inward, a movement that is counteracted partly by the fibers attached to the ribs and by the elevation of the ribs. The main muscles that elevate the ribs and enlarge the thorax are the intercostals, the scaleni, and the levatores costarum.

Ordinary respiration is brought about by the elastic recoil of the lung tissue, the stretching of the costal cartilages, and the action of the abdominal muscles.

During forced inspiration, other muscles work to increase the chest capacity. The main benefits of breathing exercises are:

1. To keep the lungs healthy by maintaining their natural elasticity.
2. To increase the intake of oxygen and the giving off of carbon dioxide.

3. To improve the function of all internal organs.
4. To benefit circulation and nourishment of the body.

The client will find deep-breathing exercises beneficial and should observe the following rules for proper breathing:

1. It is important to breathe with the mouth closed. The nasal cavities warm the air as it enters. Also, the small hairs and mucous membrane are constructed to catch any small impure particles of dust in the air and prevent them from entering the lungs. If the client has an obstruction that prevents normal breathing through the nasal passages, he or she should consult a physician without delay.
2. Deep-breathing exercises should be done in the fresh air (out of doors) when possible. Deep breathing is most beneficial when done with active exercises. An example is raising the arms and inhaling, then exhaling while lowering the arms to the sides.
3. The client may not understand the meaning of diaphragmatic (deep) breathing and may be breathing in a shallow manner. Have the client place a hand just above the waistline and inhale deeply. The abdominal region should expand as the lungs are filled with air. The client should then exhale slowly to feel the abdominal region contract as air is expelled from the lungs.

Proper breathing is an asset in developing a speaking and singing voice and is an aid to relaxation of tension. The following exercises can be done lying down or standing:

1. Inhale slowly while raising the arms forward, with palms down, to a straight position directly overhead. Exhale slowly as the arms are returned to the sides of the body. Repeat the exercise 5 to 10 times.
2. Inhale while lifting the shoulders as high as possible toward the ears. Exhale slowly while rolling the shoulders backward and down to a normal relaxed position. Repeat 5 to 10 times.
3. Place a hand on the diaphragm (area above the abdomen), and pant quickly 5 to 10 times.
4. Use the forefinger to close one nostril. Inhale slowly and deeply, then exhale. Repeat the exercise on the other nostril.

## POSTURE IMPROVEMENT

Poor posture habits cause fatigue and strain on the muscles and joints. In addition, they cause the figure of a man or woman to appear older. Good posture helps to prevent backaches, fatigue, sagging muscles, and internal problems such as constipation and poor circulation. Good posture also improves appearance in clothes and imparts a sense of well-being.

The client will welcome a few lessons in posture improvement, and these basic instructions can be given before the beginning of regular exercises. Posture problems can be detected better if the client is wearing close-fitting garments such as leotards or shorts and T-shirt. The following are indications of poor posture:

The shoulders are tense and held high and the arms appear stiff. This posture gives a shy, self-conscious look.

Knees are locked causing the back to sway and the shoulders to droop.

The back sways into an inward curve causing the hips to protrude.

The head is held forward causing the shoulders to be rounded.

Any extreme deviation of the spine may indicate scoliosis and should be brought to the attention of a physician.

**The Spine**

The spine is divided into three sections. The first seven vertebrae, the cervicals, support the head. The second section is composed of the middle 12 thoracic vertebrae. The third section of the spine is known as the lumbar region and has five lumbar vertebrae. An exaggerated inward curve of the spine is called lordosis or swayback. When the thoracic curve is exaggerated and affects the shoulders, it is called kyphosis or humpback.

Scoliosis means a lateral (toward or from the side) deviation of the spine. When an abnormality of the spine is suspected, or when there is persistent pain in any area of the back, the client should be advised to see a physician without delay.

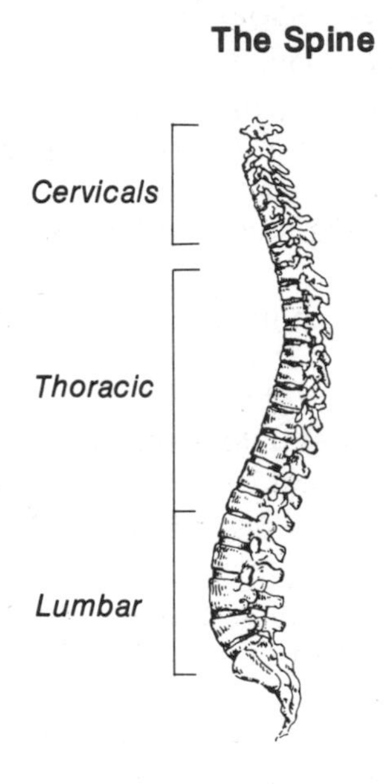


**Body Postures**

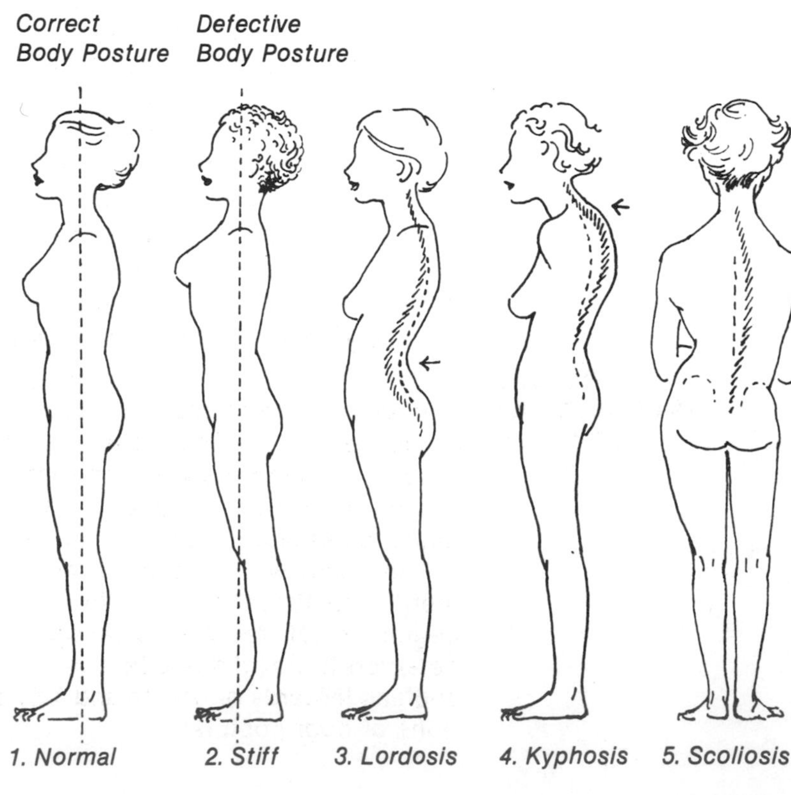


*1. Normal erect posture*

*2. Stiff rigid posture*

*3. Swayback or lordosis*

*4. Humped shoulders or kyphosis*

*5. Deviation of the spine or scoliosis*

## POSTURE CORRECTION EXERCISES

When teaching posture correction, have the client stand before a full-length mirror with a side view of the body. While looking over the shoulder into the mirror, the client should be able to detect posture faults that need attention. Normal erect posture does not mean stiff, rigid positions, whether standing, sitting, or walking. Good posture is relaxed, yet controlled. Check the following points:

1. When standing and walking, the weight should be over the balls of the feet not on the heels.
2. When walking or standing, the knees should be kept slightly flexed. Stiff knees throw the body off balance.
3. To properly align the body, the head should be lifted up from the waistline and the upper body balanced over the pelvic area. There should be no sagging of the shoulders or mid-section of the body, nor should the shoulders be held too high or thrust back.

The client should be encouraged to practice walking, standing, and sitting with correct body alignment until the correct posture feels natural and comfortable.

### Exercises for Strength, Balance, and Coordination

The best exercises for correcting faulty posture and for strengthening the back are borrowed from exercises done by ballet dancers. The following exercises will improve coordination and will strengthen the legs and back.

#### *Exercise 1—The Demi-Knee Bend Exercise for Posture*

*Starting position—Place a hand on the back of a chair or side of a door for balance (ballet dancers use a barre). The feet are placed in a comfortable stride slightly apart. The hips are kept tucked under as the pelvic area is lifted up and forward.*

*The body is slowly lowered as if to sit on the heels. This takes about 4 to 6 counts. The body is raised slowly back to a standing position. The exercise should be repeated about 4 times then increased as client becomes more comfortable and the muscles of the legs and back become stronger.*

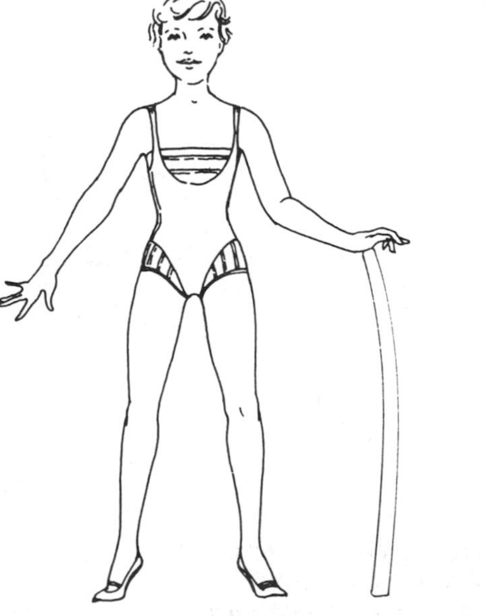

***Exercise 2—Exercise for Stretching the Waist and Back***

This exercise helps to make the muscles supple and strong. It is excellent for trimming the waistline and helps to improve posture.

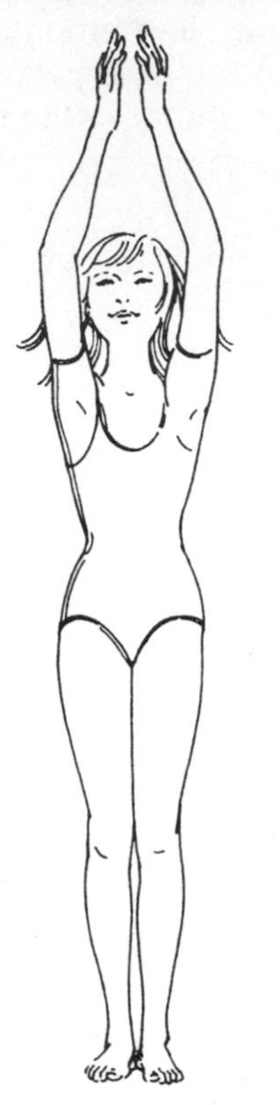

*Starting position—Stand erect with the feet in a comfortable stride with both hands overhead.*

*First count. Keeping the hands together, twist the upper body toward the right, and touch the hands to the side of the right knee. Second count. Return to the erect position. Third count. Twist the upper body to the left, and touch the side of the left knee with the hands. Fourth count. Return to the erect position. Repeat this exercise combination 5 to 10 times or more as strength increases.*

**General Warm-Up Exercises**

General warm-up exercises should be done before progressing to more active exercises. The following warm-up exercises are suitable for both men and women.

***Exercise 3—Shoulders and Arms***

*Starting position—Stand erect with feet together, arms outstretched at shoulder level.*

*First count. Rotate shoulders in a forward direction. Second count. Rotate shoulders in backward direction. Repeat 5 to 10 times forward and backward.*

**Exercise 4—Shoulders, and Upper Arms**

*Starting position—Stand erect with feet apart with hands clasped behind the neck.*

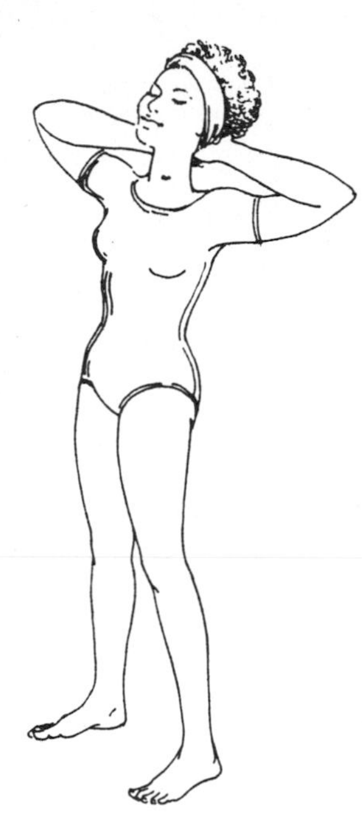

*First count. Pull head forward until the chin touches the chest. Second count. Raise the head and pull back as far as possible resisting with the arms. Repeat 5 to 10 times.*

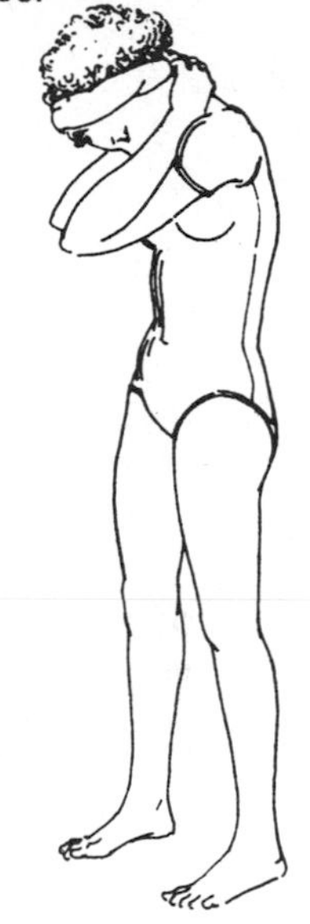

**Exercise 5—Swing and Bend**

*Starting position—Stand erect with the feet in a wide, comfortable stride with hands overhead.*

*First count. Bend over while bringing the left hand past the right foot. Keep the right hand up. Second count. Return to erect position. Third count. Bend over while bringing the right hand past the left foot. Keep the left hand up.Fourth count. Return to an erect position. Repeat the exercises 10 to 20 times. Establish a rhythm swinging the body down, to side and up again.*

**Exercise 6— The Runner**

*Starting position—Stand with feet together and arms at the sides. Run in place for 50 to 100 counts.*

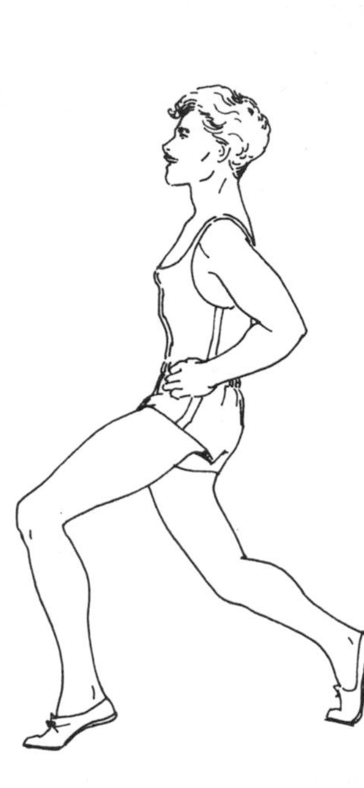

*Count fast while rotating the arms and skipping a real or imaginary rope. Count to 100. Relax and repeat the exercise.*

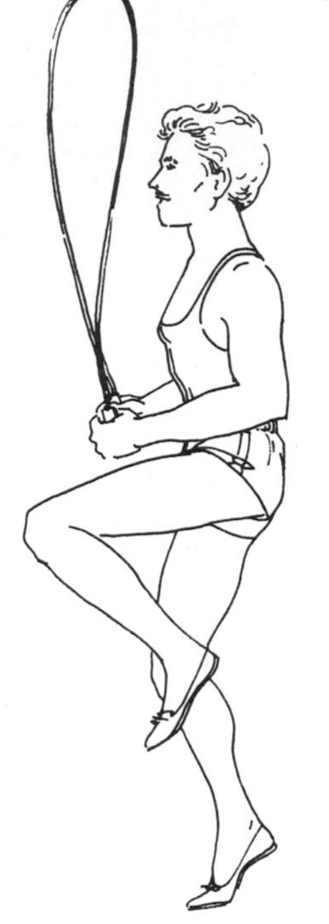

**Exercise 7— Leg Swings**

*Starting position—Stand with feet together and hands at the waist.*

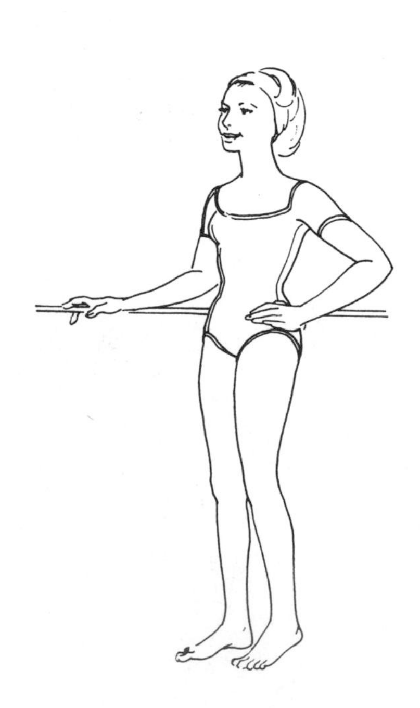

*First count. Lift the right leg as high as possible. Second count. Bring the right leg back to place (beside the left foot), and begin kicking the right leg up and down for 10 counts. Pause. Repeat the exercise with the left leg.*

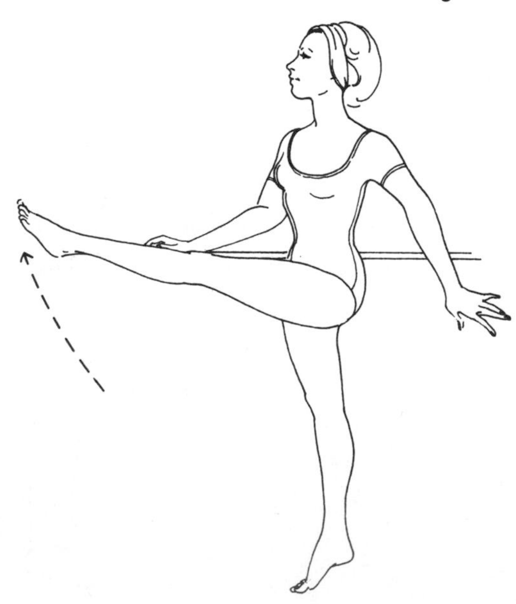

**Exercise 8—**
**Backward Leg Swing**

*Starting position—Stand with the feet slightly apart, hands at waist.*

*First count. Lift the right leg up and back as far as possible, and return it to place beside the left foot. Kick the right leg back and up for 10 counts. Pause. Repeat the exercise with the left leg.*

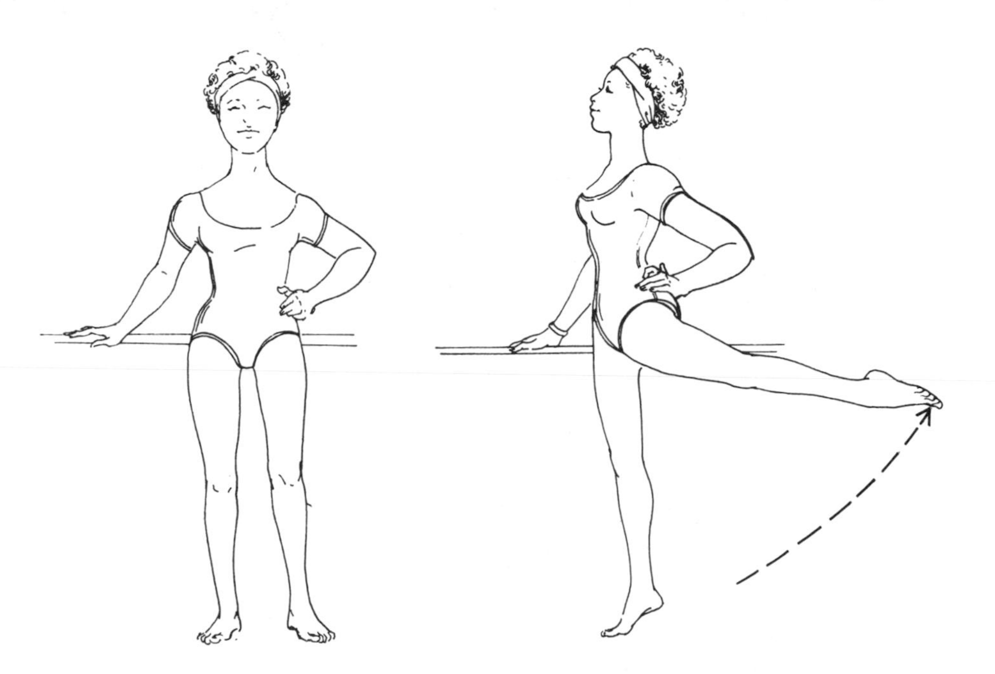

**Toning Exercises**

Toning exercises are less vigorous and can be done to cool down following more strenuous exercises.

**Exercise 9—**
**Exercise for Toning**
**Abdominal Muscles**

*Starting position—Lie flat on the back, with knees bent and feet flat on the floor. Keep arms down at sides.*

*First count. Lift both legs and perform a bicycling movement with both legs making larger and larger circles. Continue this exercise for 50 counts. Reverse the movement making larger and larger circles with both legs. Repeat for 50 counts.*

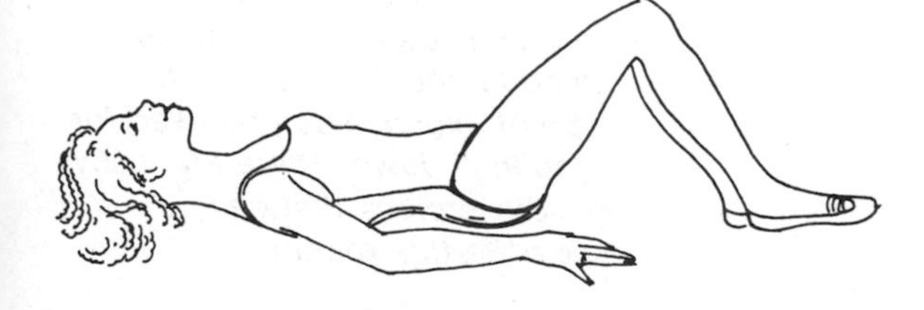

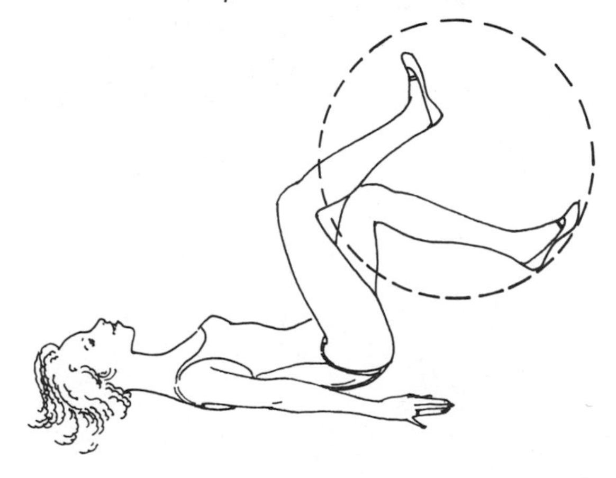

### Exercise 10—Exercise for Toning Back and Abdominal Muscles

*Starting position—Lie flat on the abdomen, with feet extended and arms outstretched to support the upper part of the body. Keep the back arched.*

*First count. Bend arms allowing the upper part of the body to lean forward. Lift the feet as high as possible and do kicking motions. Repeat the exercise for 50 counts, pause for a short rest, and repeat for 50 counts.*

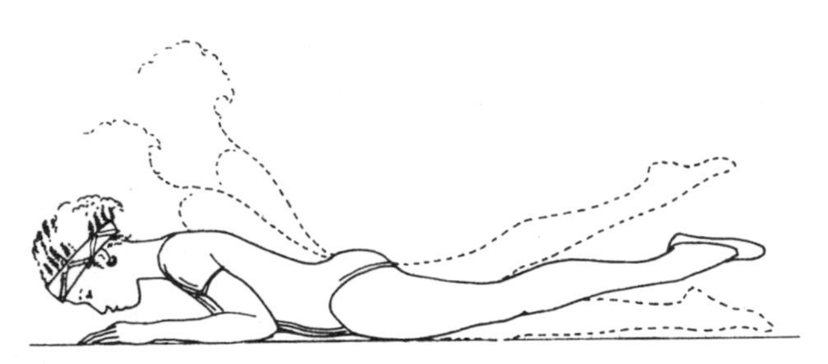

### Exercise 11—Exercise to Tone the Hips and Thighs

*Starting position—Lie flat on the floor, knees bent and arms to sides.*

*First count. Drop both knees to the right side. Second count. Roll knees to the left side. Continue rolling the knees from side to side. Keep weight on the buttocks.*

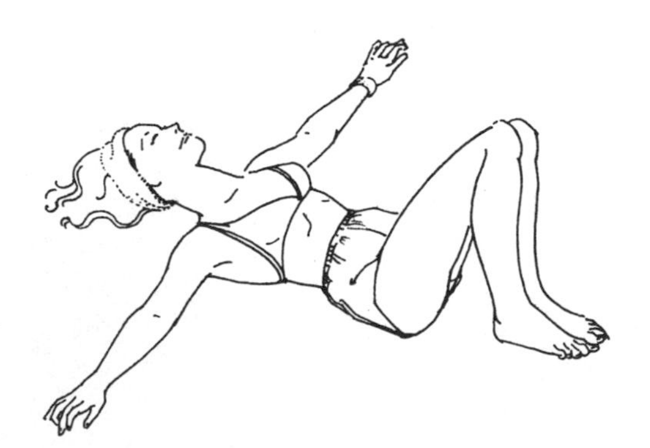

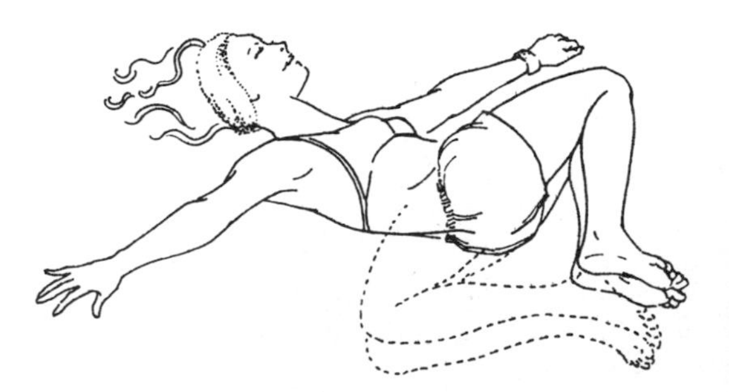

*Repeat the exercise for 50 counts, pause then continue for an additional 50 counts. This type of exercise can be used for "cooling" down. There are many good exercises that can be added to this routine.*

**Exercise 12— Leg and Abdominal Exercise**

*Starting position: Lie flat with the back flat, arms to sides and feet together.*

*First count. Lift both legs straight up and hold for 5 counts. Slowly lower the legs to the floor (5 counts).*

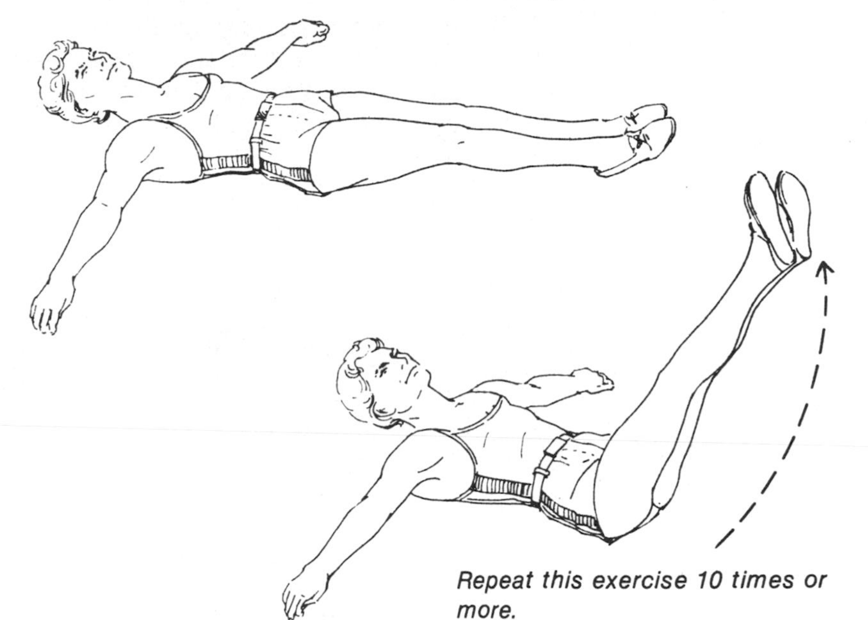

*Repeat this exercise 10 times or more.*

**Stress-Reducing Exercises**

It is better to have a vigorous daily workout, but there are times when it is just as important to take a few minutes to do relaxing exercises. Many executives have found relaxation exercises the best way to combat stress and tensions without having to go to a gym. The following exercises can be done while sitting at a desk or standing. The exercises release tension and revitalize the body.

1. Deep breathing. Inhale slowly for 5 counts. Hold the breath for 5 counts, then exhale slowly.
2. Toe to head relaxation. Sit in a comfortable chair and concentrate on relaxing the feet and ankles. Remove shoes then rotate the feet inward for 10 counts, then outward for 10 counts.
3. Point the toes and stretch the arches for 5 counts. Bring the toes toward the ankles, and hold for 5 counts. Repeat the exercise several times.
4. Raise the legs (knees straight) until they are level with the seat of the chair. Bend the knees so the feet swing apart outward and back together again. Repeat several times.
5. Sit erect with shoulders thrown back. Rotate the shoulders forward and back several times.
6. Rotate the head first to the right then to the left several times.
7. Close the eyes and massage the temples with the fingertips. Make circular movements for 10 counts.
8. Inhale slowly and concentrate on total relaxation. If possible lie down with the feet elevated for 15 minutes or longer.

## YOGA FOR BALANCE AND RELAXATION

A yogi is one who practices yoga. Yoga is a series of postures or positions to control breathing by mental concentration and muscular control. Western culture has borrowed many of these exercises from India (their point of origin) where they are practiced religiously with spiritual overtones. Yoga benefits the nervous system and helps to combat stress. It increases stamina and imparts a sense of physical and mental balance. Teachers of yoga recommend that a person practice moderation in eating and drinking. The following are just a few yoga exercises the average person may include in his or her daily exercise routine.

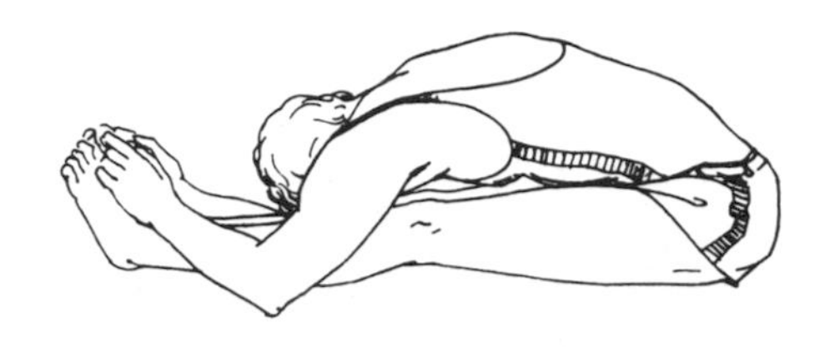

1. *Posterior stretching pose:* Sit on the floor with the feet extended. Catch hold of or touch the right big toe with the right hand and the left big toe with the left hand. Push forward to stretch and tone the back and leg muscles. While breathing deeply, fall forward over the knees. It is important for the person seriously interested in yoga to study the postures with a proficient teacher. Some postures are very strenuous and may cause strain or bodily damage if not practiced correctly.

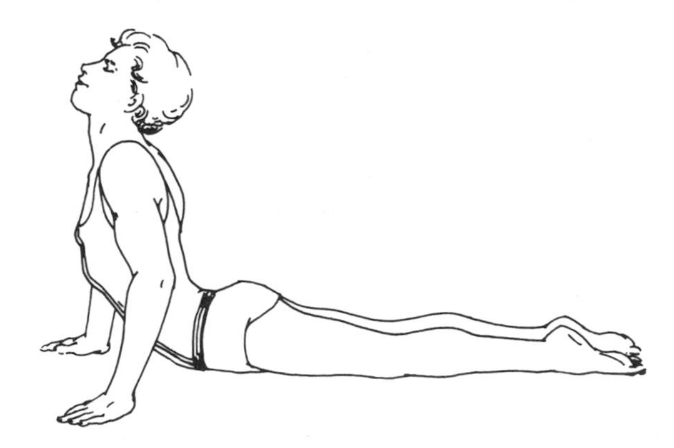

2. *Cobra pose:* Lie on the floor face down. Place the palms of the hands flat on the floor and raise the chest while bending the back as much as possible. Hold the pose, while breathing evenly, for about 10 seconds. Relax, then repeat the exercise several times. Caution: The spine should not be forced.

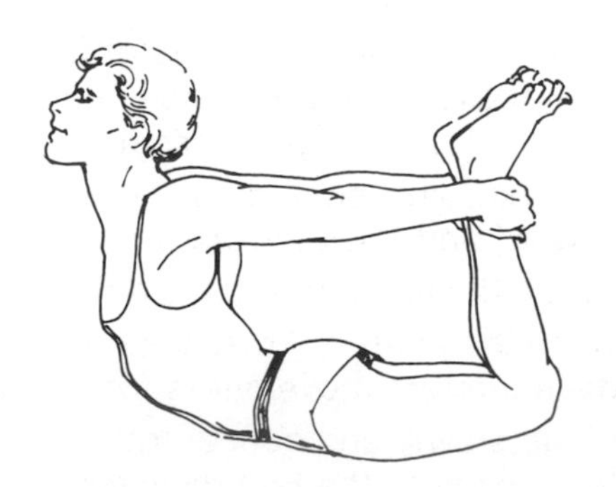

3. *Bow pose:* Lie face down on the floor then reach back and grasp the ankles, curving the back. While breathing evenly, hold the position for 5 to 10 counts. Relax and repeat several times. This exercise is excellent for strengthening the back, chest, and abdominal muscles.

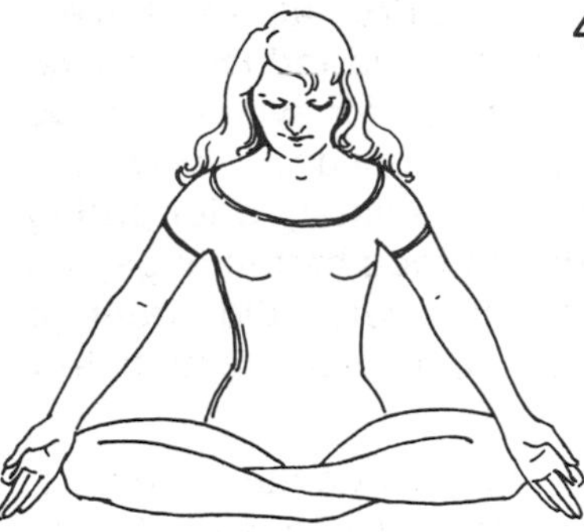

4. *The easy sitting pose:* Sit on the floor with the right leg bent at the knee and the right foot placed under the left thigh. The left leg is bent at the knee and the left foot is placed under the right thigh. The arms are extended, palms up. The spine is held erect. Breathe deeply from the diaphragm, making inhalations and exhalations the same length. This pose is used for concentration and meditation.

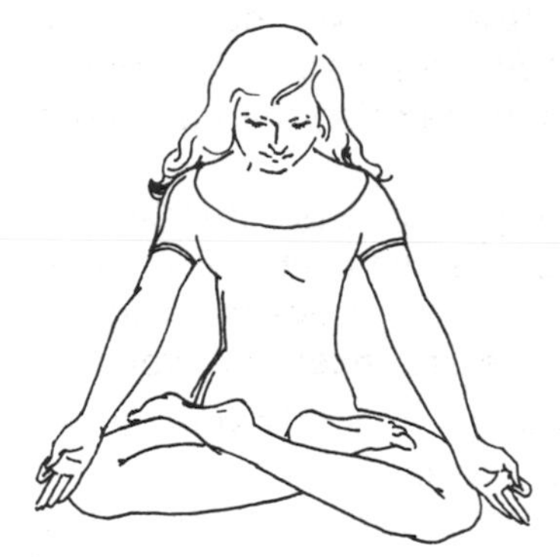

5. *The lotus pose:* This pose should not be attempted unless the body is quite supple. The right leg is bent and the right foot placed on the left thigh close to the hip joint. The sole of the foot is turned upward. The other foot is placed on the right thigh with the ankles crossed. The arms are extended, palms up at the sides of the body. Again, breathing should be deep and from the diaphragm. This pose is used for concentration and meditation. There are a number of yoga poses and positions the client may want to learn. With all yoga exercises, proper, controlled breathing is encouraged.

## PLANNING A PERSONAL FITNESS PROGRAM

Research indicates that a fitness routine should be done at least three to four times a week to achieve and maintain fitness. Body pulse rate is a measure of healthy physical exertion. Most exercise centers have heart rate monitors as part of their equipment. Users set the monitor for optimum heart-rate range during workouts. It is also practical to explain to the client how to find his or her own maximum heart rate during a regular or aerobic workout. The formula is to subtract your age from 220 and multiply it by 0.7. This will determine the optimum heart beats per minute the individual should register when working at peak performance.

To gauge the level of exertion after exercising vigorously for a few minutes, stop and count the pulse rate. Take the pulse for about six seconds then multiply that number by 10. Generally, a pulse rate between 140 and 170 per minute is healthy for the average adult.

### Weight Training

Weight-training machines are designed to place emphasis on specific muscle groups. Weight training generally concentrates on isotonic or resistance exercise. The muscle groups worked are the deltoids (shoulder muscles), the triceps and biceps (back and front of upper arms), the pectorals (the chest muscles), quadriceps (front of thighs), the gluteus maximus (muscles of the buttocks), and the abdominal muscles.

**Swimming**

Besides being refreshing, swimming is a first-rate aerobic exercise. It exercises the entire body safely and induces relaxation. It is important to observe certain rules for swimming. Do warm-up exercises before swimming and cool-down exercises after a brisk swim. Avoid swimming immediately after eating because the body needs energy to digest food before engaging in strenuous activity. Avoid jumping into very cold water or becoming chilled. It is important to dry the body off immediately after a swim.

**Walking**

Walking as part of a daily fitness routine is popular because it does not require special equipment or clothing and is a safe way to exercise. Although walking may take longer to achieve the same results as running, studies have shown that the differences are not so great. For example, a person who runs a mile in 8½ minutes burns only 26 more calories than a person walking a mile in 12 minutes.

Walking generates a lot of body heat, so it is important to wear lightweight clothing. Most walkers wear layers of light clothing such as sweater over a T-shirt then remove the sweater after warming up. Proper walking shoes are recommended.

**DAILY EXERCISE**

A daily exercise program should include general exercises as well as those for specific purposes. Exercise should be done gradually, and a record should be kept of progress and improvement. Exercise progress may be recorded in a small notebook or on exercise cards. Sample exercise card:

**Daily Exercise Record Card**

Week of ________________

Number of times I was able to do exercise on:

| No. and Name of Exercise | 1st day | 2nd | 3rd | 4th | 5th | 6th | 7th | Measurements at Beginning of week: |
|---|---|---|---|---|---|---|---|---|
| Warm-up | | | | | | | | Wt.__________ |
| etc. | | | | | | | | Chest __________ |
| | | | | | | | | Waist __________ |
| | | | | | | | | Hips __________ |
| | | | | | | | | End of Week: |
| | | | | | | | | Wt.__________ |
| | | | | | | | | Chest __________ |
| | | | | | | | | Waist __________ |
| | | | | | | | | Hips __________ |
| | | | | | | | | |
| Notes:__________ | | | | | | | | |
| | | | | | | | | |
| | | | | | | | | |

## QUESTIONS FOR DISCUSSION AND REVIEW

1. Why is exercise important when dieting for weight loss?
2. Why is it important to do warm-up exercises before doing more strenuous ones?
3. Why are cooling exercises recommended following a brisk workout?
4. Why is it necessary to have a consultation with the client before prescribing an exercise regimen?
5. What are four of the major benefits of breathing exercises?
6. What are five of the benefits of good posture?
7. What are the differences between the posture problems lordosis, kyphosis, and scoliosis?
8. Which exercises are done faster, circulatory or warm up?
9. From which country has Western culture borrowed yoga exercises?
10. Which two yoga poses are used primarily for relaxation and meditation?
11. Why is swimming recommended as a first-rate aerobic exercise?
12. Why is walking a highly popular form of exercise?

## ANSWERS TO QUESTIONS FOR DISCUSSION AND REVIEW

1. Exercise is important when dieting for weight loss because exercise firms and proportions the body as it burns calories and the excess weight is lost.
2. Warm-up exercises help to prevent muscle strain and soreness.
3. Cooling-down exercises bring body functions back to normal and help to prevent soreness and stiffness in muscles and joints.
4. A consultation with the client helps in determining the correct exercise program, gives insight into his or her health condition, and helps to prevent legal problems for the place of business and its employees.
5. The four major benefits of breathing exercises are:
   1. Healthier lungs.
   2. An increase in the intake of oxygen and the giving off of carbon dioxide.
   3. Improved function of all the internal organs.
   4. Improved circulation and nourishment of the body.
6. The five major benefits of good posture are:
   1. Prevention of backaches and fatigue.
   2. Lessening of strain on muscles and joints.
   3. Lessening or elimination of problems such as constipation.
   4. Improved circulation.
   5. Improved appearance.

7. Lordosis is a form of swayback; kyphosis affects the shoulders and is associated with humpback; scoliosis is a lateral deviation of the spine.
8. Circulatory exercises are done faster than warm-up exercises.
9. India is the country from which Western cultures borrowed yoga exercises.
10. The "easy sitting pose" and the "lotus pose" are the two yoga poses used primarily for relaxation and meditation.
11. Swimming is a first-rate aerobic exercise because the entire body can be exercised safely.
12. Walking is a popular form of exercise because it requires no special equipment and is a safe and pleasant way to exercise.

# PART VII BUILDING A SUCCESSFUL BUSINESS

# Chapter 18 Opportunities in the Massage and Fitness Field

**LEARNING OBJECTIVES**

After you have mastered this chapter, you will be able to:

1. Explain the application of rules of professionalism to business practice.
2. Explain why careful planning is important before opening a business.
3. Explain the difference between a partnership, a corporation, and a proprietorship.
4. Explain the importance of advertising to business success.
5. Describe a physical layout for a beginning business operation.
6. Explain the importance of business location to the success of a personal service business.
7. List the basic rules that apply to business administration.
8. Make a checklist of factors to consider before opening a business.
9. Explain the advantages or disadvantages of operating your own business.
10. Explain how to set goals for future business success.

**INTRODUCTION**

As the emphasis on physical fitness continues to grow, there will be more business opportunities for ethical and well-trained massage practitioners. Whether the practitioner works as an employee or aspires to managing a business, it is important to understand the responsibilities associated with doing business. The employee who understands business procedures is more valuable to the employer because he or she will be more profit oriented, more aware of the importance of good customer relations, and more involved in the overall operation of the business.

An ambitious practitioner may choose to open his or her own salon or occupy space within an established salon, clinic, or studio. The beginning practitioner who wishes to gain valuable experience may also look for employment in a health spa, on a cruise ship, in conjunction with a health facility, or as a freelance professional. Regardless of the environment in which the practitioner works, it is important to know something about business procedures. This includes keeping records for tax purposes, understanding laws and regulations, being familiar with insurance requirements, and much more.

## RULES FOR PROFESSIONAL PRACTITIONERS

Whether the practitioner works in his or her own business or for someone else, the following rules of professionalism should be observed:

1. Always present a professional appearance.
2. Maintain a sense of dignity and professionalism in your work.
3. Project a pleasant, optimistic personality.
4. Treat each client with courtesy.
5. Maintain good health habits.
6. Keep surroundings neat, clean, and attractive.
7. Follow a systematic plan and organize your work properly.
8. Space appointments so that sufficient time is allowed.
9. Keep clients' records and conversations confidential.
10. Keep accurate records of all treatments.
11. Keep an active card file and mailing list of regular and prospective clients.
12. Use professional business cards and stationery.
13. Make periodic mailings of services that are offered.
14. Be sure that all advertising represents your business in the most professional manner.
15. Let physicians and other professional people know about your work and how you may be of valuable assistance to them.
16. Make every effort to eliminate negative concepts of your business by speaking before groups, and educating the public about your work.
17. Join professional organizations that strive to upgrade, improve, and set high standards for your business.
18. Continue to promote your own personal and professional growth.
19. Work to eliminate any activities that cast unfavorable light on your business.
20. Be responsible in keeping your word and meeting your obligations.
21. Obey all laws and legal requirements regulating the practice of massage.
22. Charge a fair price for services rendered.
23. Continue to build a good reputation by your own work and conduct.
24. Recommend massage treatments only as the client requires and desires them.
25. Be loyal to your employers, associates, and clients.

## WORKING IN A SPA OR HEALTH CLUB

Today, many people integrate a spa vacation into their business schedules as a means of coping with the stress and tensions of modern life. Spas are no longer thought of as "fat" or "dry out" farms but as a means to improving health and appearance in a limited amount of time. Spa programs generally have guests concentrate on special exercises that are often followed by massage. Swedish massage and shiatsu are favorites. Well-balanced, low-calorie diets are stressed. Guests may enjoy whirlpool baths, swimming, herbal wraps, and other beneficial activities. Women clients are usually treated to makeup, haircare, and nailcare sessions.

Health club or athletic clubs offer memberships that entitle members to the use of club facilities. Some centers offer doctor-supervised physical therapy and rehabilitation services. Depending on the center, a client may be offered individualized training sessions, or the program may feature one instructor for several clients. In either case, adequate training must be given in the use of fitness apparatus so clients do not hurt themselves. Club personnel must be careful to consult with clients regarding their health and to give appropriate fitness tests before beginning a fitness program. Health club practitioners are responsible for the health and fitness of their clients. This is why legitimate businesses are anxious to hire qualified instructors and massage practitioners who know their business, are dedicated to their work, and who get along well with people.

## WORKING IN A FULL-SERVICE SALON

In recent years many full-service (beauty) salons have added additional services such as skincare (facials) and body massage. Hairdressing, manicures, facials, and the like services are given by licensed personnel. While the massage practitioner need not be a cosmetologist, he or she will need an approved (massage practitioner's) license to work in a full-service salon.

## BEGINNING IN BUSINESS

As a business owner and manager, you must have knowledge of your field, good business sense, ability to hire qualified people, and a sense of diplomacy. In addition, you must keep accurate records and understand all business procedures involved in your kind of business. You can hire tax consultants and bookkeepers to do some of the more extensive work, but it is the owner who is responsible for the success of the business.

Most people who succeed in the personal-service business gain experience by learning while working for someone else. They learn efficiency of management, motivating employees, promoting good customer relations, and numerous other business procedures. Once a practitioner has gained experience and knowledge, he or she may look for an established business to buy or manage. In this case, it is important to be sure the business has a good reputation, that it is worth the price being asked, and that it has an established clientele.

If you are beginning a new business, you will need to consider costs of equipment and everything else you will need before you can begin to generate income. As part of your business operation, you must always know where your money is being spent and operate with sufficient cash flow.

When planning a business operation, it is important to establish good credit and banking relations. Many business people rely on getting business loans when necessary in order to have sufficient working capital. It usually takes time to build clientele, so money must be available to take care of necessary expenses. A major cause of small business failure is the owner's inexperience in judging overhead expenses and having inadequate capital to carry the business through slow periods. As income and profits grow, the budget may be increased for expansion of facilities, advertising, and other areas of growth.

**Types of Business Operations**

A business may be organized as a sole proprietor, corporation, or partnership. As an individual owner, you would have all expenses, obligations, liabilities, and assets. You would receive all profits from your business and be responsible for all losses. Many people prefer being a sole proprietor if they can handle the financial and personal responsibilities involved.

A partnership may be the answer if you know someone who wants to invest and who is qualified to carry his or her share of the responsibility. The combined ability and experience of two people can make it easier to operate.

A corporation has advantages and disadvantages. It is subject to regulation and taxation by the state, and a charter must be obtained from the state in which the business operates. Management of the corporation is in the hands of a board of directors who determine policies and make decisions in accordance with the charter. Stockholders share in profits but are not legally responsible for the actions of the corporation.

**Buying an Established Business**

You may have an opportunity to buy an established business, in which case you must weigh the advantages or disadvantages. It is important to consult a lawyer who can handle all legal aspects of the transaction to the satisfaction of everyone involved. A written purchase and sale agreement will be needed. You will also need a complete inventory of all fixtures, goods, supplies, and the like as well as the value of each article that is to be part of the agreement. To avoid future misunderstandings, it is advisable to take photographs of furnishings and equipment. This will help to assure that you receive the exact items listed.

When making a lease, be sure you insert into the lease agreement any options for removing or replacing fixtures; making repairs; changing specific structures; or installing equipment, plumbing, and electrical work.

**Protecting Your Business**

You will need to have adequate insurances against fire, theft, and lawsuits. It Is also necessary to examine all records to understand the assets and liabilities of the business you are buying. An investigation should be made to determine any outstanding debts or obligations that may be held against the business.

It is a good idea to question customers as well as other business owners in the vicinity regarding the reputation of the business. Of course, you will want to know why the present owner is selling. It will not be to your advantage to buy a business that is being sold because it is failing. Generally, the owner is moving, retiring, or changing occupations.

**Location of a Business**

Another frequent cause of business failure is locating in an area that is wrong for that particular type of business. If a business is large enough to support a consistent advertising program, it may be located in an out-of-the-way, prestigious location. However, the smaller, less affluent business should be located near other active places of business in order to attract the attention of potential clients. Being near public transportation and having adequate parking facilities are important considerations.

The building in which a personal service business is located should be in good condition and in a fairly prosperous location. Cients will avoid a shabby, undesirable locale.

**Planning the Physical Layout of a Business**

The layout of a business takes careful planning in order to achieve efficiency and economy of operation. Once the building or space within a building has been decided upon, the interior must be designed. An efficient salon, studio, or clinic offering massage should have the following:

1. Adequate air conditioning and heating systems.
2. Appropriate plumbing for showers and rest rooms.
3. Adequate lighting for the entire operation.
4. An adequate dispensary.
5. Proper equipment and adequate space for its use.
6. Furniture that is appropriate, attractive, durable, and in keeping with the dignity of the business.
7. An attractive and comfortable private consultation room.

In addition to the above, an attractive and comfortable reception area is essential. Clients form either a positive or negative first impression of a business operation by the appearance of the reception area. The decor and appointments need not cost a fortune, but should give the impression that the business and the people employed there are highly professional. The reception area can be one of your best promotional tools if the client is impressed favorably and speaks well of you. If you have an attractive window, people who pass by may become interested in your services.

## Massage Business Floor Plans

When planning a massage business, all facilities must be considered. A business may be located within another business such as a hairdressing and skincare salon where the reception area, storage, rest rooms and other facilities might be shared. The basic floor plan B, the functional floor plan C, show only essential furnishings. This is often the ideal plan for the beginning practitioner.

Floor plan A, shows adequate space for a larger business that offers additional services such as hydrotherapy and exercise.

### *Floor Plans*

A. Ideal space 28' x 50'

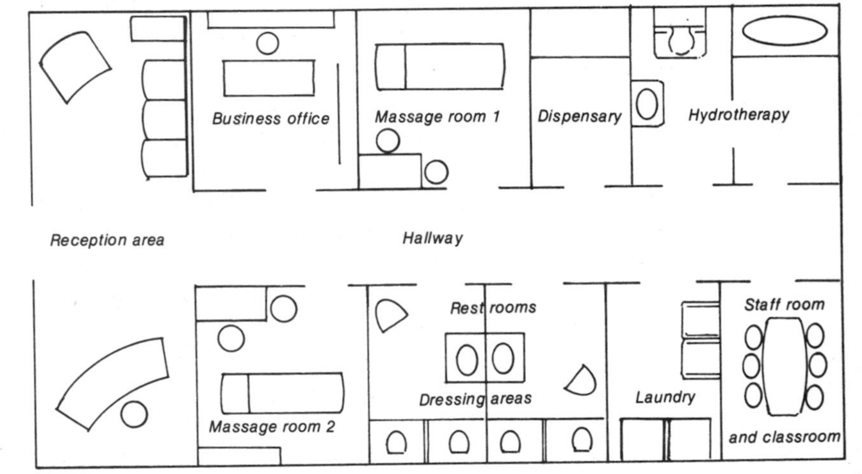


***B. Basic 10' x 12'***

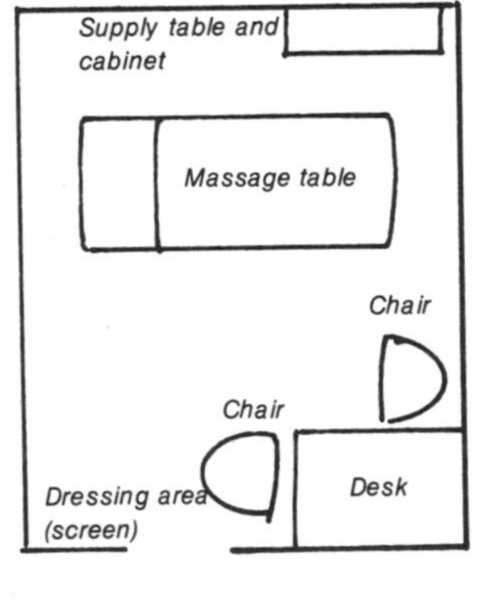


***C. Functional 12' x 16'***

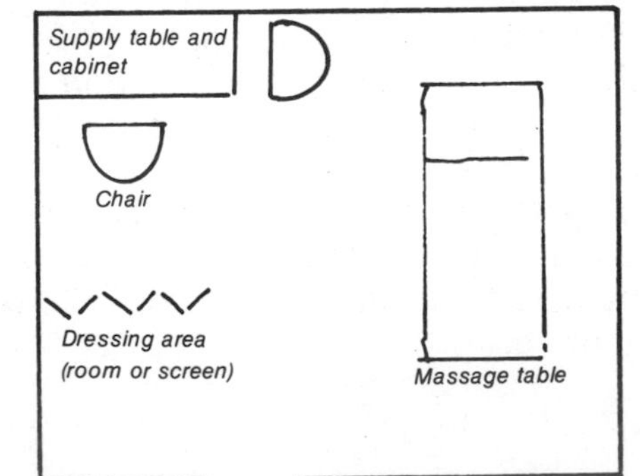

## Effective Advertising

Advertising is important to business success because it helps you reach the public. When giving personal services such as massage, it is particularly important that your advertising not be misunderstood and that it creates a favorable impression to the public. Advertising should always reflect your professional status and the quality of your services. Keeping your name before the public will be important to building your business.

The following are some suggestions that are helpful when planning your advertising program:

1. Plan your advertising budget. You must try to obtain the most effective media for the amount of money you have budgeted for advertising purposes. Newspaper advertising is generally the most economical way to reach the most people when you are opening a new business. The people in the advertising department of the paper will help you determine cost, size, and style of your ad.
2. Place a classified ad in the yellow pages of your local telephone directory. This is fairly inexpensive and is usually an effective method of advertising for personal service businesses.
3. Radio and television advertising spots are expensive, but they are highly effective.
4. Direct mail is often effective for certain locales. You may want to obtain a mailing list from a company that sells specific consumer lists.
5. You may want to have a brochure designed with a mailing envelope. Also a head and shoulder business-type photograph on a brochure helps to personalize this type of advertising.
6. You may offer to make personal appearances to give talks or demonstrations to various groups. You may offer to speak at health clubs, sports events, schools, and as a guest on a television talk show. You could act as guest instructor at a school or health facility where your type of personal services could be taught.
7. Advertising consultants are usually expensive, but if you have a flexible advertising budget, you may find that a professional consultant can save you both time and money. A good consultant will be able to help you with creative ideas for logos, letterheads, and advertising that gets your message across in the most professional, tasteful, and dramatic way.
8. Word-of-mouth advertising. Satisfied customers are still one of your most effective means of advertising. Many personal service businesses offer gift certificates, special prices to loyal customers, and even an occasional extra "no charge" product or service.

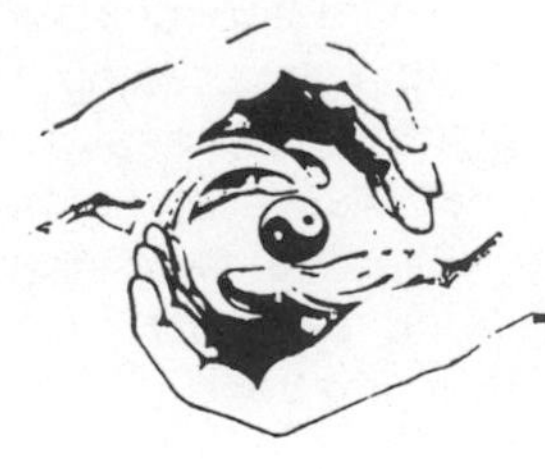

**Name of Business and Logo**

*SERVICES AND POLICIES*

Massage is a total body-mind experience. It comes in many forms. We offer a great variety.

FULL BODY MASSAGE is a wonderful way to treat yourself to the experience of deep relaxation and at the same time benefit from the effects of increased circulation, tension reduction and muscle rejuvination. It's a great way to help get rid of achey muscles or stored up tension and stresses of our busy every day life. If you feel good, a massage will make you feel even better!

MASSOTHERAPY is the choice for you if you have a specific condition that requires more directed attention.

A RUB DOWN is a quick thirty minute massage of the neck, arms, legs and back.

REFLEXOLOGY is a method of affecting the whole body by massaging the feet and finding reflexes that affect possible problem areas throughout the body. (Some reflexology is included in a full body massage and massotherapy.)

STRUCTURAL BALANCING is for you if you are a little out of whack, which usually shows up as PAIN! It uses techniques of applied kinesiology, accupressure, reflexology and others to balance muscles and relieve pain. VERY EFFECTIVE!

ABSOLUTELY NO SEXUAL MASSAGE.

*FEES*

| | | | |
|---|---|---|---|
| Full Body Massage | $. | Rub Down | $ |
| Structural Balancing | $. | Reflexology | $ |
| Massotherapy | $. | 10 Session Plan | $ |
| Children | $1.00 for every year of age | 6 Session Plan | $ |

*Discounts available for senior citizens on low fixed incomes upon request.*

PAYMENT POLICY: Cash or Check at the time of the appointment.

*MASSAGES ARE BY APPOINTMENT ONLY*

Please call our Buhl phone number to make appointments for both our Twin Falls and Miracle Hot Springs offices. If necessary you may call the Twin Falls office during office hours. We do not have a receptionist, however, we do have an answering machine so you may leave a message. The best time to talk to us in person is between 7:30-9:30 a.m. or 5:30-7:30 p.m.

OFFICE HOURS: Tuesday, Wednesday, Friday and Saturday - 9:30 a.m. to 5:30 p.m. Evening appointments available upon request.

IF YOU CANNOT KEEP AN APPOINTMENT, PLEASE NOTIFY US 24 HOURS IN ADVANCE. As of November 15 failure to cancel an unkeepable appointment will result in you being charged for that appointment.

*WHAT TO WEAR*

The best thing to wear when receiving a massage is nothing, this includes jewelry and makeup. We have private dressing areas and draping methods so that you will be covered except for those body parts which are being massaged. However wearing undergarments or a swimming suit is quite acceptable. Structural balancing or reflexology can be done with loose fitting clothes on provided they are either white or neutral in color and preferably cotton.

*BATHS*

A soak in a natural hot springs, a hot bath, whirlpool, steam or sauna are optimal choices for relaxation and cleansing the body before a massage. However, a shower is acceptable. We MUST have a clean body to work on! At the present time our Twin Falls office has no bathing facilities, so plan on bathing before you come. Remember, Miracle Hot Springs and Massage at Miracle Hot Springs are separate businesses so pay for your bath separately.

*Address and Telephone*

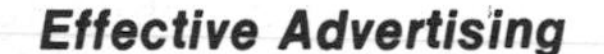
**Effective Advertising**

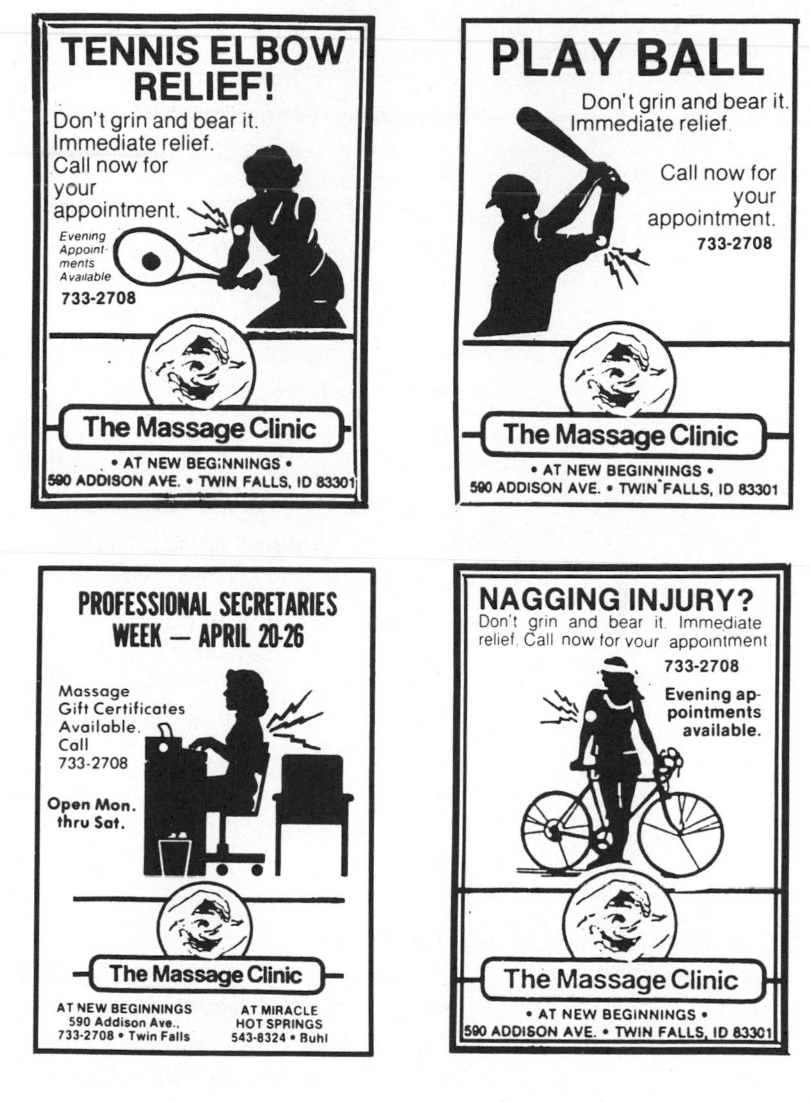


*Advertising ideas Courtesy of The Twin Falls News, Twin Falls, Idaho.*

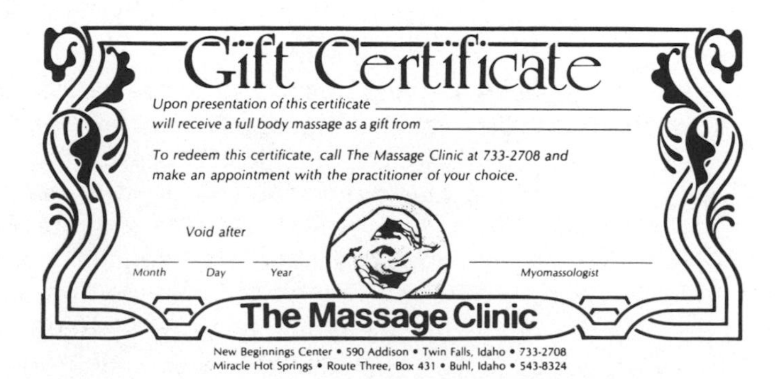

### Your Business Telephone

The business telephone is a powerful advertising tool because it is your contact with potential and steady clients. It is important that anyone placing or receiving calls know proper telephone techniques and courtesies. Your telephone number will accompany ads you place in telephone directories or newspapers and will be printed on your business cards. Therefore, the person answering your telephone should know how to do the following:

Give accurate information and encourage a potential client to make an appointment.

Make or change appointments for clients when necessary.

Take messages accurately.

Return all calls promptly.

Place orders for supplies and other items when needed.

Handle any complaints tactfully.

Remind clients of appointments or needed services.

Build good will and new business.

In addition to the above, your business telephone serves as a security instrument in calling for help in case of emergency. For the protection of your employees and clients the following information should be placed near your business telephone:

Nearest fire station.

Nearest ambulance service and hospital emergency service.

Police, local and state.

Taxi service.

Companies that provide needed services such as telephone, utilities, etc.

Names and telephone numbers of owners, managers, custodians, and employees.

Names, addresses, and telephone numbers of all clients, which are kept in a private file but available in case of emergency.

### Safety Procedures

All employees should know where exits are located and be able to instruct clients in safety procedures for leaving the areas in case of fire or other emergency. Employees should be trained in basic first-aid procedures in case of sudden illnesses or accidents.

## BUSINESS ADMINISTRATION

Business records are necessary to meet the requirements of local, state, and federal laws pertaining to taxes and employees. A good bookkeeping system is essential to the success of a business. You will need to keep records of income from both services and sales of products. Receipts, cancelled checks, and invoices should be kept in appropriate files for tax purposes. Even though businesses hire accountants, it is still important for the manager or owner to understand the system. This is why it is a plus for an inexperienced person to take training in business administration before opening a business. It is more difficult to manage a business if you don't understand the principals of sound business administration and management.

Without a proper bookkeeping system and accurate records, the owner or manager of a business would not be able to determine the progress of the business, especially the cost of doing business in relation to income. The manager of the business should see that records are kept properly for social security and withholding taxes (state, city, federal taxes) and insurance benefits. The manager should also be aware of wage and hour laws, compensation, and any other laws or regulations that apply to hiring (or firing) of employees.

**Payment Record**

Name .................................................... No. ...................

Address .................................................. Terms $..................

City & State ..........................................................................

| Date | How Paid | Paid on Account | Rec'd By | Balance | Date | How Paid | Paid on Account | Rec'd By | Balance |
|---|---|---|---|---|---|---|---|---|---|
| | | | | | | | | | |
| | | | | | | | | | |
| | | | | | | | | | |
| | | | | | | | | | |
| | | | | | | | | | |
| | | | | | | | | | |
| | | | | | | | | | |
| | | | | | | | | | |
| | | | | | | | | | |
| | | | | | | | | | |
| | | | | | | | | | |
| | | | | | | | | | |
| | | | | | | | | | |
| | | | | | | | | | |
| | | | | | | | | | |
| | | | | | | | | | |
| | | | | | | | | | |
| | | | | | | | | | |
| | | | | | | | | | |
| | | | | | | | | | |
| | | | | | | | | | |
| | | | | | | | | | |
| | | | | | | | | | |

*Payments to be made without fail.*

Instruments: .............................. Locker No. ..............................

Amount $ .............................. Amount $ ..............................

Terms ..............................

| Date | | Item | How Paid | Paid on Account | | Received By | Balance | |
|---|---|---|---|---|---|---|---|---|
| | | | | | | | | |
| | | | | | | | | |
| | | | | | | | | |
| | | | | | | | | |
| | | | | | | | | |
| | | | | | | | | |
| | | | | | | | | |
| | | | | | | | | |
| | | | | | | | | |
| | | | | | | | | |
| | | | | | | | | |
| | | | | | | | | |
| | | | | | | | | |
| | | | | | | | | |
| | | | | | | | | |

*IMPORTANT*
*Prompt and Regular Attendance Plus Diligent Effort Mean Success*

**Keep Service Records**

The service record shows the name and addresses of the client, the type of services given, the date given, the products used, results obtained, and the amount charged for each item. This helps the practitioner to render prompt and efficient service. Some clients will book the same time on a regular basis. These regular customers are the mainstay of many businesses because they can be counted on for a certain amount of regular income.

A good inventory system helps to assure that you will not run out of supplies or be overstocked on items that do not move well. Supplies to be used are classified as consumption supplies, and those to be sold are classified as retail supplies. You may need to keep records of sales tax on supplies sold.

**Business Expenses**

The largest items of expense for personal-service-type businesses are generally salaries, rent, advertising, and supplies. The following figures are suggested merely as a general guide. Such figures may vary in different locales. For example, in a large city rents are much higher than in small towns. Salaries and commissions also differ depending on the range of services offered.

| | Percent |
|---|---|
| Salaries and commissions | 30 |
| Rent | 15 |
| Janitorial and/or cleaning services | 3 |
| Utilities (light and power) | 3 |
| Telephone | 3 |
| Advertising | 4 |
| Insurance | 5 |
| Sales tax, business tax | 2 |
| Laundry | 2 |
| Repairs | 1 |
| Miscellaneous | 1 |
| Depreciation | 1 |
| Total expense | 70 |
| Net profit | 30 |

**Business Law**

In conducting business and employing help, it is necessary to comply with local, state, and federal laws and regulations. Federal laws cover social security, unemployment compensation or insurance, and tax payments on cosmetics as well as a number of other taxes. Income tax laws are covered by both the state and federal governments. State laws cover sales taxes, licenses, worker's compensation, and the like. Business owners and managers may hire a tax accountant, but they should also be familiar with these laws and regulations.

**Hiring Employees**

As an employer you are expected to be fair and honorable in dealing with employees, and you have a right to expect the same consideration from those you hire. Employees can make the differences between success and failure of a personal-service business. Clients often return to a place of business because they like the people who serve them as much, if not more, than the products and services. The following are important considerations when hiring someone to represent your place of business. The potential employee should:

1. Have the necessary licenses or other credentials required by law.
2. Set a good example by having clean, healthy personal habits.
3. Be profit conscious and willing to work hard to achieve business goals.
4. Be courteous and professional when dealing with all clients.
5. Obey all rules, regulations, and laws pertaining to the business.
6. Be willing to learn new techniques and to grow both personally and professionally.
7. Be self-motivated and industrious.
8. Be honest and ethical.

**CHECKLIST** The following is a checklist of important basics to consider before opening a business of your own. Use this checklist as a guide to important factors before opening a business.

**Capital**
Amount available
Amount required

**Organization**
Individual, partnership, corporation

**Banking**
Opening a business account
Deposits, drawing checks
Monthly statements
Notes and drafts

**Selecting a Location**
Population
Transportation facilities
Space required
Zoning ordinances
Parking

**Decorating and Floor Plan**
Interior decorating
Installing telephones
Exterior decorating

**Bookkeeping System**
Record of appointments
Receipts and disbursements
Petty cash
Profit and loss
Inventory

**Cost of Operation**
Supplies, depreciation
Rent, lights, water
Cleaning service, laundry
Salaries
Products for services
Telephone
Taxes, insurances

**Management**
Methods of building goodwill
Client courtesies, gifts
Adjusting complaints
Personnel relations
Public relations
Selling merchandise

**Telephone and Telecommunications**
Electric or other signs

**Equipment and Supplies**
Selecting equipment
Installation of equipment

**Advertising**
Planning
Direct mail
Newspaper
Radio
Television
Personal Appearances

**Legal**
Lease, contracts
Claims, lawsuits
Compliance with State, Local and Government laws
Licensing of business
Licensing of managers and practitioners

**Ethics and Professional Growth**
Courtesy
Observation of professional practices
Interaction with professional groups
Setting goals

**Office Administration**
Stationary and office supplies
Inventory

**Insurance**
Public liability and malpractice
Compensation, unemployment
Social security
Fire, theft, burglary

**Methods of Payment**
In advance
Open account
Time payments
Charge cards

**Compliance with Labor Laws**
Minimum wage law
Hours of employment

**QUESTIONS FOR DISCUSSION AND REVIEW**

1. Why is the employee who is aware of business procedures more valuable to a business?
2. How do most business owners generally gain experience?
3. What is the major cause of business failure, especially of small service-type businesses?
4. What are the three popular types of business operations?
5. Why is location of a business important to its advertising plan?
6. How does the reception area of a business serve as a promotional tool?
7. What is your first consideration when selecting an advertising media?
8. Why is the business telephone considered a powerful advertising tool?
9. Although the owner may hire a tax accountant and other professionals, why should he or she also have some training in business administration?
10. How is a business checklist helpful when planning a business?

**ANSWERS TO QUESTIONS FOR DISCUSSION AND REVIEW**

1. The employee who is aware of business procedures is more valuable because he or she is more profit oriented, more aware of the importance of good customer relations and more likely to be involved in the overall operation of the business.
2. Most successful business owners generally gain experience by working for an established business.
3. The major cause of business failure is due to owners being inexperienced in judging overhead expenses and not having enough capital to carry the business through slow periods.
4. Three popular types of business operations are sole proprietorship, partnership, and corporation.
5. The location of a business helps to determine how much and what kind of advertising is required to attract attention and to build business.
6. The reception area of a business serves as a promotional tool by creating a positive first impression of the entire business.
7. Your first consideration when selecting advertising media is your advertising budget.
8. The business telephone is a powerful advertising tool because it is your first contact with both potential clients and your steady clients.
9. The business owner or manager will find it difficult to manage a business unless he or she understands the principles of sound business administration and management.
10. A business checklist is useful as a guide to planning the steps you must take and tasks to be accomplished before opening your own business.

# Prefixes

A careful study of the following prefixes will enable you to grasp the meaning of many anatomical, medical and electrical terms or words.

**Ad:** to; toward; addition; intensification.
**Anti:** opposite; contrary.
**Auto:** self; acting upon one's self; of or by itself.
**Bi:** two; twice; double.
**Cliedo:** relation to the clavicle.
**Contra:** against; opposite; contrary.
**De:** from; down; away.
**Di:** two-fold; double; twice; separation or reversal.
**Dia:** through; apart; asunder between.
**Dis:** apart; away; asunder; between.
**Ecto:** without; outside; external.
**Endo:** inner; within.
**Epi:** upon; beside; over; among.
**Ex:** out of; from; away from.
**Hydro:** water; hydrogen.
**Hyper:** excessive; above normal; over; above; beyond.
**Hypo:** under; beneath; lower state of oxidation.
**In:** not; negation; within; inside.
**Infra:** below; lower.
**Inter:** between; among; amid.
**Leuco:** white; colorless.
**Mal:** ill; evil; bad.
**Mega:** great; extended; powerful; a million.
**Meso:** in the middle; intermediate.
**Micro:** very small; trivial; slight; millionth part of, as in the metric system.
**Mid:** the middle part.
**Mono:** uni; singly.
**Non:** not.
**Onycho:** relating to nail.
**Para:** alongside of; beyond; beside; against; near.
**Per:** through; throughout; by; for.
**Peri:** around; about; near.
**Post:** back; after.
**Pyro:** fire; prepared by fire.
**Re:** back to original or former state or position.
**Sterno:** denoting connection with the sternum (breast-bone).
**Sub:** under; below.
**Super:** over; above; beyond.
**Supra:** over; above; on top of; beyond; besides; more than.
**Syn:** along with; together; at the same time.
**Trans:** over; across; through; beyond.
**Ultra:** beyond; on the other side; excessively; exceedingly; extraordinarily; abnormally.
**Un:** not; contrary.
**Uni:** one; once.

# Suffixes

Many medical and anatomical words are of Latin origin. The following endings will enable you to tell at a glance whether they are singular, plural or possessive.

ENDINGS OF REGULAR LATIN NOUNS

| Singular: | Plural: | Possessive Singular: |
|---|---|---|
| . . . **us** —Nasus | . . . **i** —Nasi | . . . **i** —Nasi |
| . . . **a** —Ala | . . . **ae**—Alae | . . . **ae**—Alae |
| . . . **um**—Labium | . . . **a** —Labia | . . . **i** —Labii |

. . . **tis, sis:** a termination denoting inflammation of a part to the name of which it is attached; such as pityria**sis**, dermati**tis**.

. . . **al:** termination denoting belonging to, of, or pertaining to; such as nas**al**.

. . . **oma:** termination properly added to words derived from Greek roots, denoting a tumor; such as cyst**oma**.

. . . **ize:** termination forming transitive verbs; such as steril**ize**.

. . . **ive:** termination signifying relating or belonging to; such as act**ive**.

. . . **ide:** termination forming names of compounds, such as bacteric**ide**, germic**ide**.

# Glossary

This glossary has been included as a quick reference. It is not a substitute for a medical dictionary. The following medical and cosmetology dictionaries are recommended: Blakiston's Gould Medical Dictionary; Dorland's Illustrated Medical Dictionary; and Milady Illustrated Cosmetology Dictionary.

Terms that are adequately defined in the text are not always included in the glossary. The index will provide information to word sources. Dictionaries are available from Milady Publishing Corporation (A Wiley Company), 3839 White Plains Road, Bronx, New York 10467-5394.

## A

**Abdomen** *(**AB** do men):* the cavity in the body between the thorax and the pelvis.

**Abducent nerve** *(**AB** doo sent nurv):* the sixth cranial nerve; a small motor nerve supplying the external rectus muscle of the eye.

**Abduction** *(**AB** duk shon):* a movement away from the median line; to move a part outward or away from the midline of the body.

**Abductor** *(**AB** duk tor):* a muscle that draws a part away from the median line of the body.

**Abrasion** *(a **BRAY** zhon):* the scraping away of the superficial layers of the skin.

**Absorbent** *(ab **SOR** bent):* able to take up; retain moisture, as absorbent cotton.

**Accent** *(**AK** sent):* to emphasize.

**Acetic** *(a **SEE** tik):* pertaining to vinegar; sour.

**Achilles tendon** *(a **KIL** eez **TEN** don):* a tendon located just above the heel that contracts the calf muscle.

**Achroma** *(a **KRO** muh):* absence of color.

**Acid** *(**AH** sid):* a substance having a sour taste; a substance containing hydrogen replaceable by metals to form salts; having a pH number below 7.

**Acid mantle** *(**AH** sid **MAN** tel):* the natural acidity of the hair or skin which helps to retard irritation or bacterial growth.

**Acidosis** *(as i **DOH** sis):* a condition in which there is an excess of acid products in the blood or tissues, or excreted in the urine.

**Acne** *(**AK** nee):* inflammation of the sebaceous glands from retained secretions.

**Acne albida** *(**AK** nee **AL** bi duh):* milium; whitehead.

**Acne pustulosa** *(**AK** nee **PUS** choo lo suh):* acne vulgaris in which the pustular lesions predominate.

**Acne rosacea** *(**AK** nee roh **ZAY** shee a):* a form of acne usually occurring around the nose or on the cheeks, due to congestion in which capillaries become dilated and sometimes broken.

**Acne simplex** *(**AK** nee **SIM** pleks):* acne vulgaris, simple uncomplicated pimples.

**Acne vulgaris** *(**AK** nee vul **GAR** is):* acne simplex, simple uncomplicated pimples.

**Acromion process** *(a **KRO** mee on **PROH** ses):* an outward extension of the spine of the scapula, forming the point of the shoulder.

**Active assistive** *(**AK** tiv a **SIS** tiv):* joint movements in which the client assists the practitioner in specific movements of a limb.

**Active joint movement** *(**AK** tiv joint **MOOV** ment):* a motion or movements performed by the client with or without assistance from the practitioner.

**Acupressure** *(**AK YOO** press ur):* a method stemming from Chinese acupuncture that employs various methods of stimulating pressure joints to relieve pain or other physiological imbalances in the body; touch pressure.

**Acupuncture** *(**AK YOO** punk chur):* a medical practice originating in China whereby the skin is punctured at specific points with needles for therapeutic purposes.

**Acute** *(a **KYOOT**):* attended with severe symptoms; having a short and relatively short course; not chronic; said of disease.

**Adduction** *(a **DUK** shon):* a movement toward the median line of the body that involves the adductor muscle; femur, pubic bone, and hip joint; to move a part inward.

**Adductor** *(a **DUK** tur):* a muscle that draws a part toward the median line of the body.

**Adenosine triphosphate (ATP)** *(a **DEN** o seen trye **FOS** fate):* a substance involved in the release of energy for muscular and cellular activity.

**Adhesion** *(ad **HEE** zhun):* scar tissue binding together tissues that are not normally joined.

**Adipose tissue** *(**AD** i pohs **TISH** yoo):* fatty tissue; areolar connective tissue containing fat cells; subcutaneous tissue.

**Adrenal gland** *(a **DREE** nal gland):* an endocrine gland situated on top of a kidney.

**Adrenaline** *(a **DREN** a lin):* a hormone secreted by the adrenal gland; it stimulates the nervous system, raises metabolism, increases cardiac pressure and output, and increases blood pressure.

**Aeration** *(**AY** ur **AY** shun):* airing; saturating a fluid with air, carbon dioxide other gas; the change of venous into arterial blood in the lungs.

**Aerobe** *(**AY** ur obe):* an organism that requires oxygen.

**Aerobics** *(**AY** ur **O** bik):* cardio-respiratory exercise.

**Aesthetics** *(es **THET** iks):* relating to or dealing with that which is considered beautiful; also esthetics as applied to the care and beautification of the skin.

**Afferent** *(**AF** er ent):* a structure such as a blood vessel leading from the periphery to the center; bearing or conducting inward.

**Afferent fibers** *(**AF** er ent a **FEYE** burs):* the fibers that stimulate impulses to the central nervous system.

**Afferent nerves** *(**AF** er ent nurvz):* nerves that convey stimulus from the external organs.

**AIDS** *(**AYDS**):* Acquired Immune Deficiency Syndrome; a disease caused by a virus that breaks down the body's immune system causing the body to become unable to combat various infections.

**Aidosterone** *(ai **DOS** teh ruhn):* a very important regulator of metabolism of sodium and potassium.

**Alcohol** *(**AL** ko hawl):* a readily evaporating colorless liquid with a pungent odor and burning taste; a powerful stimulant and antiseptic.

**Allergen** *(**AL** er geen):* an antigen that produces an allergy.

**Allergy** *(**AL** er gee):* a disorder due to extreme sensitivity to certain food, chemicals or other substances.

**Alternating current** *(**AWL** ter nat ing **KUR** ent):* current occurring in reciprocal succession.

**Alum, alumen** *(**AL** um):* sulphate of potassium and aluminum; used as an astringent and as a styptic.

**Amino acid** *(a **MEE** no **AH** sid):* the basic structure of protein.

**Amma** *(**AH** muh):* a special procedure developed by the Chinese as part of healing massage.

**Amitosis** *(**AM** i to sis):* the direct division of a cell in which the nucleus and cytoplasm divide by simple construction without splitting of chromosomes.

**Ammonia** *(uh **MO** ny uh):* a colorless gas with a pungent odor and is soluble in water.

**Ampere** *(**AM** peer):* the unit of measurement of strength of an electric current.

**Amphiarthrosis** *(**AM** fee ahr THRO sis):* an articulation permitting little movement.

**Amylase** *(**AM** i laze):* a starch digesting enzyme.

**Anabolism** *(ah **NAB** o lizm):* constructive metabolism; the process of assimilation of nutritive matter and its conversion into living substance.

**Anaerobe** *(**AN** ur obe):* an organism that does not require oxygen.

**Anaphase** *(**AN** uh faze):* the stage of mitosis between the metaphase and telephase, in which the daughter chromosomes move apart toward the poles of the spindle to form the amphiaster.

**Anaphoresis** *(**AN** uh fo REE sis):* the process of forcing liquids into the tissues from the negative toward the positive pole.

**Anastamosis** *(a **NAS** toh MOH sis):* the joining together of structures; communication between vessels.

**Anatomical position** *(**AN** uh TOM i kul puh **ZISH** un):* the position devised by physicians, with the body standing upright, palms forward showing planes of the body.

**Anatomy** *(ah **NAHT** o mee):* the gross structure of the body; the study of an organism and the interrelations of its parts.

**Androgen** *(**AN** dro jen):* any of various hormones that control the development of male characteristics.

**Anesthetic** *(**AN** es THET IK):* a substance producing anesthesia.

**Aneurism** *(**AN** yoo RIZ um):* a condition characterized by localized dilation of a blood vessel.

**Angina** *(an **JYE** nuh):* spasmodic, severe pain frequently in the chest.

**Angular artery** *(**ANG** gew lur **AHR** te ree):* artery that supplies the lacriminal sac and the eye muscle.

**Anguli** *(**AN** gew lye):* plural of angulus: situated at an angle; corner.

**Anadrosis** *(ana **DROH** sis):* a deficiency in perspiration.

**Anode** *(**AN** ode):* the positive terminal of an electric force.

**Antagonist** *(an **TAG** uh nist):* the muscle that relaxes when a prime mover contracts.

**Antagonist reflexes** *(an **TAG** uh nist **RE** flexes):* reflexes in response to different stimuli which elicit opposing effects, such as flexion and extension of a limb.

**Anterior or ventral aspect** *(an **TEER** i or or **VEN** trul **AS** pekt):* situated before or in front of.

**Antibody** *(AN ti **BOD** ee):* a substance in the blood which builds resistance to disease.

**Antiseptic** *(AN ti **SEP** tik):* a chemical agent that prevents the growth of bacteria.

**Antitoxin** *(an ti **TOKS** in):* a substance in serum which binds and neutralizes toxin.

**Aorta** *(ay **OR** ta):* the great artery leaving the left side of the heart, and carrying blood to the various arteries throughout the body.

**Appendage** *(a **PEN** dig):* an outgrowth attached to an organ or part of the body and dependent upon it for growth.

**Apex** *(**A** pex):* the top or pointed extremity of a body.

**Appocrine glands** *(**AP** ok rin glandz):* sweat glands that produce a characteristic odor, found in the underarms and pubic areas of the body.

**Aponeurosis** *(**AP** o new RO sis):* a broad, flat tendon; attachment of muscles; a fibrous sheet or expanded tendon that serves to connect one muscle to another.

**Aqueous** *(**AH** kwee us):* watery; pertaining to water.

**Arrector pili** *(ah **REK** tor **PI** lee):* the minute, involuntary muscle fibers in the skin attached to the base of the hair follicles.

**Arteries** *(**AHR** tee reez):* vessels that convey blood from the heart to other parts of the body.

**Arteriole** *(ahr **TEER** ee ole):* one of the small terminal twigs of an artery that ends in the capillaries.

**Arthritic** *(arh **THRIT** ik):* pertaining to or affected with arthritis; inflammation of a joint.

**Articular end** *(ahr **TICK** yoo lur end):* end of bone covered with cartilage.

**Articulation** *(ahr **TICK** yoo lay shun):* joint; a connection between two or more bones, or skeletal parts, whether or not allowing any movement between them.

**Asepsis** *(ay **SEP** sis):* a condition in which pathogenic bacteria are absent; exclusion of micro organisms.

**Asphyxia** *(as **FICK** see uh):* lack of oxygen, or excess of carbon dioxide in the body causing unconsciousness.

**Asteatosis** *(**AS** tee ah TOH sis):* a deficiency or absence of sebaceous secretions, as dry scaly skin due to lack of sebum.

**Asthma** *(**AZ** muh):* a disease characterized by coughing or wheezing.

**Astringent** *(a **STRIN** jent):* a substance that causes contraction of the tissues and checks secretions.

**Athlete** *(**ATH** leet):* one trained in acts or feats of physical agility, as in sports.

**Athlete's foot** *(**ATH** leetz foot):* epidermophytosis, a form of dermatitis caused by fungus germs that thrive in moist interiors of shoes and affect the feet. Severe itching may occur with scales and small blisters.

**Athletic massage** *(ath **LET** ik ma **SAHZH**):* sports massage; massage and manipulations to improve an athlete's ability to perform, help to prevent injuries, and as an aid to restoring mobility to injured muscle tissue.

**Auto massage** *(**AW** to ma **SAHZH**):* massage of one's own muscles; massage technique for athletes and dancers or other active people who must keep their muscles supple.

**Automatic** *(aw to **MAT** ik):* working of itself without human control; self regulating.

**Autonomic** *(aw to **NOM** ik):* performed without the will; automatic.

**Autonomic nervous system** *(aw to **NOM** ik **NURV** us **SIS** tem):* the sympathetic nervous system that controls the involuntary muscles.

**Avitaminosis** *(AY vi ta mi **NOH** sis):* a condition resulting from deficiency of one or more vitamins.

**Avulsion** *(a **VUL** shun):* the forcible tearing or wrenching away of a part of the body.

**Axilla** *(ack **SIL** uh):* the armpit.

**Axillary** *(ack **SIL** ya ree):* pertaining to the axilla.

# B

**Bacteria** *(bak **TEER** i ah):* plural, bacterium: widely distributed unicellular microorganisms with both plant and animal characteristics; commonly known as germs or microbes.

**Bactericide** *(bak **TEER** e sid):* an agent that destroys bacteria.

**Bacteriology** *(bak **TEER** ee ol oh jee):* the science which deals with bacteria.

**Balance** *(**BAL** ans):* the observance of equality and equilibrium.

**Barbituate** *(baar **BITCH** U it):* a sedative or drug which can interfere with healthy body metabolism when taken in excess; a sleeping pill.

**Baths** *(baths):* practices whereby the body is surrounded by water as in a whirlpool or vapor as in a steam cabinet to achieve external cleanliness, and to stimulate skin functions.

**Belly** *(**BEL** ee):* the thicker part of a muscle; the rounded part of the abdomen.

**Bi** *(bi):* a prefix meaning two, twice, double.

**Biceps** *(**BI** seps):* a muscle having two heads; a muscle producing the contour of the front and inner side of the upper arm.

**Biceps brachii** *(**BI** seps **BRAY** kee):* muscle that flexes and supinates the forearm.

**Biceps femoris** *(**BI** seps **FEM** uh rus):* muscle that flexes the knee and rotates the leg outward.

**Bifurcation** *(**BYE** fur **KAY** shun):* the division of a structure, such as the branching of a large artery into two smaller arteries.

**Bilateral** *(bye **LAT** er ul):* affecting both sides; pertaining to or of the body.

**Bile** *(**BYE** ul):* a bitter, alkaline, greenish fluid secreted by the liver into the duodenum. It aids in digestion, emulsification and, absorption of fats and in alkalinization of the intestines.

**Bio** *(**BYE** o):* meaning life.

**Bio-mechanics** *(**BYE** o me KAN iks):* the integrated movement of the entire body.

**Blood** *(**blud**):* the red oxygen and nutriment bearing liquid, circulating in the body.

**Blood cell** *(**BLUD** cell):* any of the cells or corpuscles that constitute elements of circulating blood; an erythrocyte or a leucocyte.

**Blood count** *(**BLUD** kownt):* the number of corpuscles in a specific volume of blood.

**Blood pressure** *(**BLUD PRESH** ur):* the pressure of blood within the arteries and veins.

**Body system** *(**BOD** ee **SIS** tem):* a group of bodily organs working together to perform a bodily function.

**Body temperature** *(**BOD** ee **TEM** pe ra chur):* normal body temperature about 98.6F (fahrenheit) or 37C (celcius); the intensity of heat or cold in a living body.

**Bone marrow** *(bohn **MAR** oh):* connective tissue filling the cavity of bones.

**Boric acid** *(bo **RIK AH** sid):* acidum boricum; used as an antiseptic dusting powder or in liquid form as a wash.

**Brachial** *(**BRAY** kee ul):* the region between the elbow and the shoulder.

**Brachial artery** *(**BRAY** kee ul **AHR** tur ee):* the main artery of the upper arm.

**Brachial plexus** *(**BRAY** kee ul plex us):* the four lower cervical nerves and first thoracic nerves form the brachial plexus which controls movement of the arm by way of the median and ulnar nerves.

**Bradycardia** *(**BRAD** ee kahr DEE uh):* a lower than normal pulse rate.

**Brain** *(brayn):* that part of the central nervous system contained in the cranial cavity, and consisting of the cerebrum, the cerebellum, the pons, and the medulla oblongata.

**Bronchi** *(**BRONG** ki):* major air passageways in the lungs.

**Bronchus** *(**BRONG** us):* air tubes entering the lungs.

**Buccal nerves** *(**BUCK** ul nurvz):* nerves of the buccinator and orbicularis oris.

**Buccinator** *(**BUCK** si NAY tur):* a thin, flat muscle of the cheek, shaped like a trumpet; largest muscle of facial expression that purses the lips.

**Buffer** *(**BUF** er):* an agent that resists a change in pH.

**Bulla** *(**bool** uh):* a large bleb or blister.

**Bursa** *(**BUR** sa):* a fluid-filled sac, usually lined with a synovial membrane.

# C

**Calcification** *(**KAL** si fi KAY shun):* a process by which tissue becomes hardened due to the deposit of calcium salts.

**Calcitonin** *(**KAL** si ton in):* a hormone from the thyroid gland that assists in the deposition of calcium into bone.

**Calcium** *(**KAL** si um):* a grayish-white chemical element present in bones and teeth.

**Callus** *(**KAL** us):* an area of thick, hardened tissue.

**Calorie** *(**KAL** o ree):* a unit of heat; the amount of heat necessary to raise the temperature of water from zero to one degree centigrade; a unit of heat used to express the heat-energy producing content of foods; kilogram calorie.

**Cancellous bone tissue** *(**KAN** sell ous bohn **TISH** yoo):* spongy tissue that forms the interior of bone, the end of bone shaft and very thin bones.

**Cancer** *(**KAN** ser):* a tumor, especially a malignant growth; a disease in which growths form.

**Canker** *(**KANG** ker):* a disease that causes ulcerous sores, especially of the lips and mouth.

**Capillaries** *(**KAP** i ler eez):* minute blood vessels which connect the arteries and veins; hairlike blood vessels.

**Carbohydrate** *(**KAHR** bo HI drayt):* organic compounds such as sugars and starches, the most important being glucose which is stored in muscles and the liver as glycogen (animal starch); foods that give the body most of its energy.

**Carbuncle** *(**KAHR** bung kel):* a large circumscribed inflammation of the subcutaneous tissue that is similar to a furuncle, but is more extensive.

**Carcinogen** *(kahr **SIN** o jen):* a cancer producing substance.

**Carcinoma** *(kahr si **NOH** ma):* a cancerous growth.

**Cardiac imput** *(**KAHR** di ac **im** put):* the amount of blood pumped per minute by one ventricle; normally about 5 liters per minute in a resting subject.

**Cardiac** *(**KAHR** di ac):* pertaining to the heart.

**Cardio-vascular** *(**KAHR** di oh **VAS** kyu lar):* of or involving the heart and blood vessels.

**Carotid** *(ka **ROT** id):* the principle artery of the neck.

**Carotid arteries** *(ka **ROT** id **AHR** te reez):* arteries that serve as main sources of blood supply to the head, face and neck.

**Carpals** *(**KAHR** pal):* wrist bones; of the wrist joint.

**Cartilage** *(**KAHR** ti lij):* tough, white flexible tissue attached to bones.

**Catabolism** *(ka **TAB** o lism):* the breaking down of larger substances or molecules into smaller ones.

**Cataphoresis** *(KAT a fo re sis):* the use of positive poles to introduce a positive charged substance such as acid ph astringent solution into the skin. A technique often used in facial massage.

**Caudal** *(KAW dal):* inferior; situated under, lower or farther from the crown of the head.

**Cell** *(sel):* a minute mass of photoplasm forming the structural unit of every organized body; capable of performing all the fundamental functions of life; the basic units of all living matter of animals, plants, and bacteria.

**Cellulite** *(SEL u lit):* an anatomical and functional condition of the connective tissues that produces a gel-like substance made up of wastes, water, and some fat; generally located between the muscles.

**Cellular** *(SEL yu lar):* consisting of or pertaining to cells; having a porous texture.

**Cellulitis** *(SEL yu LIT is):* an acute inflammation of tissues.

**Celsius** *(SEL si us):* centegrade.

**Centering** *(SEN ter ing):* a term used to describe a concept of a geographical center in the practitioner's body, in the pelvic area that gives a sense of confidence and balance; a point toward which interest is directed as center of balance or gravity.

**Centigrade** *(SEN ti grayd):* a temperature scale divided into 100 degrees, 0 being the freezing point and 100 degrees boiling point of water.

**Central** *(SEN tral):* of or forming the center.

**Centrifugal movement** *(sen TRIF yu gal):* moving away from the center, thus decreasing the heartbeat and blood flow; movement often used to conclude a massage.

**Centripetal movement** *(sen TRIP e tal):* stronger movement, directed toward a center such as the heart, and following the direction of the blood current; moving toward the center of axis.

**Cephalic** *(se FAL ik):* pertaining to the head.

**Cerebro** *(se RE bro):* spinal nervous system; the system consisting of the brain and spinal cord, spinal nerves, peripheral nerves, and cranial nerves.

**Cerebellum** *(sera a BEL um):* the portion of the brain that controls movements of muscles.

**Cerebrum** *(se RE brum):* the large frontal part of the brain that controls memory, reasoning, will, and emotions.

**Cerumen** *(se ROO men):* waxlike material found in the external meatus of the ear; earwax.

**Cervix** *(SUR viks):* the neck.

**Cervical** *(SUR vi kal):* region of the neck.

**Cervical cutaneous nerve** *(SUR vi kal kyoo TAY ni us nurv):* nerves which supply skin of the lower jaw, back of ear, lateral and interior sides of neck and skin of upper anterior thorax.

**Cervical plexus** *(SUR vi kal PLEX us):* the four upper cervical nerves from the cervical plex which supplies the skin and controls movement of head, neck, and shoulders.

**Cervical vertebrae** *(SUR vi kal VUR te bra):* vertebrae of the neck axis and atlas.

**Chafe** *(chayf):* to make or become sore from rubbing.

**Chap** *(chap):* sore or cracked skin.

**Chi** *(ki or chi):* bio-force; a term used in Chinese acupuncture meaning life force energy.

**Chiropody** *(ki ROP o dee):* treatment of ailments of the feet.

**Chiropractic** *(ki ro PRAK tik):* a method of therapy based on the theory that disease is mainly due to malfunction of nerves, and may be corrected by manipulating of bodily structures, especially the spinal column.

**Chiropractor** *(ki ro PRACK tor):* one who is trained in the treatment of disease based on the theory that the disease is caused by interference with nerve functions that may be relieved or restored by manipulation of joints and spine.

**Chucking** *(CHUK ing):* a friction movement in massage accomplished by grasping the flesh firmly in one hand, and moving it up and down along the bone, while the other hand steadies the limb.

**Chyle** *(kil):* a milky fluid taken up by the lacteals in the small intestine as an aid to digestion.

**Ciatrix** *(SIX a triks):* the skin or film that forms over the wound to form a scar.

**Circular friction** *(SIR kyu lar FRIK shun):* using the hands or fingertips to make large or small circles over a part of the body.

**Circulatory system** *(SIR kyu la TO ree SIS tem):* a system of the body that controls the circulation of blood and lymph; the blood vascular system and the lymphatic systems of the body.

**Circumduction** *(SIR kum DUCK tion):* to move the distal end of an extremity in a circle while the proximal end remains fixed.

**Clavicle** *(KLAV i kul):* the collarbone.

**Clockwise movement** *(KLOK wiz):* direction moving outward and downward as the hands of a clock.

**Coccyx** *(KOK siks):* tailbone; the last bone in the vertebral column.

**Collagen** *(KOL a jen):* a protein forming the chief constituent of the connective tissues and bones; a substance from certain animals used in some types of cosmetic products.

**Collarbone** *(KO lar bohn):* the bone joining the breastbone and shoulder blade; clavicle.

**Collateral** *(ko lat e ral):* accessory or secondary; not direct; a side branch, as of a vessel or nerve fiber.

**Comedo** *(kom eh DOH):* blackhead.

**Compact tissue** *(kom PAKT TISH yoo):* tissue forming the hard bone found in shafts of long bones and along the outside of flat bones.

**Compression** *(kom PRESH on):* massage movements such as pressing, squeezing, and rubbing the skin over the underlying structures.

**Compression, digital** *(kom PRESH on DIJ i tal):* pressing movement directed into muscle tissue by the fingers.

**Compressor** *(kom PRES er):* a muscle that compresses.

**Condyle** *(KON dil):* a rounded articular surface at the end of a bone.

**Congeal** *(KON jee al):* to change from liquid to a jelly-like substance; as thickening or clotting of blood.

**Congeal plexus** *(KON jee al PLEKS us):* portions of the fourth sacral and the fifth sacral nerves from the congeal plexus which supplies the skin and muscles around the coccyx.

**Congenital** *(kon JEN i tal):* pertaining to a condition existing at birth.

**Contagion** *(KON ta jon):* transmission of specific diseases by direct or indirect contact.

**Contaminate** *(kon TAM i nat):* to make impure by contact; to taint or pollute.

**Contour** *(KON toor):* the outline of the body.

**Contractility** *(KON trak TIL i tee):* the ability of a muscle to exert force.

**Contraindication** *(KON tra in di KAY shun):* pertaining to conditions that make massage or specific treatments inadvisable.

**Convalesce** *(KON val les):* to recover health and strength gradually, after illness.

**Convalescence massage** *(KON va lez enz):* massage given by nurses or their aids to patients to stimulate blood flow, relieve sore muscles, and increase the psychological and psychological well-being of patients.

**Convolution** *(KON vo lew shun):* an elevated part of the surface of the brain.

**Coracord process** *(KOR uh koid PRO ses):* projecting part of the shoulder blade.

**Core** *(kor):* the central or most vital part of anything.

**Corium** *(KOR re um):* the dermis or true skin.

**Cornea** *(KOR nee uh):* the transparent outer part of the eyeball.

**Corneum** *(KOR ne um):* stratum corneum; horny layer of the skin.

**Coronal** *(ko **ROH** nal):* pertaining to the corona or crown of the skull.

**Coronal plane** *(kor **ROH** nal plane):* a plane parallel to the long axis of the body dividing it into a front and back portion.

**Coronary** *(**KOR** a ner e):* a term applied to vessels, nerves or attachments that encircle a part or an organ; either of two arteries of the aorta which supply blood to the heart muscle.

**Coronary occlusion** *(**KOR** a ner e uh **KLEW** zhun):* the blockage of a blood vessel supplying the heart.

**Coronary thrombosis** *(**KOR** a ner e **THROM** bo sis):* a clot in a blood vessel supplying the heart; thrombus.

**Corpuscle** *(**KOR** pus l):* a small mass of body; a minute cell; a cell found in the blood.

**Corpuscle, red** *(**KOR** pus l red):* cells in the blood whose function is to carry oxygen to the cells; erythrocytes.

**Corpuscle, white** *(**KOR** pus l whit):* cells in the blood whose function is to destroy disease germs; leukocytes.

**Cortex** *(**KOR** teks):* the outer part of an organ.

**Cortical** *(**KOR** ti kul):* pertaining to the cortex.

**Cosmetic** *(**KOS** met ik):* any external preparation intended to cleanse and beautify the skin, or hair or other part of the body.

**Counter clockwise** *(**KAUN** ter **KLOK** wise):* direction moving backward and downward as reversing the normal direction of the hands of a clock.

**Couperose** *(**KOO** per os):* a skin condition caused by glands dilated or broken capillaries.

**Cowper's glands** *(**KOU** purz glandz):* bulbourethral glands; two pea sized glands located beneath the prostate gland in males.

**Cranial nerves** *(**KRA** ne al nurvs):* nerves connected to the brain surface classified as motor, sensory, and motor-sensory nerves.

**Cranial or superior aspect** *(**KRA** ne al or soo **PEER** i or **AS** pekt):* situated higher or toward the crown of the head.

**Cranium** *(**KRA** ne um):* the top and back of the skull containing the brain.

**Cross fiber friction** *(**KRAWS FI** ber **FRIK*** shun): a deep pressure movement applied by use of the thumb, fingertips or fist to work on muscle fibers.

**Cruciate** *(**KROO** shi ate):* cross shaped; cruciale ligament.

**Cryogenic** *(**KRI** o JEN ik):* at very low temperatures.

**Cubital fossa** *(**KYOO** bi tal **FOS** ah):* antecubital fossa; the depression in front of the elbow.

**Cupping** *(**KUP** ing):* a massage movement done with the fingers of both hands almost closed into a fist, and using the perifery sides of the hands to apply light tapping movements.

**Cyanosis** *(si u **NOH** sis):* a condition that causes a bluish discoloration of the skin due to an insufficient supply of oxygen into the blood.

**Cytology** *(si **TOL** o jee):* the scientific study of cells.

# D

**Defecation** *(**DEF** e kay shun):* elimination of waste material from the bowels.

**Dehydrate** *(dee **HI** drayt):* to remove moisture content; to lose moisture.

**Deltoid** *(**DEL** toid):* region of the shoulder joint and deltoid muscle.

**Dendrites** *(**DEN** drite):* the branched part of a nerve cell that carries impulses toward the cell body.

**Dense bone tissue** *(denz bohn **TISH** yoo):* compact tissue that forms the hard bone found in shafts of long bones and along the outside of flat bones.

**Depression** *(de **PRESH** on):* to lower a part of the body, as in lowering the shoulders.

**Depressor labii inferioris** *(di **PRES** sor **LAY** be i in **FEER** i or us):* muscle of facial expressions; inverts and draws the lower lip downward.

**Diaphragm** *(**DI** a fram):* the muscular sheath between the thorax and abdomen.

**Diaphoresis** *(di a fo **REE** sis):* excessive perspiration, usually artificially produced.

**Diaphysis** *(**DIE** af i sis):* the shaft of a long bone.

**Diathermy** *(**DI** a thur mee):* medical heat treatments with high frequency current.

**Diarthrotic joints** *(**DI** a thro tik):* joints that are freely movable as ball and socket, hinge, pivot, turning head, and saddle movement.

**Diastole** *(**DI** as to lee):* the relaxation of the heart between contractions.

**Diencephalon** *(**DIE** en sef uh lon):* the portion of the brain between the cerebrum and the midbrain.

**Digestive system** *(die **JEST** tiv **SIS** tem):* a system consisting of all the structures involved in the process of digestion including the mouth, stomach, intestines, salivary and gastric glands.

**Dilator** *(di **LAY** tor):* that which expands or enlarges.

**Distal** *(**DIS** tal):* farther from the body or from the origin of a part.

**Diuresis** *(**DIE** yoo ree sis):* increased urine production.

**Diverticulum** *(DI ver **TIK** yoo lum):* a pouch leading from a main cavity or tube.

**DNA** (Deoxyribonucleic acid) *(dee **OCK** rye bo new KLEE IK **AH** sid):* a spiral shaped molecule that contains the hereditary material of the cell.

**Dorsal** *(**DOR** sal):* the posterior aspect or back of the body or organ.

**Dorsiflexion** *(**DOR** si FLEK shun):* flexion or bending the foot toward the leg.

**Draping** *(**DRAP** ing):* to arrange or cover with a cloth; the process of using sheets or towels to keep the client covered while a massage is given.

**Diuretic** *(**DIE** yoo RET ik):* a drug used to induce diuresis.

**Duodenum** *(**DEW** o dee num):* the first portion of the small intestine.

**Dura mater** *(**DEW** ruh **MAH** tur):* the outermost meninges covering the brain and spinal cord.

**Dysfunction** *(dis **FUNK** shun):* disturbed or abnormal function of an organ.

**Dystrophy** *(**DIS** truh fee):* faulty or defective nutrition.

**Dysuria** *(dis **YOO** ree uh):* painful or difficult urination.

# E

**Ecchymosis** *(**ECK** i mo sis):* a bruise.

**Echocardiogram** *(**ECK** o KAHR dee o gram):* a recording of the position and motion of the heart obtained by use of ultrasonic waves directed through the heart walls.

**Ecklampsia** *(e **KLAMP** see uh):* a disease that may occur in the later half of pregnancy, characterized by acute elevation of blood pressure, protein uria, edema, sodium retention, and convulsions.

**Ectopic** *(eck **TOP** ick):* displaced; out of place.

**Eczema** *(**EK** ze mah):* an inflammatory, itching disease of the skin.

**Edema** *(e **DEE** muh):* an abnormal accumulation of clear watery fluid in the lymph spaces of tissue; swelling.

**Efferent** *(**EF** ur unt):* carrying or conducting away.

**Efferent duct** *(**EF** ur unt dukt):* a duct that drains the secretion from an exocrine gland.

**Effleurage** *(ef **LOO** razh):* stroking movements used in massage.

**Elastin** *(i **LAS** tin):* a protein base similar to collagen, which forms elastic tissue.

**Electrotherapy** *(e **LECK** tro THER uh pee):* treatments given with the use of electrical apparatus.

**Electrovibratory massage** *(e **LECK** tro VI bra tor ry):* massage performed by means of a vibrating apparatus.

**Element** *(EL e ment):* any one of the ultimate parts of which anything is composed, as the cellular elements of tissue.

**Elevation** *(EL e VAY shun):* to lift or raise a part of the body, as raising the shoulders.

**Embolism** *(EM bo liz um):* a blood clot moving in the bloodstream.

**Emesis** *(EM e sis):* vomitus.

**Emolient** *(ee MOL ee ent):* a substance used to soften and soothe the skin.

**Emphysema** *(em fi SEE moh):* a chronic lung disease usually characterized by an extended alveoli.

**Emulsion** *(e MUL shun):* a colloidal system of one liquid dispersed throughout another.

**Enamel** *(e NAM el):* the hard, calcified substance that covers the teeth.

**Endocardium** *(EN do KAHR de um):* the lining of the heart.

**Endocrine gland** *(EN do krin gland):* ductless glands that throw secretions directly into the bloodstream.

**Endocrine system** *(EN do krin SIS tem):* the ductless glands of the body, whose secretions are released directly into the bloodstream.

**Endoderm** *(EN do durm):* the innermost of three primary germ layers which form the lining from pharynx to rectum.

**Endogenous** *(en DOJ e nus):* originating within the body.

**Endomorphy** *(EN do MOR fee):* the tendency to have a rounded, soft body. Pertaining to the endomorph body type.

**Endoplasmic reticulum** *(EN do PLAS mick ree TIK yoo lum):* microscopic tubular structures used for the transport of substances through cells.

**Endothelium** *(EN do THEEL ee um):* a membrane composed of flat, thin cells lining blood vessels, tubes, and cavities.

**Energetic manipulation** *(EN ur jet ick mul NIP yoo LAY shun):* techniques that detect imbalances in the flow of the force, energy, or vibrations in the body and effect them in such a way as to bring them back into balance or homeostasis.

**Enzymes** *(EN zim):* protein substance formed in the cell that acts as an organic catalyst to initiate or accelerate specific chemical reactions in the metabolic process while they themselves remain unchanged.

**Epicraniuis** *(ep i KAY nee us):* muscle that draws the scalp backward.

**Epidermis** *(ep i DUR mis):* the outermost layer of the skin.

**Epigastric** *(ep i GAS trick):* the abdominal region located medial to the hypochondric region of the body.

**Epiglottis** *(ep i GLOT is):* a leaf-shaped cartilage that covers the entrance to the larynx during swallowing.

**Epimysium** *(ep i MIZ ee um):* the delicate cover of muscle fibers.

**Epiphysis** *(e PIF i sis):* the ends of long bones.

**Epithelial tissue** *(ep i THEEL ee ul):* a thin protective layer that functions in the processes of absorption, excretion, secretion, and protection.

**Erectile tissue** (*e RECK til TISH yoo*): a sponge-like arrangement of irregular vascular spaces.

**Erector** *(e RECK tur):* that which draws upward.

**Erythema** *(eer i THEE muh):* a superficial redness of the skin.

**Erythrocytes** *(e RITH ro sits):* red corpuscles or red blood cells that carry oxygen from the lungs to the body cells and transport carbon dioxide from the cells to the lungs.

**Ethics** *(ETH iks):* the study of standards and philosophies of human conduct; a system or code of morals of an individual, a group, or of a profession.

**Ethmoid** *(ETH moid):* pertaining to bone supporting nasal cavities and helps to form the orbits.

**Euphoria** *(yoo FO ree uh):* an exaggerated feeling of well being; lightness.

**Eustachian tube** *(yoo STAY shee un):* the canal extending from the throat to the middle ear.

**Eversion** *(e VUR zhun):* to turn the plantar surface away from the midline.

**Excoriation** *(eks SKOHR i ay shun):* act of wearing or stripping off the skin; an abrasion.

**Excretory system** *(EK skre TOHR ee SIS tem):* a system including the skin, kidneys, bladder, liver, lungs, and large intestines, which are engaged in the process of eliminating waste products from the body.

**Exfoliation** *(eks FOH lee AY shun):* peeling or shedding of the horny layer of the skin.

**Exocrine glands** *(ECK so krin):* duct glands that possess canals leading from a gland to a particular part of the body.

**Exogenous** *(eck SOJ e nus):* originating outside the body.

**Extension** *(eck STEN shun):* a movement allowing a part to be extended; involves the rectus femoris muscle, femur, tibia, fibula, and the knee joint.

**Extensor** *(ecks STEN sur):* a muscle which extends or stretches a limb or part, or increases the angle at a joint.

**External oblique** *(ECKS tur nal o BLEEK):* muscle that compresses the viscera and flexes the thorax.

**Extravascular** *(ECKS truh VAS kew lur):* within interstitial spaces of the body.

**Extremity** *(eck STREEM i tee):* an upper or lower limb; the distal, or terminal end of a part.

# F

**Fascia** *(FASH ee ah):* fibrous connective tissue forming layers or sheets beneath the skin to enclose or connect muscles or internal organs.

**Fascia band** *(FASH ee ah band):* a delicate membrane of connective tissue covering muscles and separating their several layers of groups of layers.

**Facial nerve** *(FASH al nurv):* nerves of the muscles of facial expression.

**Fats** *(fahts):* any of various solid or semi-solid oily or greasy materials found in animal tissue, seeds, and nuts.

**Feathering** *(FETH er ing):* the technique of allowing the fingers to gently cease stroking movements as a finish to the massage movement.

**Fertilization** *(FUR ti li ZAY shun):* the union of male and female reproductive cells.

**Femoral** *(FEM o ral):* region of the femur or thigh.

**Femoral nerve** *(FEM o ral nurv):* nerve serving the region of the thigh bone or femur, the long bone extending from the pelvis to the knee.

**Femur** *(FEE mur):* thigh bone.

**Fibril** *(FI bril):* a component filament of a fiber, as of a muscle or nerve.

**Fibrin** *(FI brin):* protein threads that form the framework of a blood clot.

**Fibrinogen** *(FI brin o jen):* a protein of blood plasma.

**Fibroblasts** *(FI broh blasts):* connecting tissue cells that form in the body.

**Fibrosis** *(FI BROH sis):* the formation of fibrous or scar tissue.

**Fibrous** *(FI brus):* like fibers; made of fibers.

**Fibula** *(FIB yu la):* smaller bone of the lower leg.

**Fissure** *(FIS yoor):* a crack in the skin penetrating into the dermis.

**Flaccid** *(FLA sid):* poor muscle tone; soft and flabby.

**Flagella** *(flah JEH la):* slender, whip-like processes which permit locomotion in certain bacteria.

**Flatus** *(FLAY tus):* air or gas in the intestines or stomach.

**Flex** *(fleks):* to bend a joint or limb.

**Flexion** *(FLEKS shun):* decreasing the angle at a joint such as bending the knee or elbow.

**Follicle** *(FOL i kel):* a small secretory or sac; the depression in the skin containing the hair root.

**Foramen** *(fo* ***RAY*** *men):* an opening.

**Fossa** *(****FOS*** *uh): a shallow or hollow place in a bone.*

**Friction** *(****FRICK*** *shun):* massage strokes designed to manipulate soft tissue in such a way that one layer of tissue is moved over or against another.

**Frontal** *(****FRON*** *tul):* region of the head.

**Frontal bones** *(****FRON*** *tul bohnz):* bones that form the forehead, nasal cavity, and orbits.

**Frontalis** *(****FRON*** *tal us):* a muscle that elevates eyebrows and wrinkles skin of forehead.

**Fungus** *(****FUN*** *gus):* a vegetable parasite; a spongy growth of diseased tissue.

**Furuncle** *(****FU*** *rung kel):* a small skin abscess; a boil.

## G

**Galvanic current** *(gal* ***VAN*** *ik* ***KU*** *rent):* a constant and direct current rectified to a safe, low voltage level. Used to force chemicals through unbroken skin by a process of phoresis or ionization used in facial massage, and in the treatment of cellulite.

**Gamete** *(****GAM*** *eet):* a sex cell.

**Gamma globulin** *(****GAM*** *a GLOB yoo lin):* a blood fraction that carries antibodies.

**Gastritis** *(gas* ***TRI*** *tis):* an inflammation of the lining of the stomach.

**Gastronemius** *(gas* ***TRO*** *nee i mus):* muscle that extends the foot.

**Genetics** *(je* ***NET*** *iks):* the science that deals with the theory and variations of organisms.

**Germinative layer** *(jur* ***MI*** *nah tiv* ***LAY*** *er):* stratum; a layer of cells beneath the stratum malpighi, and is responsible for the reproduction of new cells.

**Glucocorticoid** *(****GLOO*** *ko KOR ti koid):* an adrenal cortex hormone, such as cortisol, that affects the metabolism of glucose.

**Glucagon** *(****GLOO*** *kuh gon):* a hormone produced by the pancreas.

**Gluconeogenesis** *(****GLOO*** *ko NEE o jen e sis):* the manufacture of glucose by the body from non-carbohydrate materials.

**Glucose** *(****GLOO*** *koz):* the most important carbohydrate which is stored in the muscles and liver as glycoten, animal starch.

**Gluteal** *(gloo* ***TEE*** *ul):* region of the muscles of the buttocks.

**Gluteals** *(gloo* ***TEE*** *uls):* muscles of the buttocks.

**Gluteus medius** *(****GLOO*** *tee us* ***ME*** *dee us):* rotates, abducts, and advances the thigh.

**Gluteus maximus** *(****GLOO*** *tee us* ***MAX*** *i mus):* extends, abducts, and rotates the thigh outward.

**Glycogen** *(****GLEYE*** *ko jen):* animal starch; the storage form of glucose.

**Glycolysis** *(****GLEYE*** *ko ten is):* the anaerobic breakdown of glucose to pyruvic acid.

**Golgi** *(****GOHL*** *jee):* apparatus; a cytoplasmic organelle that is essential to the export of substances manufactured by cells.

**Gonad** *(****GOH*** *nad):* a male or female sex gland, in which the reproductive cells develop; an ovary or a testis.

**Gonadotropin** *(****GON*** *ah do* ***TROH*** *pin):* a hormone from the anterior pituitary gland that stimulates the sex glands.

**Gonorrhea** *(****GON*** *uh* ***REE*** *uh):* a venereal disease characterized by discharge and a burning sensation when urinating. Transmitted by sexual contact with an infected person.

**Gooseflesh** *(****GOOS*** *flesh):* a condition often caused by cold or fright, whereby the contraction of the arrector pilorum muscles around a hair follicle causes the skin to appear bumpy.

**Gram** *(gram):* the basic unit of mass or weight in the metric system.

**Greater auricular nerve** *(****GRAYT*** *er aw* ***RIK*** *u lar nurv):* nerves of the side of the neck and ear.

**Greater occipital nerve** *(****GRAYT*** *er ock* ***SIP*** *i tul nurv):* nerves of skin over back part of the head.

**Groin** *(groin):* the depression between the abdomen and thigh.

**Gymnastics** *(jin* ***NAS*** *tiks):* a system of exercises for physical fitness originated by the Greeks.

## H

**Hamstrings** *(****HAM*** *strings):* the group of three muscles of the posterior thigh (biceps femoris, semi-membranosis, and semi tendonosis.

**Haversian Canals** *(ha* ***VUR*** *zhun* ***KUH*** *nals):* channels where branches of blood vessels penetrate to nourish bones.

**Heart** *(hahrt):* the muscular, conical-shaped organ located in the chest cavity, and enclosed in a membrane called the pericardium.

**Hemastat** *(****HEE*** *muh stat):* an instrument or clamp used to stop the flow of blood.

**Hematology** *(he muh* ***TOL*** *o jee):* the scientific study of the blood.

**Hematoma** *(****HEE*** *muh TO muh):* a swelling that contains blood.

**Hemeostasis** *(****HEE*** *mee o STAY sis):* the maintenance of normal, internal stability in an organ.

**Hemoglobin** *(****HEE*** *mo GLOH bin):* the pigment that gives red blood cells their color.

**Hemolysis** *(hee* ***MOL*** *i sis):* destruction of red blood cells.

**Hemophilia** *(HEE mo* ***FIL*** *ee uh):* a hereditary blood disease characterized by the tendency to bleed freely.

**Hemorrhage** *(****HEM*** *uh rij):* an abnormal escape of blood from vessels; bleeding.

**Hemorrhoids** *(****HEM*** *uh roid):* a tumor or dilation of veins in the anal region characterized by pain and bleeding.

**Hemostasis** *(HEE mo* ***STAY*** *sis):* stopping the flow of blood.

**Hepatitis** *(****HEP*** *uh TYE tis):* an inflammatory disease of the liver.

**Hernia** *(****HUR*** *nee uh):* the protrusion of an organ or part of an organ through the opening of the abdominal wall.

**Herpes facialis** *(****HUR*** *peez fay shee* ***AY*** *lis):* a type of herpes simplex occurring on the face, usually about the lips; it may occur in the mouth and pharynx.

**Herpes progenitalis** *(HUR peez pro* ***JEN*** *i TAY lis):* a type of herpes simplex in which vesicles occur in the genitalia.

**Herpes simplex** *(****HUR*** *peez* ***SIM*** *pleks):* a viral disorder characterized by groups of vesicles.

**Herpes simplex virus** *(****HUR*** *peez* ***SIM*** *plecks* ***VI*** *rus):* a virus that causes a variety of diseases. Symptoms often occur at irregular intervals.

**Hippocratic oath** *(****HIP*** *o krat ick ohth):* an oath incorporating a Code of Ethics for physicians; devised by Hippocrates, Greek physician, known as the father of medicine.

**Histology** *(hi* ***STOL*** *o jee):* the science of the minute structure of organic tissue; microscopic anatomy.

**Holism** *(****HO*** *liz um):* a health concept of the total cultivation of both body and mind.

**Homeostasis** *(HO mee o* ***STAY*** *sis):* a mechanism by which the internal environment of the body tends to return to normal whenever it is disturbed.

**Hormones** *(****HOR*** *mohns):* secretions produced in or by one of the endocrine glands, such as the pituitary, thyroid, and adrenals; and carried by the blood stream or body fluid to another part of the body or organ, to stimulate functional activities.

**Humerus** *(****HU*** *mer us):* upper arm bone.

**Hydrolysis** *(heye* ***DROL*** *i sis):* a chemical reaction whereby the ions of water and those of a salt form an acid and a base changing the pH of a solution.

**Hydromassage** *(**HIGH** droh ma SAHZH):* massage by means of moving water.

**Hydrotherapy** *(**HIGH** droh THERR uh pee):* the science of water treatments for external applications to the body.

**Hygiene** *(**HEYE** jeen):* the science of health; the practice of cleanliness of person and environment.

**Hyperextension** *(**HEYE** per eck STEN shun):* movement to increase the angle beyond the anatomical position; as the lifting the chin.

**Hyperglycemia** *(**HEYE** per glye SEE mee uh):* excess sugar in the blood.

**Hyperidrosis** *(**HEYE** per o DROH sis):* excessive perspiration caused by intense heat or body weakness.

**Hyperkalemia** *(**HEYE** per ka LEE mee uh):* excess potassium in the blood.

**Hyperemia** *(**HEYE** per EE mee ah):* increased blood supply to a muscle.

**Hypernatremia** *(**HEYE** per nat REE mee ah):* excess sodium in the blood.

**Hypernea** *(hye **PERN** ee uh):* rapid abnormal breathing.

**Hypertension** *(**HEYE** per TEN shun):* high blood pressure.

**Hypertrophy** *(**HEYE** per TROH fee):* abnormal growth of a part or an organ; overgrowth; abnormal muscle size.

**Hyperventilation** *(**HEYE** per ven ti LAY shun):* rapid breathing.

**Hypervolemia** *(**HEYE** per vo LEE mee uh):* abnormally high blood volume.

**Hypochrondriac** *(**HEYE** po KON dree ack):* the regions of the abdomen lateral to the epigastric region. A person with unnatural anxiety about health.

**Hypogastric** *(**HEYE** go GAS trik):* region under the stomach and inferior to the umbilical region.

**Hypopigmentation** *(**HEYE** po pig men TAY shun):* lack of melanin pigment in the skin.

**Hypotension** *(**HEYE** po TEN shun):* low blood pressure.

**Hypothalamus** *(**HEYE** po THAL a mus):* the part of the brain that regulates many visceral functions; temperature, water balance, and pituitary hormones.

**Hypothermia** *(**HEYE** po THUR mee uh):* subnormal temperature of the body; artificial reduction of temperature.

## I

**Illiac vein** *(**ILL** i ak):* vein that serves the lower part of the body.

**Immunity** *(i **MYOO** ni tee):* freedom from, or resistance to disease.

**Illum** *(**IL** i um):* largest part of the pelvic bone.

**Incontinence** *(in **KON** ti nence):* inability of a person to control elimination of urine or fecal matter.

**Indurate** *(**IN** du rayt):* to become hard, unfeeling.

**Infarct** *(in **FAHRKT**):* an area of necrosis due to lack of normal blood supply.

**Infection** *(in **FEK** shon):* the spreading of disease.

**Inferior** *(in **FEER** i or):* lower; below.

**Inflammation** *(in fla **MAY** shun):* the reaction of tissues to injury, characterized by heat, redness, swelling and pain.

**Infrared ray** *(**IN** fra RED ray):* a specific lamp using heat radiation to calm the nerves and relieve sore muscles.

**Infra-orbital nerves** *(**IN** fra OR bit tal nurvs):* nerves of the cheek and lower eyelid.

**Inguinal** *(**ING** gwi nul):* the region of the groin.

**Inorganic** *(in or **GAN** ik):* substances not characteristic of living bodies.

**Integumentary system** *(in **TEG** u men TAR ee **SIS** tem):* the skin or outer covering of the body.

**Intercostal** *(IN ter **KOS** tal):* between the ribs.

**Intercostal nerve** *(IN ter **KOS** tal nurv):* the branches of the thoracic nerves in the intercostal spaces; area between the ribs.

**Interferon** *(IN ter **FEER** on):* a protein produced by virus infected cells that helps prevent the spread of virus to other cells.

**Interstitial fluid** *(IN tur **STISH** ul **FLU** id):* fluids situated within or between the tissues of an organ or body part.

**Intracellular** *(IN truh **SEL** yoo lur):* within the cell.

**Intravascular** *(IN truh **VAS** kew lur):* within vessels of the body.

**Introflexion** *(IN tro **FLECK** shun):* inward flexion; bending inward.

**Inversion** *(in **VUR** zhun):* to turn the planter surface toward the midline; turning inward.

**Irritability** *(ir i ta **BIL** i tee):* the power of muscle cells to receive and react to stimuli.

## J

**Jacuzzi** *(**JA** kuz ee):* an unusually large tub equipped with apparatus that causes water to flow in different directions.

**Jaundice** *(**JAWN** dis):* a morbid condition characterized by yellowness of the eyes, skin, and urine.

**Jejunum** *(ji **JOO** num):* the second portion of the small intestine.

**Joint** *(joint):* a connection between two or more bones.

**Joint movements** *(joint **MOOV** ments):* manipulation of joints during massage; basic classifications of joint movements are passive and active.

**Jowl** *(jowl):* the loose part of a double chin; lower cheeks and jaw.

**Jugular** *(**JUG** yoo lur):* pertaining to the neck or throat; the large vein in the neck.

## K

**Keloids** *(**KEE** loids):* thick scars resulting from excessive growth of fibrous tissue.

**Kerating** *(**KER** a tin):* a fiber protein characteristic of horny tissue, as hair or nails.

**Keratoma** *(**KER** ah TOH mah):* a callus; a thickened patch of epidermis, caused by friction, usually on the hands and feet.

**Ketosis** *(**KEE** to sis):* a disturbance of the acid base balance of the body.

**Ki** *(ki):* a Japanese term meaning bio-force. The concept of growth and change; also Chi, Chinese concept of bio-force.

**Kinesics** *(ki **NEE** siks):* the study of body movements.

**Kinesiology** *(ki **NEE** si ol o jee):* the science of the anatomy, physiology, and mechanics of purposeful muscle movement in humans.

**Kneading** *(**NEED** ing):* petrissage; a vigorous movement in massage generally applied by squeezing, rolling, or pinching the flesh in a circular direction.

**Kyphosis** *(ki **FOH** sis):* a condition affecting posture; hunchback.

## L

**Lacrimal** *(**LAK** ri mal):* glands that produce tears.

**Lacrimal bones** *(**LAK** ri mal bohns):* a pair of bones making up a part of the orbit at the inner angle of the eye.

**Lacteals** *(lak **TEELS**):* lymphatic vessels that carry chyle, a milky emulsion of lymph and fat from the intestines to the thoracic duct.

**Lactic acid** *(**LAK** tik **AH** sid):* a waste product produced by active cells.

**Lanolin** *(**LAN** o lin):* a natural emollient and emulsifier from the oil gland of the sheep.

**Lateral aspect** *(LAT e ral AS pekt):* on the side, farther from the midline or center.

**Latissimus dorsi** *(la TIS i mus DOR si):* muscle that draws the arm backward and downward; rotates the arm inward.

**Lentigines** *(len TIJ I neez):* freckles; small brownish, yellow spots on the skin.

**Lesion** *(LEE zhun):* any abnormal change in the structure of tissue or organ due to injury or disease.

**Lesser occipital nerve** *(LES er ok SIP pi tal nurv):* nerves of the skin behind the ear and back of the scalp.

**Leucocytes** *(LOO ko sits):* white corpuscles or white blood cells produced in the spleen, lymph glands, and the red marrow of long bones. Their function is to protect the body against disease by fighting harmful bacteria.

**Leukocytosis** *(LOO koo si TOH sis):* any increased number of white blood cells.

**Levator** *(le VAY tur):* that which lifts or raises.

**Levator anguli oris** *(le VAY tur AN gew lye OR is):* muscle of facial expression at angle of the mouth.

**Levator scapula** *(le VAY tur SKAP u la):* deep muscles of the back.

**Ligaments** *(LIG a ments):* tough, fibrous bands of tissue that connect bones or support viscera.

**Lipase** *(LYE pace):* a fat-splitting enzyme.

**Lipid** *(LI pid):* a fatty substance.

**Loofah** *(LOO fah):* a fibrous fruit of the gourd family; used as a sponge when bathing to stimulate circulation and to remove dead surface cells from the skin.

**Lordosis** *(lor DOH sis):* a forward curvature of the spine; swayback.

**Lumbar** *(LUM bahr):* region of the back lying lateral to the lumbar vertebrae.

**Lumbar plexus** *(LUM bahr PLEK sus):* the first four lumbar nerves which supply the skin of the abdominal organs, hips, thighs, knees, and legs.

**Lumbar vertebrae** *(LUM bahr VUR te brae):* vertebrae in the lumbar region.

**Lymph** *(limf):* a yellowish fluid derived from body tissues, consisting of plasma and lymphocytes, conveyed to the blood stream by the lymphatic tissues.

**Lymph massage** *(limf MA sahj):* lymphatic massage; a pumping motion done with the palm of the hand pressing toward the center of the body; designed to improve metabolism by accelerating the flow of lymph, thus helping to rid the body of toxins.

**Lymph nodes** *(limf nohd):* lymph glands made of lymphoid tissue; oval or rounded masses in the shape of a bean that filter and neutralize harmful bacteria and toxic matter from lymph.

**Lymph vascular system** *(limf VAS kyoo lar SIS tem):* the body system that pumps lymph and carries waste and impurities away from cells; a system consisting of lymph glands, nodes, vessels, spleen, thymus, tonsils, and adenoids.

**Lymphatics** *(lim FAT iks):* vessels that transport lymph from the lymph spaces of the body back toward the venous blood system.

**Lymphocyte** *(LIM foh site):* a substance formed in the lymph nodes; a type of white blood cell.

**Lysosome** *(LYE so som):* a cytoplasmic organelle.

# M

**Macule** *(MAK yool):* small discolored spot or patch on the surface of the skin; freckle.

**Maltase** *(MAWL taze):* an enzyme that converts maltase into glucose.

**Mandible** *(MAN di bel):* the jawbone.

**Mandubular nerve** *(MAN dib yoo lar nurv):* nerves of lower lip and chin.

**Marrow** *(MAR oh):* the connective tissue filling the cavities of bones.

**Massage** *(ma SAHZH):* massology; the systematic manipulation of the soft tissues of the body by movements such as rubbing, stroking, kneading, pressing, rolling, slapping, and tapping for the purpose of promoting circulation of the blood and lymph, relaxation of muscles, relief from pain, restoration of metabolic balance in the body, and other benefits both physical and mental.

**Massage practitioner** *(ma SAHZH prak TISH o ner):* one who is professionally trained to practice the art and science of therapeutic massage.

**Massage systems** *(ma SAHZH SIS tems):* orderly combinations or arrangements of various massage movements into complete treatments.

**Massage technician** *(ma SAHZH TEK ni shan):* one who is trained in the art and science of massage.

**Masseter** *(MAS se tur):* muscle which pulls the mouth upward and back.

**Masseur** *(ma SUR):* a male massage practitioner.

**Masseuse** *(ma SUHZ):* a female massage practitioner.

**Massology** *(MA sol o jee):* the art and science of massage and the study and pursuit of knowledge of the subject.

**Massotherapy** *(MAS o THER uh pee):* treatment by massage.

**Mastitis** *(mas TI tis):* inflammation of the breasts.

**Mastoid** *(MAS toid):* region of the temporal bone behind the ear.

**Matrix** *(MAY tricks):* the intercellular substance of tissue; that in which something originates or takes shape.

**Matter** *(MAT er):* the substance of material things and that which is physical; occupies space, and can be perceived by the senses.

**Maxilla** *(mak SIL a):* bone of the upper jaw.

**Maxillary area nerves** *(MAK sil er ee AIR i a nurvs):* nerves of the nasal pharynx; of the teeth of the upper jaw; and of the skin of the cheek.

**Meatus** *(ME ay tus):* a passageway in the body.

**Medial aspect** *(MEE di al AS pekt):* pertaining to the middle or center, nearer to the midline.

**Median nerve** *(MEE di an nurv):* the nerve located in the center of the arm.

**Meiosis** *(MEYE oh sis):* cellular division in which the chromosome number is halved; also called reduction division.

**Melanoma** *(MEL ah noh mah):* black pigment; a malignant tumor of the skin.

**Membrane** *(MEM brayn):* a thin, pliable, sheet-like layer of tissue that covers or lines an organ, separates adjoining cavities, or connects adjoining structures.

**Meninges** *(mee NIN jeez):* the three membranes; the dura matter, pia matter, and arachnoid covering the brain and spinal cord.

**Mentalis** *(MEN tal is):* muscle which raises and protrudes lower lip.

**Meridian** *(me RID i an):* channels; pertaining to ki or energy that circulates in a network of channels and collaterals in the body.

**Mesocolon** *(MEZ o koh lon):* the mesentry connecting the colon with the posterior abdominal wall.

**Metabolism** *(me TAB o liz em):* a complex chemical and physical process that takes place in living organisms whereby the cells are nourished and carry out their various activities.

**Metacarpals** *(MET* a kahr puls): bones of the hand.

**Metaphase** *(MET ah fayz):* in biology (cell division); the middle state in mitosis, when chromosomes become aligned in the middle of the spindle.

**Metatarsals** *(MET a tahr sals):* bones of the instep of the foot.

**Metastasis** *(me **TAS** ta sis):* the transfer of diseased cells from one part of the body to another.

**Midsagittal** *(**MID** saj i tal):* a plane dividing the body or an organ into right and left halves.

**Mineral oil** *(**MIN** e ral oyl):* petroleum derivative, used as a lubricant and emollient.

**Mitochondria** *(**MIT** o kon DREE uh):* small glandular bodies found in the cytoplasm of a cell; thought to be energy producing.

**Mitosis** *(mi **TOH** sis):* in the human body, the reproduction by division of a mature cell.

**Mobile** *(**MOH** bil):* movable; not fixed.

**Mole** *(mohl):* a macule that is tan to dark brown in color, usually raised, that may or may not contain hair.

**Motor point** *(**MO** tor point):* sensitive spot on the body that readily responds to stimulation.

**Mucus** *(**MEW** kus):* a secretion produced by mucous membranes.

**Mucous membrane** *(**MEW** kus **MEM** brayn):* a type of membrane that lines body cavities that open to the outside of the body.

**Muscular** *(**MUS** kyoo lar):* relating to a muscle or the muscles.

**Muscular system** *(**MUS** kyoo lar **SIS** tem):* a body system made up of voluntary and involuntary muscles necessary for the movement of parts of the body.

**Myelin** *(**MIGH** e lin):* a fatty covering or sheath around certain nerve fibers.

**Myoblast** *(**MIGH** o blast):* a cell which develops into a muscle fiber.

**Myocardiam** *(**MIGH** o KAHR dee um):* the heart muscle.

**Myodystrophy** *(**MIGH** o DIS truh fee):* degeneration of muscles.

**Myoedema** *(**MIGH** o e DEE muh):* edema of a muscle.

**Myofibril** *(**MIGH** o FIGH bril):* a fibril found in the cytoplasm of a muscle cell.

**Myolgia** *(**MIGH** o LO jee uh):* pain in the muscles.

**Myology** *(magh **OL** o jee):* the science of the nature, functions, structures, and diseases of the muscles.

**Myopalmus** *(**MIGH** o PAL mus):* twitching and quivering of a muscle.

**Myopathic** *(**MIGH** o PATH ick):* pertaining to disease of the muscles.

**Myositis** *(**MIGH** o SIGH tis):* inflammation of muscle tissues.

**Myotasis** *(**MIGH** ot UH sis):* stretching and extending of a muscle.

**Myotrophy** *(**MIGH** ot RUH fee):* nutrition of the muscles.

# N

**Nasal bones** *(**NAY** zal bonz):* a pair of bones forming the bridge of the nose.

**Nasal nerves** *(**NAY** zal nurvs):* nerves of the skin of mucous membrane of the nose.

**Negative pole** *(**NEG** a tiv pol):* the pole from which galvanic current flows.

**Nervous system** *(ner **VUS SIS** TEM):* a system of the nerves of the body, spinal cord, and brain; controls and coordinates other body systems.

**Neuralgia** *(**NUV** ral ja):* acute pain extending along the course of one or more nerves.

**Neurodermatitis** *(nuu **RO** dur muh TYE tis):* a skin disorder generally caused by nervous anxiety.

**Neurology** *(nuu **ROL** o je):* the scientific study of nerve systems, their functions and diseases.

**Neuron** *(**NOOR** on):* the structural unit of the nervous system comprised of a nerve cell and cell processes.

**Neutral** *(**nuu** tral):* exhibiting no negative or positive properties; neither acid nor alkaline.

**Nevus** *(**NEE** vus):* a mole or birthmark.

**Non-pathogenic bacteria** *(non-**PATH** o jen ik bak **TEER** i ah):* harmless bacteria.

**Nucleus** *(**NOO** klee us):* the central part of a cell containing the hereditary material of the cell.

**Nutriment** *(**NOO** tri ment):* that which nourishes; food.

**Nutrition** *(noo **TRISH** on):* the processes involved in taking in nutriments and in assimilating and utilizing them.

# O

**Obese** *(oh **BEES**): extremely overweight; stout; fat.*

**Obesity** *(oh **BEES** i tee):* the condition of being overweight.

**Occipital** *(ocl **SIP** i tul):* pertaining to the base of the skull.

**Occipitalis** *(ock **SIP** i TAL lis):* the posterior part of the epicranius muscle.

**Occlusion** *(uh **KLEW** zhun):* a blockage.

**Olecranon** *(O **LEK** ray non):* point of elbow.

**Ophthalmic area** *(off **THAL** mick):* area of tear glands, eye membrane, skin of forehead, and nose.

**Orbicularis oculi** *(or **BICK** yoo lur is **OCK** yoo lye):* the ring muscles of the eye.

**Orbicularis oris** *(or **BICK** yoo lur is **O** ris):* muscle of expression, especially of the smile; open and closes lips; ring muscle of the mouth.

**Organelle** *(or guh **NEL**):* a discreet structure within a cell, having specialized functions, identifying molecular structures, and a distinctive composition.

**Organic** *(or **GAN** ik):* relating to an organ; pertaining to substances having carbon-to-carbon bonds.

**Orthopedics** *(**ORTH** uh PEE dicks):* the science that deals with disorders of the skeletal system.

**Oscillator** *(**OS** si LAY tur):* a mechanical or electronic device that produces electrical vibration; used in physical therapy.

**Osmosis** *(oz **MO** sis):* the diffusion of fluid through semi-permeable membrane resulting in equalization of pressure on each side.

**Ossification** *(OS i fi **KAY** shun):* formation of bone.

**Osteoblast** *(**OS** tee o blast):* a bone building cell.

**Osteology** *(**OS** tee OL uh jee):* science of anatomy, structure, and function of bones.

**Osteopath** *(**OS** tee o path):* a doctor who practices osteopathy.

**Osteopathy** *(**OS** tee OP uth ee):* a system of healing based on the theory that many diseases are the result of abnormalities of the body that may be corrected by manipulation of the affected parts.

**Osteoporosis** *(**OS** tee o po RO sis):* a disease in which there is a decrease in bone density.

**Ovaries** *(**O** vur eez):* two almond-shaped bodies that produce estrogen and progesterone, and are essential in the development of female characteristics; located in each side of the uterus.

# P

**Pain receptors** *(payn ree **SEP** torz):* sensory nerve fibers that respond to pain causing stimuli.

**Palpitation** *(PAL pi **TAY** shun):* examination of the body by means of feeling with the hand.

**Pancreas** *(**PAN** kree us):* gland that aids in the synthesis of sugar to glycogen, storage of glycogen, and conversion of glycogen to glucose in the liver; located between the first and second lumbar vertebrae behind the stomach.

**Panhidrosis** *(**PAN** hi DRO sis):* generalized perspiration.

**Papilla** *(pa **PIL** uh):* small nipple-shaped elevations.

**Papillary layer** *(**PAP** i ler ee **LAY** er):* the outer layer of the dermis.

**Parasympathetic** *(PAR uh si puh **THET** ick):* pertaining to the nervous system which balances action of the sympathetic nervous system.

**Parathyroid gland** *(par ah **THEYE** roid gland):* small endocrine gland located in or near the thyroid.

**Parietal** *(puh **RYE** e tul):* region of the head posterior to the frontal region and anterior to the occipital region.

**Parotid** *(pa **ROT** id):* situated near the ear.

**Passive** *(**PAS** iv):* not active; not performed or produced by active efforts.

**Passive joint movement** *(**PAS** iv joint **MOOV** ment):* a movement in which the practitioner moves a joint while the client's muscles are relaxed.

**Patella** *(pa **TEL** uh):* the flat, movable, oval bone in front of the kneejoint; the kneecap.

**Patellar** *(pa **TEL** ur):* region of the knee and kneecap.

**Pathogen** *(**PATH** uh jen):* a disease-producing microbe.

**Pathogenic bacteria** *(**PATH** uh jen ick bak **TEER** i ah):* harmful bacteria.

**Pathology** *(pat **HOL** uh jee):* a branch of medicine concerned with the structural and functional changes caused by disease.

**Pectoral** *(**PECK** tuh ral):* region of the breast and chest.

**Pectoralis major** *(**PECK** tuh RAL is **MAY** jur):* muscle that draws the arm downward and forward.

**Percussion** *(pur **KUSH** un):* rapid and alternate movement of the hands in a striking motion against the surface of the client's body, using varying amounts of force and hand positions.

**Pericardium** *(per i **KAHR** dee um):* the membranous sac around the heart.

**Perimysium** *(**PEER** i my SEE um):* connective tissue that holds muscle fibers together in muscle bundles.

**Periosteum** *(**PERR** ee OS tee um):* the covering of a shaft of bone.

**Peripheral nervous system** *(pe **RIF** er rahl **NUR** vus **SIS** tem):* system of nerves and ganglia that connect the peripheral parts of the body to the central nervous system. It has both sensory and motor nerves.

**Peroneal** *(**PEER** on EE ul):* pertaining to the fibular side of the leg.

**Peroneal nerve** *(**PEER** on EE ul nurv):* the nerve that receives stimuli from the skin of the lateral aspect of the leg.

**Petrissage** *(**PET** tri sazh):* compression movements such as kneading, used in massage.

**Phalanges** *(fa **LAN** jis):* pl., of phalanx; finger or toe bones.

**Pharynx** *(**FAH** rinks):* the upper portion of the digestive tube behind the nose and mouth.

**Phlebitis** *(fle **BYE** tis):* a condition characterized by inflammation of a vein accompanied by pain and swelling.

**Physiology** *(fiz i **OL** o jee):* the science of the function of an organism.

**Physiotherapist** *(**FIZ** ee o THEER uh pist):* one who practices physiotherapy.

**Physiotherapy** *(**FIZ** ee o THERR uh pee):* treatment of disease or injury by physical means such as heat, light, water, exercise.

**Pigment** *(**PIG** ment):* any organic coloring matter; as that of the red blood cells; the hair, skin, or iris of the eye.

**Pigmentation** *(pig men **TAY** shun):* coloration resulting from pigment.

**Pimple** *(**PIMP** pel):* a small elevation on the skin; a papule or small pustule.

**Pineal gland** *(**PIN** e al gland):* a gland attached to the roof of the third ventricle of the brain.

**Pituitary gland** *(pi **TOO** i ter ee gland):* the gland located in a depression just behind the point of the optic nerve crossing in the brain; produces hormones that regulate many body processes.

**Plane** *(playn):* the three anatomical sections of the body called sagittal, coronal, and transverse; and by which specific regions of the body are identified.

**Plantar flexion** *(**PLAN** tahr **FLEX** shon):* extension of the foot downward.

**Plantar nerves** *(**PLAN** tahr **NURVS**):* nerves of the feet.

**Plasma** *(**PLAZ** muh):* the fluid portion of circulating blood.

**Platelet** *(**PLAIT** lit):* a particle of the blood that is essential to the formation of clots.

**Platysma** *(pla **TIZ** muh):* subcutaneous muscle; a broad, thin muscle of the neck.

**Pleura** *(plo **OR** uh):* the serous membrane that surrounds the lungs.

**Podiatrist** *(po **DYE** uh trist):* one who treats diseases and conditions of the feet.

**Polarity** *(po lar i **TE**):* the opposite poles in an electric current.

**Polarity therapy** *(po **LAR** i tee **THERR** a pee):* a method using massage manipulation derived from both Eastern and Western massage techniques.

**Popliteal space** *(pop li **TEE** ul space):* a diamond-shaped area behind the knee-joint.

**Positive pole [P or +]** *(**POZ** i tiv pole):* the pole from which positive electricity flows.

**Posterior aspect [dorsal]** *(pos **TEER** er ur AH spekt):* situated behind or in back of.

**Practitioner** *(prak **TISH** o ner):* one qualified to practice a specific profession; a massage practitioner.

**Preeclampsia** *(pree E **KLAMP** see uh):* a type of toxemia sometimes occurring in the latter half of pregnancy; characterized by high blood pressure, edema, and sodium retention.

**Prenatal massage** *(**PREE** nay tal ma **SAHZH**):* a specific massage designed as a therapeutic aid during pregnancy.

**Prime mover** *(prim **MOV** er):* the moving muscle; when a muscle is the prime mover and contracts, its antagonist must relax.

**Progesterone** *(pro **JES** te rohn):* a female hormone.

**Prognosis** *(prog **NOH** sis):* a prediction as to the probable cause and outcome of disease, injury, or developmental abnormality in a patient.

**Pronation** *(pro **NAY** shun):* to turn the palm of the hand downward.

**Prone position** *(pron puh zi **SHUN**):* lying face downward on anterior [front] of body.

**Prophase** *(**PRO** faze):* the first stage of mitosis, in which the chromosomes are organized from nuclear materials as elongate spiremes.

**Proprioceptor** *(**PRO** pree o SEP tur):* end organ of a sensory nerve fiber located in muscle and joints.

**Protein** *(**PROH** teen):* a complex, organic substance present in all living tissue, and necessary to sustain life.

**Protoplasm** *(**PROH** toh PLAZ em):* the material basis of life; a substance found in all living cells.

**Protraction** *(**PROH** trak shun):* to move a part of the body forward, as jutting the chin forward.

**Proximal** *(**PROK** si mal):* closest to the point of attachment or organ.

**Psychologist** *(sigh **KOL** uh jist):* one who practices psychology.

**Psychology** *(sigh **KOL** o jee):* the science that studies the functions of the mind.

**Psychogenic** *(si koh **JEN** ik):* a condition caused by the emotions.

**Psychomatic** *(si koh **MAT** ik):* of or involving both the mind and the body.

**Pubis** *(**PYOO** bis):* front arch of the pelvis.

**Pulmonary** *(**PUUL** mo ner ee):* pertaining to the lungs; blood circulation from heart to lungs and back to heart.

**Pulse** *(puls):* the rhythmical throbbing of the arteries as blood courses through them, felt in the wrist at temples, and other pulse spots.

**Pulse rate** *(puls* ***RAT****):* the number of pulsations of an artery, per minute; same as heart rate. In adult females, 80 beats per minute [bpm], and in adult males, 75 [bpm] is considered normal.

**Pustule** *(****PUS*** *chool):* an elevation of the skin having an inflamed base and often containing pus.

## Q

**Quadratus** *(kwah* ***DRAY*** *tus):* a muscle having four sides.

**Quadriceps** *(****KWAH*** *dri seps):* four headed.

**Quadriceps femoris** *(****KWAH*** *dri seps* ***FEM*** *moh ris):* large extensor muscle of the leg.

## R

**Radial** *(****RAY*** *dee al):* radiating; diverging from a common center.

**Radialis** *(****RAY*** *dee ay lis):* pertaining to the radius.

**Radial pulse** *(****RAY*** *dee al pulz):* the pulse in the radial artery as felt on the wrist at the base of the thumb.

**Radius** *(****RAY*** *dee us):* the shorter bone of the forearm on the thumb side.

**Rectus** *(****RECK*** *tus):* any of various muscles that are either rectilinear in shape, oriented along, to an axis of the body or of a part.

**Reflex** *(****REE*** *flecks):* an involuntary response to an appropriate stimulus.

**Reflex action** *(****REE*** *flecks* ***AK*** *shun):* the simplest form of nerve activity; an involuntary response to a stimulus.

**Reflexology** *(****REE*** *flecks OL o jee):* a form of compression massage originating with the Chinese and based on stimulation of specific points of the body, to affect and benefit various parts of the body.

**Region** *(****REE*** *jon):* an indefinite portion or area of the body named for anatomical purposes as the lumbar region or area of the lower back.

**Regimen** *(****REJ*** *i mun):* a systematic course or plan directed toward the improvement of health or other therapeutic benefits.

**Renal** *(****REE*** *nal):* pertaining to the kidney.

**Repair** *(ri* ***PAIR****):* to restore to a healthy state.

**Reproductive system** *(****REE*** *pruh duck tiv* ***SIS*** *tem):* the system which functions to ensure continuance of the species by reproduction.

**RNA—ribonucleic acid** *(ri boh noo* ***KLEE*** *ik* ***AH*** *sid):* molecules within cells that carry the genetic pattern from DNA—deoxyribonucleic acid—to cells being formed.

**Respiration** *(res pi* ***RAY*** *shun):* the act of breathing; the process of inhaling air into the lungs and inhaling it.

**Respiratory system** *(****RES*** *pi ra TOHR ee* ***SIS*** *tem):* system of the body which includes the lungs, air passages, nose, mouth, pharynx, trachea, and bronchial tubes which lead to the lungs; the system which purifies blood through the intake of oxygen and removal of carbon dioxide.

**Reticular** *(re* ***TIK*** *yoo lar):* sponge like structure.

**Retraction** *(re* ***TRAKT*** *shun):* to move a part of the body backward; pulling back the lower jaw and chin.

**Retractor** *(re* ***TRAK*** *tor):* a device or muscle for retraction.

**Rib cage** *(rib kaj):* skeletal framework of the chest consisting of the sternum, rib cage, and the thoracic vertebrae.

**Rolfing** *(****ROLF*** *ing):* a systematic program developed from the technique of structural integration that aligns the major body segments through manipulation of the fascia or connective tissue.

**Roman baths** *(****RO*** *man baths):* public baths built by the Romans.

**Rosacea** *(roh* ***ZAY*** *shee ah):* a condition associated with excessive oilness of the skin; characterized by redness, dilation of blood vessels, papules and pustules.

**Rotate** *(roh* ***TAYT****):* to revolve or cause to revolve.

**Rotation** *(roh* ***TAY*** *shon):* movement either external, to move away from the midline; or internal, to move toward the midline.

**Rub** *(rub):* to press something against a surface and slide it to and fro.

**Rubdown** *(****RUB*** *down):* a type of massage using alcohol or powder applied with effleurage to a patient's body when a bath cannot be given, and to lower temperature when fever is present; to create a cooling effect after applications of heat, and to tone the skin.

**Rubefaction** *(****ROO*** *be fack shun):* redness of the skin.

**Ruga** *(****ROO*** *guh):* folds inside some hollow body organs, such as the stomach and bladder.

## S

**Sacral** *(****SA*** *kral):* pertaining to or located near the sacrum; the five fused vertebrae in humans.

**Sacral plexus** *(****SA*** *kral* ***PLEK*** *us):* last lumbar nerves, first sacral nerve, second sacral nerve, third sacral nerve, and a portion of the fourth sacral nerve form the sacral plexus which controls the movement of the flexor muscles of the leg.

**Sacroiliac** *(****SACK*** *ro IL ee ack):* the joint between the sacrum and the ilium.

**Sacrum** *(****SA*** *krum):* dorsal part of pelvis.

**Sagittal** *(****SAJ*** *i tul):* pertaining to a plane that divides the body into left and right portions.

**Sagittal plane** *(****SAJ*** *i tul plane):* a vertical plane or section dividing the body into the right and left halves in front to back direction.

**Saline bath** *(****SAY*** *leen bath):* a bath using salt in warm water to achieve a tonic effect by stimulating circulation.

**San-Tsau-Tou Hoei** *(****SAN*** *tsau* ***TOO*** *hoo ee ii):* a book published by the Japanese in the sixteenth century listing passive and active massage techniques.

**Saphenous nerve** *(sa* ***FEE*** *nus nurv):* the nerve accompanying a great saphenous vein of the leg.

**Sarcoma** *(sahr* ***KO*** *muh):* a malignant tumor.

**Scapula** *(****SKAP*** *yoo la):* the shoulder blade.

**Scapular** *(****SKAP*** *yoo lur):* region of the back of the shoulder or shoulder blade.

**Scarf skin** *(****SKARF*** *skin):* epidermis.

**Sciatic nerve** *(sigh* ***AT*** *ick nurv):* nerve arising from the sacral plexus and innervates the skin and muscles of both the foot and leg.

**Sclerosis** *(skle* ***RO*** *sis):* the hardening or thickening of tissue.

**Scoliosis** *(****SKO*** *le O sis):* abnormal lateral curvature of the spine; crooked spine.

**Sebaceous glands** *(se* ***BAY*** *shus glands):* glands that secrete sebum.

**Sepsis** *(****SEP*** *sis):* poisoning by bacteria.

**Septicemia** *(sep* ***TEE*** *see MEE uh):* blood poisoning.

**Sequence** *(****SEE*** *kwence):* the pattern or design of a massage; the progression of one movement into another.

**Serous membrane** *(****SEER*** *us* ***MEM*** *bran):* a membrane that lines the closed cavities of the body.

**Serratus** *(se ray* ***TUS****):* pertaining to a muscle arising or inserted by a series of processes like the teeth of a saw.

**Serratus anterior** *(se ray* ***TUS*** *an* ***TEER*** *i or):* serratus anterior muscles that elevate the ribs in inspiration.

**Serum** *(****SEER*** *um):* the clear portion of a body liquid after being separated from solids, especially that formed by the clotting of blood.

**Shiatsu** *(****SHEE*** *ah tsoo):* a Japanese word composed of shi, meaning finger, and atsu, meaning pressure of the fingers; a massage system using the fingers to follow strategic points or energy pathways to restore harmony or to treat specific conditions.

**Shingles** *(SHING uls):* a hand-over-hand style of effleurage in which one hand repeats the stroke as the previous hand completes the stroke; painful pathologic condition affecting the nervous system caused by the herpes virus, and exemplified by a blistering rash.

**Sigmoig** *(SIG moid):* shaped like the letter S.

**Sigmoid flexure** *(SIG moid FLEKS yoor):* sigmoid colon; the portion of the colon that extends from the descending colon to the rectum.

**Sinus** *(SIGN nus):* a cavity or depression; a hollow in bone or other tissue.

**Sitz bath** *(SITZ bath):* a bath using hot, tepid, or cold water and covering only the hips and pelvic region; generally given to stimulate circulation to the body region as a benefit to kidneys, bladder, bowels, and genitals.

**Skeletal** *(SKEL e tal):* pertaining to the skeleton.

**Skeletal system** *(SKEL e tal SIS tem):* the structure and hard framework upon which the other body systems depend for support and protection.

**Skin** *(skin):* the external covering of the body, and largest organ of the human body; integumentary system.

**Skin disease** *(skin di ZEEZ):* an infection of the skin characterized by a lesion, which may consist of scales and pustules.

**Soleus** *(SO lee us):* muscle that extends the foot.

**Soluble** *(SOL yoo bel):* capable of being dissolved.

**Solute** *(SOL yoot):* the dissolved substance in a solution.

**Solvent** *(SOL vent):* able to dissolve another substance.

**Spastic** *(SPAS tick):* involuntary muscle spasms.

**Sphenoid** *(SFEE noid):* pertaining to bone forming anterior part of base of cranium.

**Spinal** *(SPYE nul):* pertaining to, or situated near the vertebral column.

**Spinal cord** *(SPYE nul kord):* the portion of the central nervous system contained within the spinal or vertebral column.

**Spinal nerves** *(SPYE nul nurvs):* the nerves arising from the spinal cord.

**Spincture muscle** *(SFINK tur MUS ul):* a muscle that closes an orifice.

**Spirilla** *(spi RIL ah):* spiral bacteria.

**Spongiosis** *(spun jee OH sis):* a condition that produces a sponge-like appearance of the skin due to an increase of fluid on the cell layers.

**Sports massage** *(spohrt mah SAZH):* athletic massage; massage and manipulation to improve an athlete's ability to perform, help to prevent injuries, and as an aid to restoring mobility to injured muscle tissues.

**Spray bath** *(SPRAY bath):* the projection of two or more streams of water against the body such as a shower spray.

**Squamous** *(SKWA mus):* pertaining to carcinoma; scaly.

**Stasis** *(STAY sis):* a stoppage of the flow of any body fluid.

**Sterile** *(STER il):* free from living organisms.

**Sterilization** *(ster i li ZAY shun):* the process of making sterile; the destruction of germs.

**Sternal** *(STERN al):* pertaining to the chest, breast, breastbone.

**Sterna** *(STERN ah):* plural of stern.

**Sternocleidomastoid** *(STUR no KLYE do MAS toid):* muscle that assists in holding the head erect.

**Sternum** *(STUR num):* the breastbone.

**Steroid** *(STEER oid):* a type of hormone produced by the reproductive and adrenal glands.

**Stimulant** *(STIM yoo lant):* a product containing ingredient that speeds blood flow and metabolism.

**Stimuli** *(STIM yoo leye):* that which incites activity or responses.

**Stratum corneum** *(STRA tum KOR nee um):* horny layer of the skin.

**Stratum germinativum** *(STRA tum jur mu nah TIV um):* the deepest layer of the epidermis resting on the corneum.

**Stratum granulosum** *(STRA tum gran yoo LOH sum):* granular layer of the skin.

**Stratum lucidum** *(STRA tum LOO si dum):* the clear, transparent layer of the epidermis under the stratum corneum.

**Stratum malphigi** *(STRA tum mal PIG ee):* the germinative or innermost layer of the epidermis including the spinosum or prickle layer.

**Stratum mucosum** *(STRA tum myoo KOH sum):* mucous or malphigian layer of the skin.

**Stratum spinosum** *(STRA tum spi NOH sum):* the prickle cell layer of the skin often classified with the stratum germinativum to form the basal layer; prickle-like threads join the cells.

**Streptococcus** *(STREP to kock us):* a round microorganism that grows in chains or pairs, and is the cause of such diseases as scarlet fever.

**Stress points** *(stress poynts):* stress or alarm points generally located where a muscle ends or attaches. Location where fascia and connective tissue is most prevalent and vulnerable.

**Stress therapy** *(stress THER a pee):* massage procedure designed to alleviate tension, anxiety, and other symptoms or effects of stress.

**Stricture** *(STRIK chur):* a narrowing of a passageway.

**Stroke** *(strohk):* in massage, one of a series of movements whereby the hand, fingers, or an object is passed gently over the body.

**Stroking** *(STROHK ing):* a massage movement achieved by gliding the hand smoothly over the body surface, or over some part of the body with varying amounts of pressure or contact to achieve desired results.

**Structure** *(STRUK chur):* the way in which something is constructed or organized; the supporting framework or essential parts, as bone structure.

**Structural integration** *(STRUK chur al in te GRAY shon):* a technique that attempts to bring the physical structure of the body into alignment around a central axis.

**Subcutaneous** *(sub kyoo TAY nee us):* under the skin.

**Sucros** *(SOO krose):* an enzyme that converts sucrose to glucose and fructose.

**Sudor** *(SOO door):* sweat; perspiration.

**Sudoriferous glands** *(soo do RIF er us):* the sweat glands.

**Sudorrific** *(soo do RIF ik):* causing or inducing perspiration.

**Superficial** *(soo per FISH al):* pertaining to or being on the surface.

**Superficial fascia** *(soo per FISH al FASH ee a):* a sheet of subcutaneous tissue; tissue that attaches the dermis to underlying structures.

**Superficial stroking** *(soo per FISH al STROHK ing):* light, gentle, rhythmic stroking of the body applied in direction of the venous and lymphatic flow to produce soothing effects; pertaining to or being on the surface.

**Superfluous** *(soo PUR floo us):* more than normal; excessive.

**Superior** *(soo PEER i or):* higher in position or rank; upper.

**Supinate** *(soo PIN ate):* to turn the forearm and hand so the palmar surface is uppermost.

**Supinator** *(soo PIN a tur):* a muscle of the forearm, which rotates the radius outward.

**Supine** *(soo PIN):* lying on the back; face upward.

**Supple** *(SUP el):* flexible; bending easily; not stiff.

**Suppress** *(SOO press):* to hold back; to constrain.

**Supra** *(SOO prah):* denoting on top of; above, over, beyond, besides, more than.

**Supra-orbital nerve** *(soo PRAH or bi tal nurv):* nerve of skin of forehead.

**Suprarenal** *(soo prah REE nal):* located above the kidney; the adrenal glands.

**Supra-trochlear nerve** *(soo PRAH TROK lee ur nurv):* nerves of skin of upper eyelids and root of nose.

**Suppressor** *(**SOO** press or):* that which suppresses.

**Suppuration** *(**SOOP** yoo RAY shon):* the formation of puss.

**Surfactant** *(**SUR** fak tent):* an ingredient which is active upon the surface of the skin.

**Sutures** *(**SOO** chur):* junction of the cranial bones of the skull.

**Swedish massage** *(**SWEE** dish ma **SAHZH**):* massage movements; a series of massage movements classified as active and passive, used in therapeutic massage.

**Swedish movements** *(**SWEE** dish **MOOV** ments):* gymnastics according to a system originating in Sweden.

**Swedish shampoo** *(**SWEE** dish **SHAM** poo):* a cleansing bath applied over the entire body with a shampoo brush, bath mitt, soap, and water.

**Sympathetic nervous system** *(sim pah **THET** ik **NUR** vus **SIS** tem):* a system consisting of a double chain of tiny ganglia—masses or neurons—extending along the spinal column from the base of the brain to the coccyx.

**Sympathetic nerves** *(sim pah **THET** ik nurvz):* the fibers of the autonomic nervous system which originate in the thoracic and lumbar regions of the spinal cord.

**Synapse** *(**SIN** aps):* the point at which nervous impulse passes from one neuron to another.

**Synarthrosis** *(sin **AHR** thro sis):* a joint that permits no motion between the parts articulated.

**Synarthrotic joints** *(sin **AHR** throt ik joints):* joints that are immovable, as those in the pelvis.

**Synergetic action** *(**SIN** ur JET IK **AK** shun):* working together; the combined action or effect of two or more organs or agents, or the coordination of muscular or organ functions by the nervous system in such a way that specific movements and actions can be performed.

**Synergist** *(**SIN** ur jist):* an agent that increases the action or effectiveness of another agent when combined with it.

**Synovial fluid** *(si **NO** vee al **FLOO** id):* a lubricating fluid that functions as a preventative of friction between joints.

**Synovial membrane** *(si **NO** vee al **MEM** brayn):* membrane surrounding freely movable joints and the lining of bursa.

**Syphilis** *(**SIF** i lis):* a serious disease characterized by hard, lacerated sores; transmitted by sexual contact with an infected person.

**Systole** *(**SIS** tuh lee):* the contraction of the heart.

**Systolic blood pressure** *(sis **TOL** ik blud **PRESH** ur):* the maximum systemic arterial blood pressure during ventricular systole.

# T

**Tachyardia** *(**TACK** i **KAHR** dee uh):* abnormally rapid pulse.

**Tactile** *(**TAK** til):* of, or using the sense of touch.

**Tactile corpuscle** *(**TAK** til **KOR** puh sel):* small epidermal structures with nerve endings that are sensitive to touch and pressure.

**Talc** *(talk):* a soft mineral (magnesium silicate), used to make talcum powder; pertaining to a soft, soothing white powder used on the skin during or after some types of massage movements.

**Tapotement** *(ta **POHT** munt):* tapping movement used in massage.

**Tarsals** *(**TAHR** suls):* pertaining to the tarsus.

**Tarsus** *(**TAHR** sus):* the root or posterior part of the foot or instep; the seven bones of the instep.

**Telophase** *(**TEL** o fayze):* the final stage of mitosis in which the chromosomes reorganize to form an interstage nucleus.

**Temporal** *(**TEMP** po ral):* pertaining to or situated near the region of the temples.

**Temporal nerve** *(**TEMP** ro ral nurv):* nerve of the temporal muscle.

**Tendons** *(**TEN** donz):* sinews; white glistening cords or bands which serve to attach muscles to bones.

**Tensile** *(**TEN** sil):* of tension; tensile strength; capable of being stretched.

**Tension** *(**TEN** shon):* stretching; being stretched; the effect of forces pulling against each other.

**Tesla current** *(**TES** la current):* violet ray; heat producing current used in massage to stimulate blood circulation to an area.

**Tensor fasciae latae** *(**TEN** sur **FASH** ee ee **LA** ti):* muscle that assists in abduction, flexion, and rotation of femur.

**Tepid** *(**TEP** id):* neither hot nor cold; lukewarm.

**Terminal** *(**TUR** mi nal):* pertaining to the end.

**Testis** *(**TES** teez):* a glandular male reproductive organ which produces testosterone, the hormone which controls sex characteristics in males.

**Texture** *(**TEX** chur):* the fineness or coarseness of the skin or of a substance.

**Thalamus** *(**THAL** a mus):* a part of the brain at the side of the third ventricle that serves for transmission of sensory impulses to the cerebral cortex.

**Therapeutic** *(ther a **PYOO** tik):* pertaining to the treatment of disease, injury or other body conditions by remedial agents or methods.

**Therapeutics** *(ther a **PYOO** tiks):* the branch of medical science that deals with the healing of the body.

**Therapeutic rubdown** *(ther a **PYOO** tik rubdown):* a rubdown using oil or alcohol as part of patient care.

**Therapist, athletic** *(**THER** a pist):* a practitioner of a specific kind of therapy, as a massage practitioner.

**Therapy** *(**THER** a pee):* the treatment of disease; a treatment applied to remedy or alleviate a condition or disorder of the body.

**Thermal** *(**THUR** mal):* pertaining or relating to heat.

**Thermomassage** *(**THUR** mo ma SAZH):* massage given with the application of heat.

**Thoracic vertebrae** *(tho **RAS** ik **VUR** ti bra):* vertebrae of the thorax.

**Thorax** *(**THOHR** aks):* chest; the upper part of the body or trunk containing the lungs, heart, esophagus, and part of the trachea.

**Thrombosis** *(throm **BOH** sis):* coagulation of blood in the heart or blood vessels, forming an obstruction to circulation.

**Thrombus** *(**THROM** bus):* a clot within the heart or blood vessels.

**Thymus** *(**THEYE** mus):* part of the lymphatic system located in the upper chest cavity along the trachea; havng both lymphatic and endocrine functions.

**Thyroid** *(**THEYE** royd):* an endocrine gland producing hormones that influence metabolism and blood calcium levels.

**Thyroxin** *(theye **ROK** sin):* a hormone produced by the thyroid.

**Tibia** (*TIB i a):* shin bone.

**Tibial nerves** *(**TIB** i al nurvs):* nerves serving the leg, sole of foot, knee and foot joints.

**Tibialis anterior** *(**TIB** i al is an **TEER** i or):* a muscle of the leg.

**Tissue** *(**TISH** oo):* a collection of similar cells that carry out specific functions of the body, and comprises all body organs.

**Tissue, adipose** *(**TISH** oo **AD** i pohs):* tissue containing an abundance of fat-containing cells.

**Tissue, connective** *(**TISH** oo ko **NEK** tiv):* the tissue that binds a structure together, provides support and protection, and provides a framework for the body.

**Tone** *(tohn):* pertaining to the firmness of the skin or the muscles; not slack or sagging.

**Toner** *(**TOHN** er):* a product, such as an astringent used on the skin to stimulate blood to the surface.

**Topical** *(**TOP** i kal):* pertaining to the surface as application of oil or ointment of the skin.

**Torso** *(**TOR** soh):* the trunk of the human body.

**Touch** *(tuch):* to press or strike lightly with the hand.

**Touching** *(**TUCH** ing):* light or superficial laying of the hand on an area of the client's body as a purposeful contact to establish rapport.

**Toxemia** *(tok **SEE** mi a):* blood poisoning.

**Toxic** *(**TOK** sik):* pertaining to or caused by poisoning.

**Toxin** *(**TOK** sin):* a poisonous substance of animal or vegetable origin, especially one formed within the body by microorganisms.

**Trachea** *(**TRAY** ki a):* the windpipe.

**Trans** *(trans):* prefix: across or beyond, as transcend.

**Transverse** *(trans **VURCE**):* crosswise; at right angles to the longitudinal axis of the body or a part.

**Transverse friction** *(trans **VURCE FRIK** shon):* cross-fiber friction; a massage movement done with the tips of the fingers or thumb to assist in breaking down adhesions and roughness that form on tendon sheaths; to relieve painful tendonitis.

**Transverse plane** *(trans **VURSE** plane):* division of the body at mid-section into an upper and lower half.

**Trapezius** *(tra **PEE** zee us):* assists in moving the head, and in drawing the head backward.

**Trauma** *(**TROW** ma):* a wound, injury, or emotional shock producing a lasting effect upon a person.

**Tremor** *(**TREM** ur):* involuntary trembling or shaking.

**Tri** *(try):* a combining form meaning three.

**Triangularis** *(trye **ANG** gew la IR is):* muscle of facial expression at angle of the mouth.

**Triceps** *(**TRYE** seps):* a muscle that extends the forearm.

**Trigeminal nerve** *(trye **TEM** i nul nurv):* trifacial nerve of skin of face, tongue, teeth, and muscles of mastication.

**Trochanter** *(tro **KAN** tur):* large, bony processes on the upper end of the femur where certain muscles are attached.

**Trochlea** *(**TROCK** lee uh):* a part of a process having the nature of pully.

**Trochlea muscularis** *(**TROCK** lee uh mus kew **LAIR** is):* any anatomic attachment which serves to change the direction or pull of a muscle.

**Tsubo** *(**TSOO** - bo):* points of stimulation on the body; devised by Japanese physicians and massage practitioners.

**Tubercule** *(**TOO** ber kel):* rounded, solid elevation on the skin, or on a bone or organ.

**Tumor** *(**TOO** mur):* a swelling; an abnormal mass resulting from an abnormal multiplication of cells.

**Turbinal bones** *(**TUR** binal bohns):* a thin layer of spongy bone on either side of the outerwalls of the nasal depression.

## U

**Ulcer** *(**UL** ser):* an open sore on an internal, or external part of the body.

**Ulna** *(**UL** na):* long bone of the forearm on the little finger side.

**Ulnar** *(**UL** ner):* pertaining to the ulna or the small finger side of the arm; or medial aspect of the arm as compared to the radial lateral aspect.

**Ulnar nerve** *(**UL** ner nurv):* the nerve that effects the muscles of the little finger, the side of the arm, and the hand.

**Ultraviolet ray** *(ultra **VI** o lit ray):* shortest ray of the spectrum; used in lamps in order to stimulate circulation of blood and lymph.

**Umbilical** *(um **BIL** i kal):* region of the navel.

**Urea** *(yuu **REE** a):* a soluble, crystalline compound formed in the body, or made synthetically.

**Urinalysis** *(**YOOR** i nal i sis):* a routine examination of the urine given by a physician in order to detect infection or other problems affecting an individual's health.

**Urine** *(**YOOR** in):* a waste product of vertebrates and many invertebrates, secreted by the kidneys or other excretory structures.

**Uterus** *(**YOO** tee rus):* the organ in which a child is conceived and developed; the womb.

**Uticaria** *(**YOO** ti kar i a):* hives.

## V

**Vapor** *(**VAY** por):* the gaseous form of any substance, which is usually a liquid or a solid.

**Vapor bath** *(**VAY** por bath):* steam bath; a type of bath using vapor to induce perspiration.

**Varicose** *(**VAR** i kohs):* swollen or enlarged veins.

**Vascular** *(**VAS** kyoo lar):* supplied with blood vessels; pertaining to a vessel for the conveyance of a fluid, such as blood.

**Vascular system** *(vas **KYOO** lar **SIS** tem):* the organs in the body involved in the circulation of the blood; heart, arteries, veins and capillaries; also lymph vascular.

**Vaso-constrictor nerves** *(**VAY** zo-kon **STRIK** tur nurvs):* nerves which contract blood vessels, thereby decreasing the flow of blood to a particular area and raising blood pressure.

**Vaso-dilator nerves** *(**VAY** zo dye **LAY** tur nurvs):* nerves which expand the blood vessels, thereby increasing the flow of blood to a particular area in the body.

**Vasomotor** *(**VAY** zo **MO** tur):* pertaining to the expansion or contraction of blood vessels.

**Veins** *(vanz):* blood vessels that carry blood toward the heart.

**Vena angularis** *(**VEE** nuh ahg gew LAIR is):* the vein accompanying the angular artery.

**Vena Cava** *(**VEE** nuh **KAV** uh):* one of the two large veins which carries blood to the right auricle of the heart.

**Ventral** *(**VIN** trul):* pertaining to the anterior surface of the body or an organ.

**Ventricle** *(**VEN** tri kul):* one of the two lower chambers of the heart.

**Venule** *(**VEN** yool):* a small vein, or smallest part of a vein.

**Vertebra** *(**VUR** te bruh):* plural, vertebrae; a bony segment of the spinal column.

**Vertebral canal** *(**VUR** te brul ka **NAL**):* pertaining to the area of the vertebrae; the tube that contains the spinal cord.

**Vertebral column** *(**VUR** te brul **KOL** um):* the backbone; spinal column.

**Vertical** *(**VUR** ti kal):* long axis in erect position.

**Vesicle** *(**VES** i kel):* a small blister or sac; a small elevation on the skin.

**Viable** *(**VI** a bel):* capable of living.

**Vibration** *(vi **BRAY** shon):* a massage technique done by shaking the hands or fingers over mucous tissue in varying pressure and speed.

**Villus** *(**VIL** us):* each of the short hairlike processes on some membranes, especially on the mucous membrane of the small intestine.

**Virulent** *(**VIR** yo lent):* harmful, infectious; characterized by malignity.

**Virus** *(**VI** rus):* any class of submicroscopic pathogenic agents capable of transmitting disease.

**Viscera** *(**VIS** e ra):* internal organs.

**Visceral** *(**VIS** e ral):* relating to the viscera.

## W

**Wart** *(wort):* verruca; thickened epidermis; tumor-like.

**Wen** *(wen):* a sebaceous cyst.

**Whirlpool bath** *(**HWURL** pool bath):* the partial immersion of the body in water which is agitated to produce slight pressure; considered beneficial to circulation, soothing to muscles, and relaxing to nerves.

**White corpuscles** *(weyet **KOR** pus sels):* leucocytes; cells in the blood stream that serve as the body's defense system against infection and disease.

**Witch hazel** *(WICH **HAY** zel):* a mild lotion consisting of an alcoholic solution, and the extract from leaves and bark of the witch hazel shrub, used as a cleansing and freshening lotion.

**Wrapping** *(**RAP** ing):* a procedure by which the body is encased in wet cloth strips, coated with a substance or covered with plastic to produce weight loss, or for other effects.

## X

**Xanthosis** *(**ZAN** tho sis):* pertaining to a yellowish color of the skin.

**Xiphoid process** *(**EKS** oid **PRO** ses):* tip of sternum.

## Y

**Yin and Yang** *(yin and yang):* a Buddhist theory that demonstrates the natural process of continuous change where nothing is of itself, but is seen as aspects of the whole or as two opposites, yet complementary aspects of existence.

**Yoga** *(**YOH** ga):* a form of meditation, concentration, and exercise; a science of mind and body control; a series of postures and positions originated in India, and practiced as an aid to combating stress, increasing stamina, and imparting a sense of well being.

## Z

**Zygomatic** *(zi go **MAT** ik):* bones that help form the cheek.

**Zygomatic arch** *(zi go **MAT** ik arch):* the cheekbone; curve of the cheek.

**Zygomatic nerve** *(zi go **MAT** ik nurv):* sensory nerve; a branch of the maxillary nerve which innervates the skin in the temple area, side of the forehead, and upper part of the cheek.

**Zygomaticus major** *(zi go **MAT** i kus **MAY** jor):* muscle that pulls the mouth upward and back when laughing.

**Zygote** *(**ZI** goht):* the cell formed by the union of two gametes; the first cell of a new individual.

# Index